Equine Reproductive Physiology, Breeding and Stud Management

5th Edition

Equine Reproductive Physiology, Breeding and Stud Management

5th Edition

Mina Davies Morel

Reader in Animal Reproduction, Institute of Biological, Environmental and Rural Sciences (IBERS), Aberystwyth University. E-mail: mid@aber.ac.uk

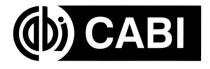

CABI is a trading name of CAB International

CABI	CABI
Nosworthy Way	WeWork
Wallingford	One Lincoln St
Oxfordshire OX10 8DE	24th Floor
UK	Boston, MA 02111
	USA
Tel: +44 (0)1491 832111	Tel: +1 (617)682-9015
Fax: +44 (0)1491 833508	E-mail: cabi-nao@cabi.org
E-mail: info@cabi.org	
Website: www.cabi.org	

A catalogue record for this book is available from the British Library, London, UK.

Library of Congress Cataloging-in-Publication Data

Names: Davies Morel, Mina C. G., author. Title: Equine reproductive physiology, breeding and stud management / Mina C.G. Davies Morel.

Description: Fifth edition. | Boston : CAB International, 2021. | Includes bibliographical references and index. | Summary: "Equine Reproductive Physiology Breeding and Stud Management, 5th Edition provides a thorough grounding in equine reproductive anatomy and physiology for equine, animal and veterinary science students"-- Provided by publisher.

Identifiers: LCCN 2020018102 (print) | LCCN 2020018103 (ebook) | ISBN 9781789242249 (paperback) | ISBN 9781789242232 (hardback) | ISBN 9781789242256 (ebook) | ISBN 9781789242263 (epub)

Subjects: LCSH: Horses--Reproduction. | Horses--Breeding.

Classification: LCC SF768.2.H67 D39 2020 (print) | LCC SF768.2.H67 (ebook) | DDC 636.1--dc23

LC record available at https://lccn.loc.gov/2020018102

LC ebook record available at https://lccn.loc.gov/2020018103

References to Internet websites (URLs) were accurate at the time of writing.

ISBN-13: 9781789242232 (hardback)
       9781789242249 (paperback)
       9781789242256 (ePDF)
       9781789242263 (ePub)

Commissioning Editor: Alexandra Lainsbury
Editorial Assistant: Emma McCann
Production Editor: Marta Patiño

Typeset by SPI, Pondicherry, India
Printed and bound in the UK by Severn, Gloucester

Dedicated to all my colleagues and students that have made my career exciting, rewarding and full of humour.

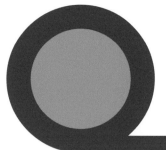

Contents

Acknowledgments

Many thanks to all those that have allowed me to use photos of their horses and studs and for giving me invaluable advice over the years. In particular, I would like to thank Prof John Newcombe, Warren House Veterinary Centre; Mr Richard Kent, Mickley Stud; Mr David Hodge, Llety Farms Stud; Dyffryn Tywi Equine Clinic; Mr Tom James, Penpompren Stud; Aberystwyth University Equine yard.

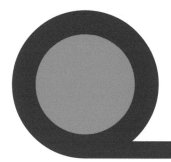

Videos for Equine Repro Phys Breeding and Stud Management

Mare Reproductive Anatomy – Chapter 1

Description of folliculogenesis, oogenesis and ovulation

- https://www.youtube.com/watch?v=-iF9dwVQUvc

Breeding Soundness Evaluation in the Mare – Chapter 8

Breeding Soundness evaluation in the mare including ultrasound examination, swabbing and uterine biopsy

- https://www.youtube.com/watch?v=dbXFTud1Dug

Breeding Soundness evaluation in the mare including ultrasound examination, vaginascopy, swabbing and uterine biopsy

- https://www.youtube.com/watch?v=srZhtfLFVFg

Management of the Mare at Mating – Chapter 10

Detecting and grading oestrus behavior in the mare

- https://www.youtube.com/watch?v=7cAxGqE84Jk&t=91s

Excerpts from a longer video describing the process of ultrasound examination in the mare

- https://www.youtube.com/watch?v=Q-xR6ez1h7I&t=7s

Management of the Mare at Mating – Chapter 10/Management of the Stallion at Mating – Chapter 16

Teasing and in hand mating of the mare and stallion

- https://www.youtube.com/watch?v=MfcsjuEuja8

In hand mating of mare and stallion

- https://www.youtube.com/watch?list=PLpQoZ2bPTsgYg9OSPJTXakP6H0U18ez8h&v=2Udq6vkb8f-w&feature=player_detailpage

Management of the Pregnant Mare – Chapter 11

The use of Colour doppler ultrasonic scanning a series of videos of the pregnant mare illustrating the uterine and embryonic blood flow (red and blue). In particular note the beating of the embryonic heart Day 23 (video 2) even clearer Days 43 and 40 (videos 8 and 9) and Day 58 (video 1); the endometrial folds within the uterus surrounding the conceptus (Video 14); clear allantois and blastocoel or yolk sac (video 5)

- https://www.youtube.com/watch?v=pmTf-_dvCdw&list=UU31zgO5a6T6xxixqcaQ0M5g&index=1

Ultrasonic scanning pregnancy diagnosis in the mare
- https://www.youtube.com/watch?v=G3UxzWmeGik

Foetal sexing in the mare
- http://www.youtube.com/watch?v=FVHfLr6it8g

Management of the Mare at Parturition – Chapter 12

The process of foaling in the mare and cesarean section
- http://www.youtube.com/watch?v=YtnRlHwTf58

Foaling in the mare followed by foal adaptation up until standing
- https://www.youtube.com/watch?v=6lGAr75WHxQ

Cesarean section in the mare
- https://m.facebook.com/story.php?story_fbid=1191828570940266&id=117440931712374

Foaling in the mare : Mutation and traction
- https://www.youtube.com/watch?v=bkhcXRnNzCs

Breeding Soundness Evaluation in the Stallion – Chapter 15

BSE Stallion, external examination of general conformation reproductive tract examination including assessing testis size plus libido assessment
- https://mediaspace.wisc.edu/media/Stallion+Breeding+Soundness+Exam/0_y41sz2rj

General Stallion Management Chapter 17

- Swiss National Stud video investigating the social interactions of stallions after group integration, the possibility of keeping stallions together
- https://www.youtube.com/watch?v=Q-xR6ez1h7I&t=7s

Foal Management – Chapter 19

Madigan squeeze technique to treat horses with Neonatal Maladjustment syndrome (NMS)
- https://www.youtube.com/watch?v=mKbwOv7eQKc

Artificial Insemination – Chapter 21

Inseminating semen into the mare

* https://www.youtube.com/watch?v=-EKWcxRdpn4

Semen collection and evaluation

* https://www.youtube.com/watch?v=O8vYiZTapPs

AI, AV preparation, semen collection, semen evaluation and insemination into the mare

* https://www.youtube.com/watch?v=ohei1K1s7As

Collecting semen from a stallion

* https://www.youtube.com/watch?v=JdhKsA-T8Lc

Semen evaluation

* https://www.youtube.com/watch?v=NCAjY1IOHTc&index=3&list=PLBPI2E05ryn-XJOcNBH-WZFT-FyKsoVs1f

Lecture/demo on semen collection and evaluation
- https://www.youtube.com/watch?v=MUB-CT6k_-o&fbclid=IwAR1x90t2gzHi3jTjaiDrRYCdnYu-RA9R1WVib6ppYfCruofSeduUAGaItdIo

The processes involved in freezing stallion semen
- https://www.youtube.com/watch?v=SgVoJB4AXPI&list=PLBPI2E05ryn-XJOcNBHWZFT-FyKsoVs1f&index=2

Semen collection in the stallion
- https://www.youtube.com/watch?v=u6gAJi4M3eA

Embryo Transfer – Chapter 22

Flushing embryos from a donor mare in preparation for embryo transfer
- https://www.youtube.com/watch?v=fLDOr04TucY

Flushing the mare, identifying the embryo and transferring the embryo into the recipient mare
- https://www.youtube.com/watch?v=78-XVxHqruA

Advanced Reproductive Technologies – Chapter 23

Intracytoplasmic injection (ICSI) in the mare, including oocyte collection, ICSI process and embryo transfer
- https://www.youtube.com/watch?v=TOlmyhamCKU

Section

A

Reproductive Anatomy and Physiology of the Mare

Section A considers the biology of breeding the mare, the anatomy of the mare, the processes involved in ova production (folliculogenesis and oogenesis), fertilization, pregnancy and parturition, and how reproductive activity is controlled in the mare. This knowledge will then enable you to understand the following sections, which apply this knowledge to breeding practice.

1 Mare Reproductive Anatomy

The Objectives of this Chapter are:

To detail the reproductive anatomy of the mare.
To enable you to understand the process of ovulation and the factors that might affect it.
To enable you to appreciate why infertility occurs and the possible treatments.
To provide you with the knowledge to understand subsequent chapters on endocrine control of mare reproduction, pregnancy, parturition and its application to breeding practice.

1.1. Introduction

The reproductive system of the mare may be considered to consist of extrinsic and intrinsic organs. The extrinsic organs are those associated with control (the hypothalamic-pituitary-gonadal axis) and the mammary glands, which are all essential in successful reproduction and will be considered in other chapters, plus the intrinsic organs, which are those that will be considered in this chapter. The reproductive tract of the mare is a Y-shaped tubular organ with a series of constrictions along its length. The wall of the tract remains largely the same throughout: the outer perimetrium (serosa layer); the central myometrium (outer longitudinal and inner circular muscle layer); and the inner endometrium (outer submucosa and the inner mucosa or epithelial cell layer) lying against the lumen of the tract. The perineum, vulva, vagina and cervix can be considered as the outer protective structures, and lie mainly within the pelvic cavity, providing protection for the inner, more vital structures: the uterus, Fallopian tubes and ovaries, which lie in the abdominal cavity and are responsible for fertilization and embryo development. Figure 1.1, taken after slaughter, shows the reproductive structures of the mare, and Figs 1.2 and 1.3 illustrate these diagrammatically. Each of these structures will be dealt with in turn in the following account.

1.2. The Vulva

The vulva (Fig. 1.4) is the external area of the mare's reproductive system, protecting the entrance to the vagina. The outer area is pigmented skin with the normal sebaceous and sweat glands along with the nerve and blood supply normally associated with the skin of the mare. The inner area, where the vulva is continuous with the vagina, is lined by stratified squamous epithelium plus mucus-secreting cells enabling it to accommodate abrasion at mating. The upper limit of the vulva (the dorsal commissure) is situated approximately 6–8 cm below the anus. Below the entrance to the vagina, in the lower part of the vulva (the ventral commissure), lie the clitoris, or clitoral body, and the three clitoral sinuses (one medial and two lateral; Fig. 1.5). These sinuses are of importance in the mare as they provide an ideal environment for the harbouring of many venereal disease (VD) bacteria, in particular *Taylorella equigenitalis* (causal agent for contagious equine metritis, CEM), but also *Klebsiella pneumoniae* and *Pseudomonas aeruginosa*. Hence, this area is regularly swabbed in mares prior to covering and, indeed, in the Thoroughbred industry such swabbing is compulsory (McAllister and Sack, 1990; Ginther, 1992; Horse Race Betting Levy Board, 2019). Within the walls or labia of the vulva lies the constrictor vulva muscle, running

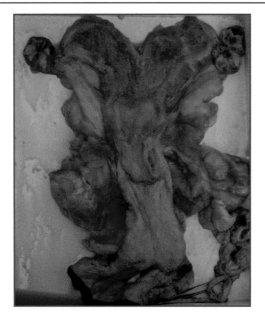

Fig. 1.1. The mare's reproductive tract after slaughter and dissection (see also Fig. 1.2).

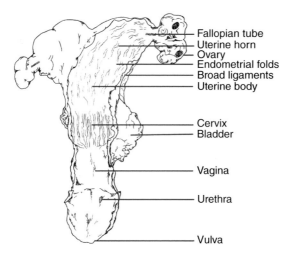

Fig. 1.2. A diagrammatic representation of the mare's reproductive tract.

just inside the ventral part of the labia is the vestibular bulb, an enlarged area of tissue thought to assist in holding the penis in place at copulation.

1.3. The Perineum

The perineum is a rather loosely defined area in the mare, but includes the outer vulva and adjacent skin along with the anus and the surrounding area. In the mare, the conformation of this area is of clinical importance, due to its role in the protection of the genital tract from the entrance of air, solids and bacteria. Mal-conformation in this area predisposes the mare to a condition known as pneumovagina or vaginal wind-sucking, in which air is sucked in and out of the vagina through the open vulva. Along with this passage of air also go environmental and faecal bacteria which bombard the cervix, exposing it to unacceptably high levels of contamination, which it is often unable to cope with (especially during oestrus when it is more relaxed and so less competent). Passage of bacteria into the higher, more susceptible parts of the mare's tract may result in bacterial infections, leading to endometritis (inflammation of the endometrium lining of the uterus, very often caused by an infection). Additionally, urovagina (collection of urine within the vagina) may also result if the reproductive tract slopes internally, further increasing the chance of bacteria breaching the cervix. Chapter 14 gives further details of the causes of VD infection in the mare, all of which adversely affect fertilization rates (McAllister and Sack 1990; Ginther, 1992; Easley, 1993; Kainer, 2011).

1.3.1. Protection of the genital tract

Adequate protection of the genital tract is essential to prevent the adverse effects of pneumovagina. This is achieved via three seals within the tract: the vulval seal, the vestibular or vaginal seal and the cervix (Fig. 1.6).

The perineal area plus the constrictor vulva and constrictor vestibular muscles in the vulval walls form the vulval seal. The vestibular seal is formed by the natural collapsing and apposition of the vagina walls, where it sits above the floor of the upper pelvic bone (ischium), in an area sometimes called the vestibulovaginal fold; plus the hymen, if still present. The tight muscle and collagen ring within the cervix form the cervical seal. On the uterine side of the cervix there are mucociliary (mucus-secreting ciliated) cells, equivalent to those in the respiratory tract, that produce a mucopolysaccharide blanket which provides a mucociliary clearance mechanism to clear debris and bacteria from

along either side of the length of the vulval lips. This muscle acts to maintain the vulval seal and to invert and expose the clitoral area during oestrus, known as winking (Kainer, 2011). Another muscle, the constrictor vestibule muscle, encircles the vulva but is dorsally incomplete allowing the considerable expansion required at parturition (Easley, 1993; Dascanio, 2011a). Lying

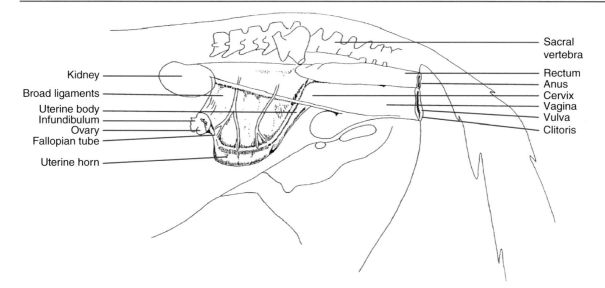

Fig. 1.3. A lateral (side) view of the mare's reproductive tract.

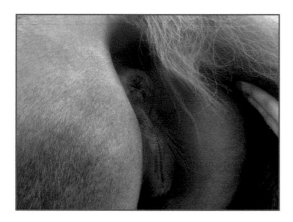

Fig. 1.4. The vulval area of the mare: in this instance, the conformation of the perineal area is poor, with the anus sunken cranially, opening up the vulva to faecal contamination. (Photo courtesy of Ms Ria McLean.)

the uterus and back through the cervix (Causey, 2007). Additionally positive abdominal pressure, typical of tight-bellied young horses or ponies, also helps to prevent the entry of air into the reproductive tract. This series of seals is affected by the conformation of an individual (Figs 1.4 and 1.7) and also by the stage of the oestrous cycle (Fig. 1.8).

The ideal conformation is achieved if around 80% of the vulva lies below the pelvic floor. A simple test can be performed to assess this. If a sterile plastic tube is

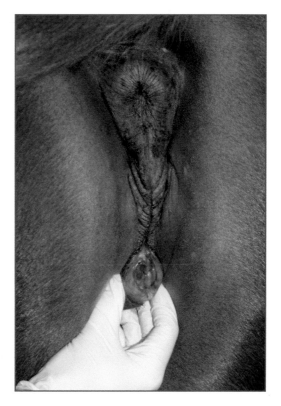

Fig. 1.5. The vulva of the mare showing the ventral commissure within which lie the clitoral body and three sinuses, one medial and one on either side.

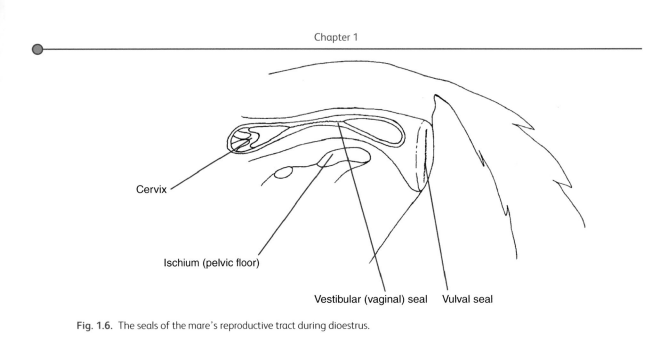

Cervix

Ischium (pelvic floor)

Vestibular (vaginal) seal   Vulval seal

Fig. 1.6. The seals of the mare's reproductive tract during dioestrus.

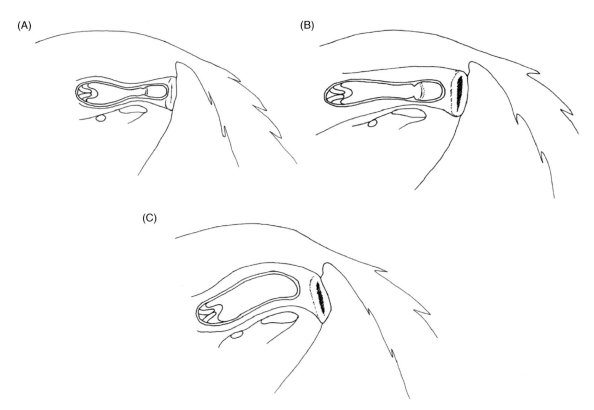

(A)

(B)

(C)

Fig. 1.7. The effect of conformation on the competence of the vulval, vestibular and cervical seals in the mare: (A) a low ischium (pelvic floor) results in an incompetent vestibular seal: in this case, the vulval seal is still competent, so infection risk is limited; (B) a low ischium results in an incompetent vestibular seal: in this case, the vulval seal is also incompetent, so infection risk is increased; and (C) an incompetent vestibular and vulval seal plus a sloping perineal area result in a significant infection risk, especially from faecal contamination.

inserted through the vulva into the vagina and allowed to rest horizontally on the vagina floor, the amount of vulva lying below this tube should be approximately 80% in well-conformed mares. This technique is illustrated diagrammatically in Fig. 8.7.

If the ischium of the pelvis is too low, the vulva tends to fall towards the horizontal plane as seen in Figs 1.4 and 1.7. This opens up the vulva to contamination by faeces, increasing the risk of uterine infection due to pneumovagina. Additionally, a low pelvis causes the vagina to slope inwards, preventing the natural drainage of urine at urination leading to urovagina, which further increases the risk of uterine infection. Lastly, negative abdominal pressure, typical of Thoroughbred type, multiparous mares with poor abdominal muscle

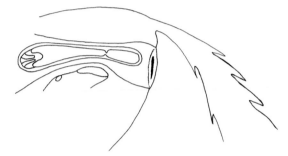

Fig. 1.8. The effect of oestrus on the competence of the vulval, vestibular and cervical seals in the mare: oestrus causes a relaxation of the seals and, therefore, an increase in infection risk.

tone, tends to draw air into the tract, especially when the mare is moving or coughs (Hemberg *et al.*, 2005). Pascoe (1979) suggested that mares should be allocated a Caslick index derived by multiplying the angle of inclination of the vulva with the distance from the ischium to the dorsal commissure. This index can then be used to classify mares into three types and so predict the likely occurrence of endometritis (Fig. 1.9).

The effect of poor conformation of the perineum area may be alleviated by a Caslick's vulvoplasty operation, developed by Dr Caslick in 1937 (Caslick, 1937). The lips on either side of the upper vulva are cut, and the two sides are then sutured together. The two raw edges then heal together as in the healing of an open wound, and hence seal the upper part of the vulva and prevent the passage of faeces into the vagina. The hole left at the ventral commissure is adequate for urination (Fig. 1.10). Short and long Caslick vulvoplasties may be performed, depending on the severity of the perineal mal-conformation and hence on the length of vulva that requires to be sutured.

The chance that a mare requiring a Caslick's operation will pass on the trait for poor perineal conformation to her offspring is reasonably high. This, coupled with the fact that the operation site has to be cut to allow natural mating and foaling, casts doubt on whether such mares should be bred. It becomes increasingly hard to perform a Caslick's operation on mares that have been repeatedly cut and resutured, as the lips of the vulva become progressively more fibrous and

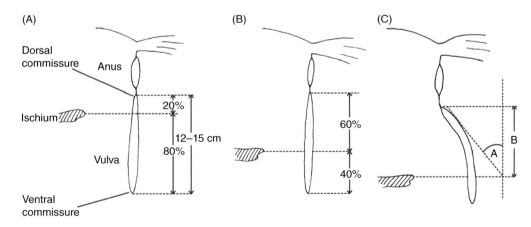

Fig. 1.9. A lateral view of the relationship between the anus, vulva and ischium, indicating: (A) type I mare with good conformation, Caslick index < 50 (b = 2–3 cm, a < 10°): no Caslick required; (B) type II mare with poor conformation, predisposing to type III in later life, Caslick index 50–100 (b = 6–7 cm, a = 10–15°): no immediate need for a Caslick but likely in later life; and (C) type III mare with very poor conformation, including vulva lips in a horizontal plane, Caslick index >150 (b = 5–9 cm, a ≥ 30°): Caslick required immediately, significant chance of endometritis and a reduction in reproductive success.

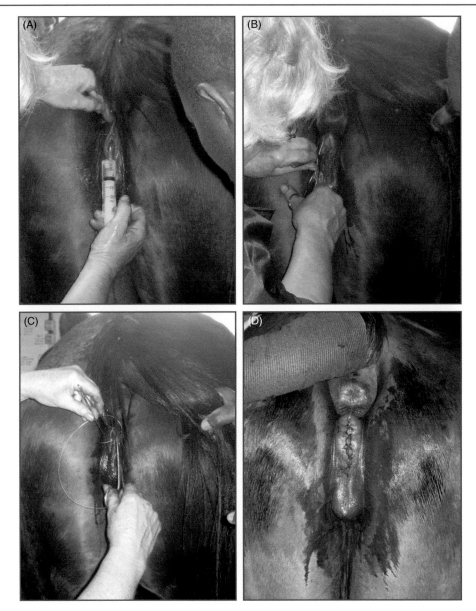

Fig. 1.10. A Caslick operation in the mare showing (A) anaesthetizing the vulval lips; (B) cutting the vulval lips; (C) suturing together the vulval lips; and (D) the finished job.

therefore difficult to suture. In such cases, a procedure termed a Pouret operation may be performed (Pouret, 1982). This is a more major operation and involves the surgical realignment of the anus and vulva (Knottenbelt and Pascoe, 2003). Other alternatives have been suggested, modified Pouret (Papa *et al.*, 2014) and vulval flap (Inoue and Sekiguchi, 2017), but are yet to be widely adopted.

Perineal mal-conformation, and hence pneumovagina and urovagina, is particularly prevalent in Thoroughbred mares. The condition tends to be exacerbated in mares with a low body condition score; multiparous, aged mares; those in fit athletic condition; and those with flat croup and/or elevated tail set. Its continued existence is in no small part due to the selection of horses for athletic performance rather than reproductive competence (LeBlanc, 1991; Easley, 1993). Recent work (McLean, 2014) indicated that up to 50% of Thoroughbred mares in the UK have had a Caslick operation.

The oestrous cycle also has an effect on the competence of the three seals. Further details of the effect of the oestrous cycle on the reproductive tract are given in Chapter 2. In summary, oestrus (period of sexual receptivity) results in the slackening of all three seals, due to a relaxation of the muscles associated with the reproductive tract, especially the cervix (Fig. 1.8). This allows intromission at covering but also decreases the competence of the reproductive tract seals and so increases the chance of bacterial invasion. In part, this is compensated for by elevated oestradiol levels characteristic of oestrus, which enhance the mare's immunological response, so reducing the chance of uterine infection, despite the increased chance of bacterial invasion.

1.4. The Vagina

The vagina of the mare is on average 18–23 cm long and 10–15 cm in diameter. In the well-conformed mare the floor of the vagina should rest upon the ischium of the pelvis, and the walls are normally collapsed and apposed, forming the vestibular seal. The hymen, if present, is also associated with this seal and divides the vagina into anterior (cranial, nearest the mare's head) and posterior (caudal, nearest the mare's tail) sections. In some texts the posterior vagina is referred to as the vestibule. The urethra, from the bladder, opens just caudal to the hymen. The walls of the vagina are muscular and include the constrictor vestibule muscle. The posterior vagina is lined by stratified squamous epithelium which accommodates abrasion at copulation whereas the anterior vagina is lined by columnar epithelium. In addition both the posterior and anterior vagina are lined by mucus-secreting cells. The muscle layer provides elasticity and its dorsal incompleteness allows the major stretching required at parturition (Fig. 1.11).

The vagina acts as the second protector and cleaner of the system. It is largely aglandular (does not contain secretory glands) but contains acidic to neutral secretions, originating from the mucus-secreting cells, the cervix and small vestibular glands situated in the posterior vagina. These acidic secretions are bacteriocidal (kill bacteria); however, they are also spermicidal (kill sperm), necessitating that sperm are deposited into the top of the cervix/bottom of the uterus at mating, to avoid the detrimental effect of the acidic conditions. The acidic conditions also attack the epithelial cell lining of the vagina, but these cells are protected by the protective mucus layer produced by mucus secretory cells. The exact composition of vaginal secretion is controlled by the cyclical hormonal changes of the mare's reproductive cycle; see Chapter 2.

1.5. The Cervix

The cervix lies at the entrance to the uterus and is a remarkably versatile structure, normally providing a tight, thick-walled sphincter, hence acting as the final protector of the system, but is also able to dilate vastly to accommodate the passage of the fetus at parturition (Figs 1.12 and 1.13). The walls of the cervix form a series of folds or crypts and are highly muscular with collagenous connective tissue cores and lined by folded columnar epithelium containing mucus-secreting cells. These crypts are continual with the uterine endometrium folds and enable the significant expansion required at parturition (Ginther, 1992; Kainer, 2011) (Fig. 1.14). In the sexually inactive, dioestrous state, the cervix is tightly contracted, white in colour and measures on average 6–8 cm long and 4–5 cm in diameter;

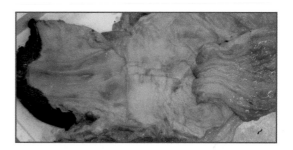

Fig. 1.11. The internal surface of the mare's vagina illustrating from the left: the vulva; the posterior vagina lined by stratified squamous epithelium; the transverse fold (position of the hymen); the anterior vagina lined by columnar epithelium; the cervix.

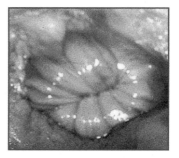

Fig. 1.12. The dioestrous cervix is retracted, presenting a tight seal against entry into the uterus

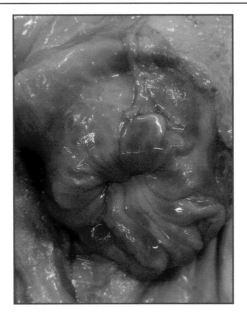

Fig. 1.13. The oestrous cervix is relaxed 'flowering' into the vagina presenting a less effective seal but facilitating the entry of the penis into the cervix for sperm deposition.

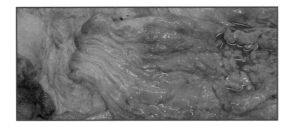

Fig. 1.14. The internal surface of the cervix and uterus illustrating the cervical folds (centre left) which are continuous with the endometrial folds that line the uterus (centre right).

cervical secretion is minimal and thick in consistency (Fig. 1.12). The muscle tone and, therefore, cervix size, along with its mucus secretion are again governed by cyclic hormonal changes (see Chapter 2). During oestrus muscle tone relaxes under the influence of increasing oestradiol, decreasing progesterone and increasing prostaglandin (PG) E (PGE) concentrations. These act on the collagen matrix, separating and dispersing the collagen fibres, which decreases tensile strength and so relaxes the cervix (Kershaw *et al.*, 2005). In addition there is an increase in secretion, so easing the passage of the penis into the entrance of the cervix. The oestrous cervix appears pink in colour and may be seen protruding or 'flowering' into the vagina (Fig. 1.13).

1.6. The Uterus

The uterus of the mare is a hollow muscular Y-shaped organ joining the cervix and the Fallopian tubes (Figs 1.1, 1.2 and 1.3). It lies in the abdominal cavity and is attached to the lumbar region of the mare by two broad ligaments, outfoldings of the peritoneum, on either side of the vertebral column. The broad ligaments provide the major support for the reproductive tract (Fig. 1.15) and can be divided into three areas: mesometrium, attached to the uterus; mesosalpinx, attached to the Fallopian tubes; and mesovarium, attached to the ovaries (Ginther, 1992).

The Y-shaped uterus is divided into two areas: the body (caudal end) and the two horns (cranial end). The body of the uterus normally measures 18–20 cm long and 8–12 cm in diameter. The two horns that diverge from the uterine body are approximately 25 cm long and reduce in diameter from 4–6 cm to 1–2 cm as they approach the Fallopian tubes. The size of the uterus is affected by age and parity, older multiparous mares tending to have larger uteri which also tend to slope

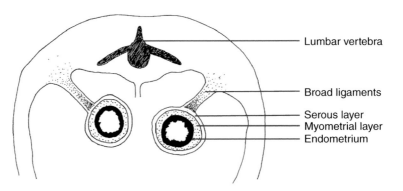

Fig. 1.15. A cross section through the abdomen of the mare illustrating the two uterine horns and supporting broad ligaments.

downwards into the abdominal cavity. The uterus of the mare is termed a simplex bipartitus, due to the relatively large size of the uterine body compared to the uterine horns (60:40 split). This differs from that in other farm livestock, where the uterine horns are more predominant. The lack of a septum dividing the uterine body is also notable (Hafez and Hafez, 2000; Frandson *et al.*, 2009). In situ the uterine walls are flaccid and intermingle with the intestine, the only lumen present being very small and that formed between the endometrial folds.

The uterine wall (Fig. 1.16), in common with the rest of the tract but most prominent here, consists of three layers: the perimetrium (an outer serosa layer) continuous with the broad ligaments; the myometrium (central muscular layer); and the inner endometrium. The central myometrial layer is particularly evident in the uterus where clearly defined outer longitudinal muscle fibres, a central vascular layer and inner circular muscle fibres can be seen. It is this central myometrial layer that allows the elasticity for expansion of the uterus during pregnancy as well as providing the force for parturition. The inner endometrium is arranged in 12–15 longitudinal folds continuous with the folds of the cervix (Figs 1.2 and 1.14) and comprises the outer epithelial cells (epithelium) and inner submucosa of endometrial connective or stroma tissue with its associated

endometrial glands and ducts (Figs 1.16 and 1.17). The submucosa can be further divided into the compact layer (stratum compactum), nearest the epithelium, and the spongy layer (stratum spongiosum), nearest the myometrium. Collagenous connective tissue cores support these endometrial folds. The activity and, therefore, appearance of the endometrial glands and the epithelial cells are dependent on the cyclical hormonal changes associated with the oestrous cycle. It is the endometrium that is responsible for supporting the early conceptus and for placental attachment and development (Ginther, 1992, 1995; Sertich, 1998; Kainer, 2011). Causey (2007) also suggested that within the uterine epithelium are mucus-secreting and ciliated cells that help eliminate bacteria, providing an additional defence against uterine bacterial invasion.

1.7. The Utero-tubular Junction

The utero-tubular junction is a constriction or sphincter formed by a high concentration of muscle cells originating from the circular myometrium of the Fallopian tube. The junction, which appears as a papilla in the endometrium, provides an abrupt connection between the end of the uterine horns and the Fallopian tubes (Fig. 1.18). Fertilization takes place in the Fallopian tubes, and the utero-tubular junction selectively allows only fertilized ova to pass through and on to the uterus

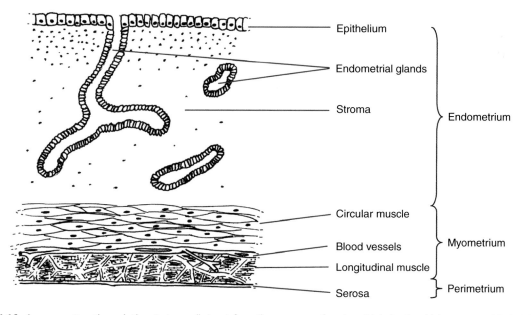

Fig. 1.16. A cross section through the uterine wall. Apart from the presence of endometrial glands, which are present in just the uterus, this cross section is the same throughout the whole of the reproductive tract.

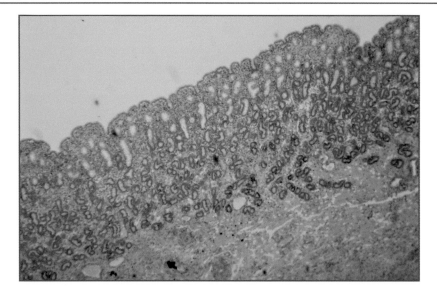

Fig. 1.17. A uterine biopsy illustrating a cross section through the uterine wall, illustrating from the top left: the outer epithelial cells of the endometrium; the endometrium stratum compactum, with a few endometrial glands; the endometrium stratum spongiosum, with a high concentration of endometrial glands; the circular muscle cells of the myometrium; and finally, in the very bottom right-hand corner, the beginnings of the longitudinal muscle cells of the myometrium.

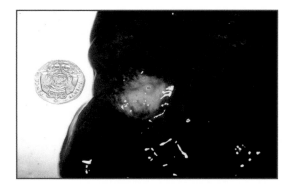

Fig. 1.18. The utero-tubular junction in the mare, as seen from the uterine horn side (the dark colour of the uterine endometrium is not natural but serves to allow easier identification of the utero-tubular junction).

for implantation and further development. Fertilized ova appear to actively control their own passage (Section 3.2) leaving the unfertilized ova on the Fallopian tube side of the junction. These then gradually degenerate (Ginther, 1992; Kainer, 2011). The utero-tubular junction may also act as a selection mechanism allowing only morphologically normal sperm to pass through to the Fallopian tube. Work by Scott *et al.* (2000) reported the presence of sperm within the folds around the utero-tubular junction for up to 4 h after mating,

suggesting that it might also act as an area for storage and then slow release of sperm, spreading the time over which sperm pass into the Fallopian tube, increasing the chance of sperm meeting the ovum at the most opportune time for fertilization.

1.8. The Fallopian Tubes

The mare has two Fallopian tubes or oviducts of 25–30 cm length, which are continuous with the uterine horns (Fig. 1.19). The diameter of these tubes varies slightly along their length, being 2–5 mm at the isthmus end (nearest the uterine horn), and gradually increasing to 5–10 mm at the ampulla (nearest the ovary). The division of the Fallopian tube between the isthmus and ampulla is approximately equal although the demarcation between the two areas is indistinct. The Fallopian tubes lie within peritoneal folds, which form the mesosalphinx part of the broad ligaments. The walls of the Fallopian tubes remain the same as the rest of the tract, but are thinner. Fertilization takes place in the ampulla region nearest the ovary, an area that is characterized by a folded epithelial layer lined with cilia or fimbrae (hair-like projections) and reduced myometrium. The cilia waft unfertilized ova into the ampulla to await the sperm and to waft fertilized ova out of the ampulla and on towards the isthmus. In contrast the isthmus has a thicker myometrial layer, contraction of which pushes the fertilized ova towards the uterotubular junction. The ampulla of each Fallopian tube ends in the infundibulum, a funnel-like opening close to the ovary (Kainer, 2011).

The infundibulum in the mare is closely associated with a specific part of the ovary, termed the ovulation fossa, which is unique to the mare and is the only site of ova release; in other mammals ovulation may occur over the whole surface of the ovary and so the infundibulum encapsulates the ovary. The infundibulum is, therefore, relatively hard to distinguish in the mare, not being so evident as a funnel-shaped structure surrounding the whole ovary. Like the ampulla, the infundibulum is lined by cilia, which again attract and catch the ova guiding them towards the entrance of the Fallopian tubes (Ginther, 1992; Kainer, 2011).

1.9. The Ovaries

The ovaries of the mare are both gametogenic (site of gamete (ova) production) and steroidogenic (site of hormone production) in function. They are evident as two bean-shaped structures normally situated ventrally to (below) the fourth and fifth lumbar vertebrae and supported by the mesovarium part of the broad ligaments. They make the total length of the reproductive tract in the mare in the region of 50–60 cm. In the sexually inactive stage, i.e. during the non-breeding season, the mare's ovaries measure around 2–4 cm in length and 2–3 cm in width and are hard to the touch owing to the absence of developing follicles. During the sexually active stage when the mare is in the breeding season, particularly during oestrus, they increase in size to around

6–8 cm in length and 3–4 cm in width; they are also softer to the touch owing to the development of fluid-filled follicles (Fig. 1.20). Older, multiparous mares tend to show larger ovaries which can be up to 10 cm in length.

The mare's ovaries are bean shaped with the convex outer surface or border of the ovary attached to the mesovarian section of the broad ligaments (Figs 1.20 and 1.21), which is the entry point for blood and nerve supply; the concave inner surface is free from attachment and is the location of the ovulation fossa. The whole ovary is contained within a thick protective layer, the tunica albuginea, except for the ovulation fossa. The tissue of the ovary in the mare is arranged as the inner cortex (active gametogenic and steriodogenic tissue) and the outer medulla (supporting tissue). Ova release at ovulation occurs only through the ovulation fossa, and all follicular and corpus luteum (CL) development occurs internally, within the cortex of the ovary (Fig 1.21). The mare differs in these aspects from other mammals, in which the medulla and cortex are reversed, ovulation occurring over the surface of the ovary and all follicular and CL development occurring on the outer borders. Rectal palpation, as a clinical aid to assess reproductive function in the mare, is not, therefore, as easy to perform as it is in other farm livestock such as the cow. However, with the advent of ultrasound, assessment of ovarian characteristics in the mare is now very accurate (see Section 10.2.2.2 Ginther, 1992, 1995; Sertich, 1998; Hafez and Hafez, 2000; Kainer, 2011).

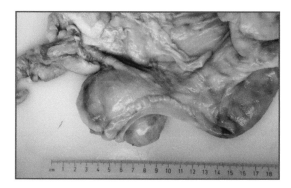

Fig. 1.19. The convoluted Fallopian tube running through the mesovarian section of the broad ligaments, from the ovary on the left to the uterine horn on the right, illustrating the broader ampulla region of the Fallopian tube (on the left) and the more wiry and narrower isthmus region to the right.

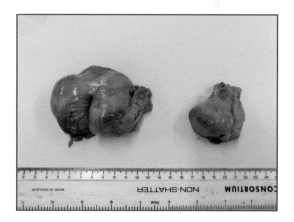

Fig. 1.20. The ovaries of the mare. Note the difference in size between the ovary on the right (inactive) and the one on the left (active). The concave surface (position of the ovulation fossa) and the convex surface (the hilus, entry point for blood and nerve supply) of the ovary are clearly seen.

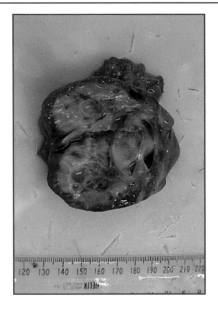

Fig. 1.21. A cross section through the mare's ovary illustrating the outer (pink) medulla (structural) and the inner (cream and grey) cortex (gametogenic and steroidogenic).

1.9.1. Folliculogenesis (follicular development), oogenesis (ova development) and ovulation

The ovary is made of two basic cell types: interstitial cells (stroma), which provide support and produce hormones (steroidogenic); and germinal cells, which provide a reservoir from which all future ova and some hormones are produced (gametogenic and steroidogenic). The number of potential ova contained within the female ovary is dictated prior to birth; subsequently, no addition to that pool of ova is made. The development of these ova to a mature enough stage to ovulate is termed oogenesis. Running in parallel to this is folliculogenesis, the development of the surrounding cells, the follicle. These very immature ova are termed oogonia (primordial germ cells); they carry a full complement of chromosomes (64) and along with their surrounding single layer of epithelial or granulosa cells are termed a primordial follicle. There are many more oogonia than an individual will use within her reproductive lifetime. It is reported that a young mare may have a pool of 35,000 primordial follicles (Draincourt *et al.*, 1982). At birth these oogonia and primordial follicles start to undergo development (oogenesis and folliculogenesis, respectively) at varying rates to form ova mature enough

to be fertilized. Folliculogenesis can be divided into two phases: stage 1, the conversion of the primordial follicle containing its oogonium into a preantral primary follicle containing an ootid; and stage 2, the final development to produce a pre-ovulatory graafian follicle containing a mature ovum (Fig. 1.22; Del Campo *et al.*, 1990; Ginther, 1992; Pierson, 1993; Hafez and Hafez, 2000; Donadeu and Pedersen, 2008; Beg and Bergfeldt, 2011). The first phase can start to occur any time after birth or even in late fetal life and these oogonia develop, within their primordial follicles, into primary oocytes surrounded by a single layer of cuboidal epithelial cells within a primary follicle. These primary oocytes, surrounded by their epithelial cells, which will become granulosa cells, undergo the first stages of meiosis. The duration of this stage 1 is unclear as the control of this first phase of folliculogenesis is not dependent upon gonadotrophic hormones (reproductive hormones produced by the anterior pituitary; Chapter 2). Hence, this is why some oogonia start the first phase of folliculogenesis before the onset of puberty. These partially developed primary oocytes increase in size and then undergo the first stages of meiosis 1 but stop at prophase 1 and are now termed ootids and are surrounded by a developing thick jelly-like layer, the zona pellucida. The surrounding cells within the primary follicle now begin to differentiate into two layers, granulosa and theca cells (Fair, 2003). The result is an ootid within a preantral follicle that now awaits puberty, when hormones secreted from the anterior pituitary drive its further development. It has been reported that follicle diameter at this stage is 2 mm (Ginther and Bergfeldt, 1993).

From puberty onwards, the second phase of oogenesis and folliculogenesis can occur where ootids develop within their primary follicles and complete the final stages of meiosis in waves, to ensure a regular supply of mature follicles is available for ovulation every 21 days during the breeding season (Ginther *et al.*, 2004b). This second phase of folliculogenesis is driven by gonadotrophic hormones and so is linked to the mare's 21-day oestrous cycle. However, not all primary follicles go on to ovulate, as many are wasted along the way, degenerating and becoming atretic; in monovular species, such as the mare, normally just one reaches the stage ready for ovulation (Davies Morel and O'Sullivan, 2001).

The length of the second phase of folliculogenesis is unclear in the mare but may be as long as 21 days. Whatever its length, the waves of second-phase oogenesis and folliculogenesis occur continually and, if they coincide with elevating hormone levels towards the end

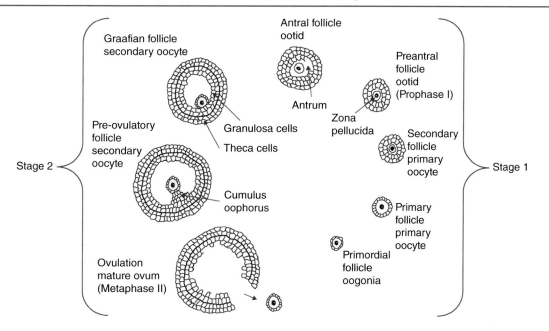

Fig. 1.22. Folliculogenesis: the development of the primordial follicle, containing an oogonium, to a mature graafian follicle, containing a mature ovum (secondary oocyte).

of the mare's 21-day cycle, will result in a pre-ovulatory or graafian follicle(s); if not, they become atretic (Ginther *et al.*, 2001, 2003). As the preantral follicle is driven by these hormones, the surrounding epithelial cells differentiate into vascularized theca cells and follicular epithelial or granulosa cells which secrete follicular fluid, filling the cavity surrounding the ootid. The follicle is now termed an antral or tertiary follicle as the fluid-filled antrum or space becomes apparent. The follicle grows in size as fluid accumulation increases. The ootid itself also continues to increase in size and completes meiosis I; it is now termed a secondary oocyte and has a haploid number of chromosomes (32). The secondary oocyte becomes associated with one inner edge of the follicle and lies on a mound of granulosa cells called the cumulus oophorus. The cells surrounding the rest of the follicle are now organized into two clear cell populations: the theca cells, the inner layer of which is vascularized (theca interna) supplying nutrients and endocrine control, whereas the outer layer is not (theca externa); and immediately inside these inner theca layers is the granulosa layer. These antral follicles continue to develop, and are termed graafian follicles, within which the secondary oocyte starts meiosis II but is arrested at the metaphase II stage; meiosis is only completed at, or if, fertilization takes place. The end of

this second phase results in a mature ovum (metaphase II) ready for ovulation, within a pre-ovulatory or graafian follicle (Figs 1.23–1.24).

During this second phase of folliculogenesis the follicle develops hormone receptors, initially follicle-stimulating hormone (FSH) receptors and then luteinizing hormone (LH) receptors. These receptors allow it to develop in synchrony with the oestrous cycle (Chapter 2). Three stages can be identified within this second stage of folliculogenesis: recruitment (recruitment of small antral follicles from the ovarian pool); selection or emergence (the selection or emergence of a few of these small selected follicles to undergo further development); and dominance (identification of one, possibly two, follicles that will go on to ovulate). The successful development of follicles through these three stages depends at least in part on their ability to react to increasing FSH, LH and oestradiol levels. Although the exact mechanisms are unclear (Fay and Douglas, 1987; Roy and Greenwald, 1987; Gastal *et al.*, 1999) it is evident that the recruited oocytes and their surrounding granulosa cells work as an autonomous unit. The granulosa cells produce growth factors, such as inhibin and insulin-like growth factor (IGF) in response to increasing FSH concentrations, which act to regulate oogenesis. The oocyte in turn produces growth factors such as

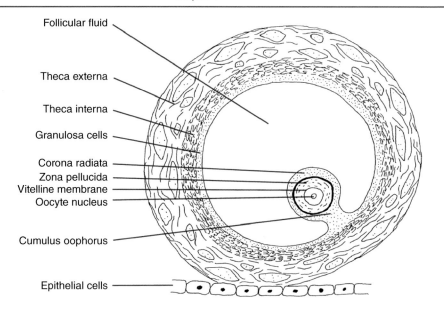

Follicular fluid

Theca externa

Theca interna

Granulosa cells

Corona radiata
Zona pellucida
Vitelline membrane
Oocyte nucleus

Cumulus oophorus

Epithelial cells

Fig. 1.23. The mature graafian follicle containing an ovum.

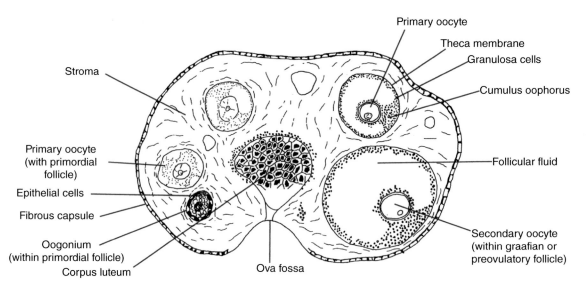

Primary oocyte

Theca membrane

Granulosa cells

Cumulus oophorus

Stroma

Follicular fluid

Primary oocyte
(with primordial
follicle)

Epithelial cells

Fibrous capsule

Secondary oocyte
(within graafian or
preovulatory follicle)

Oogonium
(within primordial follicle)

Corpus luteum

Ova fossa

Fig. 1.24. A diagrammatic representation of follicular development and ovulation within the ovary.

bone morphogenic protein 15 (BMP15), basic fibro-blast growth factor (bFGF) and growth differentiation factor 9 (GDF9) which drive the proliferation of the surrounding granulosa cells (Eppig, 2001; Nilsson et al., 2001; Fair, 2003; Knight and Glister, 2006). However, not all follicles that go through recruitment and selection actually go on to ovulate, many becoming atretic before the dominance stage.

Selection of follicles from the recruited pool is governed by their dependence on FSH. As FSH drives follicles to increase in size, the granulosa cells produce increasing amounts of oestrogen (see Chapter 2) plus inhibin. These in turn act systemically, via the anterior pituitary, to suppress the release of FSH resulting in the release of LH becoming dominant. Local feedback also governs selection, inhibin acting locally to increase LH receptors on the granulosa cells and local growth factors such as IGF further driving folliculogenesis (Beg and Ginther, 2006; Ginther *et al.*, 2008; Aerts and Bols, 2010a,b). In essence a race then exists between selected follicles as to which will become dominant.

Dominance or divergence of a dominant follicle is evident about 3–4 days before ovulation (Ginther *et al.*, 2004b, 2007b; Beg and Bergfeldt, 2011). As follicles grow they develop LH receptors, and LH takes over as the driver of final folliculogenesis. So the largest follicles now rely on LH for development, not FSH, so allowing them to continue to grow despite declining FSH levels. Hence the other now subordinate follicles, that still rely on FSH for development, begin to regress and become atretic as FSH concentrations decline. A deviation of the dominant follicle from subordinate follicles becomes increasingly evident. This dominance is further enhanced as the dominant follicle continues to produce controlling factors, in particular inhibin that actively inhibits the development of the subordinate follicles. It has been reported that 99% of follicles regress and so never ovulate (Gastal *et al.*, 1999; Ginther *et al.*, 2001). In the mare, when follicles reach around 3.5 cm in diameter this appears to be a critical stage, and follicles of this size are very likely to become the dominant follicles destined for ovulation (Ginther *et al.*, 2002; Gastal *et al.*, 2004). The number of dominant follicles that develop to a stage appropriate for ovulation depends on several factors including breed. In native ponies it is very rare for more than one follicle to develop to a stage appropriate for ovulation. Multiple follicles are more common in riding-type horses; it is reported that up to 25% of Thoroughbreds show two or more dominant follicles, which may develop and ovulate, resulting in multiple ovulation (Section 2.4.5; Davies Morel and O'Sullivan, 2001; Davies Morel *et al.*, 2005; Ginther *et al.*, 2009b).

In those follicles destined to ovulate, follicular diameter may now remain static and the follicles appear to move within the stroma of the ovary and so orientate themselves to await ovulation through the ovulation fossa. As ovulation approaches, a bulge at the apex of the follicle appears in the ovulation fossa, and the granulosa cells lining the follicle begin to detach from the underlying theca cells in readiness for ovulation (Gastal *et al.*, 2006). Ovulation of the mature follicle occurs in two stages (follicular collapse and ovum release), which normally (99% of occasions) occur concurrently (Ginther, 1992; Pierson, 1993; Hafez and Hafez, 2000). The whole process may take from a matter of seconds

up to a few hours, with ova release occurring at the later stages of ovulation (Ginther *et al.*, 2007a,b). The ova and follicular fluid are released through the ovulation fossa to be caught by the infundibulum and passed down the Fallopian tube for potential fertilization. Pre-ovulatory follicle diameter normally varies from 3.5 to 4.5 cm; however, ovulation of follicles of diameter outside this range does occur (Sirosis *et al.*, 1989; Ginther and Bergfeldt, 1993). The size of the pre-ovulatory follicle is relatively consistent within a mare (Jacob *et al.*, 2009) but varies with breed, ponies being smaller than larger heavyweight mares (Dimmick *et al.*, 1993; Newcombe, 1994a); season, spring larger than summer (Ginther, 1990b); body condition, lean condition smaller than average condition (Gastal *et al.*, 2004); and age (Ginther *et al.*, 2009a). Ovulation primarily occurs at oestrus; however, additional dioestrus ovulations are not uncommon in mares (Ginther, 1992; Davies Morel *et al.*, 2005). After the release of the ovum and follicular fluid, the old follicle collapses and the theca membrane and the few remaining granulosa cells become folded into the old follicular cavity. Bleeding from the theca interna occurs into the centre of this cavity, forming a clot. This clot, the theca cells and any remaining granulosa cells form the CL (or yellow body). Blood capillaries and fibroblasts then invade the CL. It is initially a reddish-purple colour (corpora haemoragicum); however, as it ages it becomes browner in colour and, if the mare is not pregnant, regresses and shrinks to yellow then white (corpora albucans) as it becomes non-functional. Figures 1.25–1.28 show cross sections through a mare's ovary, illustrating the presence of developing follicles and CL. The luteal tissue is then

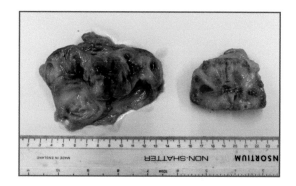

Fig. 1.25. A cross section taken along the long (convex) side of the two ovaries pictured in Fig. 1.20. Note in the active ovary (on the left) the large follicle (hollow or space at the bottom) and the remains of an old corpus luteum (area in the centre).

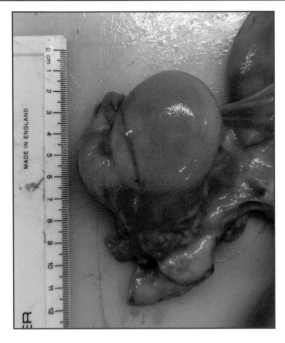

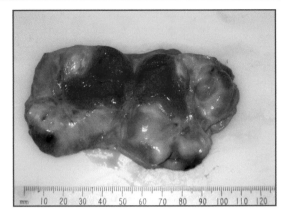

Fig. 1.28. A cross section taken along the long (convex) side of an active ovary illustrating a large red corpus luteum at the top centre of the ovary.

to maximize the chance of fertilization and subsequent maintenance of the resulting conceptus in a sterile environment, but also to expel that conceptus successfully at term.

Fig. 1.26. An ovary illustrating a large (5.5 cm) pre-ovulatory follicle.

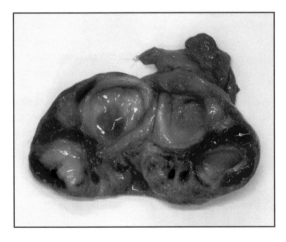

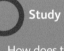

Fig. 1.27. A cross section taken along the long (convex) side of an active ovary illustrating the presence of a large pre-ovulatory follicle (3 cm in diameter) in the centre of the ovary, and smaller, possibly regressing follicles, bottom left and right.

gradually replaced with scar tissue. (Ginther, 1995; Sertich, 1998; Hafez and Hafez, 2000; Bergfeldt and Adams, 2011a).

1.10. Conclusion

It can be concluded that the reproductive tract of the mare is a remarkably versatile system, evolved not only

Study Questions

How does the mare's reproductive tract ensure an appropriate sterile environment for sperm and embryo/fetal survival?

Detail the process by which the mare's ovary provides a regular supply of ova for release at ovulation.

How does the anatomy of the mare's ovary impact on the process of ovulation in comparison to other mammals?

Detail the recruitment, selection and dominance of follicles and how this ensures in most mares that only one ovum is released at ovulation.

Suggested Reading

Ginther, O.J. (1992) *Reproductive Biology of the Mare, Basic and Applied Aspects*, 2nd edn. Equiservices, Cross Plains, Wisconsin, pp. 642.

Bergfeldt, D.R. (2000) Anatomy and physiology of the mare. In: Samper, J.C. (ed.) *Equine Breeding Management and Artificial Insemination*. W.B. Saunders, Philadelphia, Pennsylvania, pp. 141–164.

Hafez, E.S.E. and Hafez, B. (2000) *Reproduction in Farm Animals*, 7th edn. Williams and Wilkins, Baltimore, Maryland, pp. 509.

LeBlanc, M.M., Lopate, C., Knottenbelt, D. and Pascoe, R. (2004) The mare. In: Knottenbelt, D., LeBlanc, M., Lopate, C. and Pascoe, R. (eds) *Equine Stud Farm Medicine and Surgery*. W.B. Saunders, Philadelphia, Pennsylvania, pp. 113–211.

Frandson, R.D., Wilke, W.L. and Fails, A.D. (2009) *Anatomy and Physiology of Farm Animals*. 7th Ed. Wiley-Blackwell.

Beg, M.A. and Bergfeldt, D.R. (2011) Folliculogenesis. In: McKinnon, A.O., Squires, E.L., Vaala, E. and Varner, D.D. (eds) *Equine Reproduction*, 2nd edn. Wiley-Blackwell, Philadelphia, London, pp. 2009–2019.

Dascanio, J. (2011) External reproductive anatomy. In: McKinnon, A.O., Squires, E.L., Vaala, W.E., Varner, D.D. (eds) *Equine Reproduction*, 2nd edn. Wiley-Blackwell, Philadelphia, London, pp. 1577–1582.

Kainer, R.A. (2011) Internal reproductive anatomy. In: McKinnon, A.O., Squires, E.L., Vaala, W.E. and Varner, D.D. (eds) *Equine Reproduction*, 2nd edn. Wiley-Blackwell, Philadelphia, London, pp. 1582–1597.

Senger, P.L. (2011) Pathways to Pregnancy and Parturition, 2nd edn. Current Conceptions Inc., Redmond, Oregon.

2 Control of Reproduction in the Mare

The Objectives of this Chapter are:

To detail how the function of the reproductive system of the mare is controlled.
To enable you to understand how folliculogenesis and ovulation is controlled and the factors that might affect it.
To enable you to appreciate why infertility may occur.
To provide you with the knowledge to understand subsequent chapters on manipulation of the mare's reproductive activity and breeding management.

2.1. Introduction

The mare is naturally a seasonal breeder, showing sexual activity only during the spring, summer and autumn months. This is termed the breeding season; the reminder of the year is the non-breeding season or anoestrus. On average, the breeding season lasts from April until October in the northern hemisphere and from October to May in the southern hemisphere (8–12 cycles), although there is significant variation between mares. Breed of the mare, nutrition and body condition also have an effect on breeding season and it is not unknown for well-fed stabled horses to show regular oestrous cycles throughout the non-breeding season (Malpaux *et al.*, 2001; Thompson, 2011). During the breeding season, the mare shows a series of spontaneous oestrous cycles (polyoestrus) at regular 21-day intervals during which she spontaneously ovulates, regardless of being mated; she is, therefore, termed a seasonal polyoestrous spontaneous ovulator. Figure 2.1 illustrates the major milestones in the mare's reproductive life. The reproductive efficiency of the mare and her ability to produce a foal every year has a significant economic impact on the breeding industry and as such quite a lot of work has been carried out on understanding the control of reproduction in the mare. This work will be summarized in this Chapter.

2.2. Puberty

The mare's oestrous cycles commence at puberty. The exact timing of puberty depends on the criteria used to classify puberty but this usually includes first behavioural oestrus, first ovulation as determined by elevated progesterone levels and/or the presence of a corpus luteum (CL). Using these criteria, the time of puberty has been reported to be 14 months (ranging from 8 to 27 months) (Brown-Douglas *et al.*, 2004; Cebulj-Kadunc *et al.*, 2006). The factors that affect the timing of puberty include: date of birth (Wesson and Ginther, 1981; Brown-Douglas *et al.*, 2004), nutritional status, body weight (Nogueira *et al.*, 1997), breed (Lucas *et al.*, 1991) and possibly social environment such as stallion proximity (Eilts, 2011).

2.3. The Oestrous Cycle

Each cycle lasts on average 21 days (range 20–22 days). Each 21-day cycle is a pattern of physiological and behavioural events under hormonal control and can be divided into two periods according to the mare's behaviour: oestrus, when the mare is sexually receptive, normally 5–6 days; and dioestrus, when she will reject sexual advances, normally 15–16 days. On either side of truly receptive oestrus two other phases have been suggested: pro-oestrus, as the mare comes into oestrus; and metaoestrus, as the mare goes out (Aurich, 2011a,b;

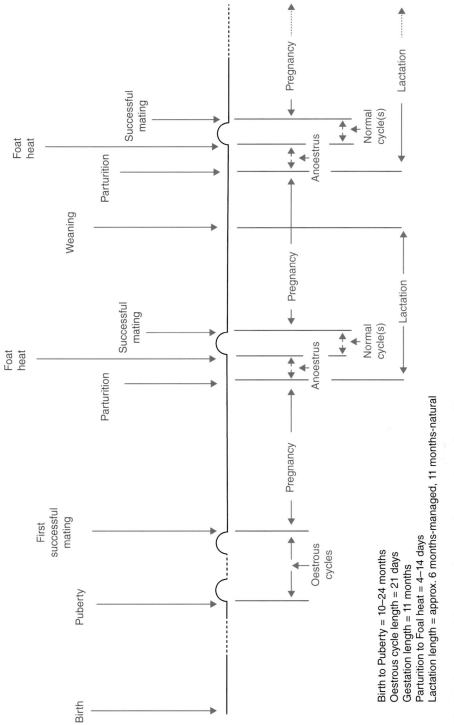

Fig. 2.1. A summary of the major milestones of the mare's reproductive life.

Birth to Puberty = 10–24 months
Oestrous cycle length = 21 days
Gestation length = 11 months
Parturition to Foal heat = 4–14 days
Lactation length = approx. 6 months-managed, 11 months-natural

Yoon, 2012; Satué and Gardón, 2013). The exact times of these periods vary considerably between individuals and with season and age, tending to be longer in the transition periods into and out of the breeding season and in older mares (McCue and Ferris, 2011). In general, any variation in cycle length is due to a variation in the oestrous phase, rather than by dioestrus. For example, a cycle length of 20 days is likely to be due to 15 days dioestrus and 5 days oestrus, whereas in a mare showing a 26-day cycle the respective times would be 15 and 11 days (Ginther et al., 2004a; J. Newcombe, Wales, 2019, personal communication). Ovulation normally occurs 24–36 h before the end of oestrus and is denoted by day 0. Days 1–21 then denote the remainder of the cycle until ovulation recurs (Ginther, 1992; McCue et al., 2011a). The cycle may also be divided according to ovarian physiology and function into: luteal (CL dominant and equivalent to dioestrus); and follicular (follicle development is dominant and equivalent to oestrus) phases.

Oestrous cycles continue throughout the mare's lifetime, although they may become more irregular in extreme old age, and only cease during the non-breeding season (Vanderwall et al., 1993). The mare is an efficient breeder, showing oestrous cycles during lactation, unlike some other seasonal breeders such as the ewe; she is, therefore, capable of being pregnant and lactating at the same time (Fig. 2.1). The mare shows her first oestrus after foaling, often within 4–10 days; this oestrus is termed her foal heat. After the foal heat, the mare may start to show her regular 21-day cycles, but in many cases (owing to the effects of lactation) it takes a while for the system to settle down to a regular pattern again (Ginther, 1992; Watson et al., 1994b; McCue and Ferris, 2011).

For ease of understanding, the following discussion on the oestrous cycle of the mare has been divided into two sections – physiological and behavioural changes – although these are very much interrelated.

2.4. Physiological Changes

The major physiological events associated with reproductive activity in the mare are endocrine changes, which in turn govern and drive the other physiological changes, as well as her behavioural activity.

2.4.1. Seasonality

The mare is a seasonal breeder which is primarily driven by photoperiod, although nutrition and body condition, environmental temperature, age, breed and close association of stallions also play a more minor role (Sharp, 2011b). Although photoperiod is the main controller of seasonality, it is evident that even in constant photoperiod the mare displays a spontaneous circannual (yearly) endogenous (naturally occurring) rhythm of reproductive activity and non-reproductive activity (Nagy et al., 2000; Murphy, 2019). Photoperiod and the other environmental cues act to entrain this natural circannual pattern so that foals are born at the most opportune time – spring. In latitudes where photoperiod does not change significantly throughout the year, other environmental cues, in particular nutrition, play a greater role in entraining the natural circannual rhythm; hence, mares in the tropics tend to enter the breeding season in the rainy season when food is plentiful (Dowsett et al., 1993; Daels et al., 2000; Murphy, 2019). The timing of the onset of the breeding season is remarkably consistent within a mare and groups of mares year on year, but the end of the breeding season is much more variable; this may indicate different control mechanisms for the start and end of the season.

2.4.1.1. Photoperiod

Photoperiod (day length) is perceived by the retina of the eye which sends a neural message to the suprachiasmatic nucleus of the hypothalamus via retinohypothalamic projections. The message then passes again via neural stimulation although the paraventricular nuclei and midbrain to the superior cervical ganglion. Nerve axons from the superior cervical ganglion then terminate close to the pinealocytes in the pineal gland at the base of the brain, which under appropriate conditions secrete the neurotransmitter norepinephrine. Norepinephrine acts on the pinealocytes to drive the conversion of tryptophan to serotonin and then to the hormone melatonin, which controls the activity of the hypothalamic–pituitary–ovarian axis, which in turn is responsible for controlling reproduction (Section 2.4.2; Nagy et al., 2004; Karasek and Winczyk, 2006; Sharp, 2011a; Zhao et al., 2019). Recent research has underlined the vital role played by the suprachiasmatic nuclei as the key biological timekeeper or clock, driving numerous circadian (daily) rhythms, not only reproductive function, acting as a self-sustaining master oscillator. This self-sustaining master oscillator continues to act as a regular biological clock, regardless of external factors, although it can be affected or entrained by external stimuli such as photoperiod (Reppert and Weaver, 2002; Takahaski, 2004; Kalsbeck et al., 2007; Murphy,

2019). Melatonin is produced nocturnally (at night) by the pineal gland, and under the influence of short day lengths dominates the reproductive system, inhibiting the activity of the axis (Diekman *et al.*, 2002). As day length increases, inhibition of the axis is slowly removed, gradually allowing gonadotrophin-releasing hormone (GnRH) to be produced by the hypothalamus, so driving luteinizing hormone (LH) and to a lesser extent follicle-stimulating hormone (FSH) production by the anterior pituitary (Sharp, 2011a; Thompson, 2011). Melatonin is secreted by the pineal gland in two phases: photophase (daytime) and scotophase (night time). It therefore demonstrates a circadian (daily) as well as circannual (yearly) variations in secretion, with the highest levels of secretion being evident during the scotophase (Cleaver *et al.*, 1991; Sharp, 2011a). The means by which melatonin then controls the hypothalamus and anterior pituitary is unclear. It may act directly, as melatonin receptors have been identified on the hypothalamus and anterior pituitary (Nonno *et al.*, 1995; Van Gall *et al.*, 2002). However, others have suggested the involvement of dopamine and/or endogenous opioids including β endorphin as intermediaries (Kilmer *et al.*, 1982; Aurich *et al.*, 1994, 1995; Guerin and Wang, 1994; Besognek *et al.*, 1995; Daels *et al.*, 2000). Of these, dopamine appears to be the main contender and is reported to be positively correlated with melatonin and negatively correlated to LH, and hence evident only in low concentrations in cerebrospinal fluid during the breeding season (Melrose *et al.*, 1990; Nagy *et al.*, 2000). Most recently Castle-Miller *et al.* (2017) have reported the presence of a vascular endothelial growth factor produced in the region of the pituitary that detects melatonin, so perhaps this growth factor has a role to play in translating the message of melatonin by affecting pituitary blood supply and therefore function.

Prolactin (another major seasonally affected hormone) is secreted by the pituitary (Thompson *et al.*, 1994; Aurich *et al.*, 2002). It is suggested by some to be responsible in the horse for non-reproductive seasonal changes such as changes in metabolic rate and increase in the food conversion efficiency during the winter months (a time of food deprivation), also in hoof and pelage (coat) growth. Especially evident in the more native breeds, this demonstrates an innate ability of the equine body to anticipate environmental conditions and respond accordingly. As might be expected, therefore, exposing mares in the non-breeding season to 16 h light per day causes an increase in prolactin concentrations (Evans *et al.*, 1991). Prolactin was previously thought, therefore, to translate primarily the changes in day length to seasonal changes in non-reproductive physiology, with only a limited effect on reproductive seasonality. However, other work suggests that prolactin may have a role to play in controlling breeding as increasing concentrations of prolactin are seen as LH rises at the beginning of the breeding season (Ginther, 1992) and prolactin receptors have been identified in ovarian tissue (King *et al.*, 2005; Morresey, 2011a). Prolactin appears to be primarily regulated by the inhibitory effect of the neurotransmitter dopamine. As such, during the non-breeding season, high dopamine concentrations appear to inhibit prolactin production, which in turn may already reduce stimulation of the follicle and hence follicle growth, ovulation and CL function at the same time as inhibiting LH and FSH production in its role as a translator of melatonin's negative effect on the hypothalamus (Cross *et al.*, 1995; Bennett *et al.*, 1998; King *et al.*, 2004; Williams *et al.*, 2012). Melatonin and prolactin release and affect appear to be opposite but very much related.

It is also interesting to note that the circadian rhythm may affect reproduction on a daily, as well as an annual, basis. The majority of mares are reported to ovulate during the scotophase (night time) (Witherspoon and Talbot, 1970).

The link or exact mechanism by which light via melatonin, prolactin and neurotransmitters such as dopamine interact in the horse is unclear and is an area requiring further investigation (Evans *et al.*, 1991; Nequin *et al.*, 1993; Besognek *et al.*, 1995; Morresey, 2011a).

2.4.1.2. Environmental conditions, temperature, nutrition and stallion proximity

The onset of the breeding season is reported to be closely correlated to environmental temperature, so an early, warm spring is normally associated with an earlier start to the breeding season (Guerin and Wang, 1994; Ginther *et al.*, 2004a).

Nutritional intake also plays a role: a high energy intake shortens the interval to first oestrus of the season (Kubiak *et al.*, 1987). Increasing protein intake also appears to have a similar effect (Van Niekerk and Van Heerden, 1997; Nagy *et al.*, 2000). This can be seen in practice where oestrous activity of anoestrous mares is advanced, and somewhat synchronized, by turnout on to lush pasture (Carnevale and Ginther, 1997). A nutritional effect may also account for the later onset of breeding in lactating mares and older mares, both of which have a higher nutritional requirement than non-lactating mature mares (Heidler *et al.*, 2004).

Housing mares in close proximity to stallions has also been associated with advancement in the start of the breeding season, although whether this is due to an auditory, olfactory or visual cue is unclear (Guerin and Wang, 1994).

Finally, stress has been implicated in reducing reproductive hormone release and hence reproductive function (Breen and Karsch, 2006). This negative effect of stress on reproductive function will be an underlying theme in Parts C and D of this book when management of breeding stock is discussed.

2.4.1.3. Mare body condition

Body condition, as well as nutrition, is reported to affect the timing of the onset of breeding (Vecchi *et al.*, 2010). Work by Gentry *et al.* (2002a,b) demonstrated that mares in high body condition demonstrate more ovarian activity (indicated by follicle size), when monitored in January, than those in a poor condition regardless of nutritional intake. Similarly, when challenged with GnRH those mares in high body condition reacted immediately with a significant release of LH, whereas those in low body condition hardly reacted at all. It is not surprising, therefore, that mares in better body condition (3–4, on a scale of 0–5) are reported to ovulate earlier than mares in poor body condition (Henneke *et al.*, 1984; Van Niekerk and Van Heerden, 1997). The perception of body condition by the hypothalamus is suggested to be via circulating concentrations of free fatty acids, glucose and leptin (Fitzgerald *et al.*, 2002; McManus and Fitzgerald, 2003; Gamba and Pralong, 2006). Kubiak *et al.* (1987) even suggested that 15% body fat content is the important figure and that, below this, onset of oestrus is delayed.

2.4.1.4. Mare age

Age also appears to moderate the breeding season: young mares, up to about 5 years of age, are reported to start breeding at a similar time to mature mares but to cease breeding on average 2 months earlier. At the other end of the age range, mares 15 years or older appear to commence breeding later but cease at the same time as younger mature mares (Wesson and Ginther, 1981; Ginther *et al.*, 2004a,b).

2.4.1.5. Mare breed

Finally, mare breed also has an effect on the timing of the breeding season. The more native-type, cold-blooded horses (mainly ponies) tend to have shorter, more distinct breeding seasons that commence later in the year than the more hot-blooded horses (Ginther, 1992).

In general, intensively managed, well-fed Thoroughbred and Warmblood-type sports horses start their breeding season the earliest and have the longest breeding season. Extensively kept, semi-feral/feral ponies have the shortest season, starting later and finishing earlier.

2.4.2. Endocrinological control of the oestrous cycle

The endocrinological control of the oestrous cycle is governed by the hypothalamic–pituitary–gonadal axis (Fig. 2.2), a similar axis to that which controls stallion reproduction; the gonads in the case of the mare are the ovaries.

When environmental cues allow, inhibition of the hypothalamus, evident in the non-breeding season, is lifted and GnRH, the first hormone in the cascade of hormones through the hypothalamic–pituitary–ovarian axis, is produced.

2.4.2.1. Gonadotrophin-releasing hormone

GnRH is a neuro-decapeptide (made up of ten amino acids) and is produced by the hypothalamus as part of a larger molecule, prepro-GnRH. Once released, it passes via the hypophyseal portal vessels to the median eminence, which is part of the pituitary stalk and so connects the hypothalamus with the pituitary. In the medial eminence it is stored as granules to be split into its two component parts: inactive GnRH associated peptide (GAP) carrier protein (56 amino acids) and active GnRH (ten amino acids) which then pass to the anterior pituitary where they take effect (Eagle and Tortonese, 2000; Clarke and Pompolo, 2005; Alexander and Irvine, 2011a). In common with other reproductive hormones, GnRH release is tonic and episodic or pulsatile in manner (Fig. 2.3). Tonic secretion describes the background continual level of secretion, whereas episodic secretion is the secretion superimposed upon this as a series of pulses or episodes of higher levels. Both the level of tonic secretion and the amplitude (amount released in each pulse) and frequency (rate of episodic release) of episodes can vary throughout the cycle. An increase in episode amplitude, frequency or tonic

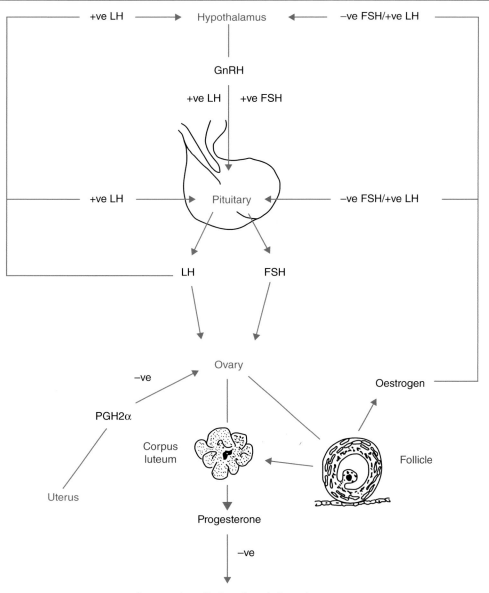

Fig. 2.2. The hypothalamic–pituitary–ovarian axis that governs reproduction in the mare. GnRH, gonadotrophin-releasing hormone; LH, luteinizing hormone; FSH, follicle-stimulating hormone; PGF2α, prostaglandin F2α.

secretions causes an increase in average hormone concentrations. There is suggestion, particularly from work in sheep, that GnRH may be released from two centres in the hypothalamus, the tonic centre and the surge centre. The tonic centre primarily drives tonic episodic release, mainly during dioestrus, and the surge centre is responsible for the large pre-ovulatory hormone increases (Sections 2.4.2.2 and 2.4.2.5). During periods of no sexual activity, GnRH episodic release may be one to four pulses per day, while during sexual activity these may rise to two pulses/h on top of elevated tonic secretion (Satué and Gardón, 2013).

Eighty per cent of GnRH released is passed directly down the hypophyseal portal vessels, to have an effect

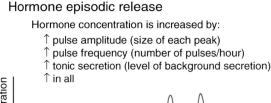

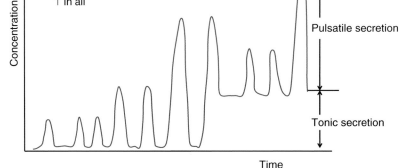

Fig. 2.3. The typical tonic and episodic or pulsatile secretion of reproductive hormones.

on the anterior pituitary (adenohypophysis), with 20% passing back to the central nervous system (CNS) to affect behaviour (Melrose *et al.*, 1994). The level of GnRH in the mare's circulatory system is, therefore, relatively low, as its passage to the anterior pituitary is directed along these specialized portal vessels. Hence measuring GnRH concentrations in a blood sample only gives limited information on GnRH release by the hypothalamus. In response to GnRH the anterior pituitary produces the gonadotrophins (hormones that affect growth and development (troph) of the ovaries (gonad)) FSH and LH, the target organs for which are the ovaries (Alexander and Irvine, 2011b). GnRH, however, appears to have a differential effect on LH and FSH, having a greater control on LH secretion than on FSH; lower episodic release (pulse frequency) favours FSH secretion, and higher episodic release favours LH secretion (see Sections 2.4.2.2 and 2.4.2.5; Watson *et al.*, 2000; Ginther *et al.*, 2004a; Elhay *et al.*, 2007; Alexander and Irvine 2011a; Satué and Gardón, 2013). The effect of GnRH on the activity of the anterior pituitary is governed not only by the levels of GnRH reaching it but also on the number of receptors for GnRH on the anterior pituitary, both of which vary with the oestrous cycle (Rispoli and Nett, 2005). GnRH is itself controlled by season, as discussed previously, but also by feedback from a number of hormones: LH, FSH, progesterone, inhibin and oestrogen, although this may be indirect via neurotransmitters such as opioids or kisspeptin acting as intermediaries (Sections 2.4.2.2.–2.4.2.6;

Magee *et al.*, 2009; Okamura *et al.*, 2013). GnRH concentrations will also increase in response to sexual stimulation (Section 10.2.2.1) and can be affected by body condition, nutritional intake and stress (Alexander and Irvine 2011a).

2.4.2.2. Follicle-stimulating hormone

FSH is part of the glycoprotein hormone family in common with LH, thyroid stimulating hormone (TSH) and equine chorionic gonadotrophin (eCG) and is made up of two subunits: α subunit which is species specific and so is the same within each species for FSH, LH, TSH, eCG, etc; and β subunit which confers the biological activity and so is different within a species for FSH, LH, TSH, eCG, etc. (Alexander and Irvine, 2011b). FSH is produced by the anterior pituitary and, as its name suggests, is responsible for the stimulation of follicle development with receptors primarily on the granulosa cells. Along with LH it is one of the two major gonadotrophins or gonadotrophic hormones that drive the development of the gonads in the mare.

FSH is secreted into the general circulatory system and initially was reported to have a biphasic mode of release, with elevated levels at days 10–11 mid-luteal phase and again just prior to ovulation (Fay and Douglas, 1987; Bergfeldt and Ginther, 1993). However, it is now thought that the biphasic release was an artefact of the sampling protocols, particularly the infrequent sampling, which – in a hormone that is known to be episodic in its release – gave erroneous results. All reproductive hormones are episodic in their release and so frequent sampling protocols are required for meaningful results. More recent work suggests that these two peaks are in fact a single period of elevated FSH during dioestrus and that, although FSH concentrations do significantly rise during late dioestrus, in line with maximum follicle development they then drop significantly as ovulation approaches (Irvine *et al.*, 1998). This supports the theory that stage 2 folliculogenesis is relatively long in the mare (Section 1.9), the preantral primary follicle requiring time to react to FSH and develop. As discussed previously (Section 1.9.1), deviation of follicles and emergence of a dominant follicle occurs towards the end of stage 2 folliculogenesis, and the means by which the dominant follicle retains its dominance is by switching its reliance for development on FSH to LH, and by suppressing FSH release via increasing production of inhibin and oestrogens which act on the hypothalamus. This results in an increase in GnRH episodic release which in turn causes a decline in circulating FSH by favouring LH release. This reduction in FSH arrests the development of the subordinate follicles and reinforces the dominance of the dominant follicle. Hence, at ovulation, FSH levels are low (Evans *et al.*, 2002; Ginther *et al.*, 2005; Alexander and Irvine, 2011b). Although FSH release is partly controlled by GnRH (Section 2.4.2.1) the effect

of GnRH on FSH is less than on LH (Gulliaume *et al.*, 2002). Indeed, episodic release of FSH (although at a reduced tonic level) is seen throughout the non-breeding season. This suggests that FSH release may be somewhat independent of GnRH, and that GnRH just acts to effect this endogenous rhythm. It appears, therefore, that both LH and FSH are somewhat driven by GnRH but that they predominate at different times of the cycle, FSH in the mid- to late-luteal phase (dioestrus) and LH in the follicular phase (oestrus). This is a challenge to reconcile, but can be explained by the different effects of GnRH on FSH and LH release via a variation in episodic release. Low-frequency episodic release of GnRH, typical of dioestrus, drives the anterior pituitary to produce FSH and – as episodic release of GnRH increases as oestrus approaches – the anterior pituitary switches to the production of LH (Turner and Irvine, 1991; Burger *et al.*, 2004; Clarke and Pompolo, 2005). Negative feedback on FSH release is primarily via the ovarian steroids progesterone and oestrogen, and via glycoprotein hormones, in particular inhibin (see following sections) plus follustatin that act on the hypothalamus and anterior pituitary (Sections 2.4.2.3.–2.4.2.6.; Padmanabhan *et al.*, 2002; Gastal, 2009).

Figure 2.4 illustrates plasma FSH concentrations. This graph, and the subsequent graphs illustrating plasma hormone concentrations, has been

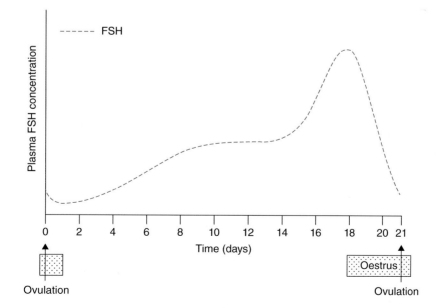

Fig. 2.4. Variations in the relative plasma concentrations of FSH in the non-pregnant mare. FSH, follicle-stimulating hormone.

drawn to give an appreciation of the relative (rather than absolute) hormone concentrations. As with GnRH, all the hormones discussed here in relation to reproduction are secreted in a tonic and pulsatile fashion. The following series of graphs indicates the average hormone concentrations. Absolute levels reported vary considerably between different scientific reports. Where known, concentrations are discussed within the text.

2.4.2.3. Inhibin, activin and follistatin

Both inhibin and activin are glycoproteins consisting of two or three subunits (α, βA, βB) respectively (Alexander and Irvine, 2011b) and are produced by the granulosa cells of the developing follicle under the influence of FSH (Nagamine et al., 1998). It appears that the decline in FSH prior to ovulation is brought about, at least in part, by the increasing secretion of inhibin by large follicles as they near ovulation (Tanaka et al., 2000; Morresey, 2011a). Inhibin concentrations therefore peak at ovulation (Nambo et al., 2002), acting specifically as a negative feedback on FSH production by modulating the anterior pituitary response to GnRH, in the form of reducing FSH secretion (Roser et al., 1994; Watson et al., 2002a,b).

Activin has also been isolated in follicular fluid and is reported to have a similar, but positive, feedback effect, again specifically on FSH secretion (Piquette et al., 1990; Nett, 1993b; Morresey, 2011a). Activin has been reported to drive granulosa cell steroidogenesis (oestrogen production, Section 2.4.2.4) and suppress luteinization either directly, or via its positive effect on FSH production (Knight and Glister, 2001).

Follustatin is a protein that binds to the β subunits of inhibin, but particularly to that of activin, disrupting activin's binding to its receptor and so its effect. Follustatin, therefore, drives a reduction in FSH and, with it, follicular development (Padmanabhan et al., 2002; Phillips, 2005).

Inhibin activin and follustatin appear, therefore, to be very much involved in the development of a dominant pre-ovulatory follicle which then suppresses other follicles, so enhancing its/their own dominance and chances of ovulation (Section 1.9.1).

2.4.2.4. Oestrogen

Oestrogens are steroid hormones produced by the developing follicle. As the follicles develop, they secrete oestrogens which are responsible for the behavioural changes in the mare associated with oestrus and sexual receptivity (Section 2.5; Belin et al., 2000). The major oestrogen is oestradiol-17β, an ovarian steroidal oestrogen produced from cholesterol by an interrelationship between the theca and the granulosa cells within the developing follicle (Fig. 2.5). The theca cells, which primarily have LH receptors and so are driven by rising LH concentrations, convert androgen precursors such as cholesterol to progesterone/17a hydroxyprogesterone, which diffuses across to the neighbouring granulosa cells. The granulosa cells, which primarily have FSH receptors and so are driven by rising FSH concentrations, then convert progesterone to oestradiol-17β (Christensen, 2011a). Additionally, this final conversion within the granulosa cells depends upon the enzyme aromatase, whose activity is FSH-dependent. Oestradiol-17β is secreted into the main circulatory system and 24–48 h prior to ovulation reaches a peak of 10–15 pg ml^{-1}; levels then start to decline, dropping to basal levels at 24–48 h post-ovulation, marking the end of oestrus (Daels et al., 1991a). This decline in oestrogen secretion is associated with the release of the granulosa cells into the follicular fluid as part of the ovulation process (see Section 1.9.1), leaving the theca cells to produce progesterone, but no granulosa cells, for the conversion of progesterone to oestradiol-17β (Tucker et al., 1991).

As FSH levels rise, follicle size increases; as follicle size increases, theca and granulosa cell populations increase, developing more receptors to LH and FSH, respectively, and so oestradiol levels also increase. Oestradiol, in turn, then feeds back on the hypothalamus to increase GnRH episodic release, so suppressing FSH and favouring LH release (Section 2.4.2.2; Ginther et al., 2006). Hence, FSH drives initial follicle development and the beginning of oestradiol production. FSH levels then decline as the dominant follicle approaches ovulation and it becomes increasingly reliant on the increasing levels of LH for its continued development. As FSH declines, LH concentration takes over as the prime driver of follicle development and so of oestradiol production. Oestradiol levels reach a peak, and along with it peak oestrous behaviour, as FSH levels begin to decline. At the same time the positive feedback of oestradiol on LH production drives rising LH levels ready for ovulation (Sections 2.4.2.2 and 2.4.2.5). This ensures that maximum follicular development, in readiness for ovulation, is synchronized with oestrous behaviour (Fig. 2.6; Garcia et al., 1979; Ginther, 1992; Nett, 1993a; Weedman et al., 1993).

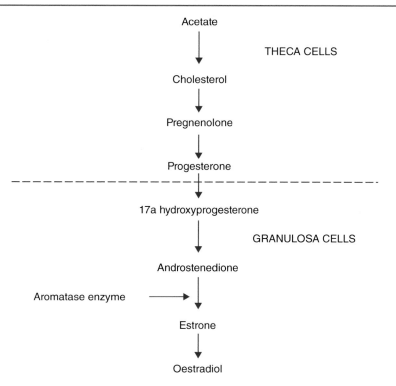

Fig. 2.5. Conversion of androgen precursors such as cholesterol to progesterone and oestrogens in the theca and granulosa cells of the equine follicle.

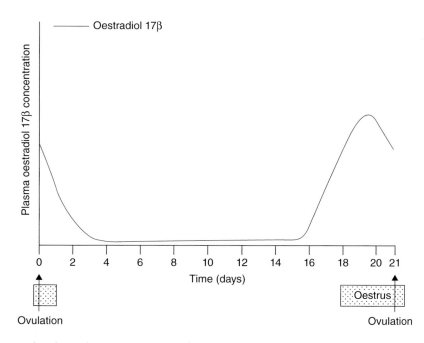

Fig. 2.6. Variations in the relative plasma concentrations of oestradiol in the non-pregnant mare.

2.4.2.5. *Luteinizing hormone*

LH, like FSH, is a glycoprotein (Section 2.4.2.2). As its name suggests LH is responsible for the luteinization (ovulation) of the dominant follicle and its conversion to a CL. LH, like FSH, is secreted by the anterior pituitary. At oestrus, both tonic and pulsatile release of LH rise to a prolonged peak (Fig. 2.7). However, it is the increase in episodic pulse frequency and amplitude that is largely responsible for peak LH concentrations. As discussed previously (Sections 1.9.1 and 2.4.2.2), receptors for LH on the theca cells of the dominant follicle increase in number as ovulation approaches. Increasing LH thus drives the later stages of follicle development as well as androgen precursor (progesterone/17a hydroxyprogesterone) production by the theca cells, which diffuse across to the granulosa cells for conversion to oestradiol-17β. Oestradiol-17β then drives oestrous behaviour but also drives LH release (Section 2.4.2.4). Thus oestradiol-17β and LH form a continual positive feedback loop on each other that culminates in a peak of LH that drives ovulation which then results in the loss of the granulosa cells (that produce oestradiol-17β) and so break the feedback loop (Robinson *et al.*,1995; Greaves *et al.*, 2000). Additionally, as rising LH levels induce increasing oestradiol-17β secretion, this further ensures the synchronization of final follicular development, ovulation and oestrous behaviour (Ginther and Bergfeldt, 1993). LH levels begin to rise from their basal levels of less than 1 ng ml^{-1}, with a pulse frequency of 1.4 pulses 24 h^{-1}, several days before the onset of oestrus. They then reportedly reach a peak of 10–16 ng ml^{-1} just after ovulation and then decline to basal levels within a few days (Whitmore *et al.*, 1973; Pantke *et al.*, 1991; Alexander and Irvine, 2011b). It has been suggested by some that LH not only drives final follicular development and induces ovulation, but is also involved in the formation and establishment of the CL, possibly explaining why peak concentrations are not reached until just after ovulation (Irvine and Alexander, 1997; Ginther and Beg, 2012). LH declines from peak concentrations to low dioestrous levels within a few days of ovulation (Pantke *et al.*, 1991; Irvine and Alexander, 1993a, 1994; Aurich *et al.*, 1994; Alexander and Irvine, 2011b; Fig. 2.7). Although LH is considered to be the prime cause of ovulation in the mare it is noteworthy that, unlike other farm livestock, ovulation can also occur in dioestrus when LH concentrations are low.

LH release is controlled by GnRH, levels of LH having a much closer correlation to levels of GnRH than do FSH concentrations (Irvine and Alexander 2011a,b). In addition, progesterone produced by the

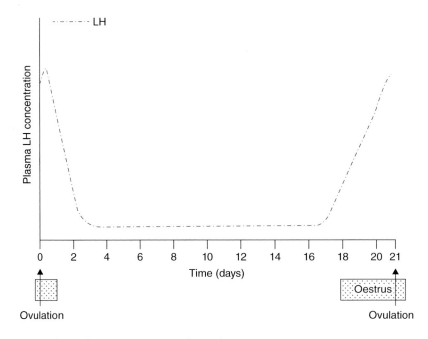

Fig. 2.7. Variations in the relative plasma concentrations of LH in the non-pregnant mare.

CL also has a negative feedback effect on LH by reducing the pulse frequency of GnRH release, so favouring FSH rather than LH release. Oestrogens also have a positive feedback effect, but exactly how this occurs is unclear. It is likely to be due to increasing GnRH release by the hypothalamus favouring LH as opposed to FSH release by the pituitary, and/or increase in LH production due to increasing GnRH receptors on the anterior pituitary. This positive feedback of oestradiol on LH, followed by increasing oestradiol production as follicle development increases, results in a self-perpetuating positive feedback loop increasing LH and culminating in the pre-ovulatory LH peak (Greaves et al., 2000; Ginther et al., 2006).

2.4.2.6. Progesterone

Progesterone and related progestogens are steroid hormones derived from cholesterol (Fig. 2.5). Progesterone is produced by the theca cells of the follicle and also, most importantly, is produced by the CL that results from ovulation. At ovulation, granulosa cells are lost, leaving the theca cells. These convert into luteal cells but continue to produce progesterone which is released into the circulation. Progesterone levels, therefore, rise 24–48 h post-ovulation. Maximum concentrations $(10–15 \text{ ng ml}^{-1})$ are reached 5–6 days post-ovulation

and are maintained until days 13–16 of the oestrous cycle (Ginther et al., 2016b). Progesterone levels are higher in multiple-ovulating mares (Nagy et al., 2004). If the mare has not conceived, progesterone levels drop dramatically around day 15–16 of the cycle, 4–5 days prior to the next ovulation, to basal levels (< 1.0 ng/ml) again during oestrus (Fig. 2.8; Nagy et al., 2004; Lofstedt, 2011a).

Progesterone works in opposition to oestradiol in affecting the mare's physiology, inhibiting the release of gonadotrophins (FSH and LH) in most farm livestock and preparing the genital tract for pregnancy, as well as suppressing oestrous behaviour. Of the two hormones, progesterone appears to be the most dominant (Pycock et al., 1995; Vanderwall, 2011). Oestrus and ovulation cannot begin, therefore, until progesterone levels have fallen to below 1 ng ml^{-1}. However, the block to gonadotrophin release in the mare is not so complete. Elevated progesterone levels appear to have an inhibitory effect on the release of LH, preventing any rise in LH (and hence ovulation) until progesterone levels decline. However, progesterone does not seem to have such an inhibitory effect on FSH. Indeed, as discussed previously, FSH levels are elevated during the mid- to late-luteal phase despite elevated progesterone concentrations (Sections 2.4.2.2 and 2.4.2.5).

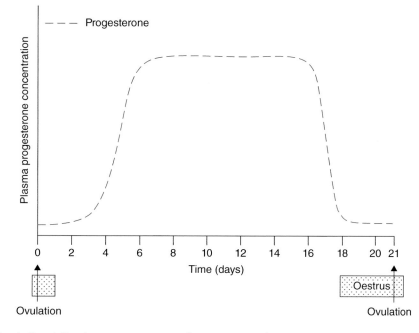

Fig. 2.8. Variations in the relative plasma concentrations of progesterone in the non-pregnant mare.

The prime role of progesterone is to prepare the genital system for pregnancy. Under its influence uterine and cervical tone increases, as do uterine oedema and the activity of the endometrial glands. The endometrial glands increase their secretion of histotrophe, in particular increasing the concentration of proteins (for example uteroferrin) in readiness to support the expected pregnancy (Ellenberger *et al.*, 2008; Hayes *et al.*, 2008; Bergfeldt and Adams, 2011a). Progesterone also blocks oestrous behaviour, which is not required if the mare conceives successfully. However, if the mare fails to conceive, progesterone levels must decline in order to allow the mare to return to oestrus and for LH levels to rise and cause ovulation on day 21. The decline in progesterone occurs in the absence of a message of pregnancy (Section 3.3.1.1.). In the presence of a conceptus, progesterone secretion is maintained; if no conceptus is detected around days 14–15 the mare's system automatically assumes there is no pregnancy. In response to this the uterus produces prostaglandin (PG) F2α (PGF2α).

2.4.2.7. Prostaglandin F2α (PGF2α)

Prostaglandins are lipid compounds derived from fatty acids and contain 20 carbon atoms. There are numerous prostaglandins with a wide range of roles; however, the major prostaglandin involved in reproduction is PGF2α with PG E (PGE) playing a more limited role (Stout, 2011). PGF2α is primarily responsible for the luteolysis (destruction) of the CL in order to allow oestrus and ovulation to reoccur, although it has been suggested that it may also pay a role in ovulation, driving follicular wall rupture (Weems *et al.*, 2006; Newcombe *et al.*, 2008; Ginther, 2012; Santos *et al.*, 2013). Prostaglandins are labile and rapidly broken down so difficult, therefore, to measure in the peripheral circulatory system because of their short half-life. However, PGF2α has a metabolic breakdown product – PG F metabolite (PGFM) – which has a longer half-life and so is easier to measure. As a metabolite of PGF2α, it closely mimics changes in PGF2α concentration. Using levels of PGFM as a guide, it can be seen that PGF2α levels rise to a peak of 40–50 pg ml^{-1} between days 14 and 16 post-ovulation, immediately before progesterone levels start to decline (Aurich and Budik, 2015; Ginther *et al.*, 2016a,b; Fig. 2.9). In mares that are pregnant, no such rise is detected. PGF2α is secreted by the uterine endometrium in the absence of a message of pregnancy. PGF2α production is driven by oxytocin which binds to receptors on the

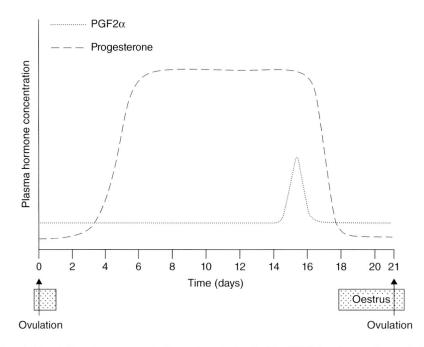

Fig. 2.9. Variations in the relative plasma concentrations of prostaglandin F2α (PGF2α) and progesterone in the non-pregnant mare.

endometrium. Oxytocin is itself also driven by PGF2α, forming a self-perpetuating positive feedback loop which culminates in the peak release of PGF2α that causes luteolysis (Section 2.4.2.8; Vanderwall *et al.*, 1998; Stout *et al.*, 2000; Rebordao *et al.*, 2017). It has been suggested that there are two aspects to PGF2α-induced luteolysis: (i) development of uterine oxytocin receptors from 10 days after ovulation onwards, allowing the uterus to be responsive to oxytocin; and (ii) up-regulation of the cyclooxygenase 2 enzyme, which is key in PG synthesis, and which occurs 13–15 days after ovulation, so enabling uterine production of PG2α (Boerboom *et al.*, 2004; Stout, 2011).

Importantly, PGF2α reaches the ovary where it causes luteolysis of the CL via the main circulatory system, and not by a local counter-current transport system, as seen in the ewe and cow (Ginther and First, 1971). This has consequences for relative dose levels of exogenous (injected) PG required to induce luteolysis when manipulating the cycle (Section 9.5.2.2; Stout, 2011).

Luteolysis and the resulting decline in progesterone levels, in response to PGF2α secretion, remove any inhibition of gonadotrophin release, allowing the hormone changes (increasing FSH, LH and oestrogen) associated with oestrus and ovulation to commence.

2.4.2.8. Oxytocin

Oxytocin is a neuropeptide produced primarily by the posterior pituitary, but also by the endometrium, and also possibly by the CL (Behrendt-Adam *et al.*, 2000; Stout *et al.*, 2000; Watson *et al.*, 2000). Oxytocin has many roles: classically it is an activator of smooth muscle, but with regard to the oestrous cycle it appears to have a role in luteolysis. Endometrial oxytocin receptors vary with the stage of the cycle, beginning around 10 days after ovulation and being most abundant at 14–17 days (LeBlanc *et al.*, 1994; Stout *et al.*, 1999). At this stage oxytocin, which in the mare appears to be primarily secreted by the endometrium itself, binds to the endometrium and drives PGF2α production (Starbuck *et al.*, 1998; Stout *et al.*, 2000). Oxytocin seems to be produced by the CL in other livestock, such as the ewe, but there is some doubt about whether this also occurs in the mare (Stevenson *et al.*, 1991). If a pregnancy is present in the uterus, the development of oxytocin receptors is inhibited and so any oxytocin produced is unable to have an effect and PGF2α release is significantly reduced (Tetzke *et al.*, 1987; Nett, 1993b; Lamming and Mann, 1995; Hansen *et al.*, 1999).

Oxytocin plasma concentrations are also reported to be slightly elevated until after ovulation and are thought to be involved in uterine contractility and expulsion of exudates post-mating (Section 2.4.3). Figure 2.10 gives a summary of all the major hormone changes during the mare's oestrous cycle.

Table 2.1 is a summary of the major events that occur in the mare's oestrous cycle.

2.4.3. Physiological changes of the genital tract

In addition to the cyclical changes in hormone concentration, changes in the mare's reproductive tract may also be observed; these are driven by the fluctuations in hormone levels. During the luteal phase (early and mid-dioestrus), under the influence of increasing progesterone and decreasing oestradiol, the uterus appears more toned. The epithelial cells appear cuboidal; and the endometrial glands become more active and secretory, appearing vacuolated (with an obvious lumen) while progesterone is dominant (Fig 2.11b). During the follicular phase (oestrus), when oestrogen is dominant, the uterus appears flaccid; the epithelial cells columnar; and the endometrial glands less active and secretory, and so non-vacuolated (Fig. 2.11a). During dioestrus, in the preparation for pregnancy, the relative concentrations of components within the endometrial gland's secretions (hystertroph) also change, with a higher protein concentration, particularly increased secretion of uteroferrin, uterocalin and uteroglobulin (Ellenberger *et al.*, 2008). Ultrasonic scanning also shows a typical 'cartwheel'-like cross section image of the uterus, caused by oedema within the endometrial folds, apparent during the late follicular phase/beginning of oestrus, as progesterone levels decline and oestradiol levels increase (Figs 2.12 and 10.16; Bragg Weber *et al.*, 2002). Leucocyte concentrations within the uterus also vary, increasing during oestrus due to elevated oestradiol concentrations, and so helping to combat infection at a vulnerable time (Pycock, 2000).

Uterine myometrial (muscle cell) contractility also varies with the cycle, being more active during the follicular phase/oestrus. This activity encourages the expulsion of uterine exudates, as well as excess sperm and seminal plasma if the mare is mated, which is particularly important at a time when the tract is most vulnerable to uterine infection. This contractility is caused by elevated localized oxytocin levels. Failure of uterine myometrial contraction leads to post-coital endometritis (Section 14.3.5.3).

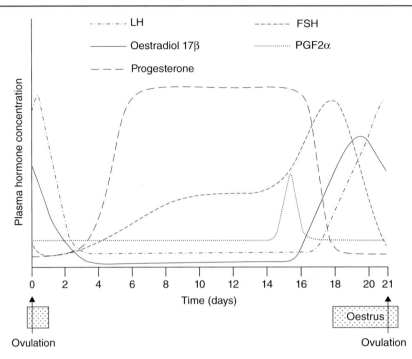

Fig. 2.10. A simplified summary of the major plasma hormone concentration changes during the oestrous cycle of the non-pregnant mare. LH, luteinizing hormone; FSH, follicle-stimulating hormone; PGF2α, prostaglandin F2α.

In general, the changes within the uterus result in an increase in uterine wall thickness and tone, as well as secretory activity, as the mare goes into the luteal phase/dioestrus in preparation for the implantation of the expected embryo. If pregnancy does not occur, luteolysis results in a reduction of the thickness of the uterine wall and a reversal of these changes during the follicular phase/as oestrus approaches.

Cervical changes also occur within the oestrous cycle. Cervical appearance, as viewed by a vaginascope or endoscope, can be used as a diagnostic aid in assessing reproductive activity. During dioestrus, the cervix is tightly closed, forming a tight seal against entry into the uterus. Its appearance is white, firm and dry. During oestrus, the cervix relaxes, opening the cervical seal to allow entry of the penis at mating. During oestrus, the cervix appears moist, red and dilated as the secretions of the uterine epithelial cells and cervical cells increase (Warszawsky *et al.*, 1972). The presence or absence of these secretions within the vagina is also indicative of the stage of the oestrous cycle. For example, it is often very hard to insert a vaginascope into the vagina of a dioestrous mare, due to the thick, sticky nature of the

secretions (Ginther, 1992; Lofstedt, 2011a; McCue *et al.*, 2011a).

2.4.4. Variations in cyclic changes

The mare is notorious for variations or abnormalities in her oestrous cycle. This is in contrast to other farm livestock which have been specifically bred over time for their ability to reproduce rather than perform athletically.

A wide variation in the length of the follicular phase and associated oestrus is evident among mares, the extremes being reported to be between 1 and 50 days. In general a variation can be seen with the time of year, longer and less-distinct oestrous periods being evident during the beginning and end of the breeding season (Christensen, 2011a). Nutritional intake also causes variation in oestrus length. When nutrition is limited oestrus tends to be longer and less distinct, making it less likely that the mare will conceive during such a non-ideal time. This effect of poor nutrition may be an additional signal to the mare, indirectly indicating seasonal and, therefore, day length changes (Daels and Hughes, 1993b). Mare age has also been reported to affect the length of oestrus with older mares (> 20 years of age) having longer cycle lengths due to an increase in

Table 2.1. A summary of the major events that occur in the mare's oestrous cycle.

Day 0	Ovulation
	LH rising
	FSH basal
	Oestradiol falling
	Oestrus
Day 1	LH peak
	Metaoestrus
Day 2	Oestrus ends
	Dioestrus begins
	LH declining
	FSH basal
	Oestradiol basal levels
	Progesterone rising
Day 5	Progesterone at maximum
Day 9	FSH rising
Day 15	PGF2α peak
	Progesterone begins to fall
Day 16	Progesterone falling
Day 17	FSH peak
Day 18	FSH falling
	Progesterone basal
	Oestradiol rising
	Pro-oestrus
	LH rising
Day 20	Progesterone basal
	LH rising
	Oestradiol reaching a peak
	Oestrus
Day 21/0	OvulationLH rising
	FSH basal
	Oestradiol failing
	Oestrus

LH, luteinizing hormone; FSH, follicle-stimulating hormone; PGF2α, prostaglandin F2α.

the follicular phase/oestrus (Vanderwal *et al.*, 1993; Carnevale *et al.*, 1994; Wilsher and Allen, 2003). Finally, several other more rare factors have been associated with abnormal follicular phase/oestrous length including: Cushing's disease (Love, 1993; Dybdal *et al.*, 1994; Masko *et al.*, 2018); granulosa cell tumours (McCue, 1992) and persistent endometrial cups after foaling or abortion (Steiner *et al.*, 2006).

The length of dioestrus also varies between mares, with the extremes being 10 days to several months. This delay is termed prolonged dioestrus; it prevents the mare returning to oestrus and ovulation, and has been reported to occur in up to 18% of mares (Kerschen, 2019). Prolonged dioestrus is normally due to one of three factors: first, a silent ovulation – ovulation occurred but it was not accompanied by oestrus, giving the impression that the mare has been in dioestrus for a prolonged period of time (Hughes *et al.*, 1975a); second, inactive ovaries – usually associated with the transition into or out of the non-breeding season or true anoestrus (McCue and Ferris, 2011); or, third, the existence of a persistent CL – a CL that has not reacted to PGF2α or has not received enough PGF2α to elicit a response. A persistent CL may have a number of causes, including endometritis (Stabenfeldt *et al.*, 1979); endotoxemia (Fredriksson *et al.*, 1986); cervical or uterine manipulation (McCue *et al.*, 2008a); embryo or pregnancy loss (McCue and Ferris, 2011); luteinized anovulatory follicles; age (McCue and Squires, 2002); and stress (Liptrap, 1993).

Other variations with the cycle do occur, the most noteworthy being ovulation in dioestrus (Newcombe, 1997). LH is normally released in a low episodic fashion (1–4 ng ml⁻¹) during dioestrus; occasionally these episodes appear to cause mid-cycle ovulation (Hughes *et al.*, 1985; Ginther, 1990a,b). This evidence of dioestrus rises in LH and, as discussed earlier, the elevated FSH concentration mid-cycle indicates that, unlike many other species, progesterone does not serve to completely block gonadotrophin release in the mare. The converse, but much less common, is oestrus with no ovulation; this has been reported, normally in mares out of the breeding season (Hughes *et al.*, 1985; Daels and Hughes, 1993b). As mentioned previously, foal heat may occur as early as 4 days post-partum, and mating on the foal heat is often less successful, as fertility rates are normally low. Additionally, the oestrous cycles following this foal heat are often irregular, showing prolonged oestrus and/or dioestrus, until steady cyclicity is achieved (Blanchard and Varner, 1993a; Camillo *et al.*, 1997).

The causes of many of these variations can be attributed to managerial or environmental influences such as nutrition, temperature and day length. Occasionally they are due to genetic faults, lactational effects or embryonic death.

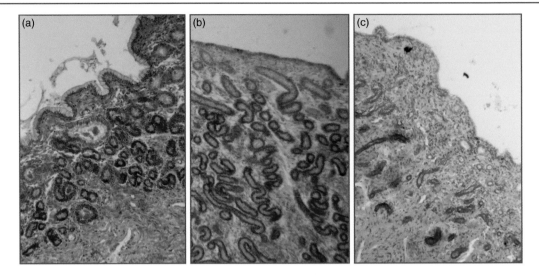

Fig. 2.11. A histological view of the mare's uterus at (a) follicular phase; (b) luteal phase; (c) anoestrus. Note in particular the difference in the size of the epithelial cells (tall and columnar during the follicular phase, shorter and cuboidal during the luteal phase) and the activity of the endometrial glands indicated by the absence (inactive – follicular phase) or presence (active – luteal phase) of lumen. In the anoestrous mare the epithelial cells are cuboidal and the endometrial glands inactive (photo courtesy of Dr Maithe Rocha Monteiro de Barros).

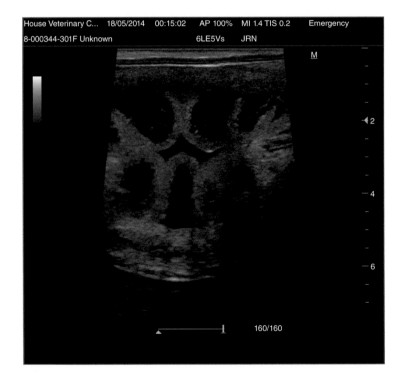

Fig. 2.12. An ultrasonic scanning image of the cross section through the uterus of a mare as she approaches oestrus (follicular phase): the dark areas is the oedema collected within the endometrial folds which occurs as oestradiol levels increase and progesterone levels decrease. Note the small amount of luminal fluid (dark area where the oedematous endometrial folds meet) (photo courtesy of Professor John Newcombe).

2.4.5. Multiple ovulation

Multiple ovulations – the release of more than one ovum per oestrus – are increasingly common in intensively bred mares. Release of the ova may occur within oestrus (synchronous) or occur over time, including early dioestrus (asynchronous). Sperm survival times of up to 7 days and ovulations occurring up to 6 days apart have been reported, indicating the potential for fertilization and the yield of viable embryos (Newcombe and Cuervo-Arango (2008). However, the more distant over time the ovulations occur, the less likely the chance of fertilization, and those occurring more than 3 days apart rarely result in multiple conceptuses. The reported incidence of multiple ovulations in mares is very variable at 0.83–42.8% (Ginther, 1982; Newcombe, 1995; Davies Morel and O'Sullivan, 2001; Davies Morel *et al.*, 2005). The issue of multiple ovulations and multiple pregnancies presents many dilemmas and is of significant economic importance to horse breeders; it is considered further in Section 3.2.4.2.

2.5. Behavioural Changes

Cyclical, hormonal changes govern the mare's behavioural patterns (i.e. oestrus and dioestrus); elevated oestradiol concentrations in the absence of progesterone, stimulating behavioural centres of the brain and causing the mare to express oestrous behaviour (Crowell-Davis, 2007). GnRH also plays a minor role in oestrous behaviour, as considered previously (Irvine and Alexander, 1993b). There are many variations between individuals in the extent and strength of behavioural changes. Details of the signs of oestrus, their interpretation and mating behaviour are given in Chapter 10. A summary of the major behavioural changes is given below.

2.5.1. Oestrus initiated by elevated oestradiol and low progesterone concentrations

Signs of oestrus in the presence of a stallion (Figs 10.2 and 10.3):

* docility;
* urination stance;
* lengthening and eversion of the vulva;
* exposure of the clitoris (winking);
* tail raised;
* urine bright yellow with a characteristic odour; and
* acceptance of the stallion's advances.

2.5.2. Dioestrus evident in the absence of oestradiol and presence of progesterone

Signs of dioestrus in the presence of a stallion (Fig. 10.5d):

* hostility; and
* rejection of the stallion's advances.

2.6. Conclusion

The prime aim of the control mechanisms for the female reproductive system is to synchronize the physiological and behavioural events associated with oestrus and ovulation, in order to synchronize mating with ovulation and so achieve fertilization, and subsequently to synchronize embryo and uterine development.

Study Questions

With the aid of a diagram detail the roles played by the hypothalamus, pituitary and gonads in the control of mare reproduction.

Discuss the mechanism by which ovulation is synchronized with oestrous behaviour in the mare.

If a mare is not mated, or mating does not result in conception, how does nature ensure that the mare has another chance to conceive?

Discuss how the environment affects reproductive activity in the mare.

Suggested Reading

Daels, P.F. and Hughes, J.P. (1993) The normal estrous cycle. In: McKinnon, A.O. and Voss, J.L. (eds) *Equine Reproduction*. Lea and Febiger, Philadelphia, Pennsylvania, pp. 121–132.

Ginther, O.J., Beg, M.A., Bergfeldt, D.R., Donadeu, F.X. and Kot, K. (2001) Follicle selection in monovular species. *Biology of Reproduction* 65, 638–647.

Crowell-Davis, S.L. (2007) Sexual behavior of mares. *Hormones and Behaviour* 52, 12–17.

Youngquist, R.S. and Threlfall, W.R. (2007) Clinical Reproductive Anatomy and Physiology of the Mare. In: Youngquist, R.S. and Threlfall, W.R. (eds.) *Large Animal Theriogenology*. Saunders Elsevier, St Louis, Missouri, pp. 47–67.

Aurich, C. (2011) Reproductive cycles of horses. *Animal Reproduction Science* 124, 220–228.

Alexander, S.L. and Irvine, C.H.G. (2011) GnRH. In: McKinnon, A.O., Squires, E.L., Vaala, E. and Varner, D.D. (eds) *Equine Reproduction*, 2nd edn. Wiley-Blackwell, Philadelphia, London, pp. 1608–1618.

Alexander, S.L. and Irvine, C.H.G. (2011) FSH and LH. In: McKinnon, A.O., Squires, E.L., Vaala, E. and Varner, D.D. (eds) *Equine Reproduction*, 2nd edn. Wiley-Blackwell, Philadelphia, London, pp. 1619–1630.

Lofstedt, R.M. (2011) Diestrus. In: McKinnon, A.O., Squires, E.L., Vaala, E. and Varner, D.D. (eds) *Equine Reproduction*, 2nd edn. Wiley-Blackwell, Philadelphia, London, pp. 1728–1731.

Satué, K. and Gardón, J.C. (2013) A Review of the Estrous Cycle and the Neuroendocrine Mechanisms in the Mare. *Journal of Steroids and Hormonal Science* 4, 115.

3 Pregnancy

The Objectives of this Chapter are:

To detail the anatomy of pregnancy in the mare.

To enable you to understand the processes involved in fertilization, and in embryo and fetal development.

To enable you to understand the process of placentation and so appreciate the vital role the placenta plays in the survival of pregnancy and the implications of placental structure on early post-natal life.

To enable you to appreciate why pregnancies can fail, and possible preventions and treatments.

To detail how the mare accommodates and supports a pregnancy and the hormones involved in that support.

To provide you with the knowledge to then understand subsequent chapters on managing the pregnant mare and the application to breeding practice.

3.1. Introduction

This Chapter considers both the anatomy and physiology of pregnancy followed by the control of pregnancy. It has been divided as such for ease of understanding but the two are integral to each other. Similarly, for ease of understanding, the anatomy of pregnancy is divided into four main sections: fertilization, early embryo development, placentation and organ growth. Each section will be discussed, along with the vital role all factors play in ensuring successful fertilization and subsequent maintenance of the pregnancy.

3.2. Anatomy and Physiology of Pregnancy

3.2.1. Fertilization

Fertilization relies on the successful accomplishment of a number of things: the release of the ovum along with the deposition of sperm into the female tract followed by sperm capacitation, sperm binding to the ovum's zona pellucida, acrosome reaction, sperm penetration of the zona pellucida, and finally binding and fusion with the ovum vitelline membrane (Fig. 3.1).

The ovum is released by the follicle through the ovulation fossa into the infundibulum and is directed down the Fallopian tube by the cilia lining, where it waits in the ampulla region, that nearest the infundibulum, for the arrival of the sperm. It is unable to pass through the utero-tubular junction until it has been fertilized (Allen *et al.*, 2006).

The sperm, having been ejaculated into the top of the cervix/bottom of the uterus, make their way up through the uterus to the utero-tubular junction. They move by means of contractions of the female tract and the driving action of their own tails, and many are lost along the way (Campbell and England, 2006; Katila, 2011).

On arrival at the utero-tubular junction, they pass through to the Fallopian tube and, if the timing is correct, meet a newly released ovum in the ampulla. It appears that only morphologically normal sperm can pass through to the Fallopian tube and that the utero-tubular junction may act as a reservoir and slow-release mechanism, helping to ensure the arrival of the sperm is synchronized with ova release and the most opportune time for fertilization (Scott *et al.*, 2000). Sperm with intact acrosome and plasma membranes appear to be preferentially attached to oviductal epithelium in this area, helping to filter out non- or sub-viable sperm. In addition, attachment to oviductal epithelium appears to arrest sperm senility, ensuring sperm are viable for longer and so increasing the chance of synchronizing the meeting of a viable ovum and sperm (Thomas *et al.*, 1994; Scott 2000). Once an ovum has

been released into the Fallopian tube, sperm appear to be attracted towards it by chemical attractants produced by the corona radiata cells (that replaced the cumulus oophorus cells) surrounding the ovum awaiting fertilization (Hunter, 2008).

As the sperm pass up through the female tract, they come in contact with uterine secretions. These induce a capacitation response, the first of two activation processes in the acrosome region of the sperm head that are essential before sperm are capable of fertilizing an ovum (Fig. 3.2). Where exactly within the female reproductive tract capacitation occurs is somewhat disputed,

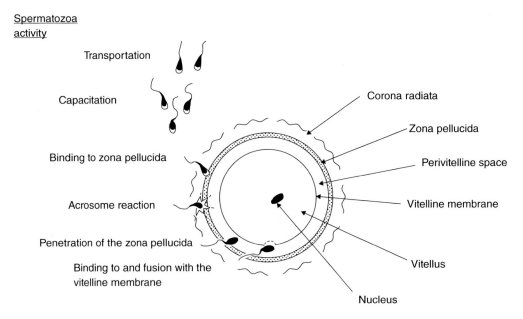

Fig. 3.1. The equine ovum prior to fertilization, also illustrating the changes to the sperm required for successful fertilization.

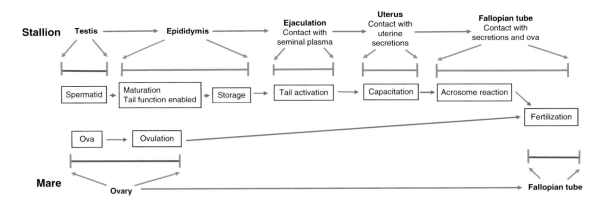

Fig. 3.2. The life cycle of the sperm and ovum from release to fertilization.

although recent work indicated that, in the mare, the oviductal cells are able to drive capacitation (Leemans *et al.*, 2016a,b, 2019). Wherever it occurs, capacitation is essential, as it activates the enzymes within the acrosome region and so enables the sperm to penetrate the corona radiata and access the zona pellucida surrounding the ovum (Yanagimachi, 1989; Suarez and Ho, 2003). Successful capacitation is a challenge in *in vitro* fertilization. Capacitation appears also to drive hyperactivation of the sperm tails, so driving them to stick to and then penetrate the outer layers of the ovum (Fig. 3.1; Gadella *et al.*, 2001; Amann and Graham, 2011; Ball, 2011a).

Hyperactivated sperm then bind to the zona pellucida of the ovum and, by means of the whipping action of their tails, penetrate through the zona pellucida to attach to receptors on the vitelline membrane. During this they undergo the second sperm-head activation process (the acrosome reaction) essential to enable fertilization (Bailey, 2007; Varner and Johnson, 2007). The glycoproteins within the zona pellucida appear to be responsible for driving the acrosome reaction, as a result of which the membrane of the sperm head alters and acrosomal contents including enzymes such as hyaluronidase are released (acrosomal exocytocis). This allows the sperm head to then bind to and fuse with the vitelline membrane of the ovum (Meyers, 2011). This fusion also initiates the release of sperm factors (PLCζ), which drive the release of calcium from oocyte stores. This calcium is then taken up again by these stores, and again released, causing calcium oscillations which drive the ovum's final meiotic division, resulting in three polar bodies and the single ovum nucleus (Saunders *et al.*, 2002; Rivera and Ross, 2013). The nuclei of the sperm decondense and fuse with the ovum nucleus (often termed the pronuclei), their haploid (32) complement of chromosomes now uniting to give the full diploid (64) of the new individual. This newly combined genetic material now dictates all the characteristics of the new individual (Bezard *et al.*, 1989; Grondahl *et al.*, 2011). There is some variation in the reported length of time that the equine ovum remains viable; figures varying between 4 and 36 h have been reported.

In order to ensure the successful fusion of one male pronucleus and one female pronucleus, it is essential that only one sperm penetrates the vitelline membrane of the ovum. Polyspermy (penetration by more than one sperm) is prevented by an instantaneous block, termed the cortical reaction, which occurs as soon as one sperm binds to the vitelline membrane. This instantaneous response is not fully understood, but is likely to involve a chemical reaction (the cortical reaction) which forces release of the contents of the cortical granules within the zona pellucida. This alters the chemical nature of the zona pellucida, enforcing an instantaneous vitelline block and making the vitelline membrane impenetrable to further sperm (Ginther, 1992b; Crozet, 1993; Flood, 1993).

3.2.2. Early embryo development

Day 1

Twenty-four hours after fertilization the fertilized ovum, now termed a zygote, has divided by mitosis (growth by cell division) into two cells. This is also called cleavage, with the stage of cleavage referring to the number of cells evident per embryo (Bezard *et al.*, 1989; Betteridge, 2011). At this stage, the outer gelatinous corona radiata layer is lost and the fertilized ovum, still within the zona pellucida, continues to divide into four (48 h), eight (72 h) 12 (96 h), etc. (Bezard *et al.*, 1989).

Day 4

At 4 days old it is a bundle of 12–16 cells, again still contained within its zona pellucida, and is now termed a morula (Fig. 3.3). It was initially thought that all these cells within the morula were identical. This may well still be the case, but recent work suggests that a polarization of cells may exist; that is, asymmetrical distribution of cells in the morula, linked to the oval shape of the equine embryo at this stage. This is of interest, as disruption of this asymmetry may be one of the reasons why advanced reproductive techniques (ART) are not very successful (Chapter 23; Betteridge, 2007).

At this stage the total volume and external size of the bundle of cells has not changed from the two-cell zygote stage. The cytoplasm of the original ovum has either been divided up between all the cells in the morula or used for energy. Nevertheless, the amount of genetic material has dramatically increased, giving a full identical complement to all cells of the morula. This stage is also critical, as the ability to function at this level so early on has consequences for embryo survival and the long-term survival and health of the future adult horse, and even the health of subsequent offspring from that adult horse. These appear to be irrevocably affected by the epigenetic results of metabolic interactions between the embryonic genome and the environment, including the ovum follicular environment

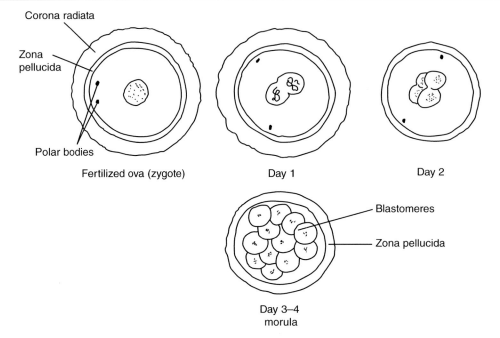

Fig. 3.3. The developmental stages from fertilized ovum to morula in the equine conceptus, illustrating the loss of the gelatinous outer layer by day 2.

(Duranthan *et al.*, 2008; Leese *et al.*, 2008; Pantaleon *et al.*, 2008; Betteridge, 2011).

As the cells continue to divide, the morula makes its way towards the utero-tubular junction by anticlockwise rotational swimming and possibly by contraction of the Fallopian tube myometrium. At this stage (day 4), the morula begins to secrete low levels of PGE, which causes relaxation and/or contraction of the myometrial smooth muscle. The localized nature of secretion by the conceptus results in its movement through the Fallopian tube and the relaxation of the utero-tubular junction sphincter, so allowing the conceptus to pass through and on into the uterus (Allen *et al.*, 2006). Fertilized ova, therefore, pass through to the uterus, overtaking on their way any unfertilized ova from that or previous ovulations. Any ovum not fertilized may take several months to degenerate (Ball and Brinsko, 1992; Robinson *et al.*, 2000; Stout and Allen, 2001). This cell division and PGE production require considerable energy metabolism in very young embryos.

Day 5

At days 5–6 the embryo is found within the uterus (Allen *et al.*, 2006), the endometrium of which undergoes significant ultrastructural and histological changes to accommodate the embryo (Caballeros *et al.*, 2019). At this stage a thin acellular glycoprotein layer, termed the capsule (see Section 3.2.2.1), appears in the perivitilline space between the trophectoderm (outer layer of the morula) and the zona pellucida (Oriol, 1994; Stout *et al.*, 2005; Betteridge, 2007). From day 6, the total size of the embryo starts to increase; this helps to force the thinning of the zona pellucida, which eventually breaks. The embryo then hatches through this break and is left surrounded by just its capsule. At this time, having lost its zona pellucida, the conceptus starts to derive nutrients for its growth and cell division from the surrounding uterine secretions, as by this stage it has used up all its own reserves. The provision of such additional nutrients allows a further increase in size. The morula is now in its mobility phase, floating freely within the uterus (Section 3.2.3.1), deriving all its nutritional requirements from secretions of the endometrial glands which produce uterine histotroph (uterine milk), the composition of which varies to match the requirements of the developing conceptus (Betteridege, 2007; Camozzato *et al.*, 2019).

Day 8

At day 8, the cells of the morula become differentiated (organized) and three distinct areas can be identified:

the embryonic disc (shield or mass) at one pole, the blastocoel and the trophoblast (Fig. 3.4). The morula is now termed a blastocyst.

These three areas go to form the embryo proper (the inner cell mass that goes to form the embryonic disc), the yolk sac (blastocoel) and the placenta (trophoblast). This cell differentiation marks the beginning of the switching on and off of various genes, cells then becoming destined to pursue set lines of development. Prior to this differentiation, all cells in theory were capable, if extracted from the morula, of each developing into new identical individuals as none of their genes had been switched off. After differentiation, this is no longer possible, as certain cells have been given the message to only pursue set lines of development. The mechanism behind this switching on and off of genes and its trigger are unknown in the horse. It is important to note that, at this differentiation stage, the conceptus is very susceptible to external physical effects such as mechanical damage, drugs, other chemicals, disease and radiation. These can disrupt the differentiation process, resulting in deformities, abnormalities and a high risk of abortion or reabsorption.

The equine embryo is unique in being free-living within the uterus for up to 18 days from arrival in the uterus to final implantation; this period of time is termed the mobility phase (Section 3.2.3.1).

Day 9

Day 9 marks further the differentiation to give two germ layers (cell layers) within the trophoblast and the embryo. In the trophoblast, the ectoderm consists of the outer blastocyst cell layers; and the endoderm consists of the inner cell lining (Fig. 3.5).

In most mammals the endoderm originates from the inner cell mass (embryonic disc) and grows and develops, working its way around to line the inside of the trophoblast to give a complete inner layer. In the mare it has been reported that, rather than originating from the inner cell mass, the endoderm cells originate from sporadically distributed colonies throughout the inner part of the trophoblast. These colonies then spread and join up to form a complete endoderm layer (Enders *et al.*, 1993). However it occurs, the endoderm and ectoderm together then encircle the conceptus and form the bilaminar (two layer) yolk sac wall and provide the means by which the embryonic disc receives its nourishment from the surrounding uterine secretions. The blastocoel, or fluid-filled centre, sometimes termed the yolk sac and acts as a temporary nutrient store (Fig. 3.5). This remains the major source of nutrients to the embryo until implantation or fixation occurs.

Day 11

Between days 11 and 16 (Figs 3.6 and 3.7) the conceptus goes through a period of rapid growth followed by one of steadier growth (Betteridge, 2011). Nutrition for this expansion is still provided by the uterine secretions via the yolk sac. However, the yolk sac undergoes changes unique to the equine conceptus in becoming hypotonic; as such, passage of fluids and nutrients into

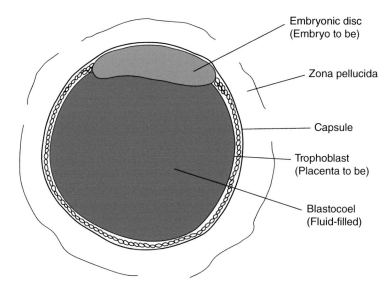

Embryonic disc (Embryo to be)

Zona pellucida

Capsule

Trophoblast (Placenta to be)

Blastocoel (Fluid-filled)

Fig. 3.4. The equine blastocyst at day 8 post-fertilization, showing the differentiation of three areas.

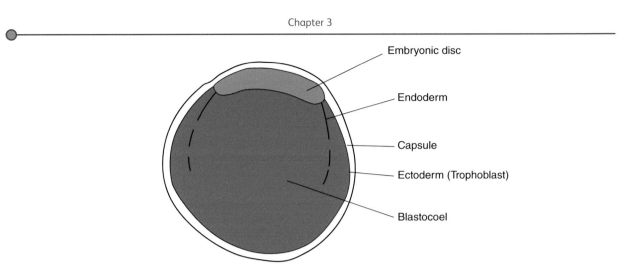

Fig. 3.5. The equine conceptus at day 9 post-fertilization, illustrating the differentiation of the ectoderm and endoderm layers.

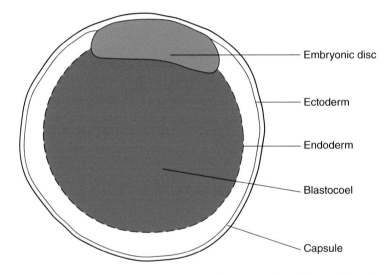

Fig. 3.6. The equine conceptus at day 12 post-fertilization, illustrating the blastocoel or yolk sac, which at this stage provides a store for the nutrients required by the developing conceptus.

the yolk sac from the surrounding uterus must be via active transfer and no longer by passive transfer along an osmotic gradient (Crews *et al.*, 2007; Budik *et al.*, 2008).

Day 14

At day 14, when the conceptus has reached 13–15 mm (Table 11.1) in diameter, the mesoderm or third germ-cell layer begins to develop. It develops progressively between the ectoderm and endoderm, in the centre of the yolk sac wall. This trilaminar (three layer) yolk sac wall works its way down from the embryonic disc,

transforming the bilaminar yolk sac wall, until it encloses the whole blastocyst (Bergfeldt and Adams, 2011b). The junction of these two areas – the line delineating the limit of mesoderm migration – is called the sinus terminalis (Figs 3.8 and 3.9; Allen *et al.*, 2011). These three germ-cell layers are also evident within the embryo itself and are the cell layers from which all subsequent placental and embryonic tissue development originates. In the case of the placenta, the ectoderm forms the outer cell layers nearest the uterine epithelium; the mesoderm forms the blood vessels and nutrient transport system within the placenta; and the endoderm forms the inner cell lining that will become the allantoic sac.

Day 16

At day 16, when the conceptus is 15–20 mm in diameter (Fig. 3.8 and Table 11.1), folds appear in the outer cell layers, and the beginnings of the protective layers that will surround the embryo become evident. The ectoderm folds over the top of the embryonic disc, taking the mesoderm with it. The outer layer of these folds is now made up of the ectoderm plus a mesoderm layer and is termed the chorion. At this stage, embryonic movement slows as the embryo becomes clamped at the base of the uterine horn (Section 3.2.3.1; Waelchi *et al.*, 1996).

Day 18

By day 18, the embryo has stopped moving and has become fixated at the junction of the uterine body and one uterine horn. The two ectoderm folds fuse, producing a fluid-filled protective space for the embryonic disc; this is the amniotic sac containing the amniotic fluid (Figs 3.8 and 3.9).

The membrane encompassing the amnion and separating it from the surrounding allantoic fluid (discussed later) is termed the allantoamniotic membrane. Initially, the amnion is visible as a clear fluid-filled bubble surrounding the embryo. As pregnancy progresses, it tends to collapse and lie close to the fetus. Through-

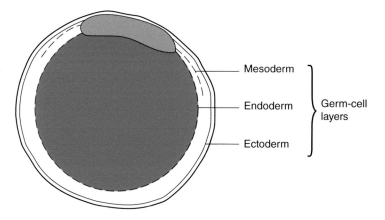

Fig. 3.7. The equine conceptus at day 14 post-fertilization, illustrating the developing mesoderm, which forms the blood vessels and nutrient transport system of the conceptus.

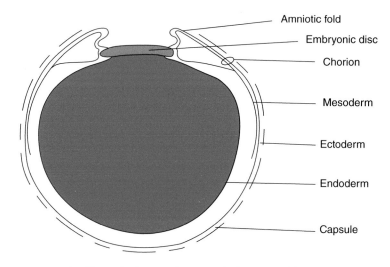

Fig. 3.8. The equine conceptus at day 16 post-fertilization, illustrating the formation of the amniotic folds over the embryonic disc.

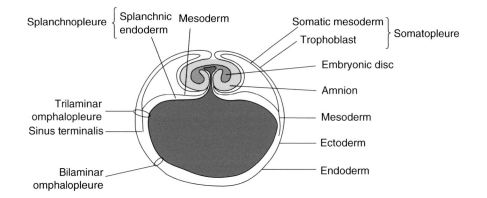

Fig. 3.9. The equine conceptus at day 18 post-fertilization, illustrating the near completion of the amniotic sac surrounding the embryonic disc. The trilaminar omphalopleure is shown, nearest the embryo, consisting of the endoderm, mesoderm and ectoderm, and the bilaminar omphalopleure, into which the mesoderm has not yet spread.

out the embryo's life in utero the amniotic sac provides a clean and protective environment in which it can develop. The source of its surrounding amniotic fluid is not clear. However, its composition is very much like blood serum, and exchange of fluids between the amniotic sac and the kidneys, intestine and respiratory tract is known to occur. The fetus in later stages appears to breathe in and swallow its surrounding amniotic fluid. The volume of amniotic fluid surrounding the fetus is about 0.4 l at 100 days post-fertilization and increases to 3.5 l at full term.

During this time the mesoderm continues to spread between the ectoderm and endoderm and does not completely enclose the conceptus until day 35 or later (Allen *et al.*, 2011).

3.2.2.1. The equine capsule

The equine conceptus is relatively unique in having a thin acellular glycoprotein/glycocalyx mucin-like capsule which develops around the conceptus at day 5. It is certainly present until day 20 and possibly even as late as day 35 of pregnancy (Fig. 3.10; Enders and Lui, 1991). This capsule appears in the perivitelline space between the trophectoderm and the zona pellucida (Fig. 3.4; Oriol, 1994). The function of this capsule is unclear. It may have a protective role in that it is strong enough to retain the spherical shape of the conceptus up until implantation. It may have an additional role in embryo mobility; by preventing the adhesion of the embryo to the endometrium it allows the prolonged mobility phase characteristic of the equine conceptus (Stout *et al.*, 2005). It may also have a role in driving embryo expansion, which occurs from day 5 (Crossett

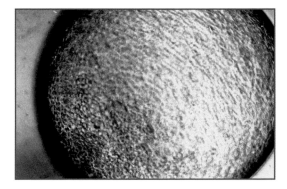

Fig. 3.10. A view of the surface of an equine embryo illustrating the outer trophoblastic cells. The capsule is evident as a clear area encircling the whole conceptus. (Photo courtesy of Ms Alison Crook.)

et al., 1995). From day 6, the conceptus increases in size; this forces a thinning of the zona pellucida, which eventually breaks. The embryo then hatches and is left surrounded by just its capsule (Stout *et al.*, 2005). At this time (day 6), the conceptus starts to derive nutrients from the surrounding uterine secretions, and so the capsule may also act to transfer nutrients from the uterus to the yolk sac. By nature of its negative electrostatic charge, and unusual glycocalyx configuration, the capsule is sticky to proteins within the surrounding uterine secretions (Oriol *et al.*, 1993; Allen *et al.*, 2011). The capsule, therefore, attracts a whole host of proteins and other components as it moves through the uterus during the period of embryo mobility. These then diffuse, or are actively transferred by carrier proteins such as lipocalin and uterocalin, across the capsule into the yolk sac to provide nutrients for the growing conceptus (Crossett *et al.*, 1998; Suire *et al.*, 2001; Quinn *et al.*, 2007; Hayes *et al.*, 2008) and may also act to drive conceptus growth (Stewart *et al.*, 1995). The provision of such nutrients is essential and provides the only source of nutrition until full implantation. The morula is now in its mobility phase, floating freely within the uterus (Section 3.2.3.1), deriving all its nutritional requirements from uterine histotroph (Camozzato *et al.*, 2019). The mechanism by which the capsule is lost around day 20 is unclear; it may be via enzymatic action (Oriol *et al.*, 1993), or by mechanical rupture due to the continual growth of the conceptus in the absence of continued capsule growth (Denker *et al.*, 1987; Betteridge, 2011).

From day 20 onwards, when the conceptus is 30–40 mm in diameter (Table 11.1), it is increasingly evident that embryology can be dealt with in two sections: placentation and organ development.

3.2.3. Placentation

The placenta has three major functions: (i) protection; (ii) regulation of fetal environment, in the form of nutrient intake and waste output; and (iii) production of hormones modifying the environment to ensure the continuation of the pregnancy. The placenta develops from the extraembryonic membranes, the trophoblast of the blastocyst. The first source of nutrients and, therefore, a form of primitive placenta, is the yolk sac or blastocoel. This provides both a temporary store and a transport system for nutrients derived from uterine secretions which have attached to, and then diffused across, the capsule; reliance on uterine secretions is termed histotrophic nutrition.

Day 14 sees the first evidence of blood vessels developing in the centre of the yolk sac wall within the spreading mesoderm. These will become the blood system of the placenta. By day 18 the vitelline artery, carrying blood away from the embryo, and the vitelline vein, carrying blood towards the embryo, are identifiable and continuous with the mesoderm spreading between the ectoderm and endoderm.

On day 20, an outpushing of the embryonic hindgut can be seen. This is termed the allantois and continues to grow with the conceptus. This sac is filled with allantoic fluid; the allantoic membrane fuses with the trophoblast cells of the endoderm, ectoderm and advancing mesoderm to form the allantochorionic membrane or placenta (Figs 3.10–3.15; Allen *et al.*, 2011).

The allantoic fluid consists of secretions of the allantochorion, along with urinary fluid, which is excreted from the fetal bladder via the urachus within the umbilical cord.

By day 45 the allantois is complete and its volume is approximately 100 ml, increasing to around 8.5 l by day 310, a considerably larger volume than seen in the amniotic sac (Morresey, 2011b). The allantoic fluid increases in volume as the fetus grows, producing more

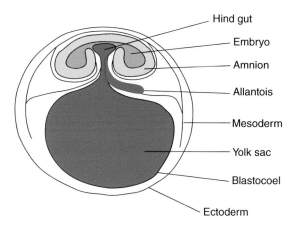

Fig. 3.11. The development of the equine placenta at day 20 post-fertilization, illustrating the development of the allantois (allantoic sac).

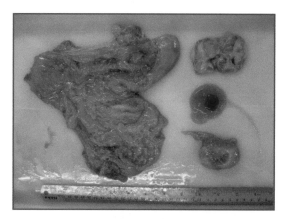

Fig. 3.12. The equine conceptus at day 35–40 alongside the ovaries and uterus from which it was dissected. Note the spherical nature of the conceptus and the embryo sitting within its amniotic sac surrounded by the enlarging allantoic sac and decreasing yolk sac. The sinus terminalis, the extent to which the mesoderm has extended, can be seen as a constriction around the conceptus.

waste fluid to be stored (Fig. 3.14). During the first trimester (3–4 months), it is clear yellow in colour, changing to brown/yellow as pregnancy progresses.

This developing allantoic sac moves over the top and then surrounds the embryo as its contents increase, forcing the embryo to one pole of the blastocyst and reducing, as it goes, the extent of the yolk sac. By day 50 the yolk sac remains only as a remnant within the umbilical cord. Hence, as the allantoic sac increases in size, the umbilical cord becomes increasingly evident. The attachment point of the umbilical cord normally cor-

responds to the position of initial implantation, the junction of the uterine horn and body. It consists of two vitelline (umbilical) arteries, one vitelline vein and the urachus plus supporting and connective tissue. The arteries and veins are responsible for blood transfer to and from the placenta to the fetal system, and the urachus transfers waste products from the fetal bladder to the allantois; as such, it extends no further than the allantois and does not reach the placenta (Fig. 3.15; Allen *et al.*, 2011).

As the fetus develops, its nutrient demand increases. The nutrients provided via the yolk sac and uterine hystotroph are soon not enough to meet this demand; thus, a more intimate relationship needs to develop between the mother and the embryo, and so its period of mobility ceases and it begins to implant. This occurs as a very gradual process from day 16 onwards, from which point the movement of the conceptus slows and it becomes clamped, normally at the base of one of the uterine horns. It now begins to derive increasingly more nutrition directly from the uterine endometrium. Initially the amount of nutrition obtained in this way is very limited, but increases over time, and so the yolk sac continues to function as a nutrient store for a reasonable length of time. At this stage the capsule begins to degenerate, although remnants have been reported as late as day 35 (Enders *et al.*, 1993; Oriol, 1994).

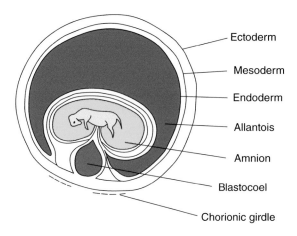

Fig. 3.13. The further development of the equine placenta at day 40 post-fertilization. The allantois now dominates the conceptus.

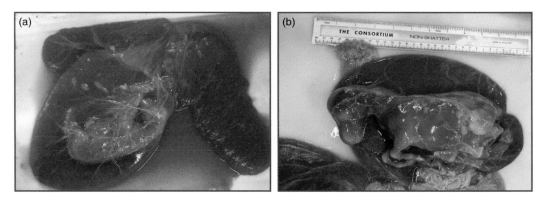

Fig. 3.14. The equine fetus at approximately 100 days of gestation, illustrating: (a) the fetus lying within its amniochorion (forming the amniotic sack) which in turn is lying within the allantochorion (placenta; forming the allantoic sack); and (b) the fetus lying just within its amniochorion (amniotic sack), the allantochorion having been removed. Note that the allantochorion mimics the shape of the uterus as it has attached to the whole uterine surface. The fetus is lying predominantly within the allantochorion from within the uterine body and partly within the allantochorion from one of the uterine horns (right), this is termed the gravid horn. Top of the photograph is the smaller part of the allantochorion that would have come from the non-gravid horn. (Photo courtesy of Tag Dillon.)

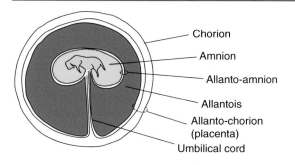

Fig. 3.15. The placental arrangement of the equine conceptus near term.

3.2.3.1. *Embryo mobility and fixation*

The period of embryo mobility in the mare is relatively long, and lasts until days 16–18 of pregnancy, during which time the conceptus moves freely within and between the uterine horns and body (Gastal *et al.*, 1996; Stout and Allen, 2001; Allen and Wilsher, 2009). Mobility is essential to provide maximum contact between the trophoblast and the uterine endometrium owing to the unusual spherical (as opposed to elongated) equine conceptus. This contact is, in turn, essential for the maternal recognition and continuation of pregnancy, and any restriction to this mobility puts the pregnancy at risk (Section 3.3.1.1). Conceptus mobility is caused by uterine myometrial contractions (uterine contractility), which is controlled by an interplay between localized secretion of prostaglandin (PGE and PGF2α) by the conceptus and progesterone secreted by the CL. Providing the uterine environment is dominated by circulating progesterone, PGE and PGF2α secreted by the conceptus cause localized uterine contractility, driving movement of the conceptus (Stout and Allen 2002; Stout, 2016). Implantation follows the period of mobility and can be divided into four stages: precontact immobilization, apposition, adhesion/implantation and endometrial invasion (Fig. 3.16). The last stage, endometrial invasion, does not occur in horses (Bazer *et al.*, 2009, 2012). By days 16–18 embryo movement slowly reduces, resulting in stage 1 precontact immobilization. This occurs because of a number of factors. First, the increasing conceptus size within an ever-reducing uterine lumen makes movement harder. The size of the uterine lumen reduces as the endometrial folds increase in size with increasing oestrogen levels around days 25–30 (Section 3.3.1.4). Immobility is also encouraged by an increase in Na and Cl ion

concentrations within the conceptus changing the conceptus osmolarity, plus the fluid and electrolyte exchange with the surrounding uterine fluid. Finally, uterine contractility decreases as the blastocyst slowly reduces its PG production (Griffin and Ginther, 1990; Gastal *et al.*, 1996). The site of implantation is normally the junction of the uterine horn and body, and appears to be independent of the site of ovulation (Silva *et al.*, 2005) and more likely to occur in the junction contralateral (opposite) to the previous year's pregnancy (Davies Morel *et al.*, 2009; Sharma *et al.*, 2010); implantation elsewhere may compromise the pregnancy.

Areolae

The first very tentative and easily dislodged identifiable contact between mother and fetus occurs around days 18–20 via areolae. These areolae are tufts of allantochorion which break through the now degenerating capsule and invade the mouths of the uterine endometrial glands and encircle the conceptus at the limit of the extent of the spread of the mesoderm, the bilaminar ophalopleure. The development of these areolae is driven by growth factors such as insulin-like growth factor II (IGFII) and they provide a more efficient method of absorption of uterine histotroph directly from the mouths of the endometrial glands (Allen, 2001a; Morresey, 2011b). This may be considered to be the second stage of implantation, the apposition phase.

Chorionic Girdle

About 8 days (day 25 of pregnancy) after the embryo has become stationary in the uterus, the third stage of implantation – adhesion – begins. At this stage a thickening appears on the outer trophoblast (allantochorion) forming a band of shallow folds where the enlarging allantois butts up against the shrinking yolk sac (De Mestre *et al.*, 2011). This is the chorionic girdle. Cells within this girdle elongate to form ridges of 6–8 mm in width and, at around day 35, some begin to invade through the now broken capsule down the endometrial glands and into the uterine endometrium. This girdle forms in an area of the conceptus similar to the areolae at the limit of the spreading mesoderm, where the bilaminar omphalopleure meets the trilaminar ophalopleure, and where the yolk sac is gradually being restricted by the developing allantois (Fig. 3.17). The growth of the chorionic girdle is likely to be governed in part by IGF such as IGF II (Enders and Lui, 1991; Enders *et al.*, 1993). This attachment is again initially only very

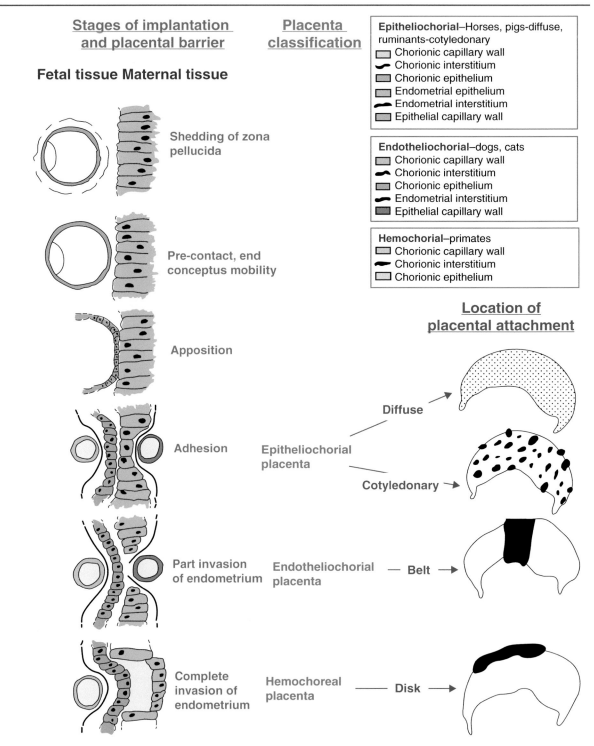

Fig. 3.16. An illustrative representation of the four stages of implantation and placentation in horses and other mammals.

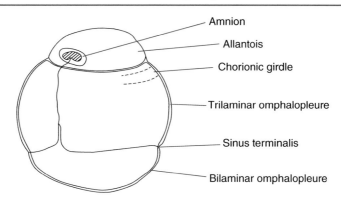

Amnion

Allantois

Chorionic girdle

Trilaminar omphalopleure

Sinus terminalis

Bilaminar omphalopleure

Fig. 3.17. The equine conceptus at day 25 post-fertilization, illustrating the position of the chorionic girdle attachment.

tenuous; however, it provides an increasingly significant exchange unit (Enders *et al.*, 1993). At days 36–37 the chorionic girdle is in the middle of invading the endometrium and is well attached to the endometrium in places. By day 38 invasion across the whole of the chorionic girdle is well under way. As the fetal chorionic girdle cells migrate into the maternal endometrium they begin to transform into binucleate hormone-producing cells which will eventually become the endometrial cups; the chorionic girdle and hence the conceptus then detaches from the endometrium as the chorionic girdle cell migration is completed.

Initially it was thought that this freed the conceptus to migrate again within the uterus. However, this is now thought to be unlikely, as the trophoblast cells have already begun to develop the preinterdigitation that will eventually form the true placental attachment, and the conceptus is held in place by its increasing size and the decreasing uterine lumen size. The exact time of takeover by, and the lifespan of, the endometrial cups may vary. It may occur later in older mares and survive longer in matings between close relatives (Carnevale and Ginther, 1992).

This invasion of fetal tissue into the maternal endometrium is akin to invasion of foreign material into the maternal tissue as fetal tissue is 50% paternal in origin. The question then remains as to why the maternal tissue does not reject the invading chorionic girdle tissue as it would any foreign body. This presents an immunological puzzle. Several hypotheses have been presented to try to explain this, including: the presence of a physical barrier between the maternal and fetal tissue; the inability of the conceptus to express antigenic molecules (immunologically naïve); the inability of the mare to mount an immunological response during pregnancy (immunologically inert); or that the uterus is a privileged site allowing such

invasion to occur. The exact answer is unclear; however, it is known that the mare does initially raise antibodies to the invading chorionic girdle cells (Allen, 2001a); chorionic girdle and endometrial cup tissue is major histocompatability complex (MHC) class 1 positive, causing a maternal immune response (Maher *et al.*, 1996). If this is the case then this sheds doubt on all the four theories suggested above. However, it is also known that this immune reaction does not continue unabated, for if it did the conceptus would never be able to implant and survive. The maternal immune reaction appears to be down-regulated over time by the invasion of T cells from the base of the endometrial cups. It is proposed that the endometrial cups may therefore exist as a 'sacrificial lamb', the slow rejection of which then allows the pregnancy to continue unchallenged. Fetal trophoblast outside the areas of the chorionic girdle/endometrial cups is MHC class 1 negative and so does not induce an immune response (De Mestre *et al.*, 2010). More recent research suggests the involvement of a preimplantation factor (PIF) in many mammals as a modulator of maternal immune response (Paidas *et al.*, 2010; Barnea *et al.*, 2012); however, the involvement of PIF in equine pregnancy is less clear (Nash *et al.*, 2018).

At this stage endometrial gland histotroph remains the main source of nourishment to the conceptus. Endometrial gland activity is presumably being driven by oestrogens and growth factors secreted by the conceptus in order to support its increasing growth (Section 3.3.1.1; Choi *et al.*, 1995; Lennard *et al.*, 1995; Camozzato *et al.*, 2019).

Endometrial Cups

The invading chorionic girdle cells stream down into the lumen of the endometrial glands and break through into the stroma of the endometrium. At day 40 they suddenly stop migrating, enlarge and tightly pack together within the endometrial stroma, forming a series of pale raised areas on the surface of the endometrium encircling the conceptus; these are termed endometrial cups (Fig. 3.18; Enders and Lui, 1991; Allen and Stewart, 1993; De Mestre *et al.*, 2011). These endometrial cups, 1–6 cm in length and 1–2 cm in width, are now completely contained with the endometrial tissue and no longer have any attachment to the conceptus. They secrete the hormone eCG, sometimes referred to as pregnant mare serum gonadotrophin (PMSG), which is essential for the maintenance of early pregnancy. eCG will be discussed in detail in Section 3.3.1.3.

Between days 60 and 70 the endometrial cups reach their maximum size and eCG production. By around day 90, the endometrial cups can clearly be seen degenerating and sloughing away from the uterine endometrium. The reason for this seeming rejection is not fully understood but, as previously discussed, the endometrial cups may act as a 'sacrificial lamb', their immunological rejection allowing the downgrading of the maternal immune response to the conceptus and so allowing the pregnancy to continue unchallenged (Asbury and LeBlanc, 1993). The duration of the endometrial cups is very variable, being longer in sibling matings, primiparous mares (mares not previously pregnant) and foal-heat matings, although in all mares they are normally no longer present after day 120 (Bell and Bristol, 1991; Koets, 1995; Wilsher and Allen, 2011a; Antczak *et al.*, 2013). The remains of these sloughed-off endometrial cups may be reabsorbed during the remainder of the pregnancy or they may be seen in the placenta at birth as invaginations or pouches in the allantochorion.

3.2.4. Placenta

From day 40 onwards the conceptus loses its spherical shape as the allantochorion spreads up into the gravid (pregnant) horn and down into the uterine body. By day 90 it has spread throughout the uterus (Figs 3.19 and 3.20). During this time the fetal allantochorion takes on a velvety appearance, created by fine microvilli over its entire surface (hence why the equine placenta is termed diffuse). It attaches to the entire uterine epithelium over the whole surface of the uterus apart from the utero-tubular junction and where the placenta abuts the cervix (Tamilselvan *et al.*, 2015). This attachment begins between days 45 and 70 and gradually becomes firmer over the next 100 days, being fully attached by

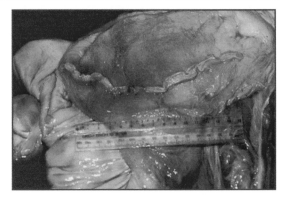

Fig. 3.18. The remains of the endometrial cups can be seen in a band running across the uterine endometrium.

day 150. These microvilli organize themselves into discrete microscopic bundles or tufts which invade into receiving invaginations in the uterine epithelium. The bundles of microvilli are termed microcotyledons, and their attachment develops over a period of time, being fully complete and functional by day 150 (Fig. 3.21; MacDonald *et al.*, 2000).

An attachment is formed between the fetus and the mother. The equine placenta is relatively thick, with six cell layers and four basement membranes. The three cell layers on the fetal side are mesoderm (chorionic capillary vessel wall), endoderm (chorionic interstitium or connective tissue) and ectoderm (chorionic epithelium or allantochorion); and the three on the maternal side are endometrial epithelium, endometrial interstitium (connective tissue) and endothelium (epithelial capillary vessel wall). The equine placenta is therefore termed epitheliochorial and covers the whole surface of the uterus, except the cervix (the cervical star) and the two utero-tubular junctions (Figs 3.15, 3.16 and 3.22; MacDonald and Fowden, 1997; Wilsher and Allen, 2003, 2011b; Carter and Enders, 2013). The placenta now becomes the prime site for nutrient uptake to, dissipation of waste from and gaseous exchange between mare and conceptus. This is termed haemotrophic exchange. However, it is evident that the areolae, covering the mouths of the endometrial glands as they open between the microcotyledons, persist. The trophoblastic cells in these areolae become phagocytic, continuing to absorb histotroph throughout pregnancy (Allen *et al.*, 2007a); this is termed histotrophic exchange and is reported to be a more important source of nutrition in the mare than in other placental groups (Enders and Carter, 2006; Carter and Enders, 2013).

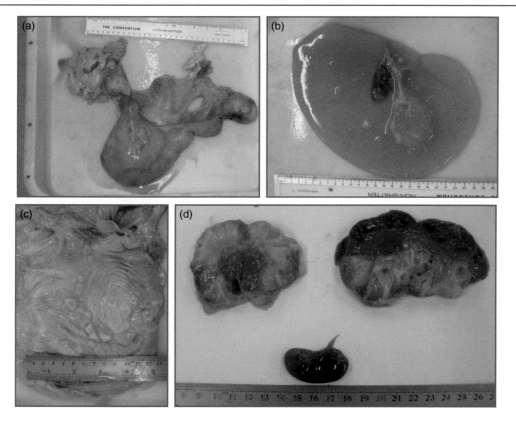

Fig. 3.19. The equine conceptus at Day 70-80 of pregnancy illustrating (a) the undissected uterus with clear difference in size between the gravid (pregnant) and non-gravid (non-pregnant) horns; (b) the conceptus with the fetus lying within its amniotic and allantoic sac; (c) the endometrial cups encircling the junction between the uterine horn and the uterine body; and (d) the fetus within its amniotic sac alongside the dissected ovaries showing a number of corporea lutea.

The presence of the microcotyledons serves to increase the surface area of the placenta and, therefore, the area for nutrient and gas exchange. Within each microcotyledon, the maternal and fetal blood supply systems come in close proximity, allowing efficient diffusion.

However, the thickness of the placental attachment prevents the diffusion of large molecules such as immunoglobulins (large protein molecules); hence the attainment of passive immunity in the foal by diffusion of immunoglobulins across the placenta is very limited. Passage via colostrum is, therefore, of utmost importance in the mare, as will be discussed in further detail in Chapters 12 and 19. The thickness and arrangement of the placenta vary in different mammals. In general, though, the thicker the placenta the less efficient is the transfer of passive immunity in utero, and hence the greater the reliance

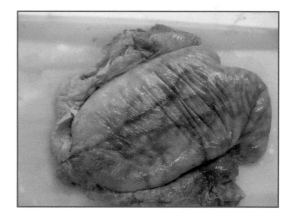

Fig. 3.20. A pregnant mare's uterus in later pregnancy illustrating the spread of the placenta into the two horns although one (the top non-gravid horn) is still slightly smaller than the horn containing the fetus (the lower gravid horn).

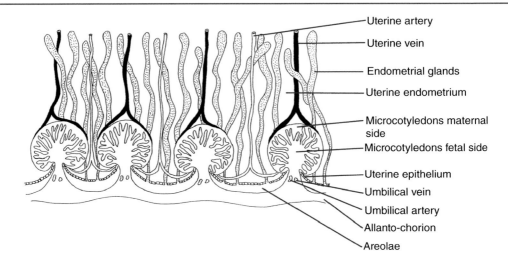

Fig. 3.21. Equine placental microcotyledons in the fully developed placenta.

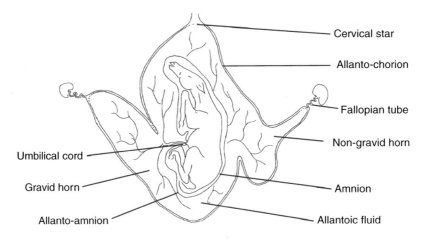

Fig. 3.22. The equine fetus and placenta near term.

on colostrum. However, a thicker placenta as seen in the mare has the advantage of providing extra protection to the fetus from harmful maternal blood-borne factors.

3.2.4.1. Placental efficiency

Despite the thickness of the placenta, nutrient and gaseous exchange across the mare's placenta is relatively efficient when compared to other farm livestock. This is due to the diffuse nature of the equine placenta (attachment to the uterus over the whole surface of the placenta) compared to the cotyledonary nature (attachment to the uterus just at discrete areas) of ruminant placentas.

However, it must be remembered that measurements taken on placental efficiency involve the acute catheterization of the umbilical arteries, and hence the technique itself may affect the results obtained. Silver *et al.* (1973) demonstrated the relative efficiency of the mare's placenta, as changes in maternal blood oxygen, glucose, free fatty acid and lactate concentrations were mimicked more closely by changes in the fetal blood concentration than in sheep. It may well be deduced, therefore, that blood-borne factors affecting the mare will have a greater effect on the fetus than is evident in ruminants, although such an association has yet to be confirmed.

As pregnancy progresses, the maternal epithelium stretches as the conceptus and uterus increase in size. As a result, the placenta also stretches and becomes thinner, and hence the resistance to gaseous and nutrient exchange decreases, the placenta becoming more efficient as the demands of the fetus increase. In addition, although the extent of the placenta is fixed by days 100–150, it is reported that the placental microvilli elongate and branch after day 275 of pregnancy and that this results in a twofold increase in glucose uptake during the last trimester, helping to accommodate increased fetal demand (Fowden *et al.*, 2000). By full term, the placenta of a 15–16 hh (400–500 kg) horse weighs 4–5 kg. Its macroscopic surface area is approximately 1.5 m^2 but, if the entire microscopic surface of the microcotyledons is included, the area is 40 m^2 and it is about 1 mm thick (Wilsher and Allen, 2003). The foal's birth weight is directly proportional to the surface area of the placenta, as this is the limiting factor controlling nutrient and gas exchange and hence their availability to the developing fetus, and may have long-term consequences for post-natal as well as pre-natal growth (Wilsher and Allen, 2003; Allen *et al.*, 2004). The surface area of a placenta may be restricted for several reasons, including mare age and parous number (MacDonald *et al.*, 2000; Wilsher and Allen, 2003; Klewitz *et al.*, 2015), breed (Robles *et al.*, 2018) and size (Allen *et al.*, 2002b, 2004), plus the presence of multiple pregnancies.

3.2.4.2. Multiple pregnancies

Multiple pregnancies in the mare are almost always dizygotic, originating from multiple ovulations, as opposed to monozygotic or identical twins originating from the splitting of a single conceptus (Newcombe, 2000b; Govaere *et al.*, 2009). Multiple pregnancies are an increasing problem in stud management, especially in intensively bred horses such as the Thoroughbred (Section 11.3). The incidence of multiple ovulations, which have the potential to result in multiple conceptuses in the Thoroughbred, is 20–25%, the vast majority of which are twins (Davies Morel and O'Sullivan, 2001; Davies Morel *et al.*, 2005). Of this potential number of twins, significant natural reduction to one conceptus does occur. Seventy per cent of twins are initially unilateral (both in the same uterine horn), of which 85% naturally reduce; 30% are bilateral (one conceptus in each horn), none of which naturally reduce (Ginther, 1989a,b; Ginther and Griffin, 1994). If twins do develop to the placentation stage, the area of

the uterus available for each placenta is restricted by the presence of the other fetus (Figs 3.23 and 3.24). If the division of uterine surface area available to each twin is equal, then both twins have an equal chance of survival, although this is rare and their birth weights will be reduced owing to the small placental size causing placental insufficiency. If the division is unequal, then the smaller one may cause the whole pregnancy to abort or, if the pregnancy is not well advanced, it may die and become mummified. If mummification occurs, the pregnancy may well continue; if this occurs after around days 100–150 the placenta of the larger surviving fetus cannot expand and attach to the uterine surface originally occupied by the now dead fetus, as the extent of placental attachment has already been fixed. At term, therefore, a single foal will be born, but with a reduced birth weight due to placental restriction (McKinnon, 2011).

3.2.4.3. Placental blood supply

As mentioned previously, the mesoderm of the blastocyst surrounding the yolk sac forms the first placental blood supply from the fetus. Early in pregnancy, a clear network of blood vessels can be identified within the trilaminar omphalopleure, with two major vessels connecting the network to the rudimentary heart. Additional pathways develop to feed areas of considerable growth. Hence, when the yolk sac degenerates and the

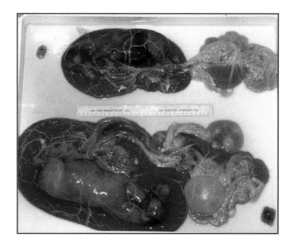

Fig. 3.23. Fetuses of a twin pregnancy dissected out at post-mortem. The different size of the twins is evident as a result of placental restriction of the smaller twin. If left to go to term, the smaller twin would eventually have died and probably have caused the abortion of the whole pregnancy.

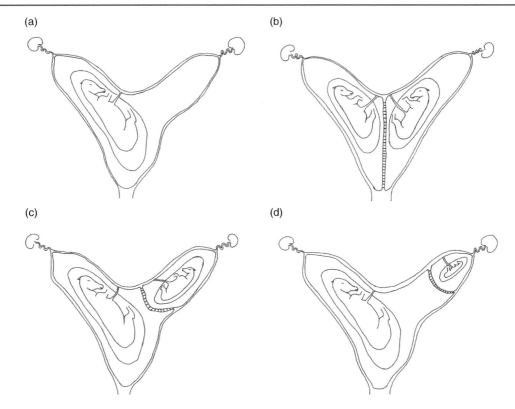

Fig. 3.24. Placental configurations in the equine singleton and twin pregnancies: (a) singleton; (b) equal split (50%:50%); (c) unequal split (60%:40%); and (d) unequal split (80%:20%).

nutrient supply to the fetus is taken over by the allanto-chorionic placenta, a well-formed network of blood vessels within the allantochorion already exists. This fine network enlarges and invaginates into the microcotyledons of the placenta (Wilsher and Allen, 2011b). Each microcotyledon is supplied on the fetal side by several arteries, but exit back to the fetal heart is via a single vein. This arrangement slows down the flow of blood through the microcotyledons and encourages more efficient diffusion and gas exchange. The oxygenated and nutritionally replenished blood returns to the fetal heart by the umbilical vein (Fig. 3.25). The umbilical cord, therefore, contains two fetal arteries and one fetal vein plus the urachus from the bladder (Whitwell, 1975; Whitwell and Jeffcote, 1975).

It should be remembered that in the fetus, because of the bypass of the non-functional lungs, deoxygenated blood is carried to the placenta via arteries and oxygenated blood is passed back to the heart via the veins (Fig. 19.7).

On the maternal side a very similar arrangement exists. Oxygenated and nutritionally enriched blood approaches the microcotyledons in a fine network of arteries, but the drainage back to the maternal system is also via a single vein, again slowing down the passage of blood and increasing the efficiency of nutrient and gaseous exchange. This transfer across the utero–fetal placental barrier can be compared in many ways to the gaseous exchange within the mammalian lung.

3.2.5. Organ development

Organ development arises from the reorganization of cell populations within the embryonic disc itself. This organization is related to that which occurs in placentation, previously discussed. This can be divided into two basic sections: gastrulation and neuralation. The former can be subdivided into segregation, delamination and involution. Further accounts of organ development can be found in Betteridge *et al.* (1982), Flood *et al.* (1982), Enders *et al.* (1988), Betteridge (2007, 2011) and Gaivao *et al.* (2014).

3.2.5.1. Gastrulation

Gastrulation is defined as the organization of the embryo into three germ layers: ectoderm, mesoderm and endoderm. This primarily involves the cells of the embryonic disc but also those of the placental tissue. The first stage of gastrulation is segregation, during which the central blastomeres or cells of the embryonic disc organize themselves into smaller outer and larger inner blastomeres (Fig. 3.26).

The larger blastomeres collect underneath the disc and migrate in two directions. First, they may migrate to line the remaining ectoderm of the blastocyst, forming the endoderm. Second, they migrate within the embryonic disc, creating at day 12 the first asymmetry, a thicker area at the caudal end (future tail end) and a thinner area at the cranial end (future head end; Fig. 3.27; Gaivao *et al.*, 2014).

The second stage of gastrulation is termed delamination. This commences at day 12 and marks the first evidence of epiblast cells, hypoblast cells and the primitive gut.

The epiblast cells are those of the embryonic disc. The hypoblast cells are the migrating endoderm, although as discussed previously (Section 3.2.2) the endoderm cells that form the trophoblast in the equine conceptus may originate from sporadically distributed colonies rather than migration from the embryonic disc (Enders *et al.*, 1993). Within this ring of endoderm

cells lies the yolk sac or blastocoel (Figs 3.5 and 3.27). At day 14, a change in this embryonic disc becomes evident. This change forms the beginning of the primitive streak identified within the epiblast cells. At this stage, it is about 1 cm in length (Gaivao *et al.*, 2014).

The third and last stage of gastrulation is involution, when the epiblast cells move inwards to the centre of the caudal end of the disc (Fig. 3.28). At this stage, three types of cells – ectoderm (epiblast cells), mesoderm and endoderm (hypoblast cells) – are evident within the embryonic disc, as seen in the extraembryonic tissue (Fig. 3.7). These three cell layers will go to form all the main body structures.

The moving ectoderm or epiblast cells reappear as mesoderm between the ectoderm and the hypoblast cells or endoderm. As the cells move through to the lower level they leave a depression in the upper surface of the epiblast. These migrating epiblast cells tend to move in greater concentrations at the caudal end of the primitive streak, making it wider. The primitive streak so formed makes the future longitudinal axis of the embryo (Fig. 3.28).

At day 15, epiblast cell movement tends to slow down; the slight indentation along the longitudinal axis of the primitive streak becomes deeper, as cells continue to move out from underneath to form the mesoderm and are not replaced by migrating epiblast cells above.

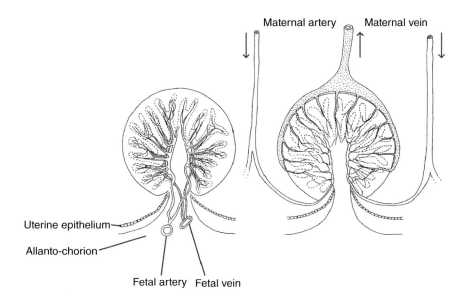

Fig. 3.25. Venous and arterial blood supplies to the microcotyledons within the equine placenta, allowing the transfer of nutrients and waste products from the maternal (right) to the fetal (left) system and vice versa.

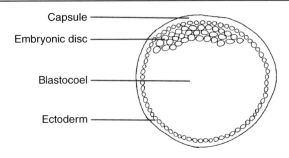

Fig. 3.26. Day 9, segregation in the equine conceptus, illustrating the larger inner blastomeres and smaller outer blastomeres within the embryonic disc.

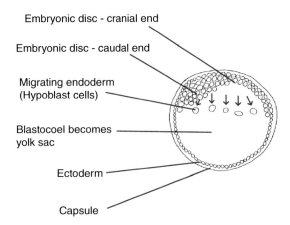

Fig. 3.27. Day 11, segregation in the equine conceptus, indicating the migration of the large blastomeres from the lower part of the embryonic disc to form the thicker caudal and thinner cranial end of the embryonic disc and possibly line the remaining ectoderm.

This deep groove is now termed the primitive groove. The cells associated with the primitive groove are termed node cells, to differentiate them from the cells of the remainder of the embryo. At day 16, these node cells can be identified as precursors of future body organs. The ectoderm node cells form the neural plate, running the length of the top of the primitive groove, the cranial end of which goes to form the head. The spreading mesoderm in the immediate vicinity of the neural plate goes to form the somites, or body trunk, and the mesoderm immediately below the primitive groove goes to form the notochord (spine and CNS). Finally, the wide caudal end forms the tail end of the embryo (Fig. 3.29; Betteridge, 2011b; Gaivao *et al.*, 2014).

The process of gastrulation is now completed, the major cell blocks are identifiable and the longitudinal axis of the embryo is determined.

3.2.5.2. Neuralation

The next stage, termed neuralation, involves the development of the CNS, gut and heart. Day 16 sees three major changes. First, the ectoderm near the neural plate thickens and two neural folds develop on either side of the neural plate. The neural plate becomes depressed and the neural folds fold over, join and then fuse to enclose a hollow tube, the spine-to-be and CNS-to-be (Fig. 3.30; Gaivao *et al.*, 2014). Second, the mesoderm on either side of the neural plate organizes itself into 14 somites (future muscle blocks). Third, at the cranial end of the neural plate, an increase in cell growth above the surface becomes apparent, with an accompanying increase

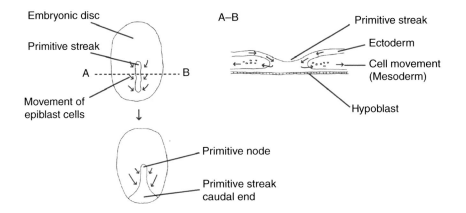

Fig. 3.28. Day 14, involution of the equine conceptus. A bird's-eye view of the embryonic disc, along with a cross-sectional view through A–B, illustrating the passage of ectoderm cells through the primitive streak to reappear between the ectoderm and endoderm, forming the mesoderm. Further cell movement results in the flattening of the caudal end of the primitive streak.

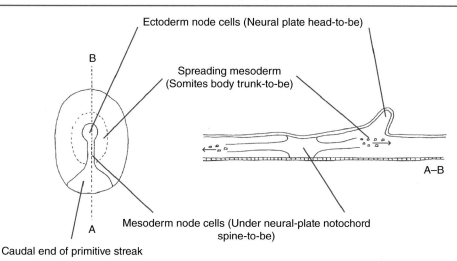

Ectoderm node cells (Neural plate head-to-be)

B

Spreading mesoderm
(Somites body trunk-to-be)

A–B

Mesoderm node cells (Under neural-plate notochord
spine-to-be)

A

Caudal end of primitive streak

Fig. 3.29. Day 15, completed gastrulation in the equine conceptus. A bird's-eye view and cross-sectional view through A–B of the embryonic disc. The formation of the head from the cranial end of the primitive groove is illustrated, along with the somites, or body trunk, formation from the mesoderm in the immediate vicinity of the primitive groove and the spine and central nervous system (CNS) formation from the mesoderm immediately below the primitive groove.

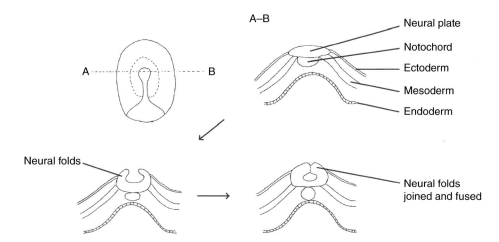

A–B

A   B

Neural plate

Notochord

Ectoderm

Mesoderm

Endoderm

Neural folds

Neural folds
joined and fused

Fig. 3.30. Days 16–17, neuralation of the equine conceptus. The ectoderm near the neural plate thickens and two neural folds develop on either side of the neural plate and join to enclose a hollow tube, the future spine and central nervous system.

in the length of the neural plate. This cell growth folds over to form the head process, heart and pharynx.

By day 18, lateral folds are beginning to develop on either side of the head process. As cells move into this area and cell division increases, the cranial end of the neural plate lifts away from the underlying tissue (Figs 3.31 and 3.32).

These lateral folds move down from the cranial end to the caudal end, lifting the whole body away from the underlining tissue (Fig. 3.32).

This lifting away from the remaining tissue leaves just one attachment point in the centre, the first evidence of the umbilical cord. The embryo continues to lift off the underlying tissue and the head and tail processes fold back down to give the embryo its characteristic C-shape configuration (Gaivao *et al.*, 2014). At this stage two more somites are evident, making 16 in total.

The gut tube also now begins to develop from the pharynx fold by closure of the endoderm folds, in a way similar to that by which the neural tube was formed from folds in the ectoderm of the neural plate. The hindgut of the fetus now extends out into the blastocoel to form the allantois, as illustrated in Fig. 3.11, and blood is also now evident in the lumen of the tubular heart (Cottrill *et al.*, 1997), which can be seen to beat from day 21 (Ginther and Griffin, 1994).

The embryo now lies away from the underlying placental tissue, and is connected directly to the placenta only by the umbilical cord, which contains a blood system derived from the mesoderm along with supporting connective tissue. The embryo now has an identifiable neural tube, the forerunner of the CNS, and a head process with enlarged neural tube, the brain-to-be. Its pharynx and gut tube are also present, as are the somites, or body muscle blocks. Therefore, by day 23, all

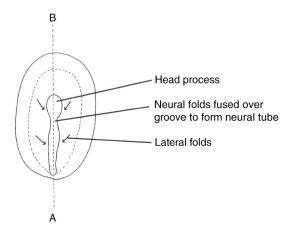

Fig. 3.31. Day 18, neuralation of the equine conceptus. A bird's-eye view of the embryonic shield, illustrating cell movement in towards the cranial end of the neural plate, which subsequently lifts away from the underlying tissue.

the basic bodily structures are evident, although only in a rudimentary form (Betteridge, 2011).

3.2.5.3. *Organ growth*

From day 23 onwards, development is in the form of fine differentiation and organ growth. By day 40, all the main body features such as limbs, tail, nostrils, pigmented eyes, ears, elbows and stifle regions, and eyelids are evident, and the embryo is now termed a fetus (Betteridge, 2011; Bergfeldt and Adams, 2011b). By days 55–60 the fetus is clearly horse-like with an elongated umbilical cord allowing the fetus to be active (Allen and Bracher, 1992). Days 39–45 herald sexual differentiation and evidence of external genitalia. At day 100 the fetal gonads start a remarkable increase in size, reaching a maximum at days 200–240 after which they regress to normal size at birth, the weight of fetal testes and ovaries being equivalent and developing to the following pattern (Douglas and Ginther, 1975):

- Day 80 – 1.4 g
- Day 140 – 18.7 g
- Day 200 – 48.0 g
- Day 320 – 31.4 g

The increase and decrease in size are due to a proliferation and degeneration of interstitial cells (Walt *et al.*, 1979) and appear to correspond to the period of masculinization or feminization of the fetus. The reason for the relatively large size of the fetal gonads in the horse is unclear, but may be related to the secretion of significant levels of oestrogen at this time.

At this stage, most of the development is complete and increase in growth now occurs (Fig. 3.33). At day 60 the eyelids close and finer eye development occurs, teats are present and the oral palate is fused. Day 160 sees the first evidence of hair around the eyes and muzzle and, by

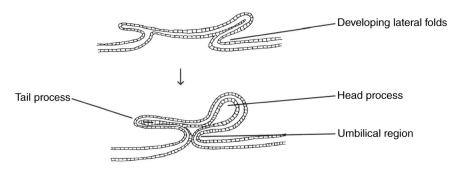

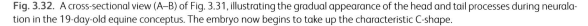

Fig. 3.32. A cross-sectional view (A–B) of Fig. 3.31, illustrating the gradual appearance of the head and tail processes during neuralation in the 19-day-old equine conceptus. The embryo now begins to take up the characteristic C-shape.

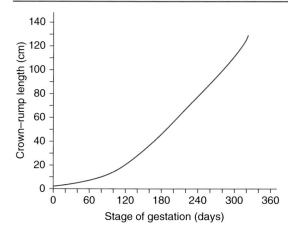

Fig. 3.33. The increase in fetal crown–rump length throughout gestation. (Adapted from Evans and Sack, 1973; Ginther, 1992.)

day 180, hair has begun to develop at the tip of the tail and the beginnings of a mane are evident. By day 270, hair covers the whole of the body surface (Table 3.1).

From day 150 onwards the hippomane, an accumulation of waste minerals within the allantois, becomes apparent. The hippomane increases in size with pregnancy (Fig. 3.34). From day 320 onwards, the testes in the male fetus may descend through the inguinal canal; however, this does not occur in all colt fetuses, as some drop neonatally.

The main milestones in equine fetal development are summarized in Table 3.1 (Ginther, 1995; Reef, 1998; Sertich, 1998).

Full term (normally at 320 days in ponies and up to 2 weeks later in Thoroughbred and riding-type horses) heralds the birth of a very well-developed fetus, typical of a preyed-upon, plain-dwelling animal. At birth foals are capable of all basic bodily functions, including running, within 30–60 min. Details of the foal's adaptation to the extrauterine environment are given in Chapter 19.

3.3. Endocrinology of Pregnancy

When examining the endocrinological control of pregnancy in the mare, gestation can be divided into two stages: early (fertilization to day 150) and late (day 150 to full term).

3.3.1. Early pregnancy

After fertilization it takes 5–6 days for the conceptus to migrate down through the utero-tubular junction and into the uterus, where it exists by deriving nutrients

Table 3.1. Summary of the major milestones for fetal development throughout pregnancy.

Day of gestation	Major milestones
1	Zygote, two cells
4	Morula, 16 cells plus
5	Capsule formation
6	Hatching of morula
8	Blastocyst, differentiated into embryonic mass, blastocoel and trophoblast
9	Ectoderm and endoderm germ layers evident, gastrulation begins
11	Segregation giving first embryonic asymmetry, caudal and cranial ends evident
12	Delamination, epiblast cells, hypoblast cells and primitive gut evident
14	Mesoderm evident, primitive streak appearing, involution commencing
15	Primitive streak now evident as a groove
16	Neuralation starts, folds leading to the formation of the amnion seen, first blood vessels evident in mesoderm, chorionic vesicle 2–4 cm diameter
18	Vitelline artery and vein identifiable, fetus begins to take on characteristic C-shape
20	Allantois forming from outpushing of the fetal hindgut, chorionic vesicle oval in shape (2.5–4.5 cm diameter), eye vesicle and ear present. Capsule begins to degenerate
21	Amnion complete
23	All basic bodily structures evident, although in rudimentary state
25	Chorionic girdle, first evident attachment of fetus
26	Forelimb bud seen, three branchial arches present, eye visible
30	Genital tubercle present, eye lens seen
36	Rudimentary three digits seen on hoof, facial clefts closing, eyes pigmented and acoustic groove forming
40	Endometrial cups forming, ear forming, nostrils seen, eyelids seen, all limbs evident and elbow and stifle joint areas identifiable, chorionic vesicle 4.5–7.5 cm diameter
42	Ear triangular in shape, mammary buds seen along ridge

(Continued)

Table 3.1. Continued.

Day of gestation	Major milestones
45	External genitalia evident, allantoic sac volume 110 ml
47	Palate fused
49	Mammary teats evident
55	Ear covers acoustic groove, eyelids closing
60	Chorionic vesicle 13.3 × 8.9 cm
63	Eyelids fused, fine eye development occurring, hoof, sole and frog areas of hoof evident
75	Female clitoris prominent
80	Scrotum clearly seen
90	Endometrial cups degenerate, chorionic vesicle 14 × 23 cm
95	Hoof appears yellow in colour
112	Tactile hairs on lips growing
120	Fine hair on muzzle, chin and eyelashes beginning to grow, eye prominent and ergot evident
150	Full attachment of placental microcotyledons, eyelashes clearly seen, enlargement of mammary gland
180	Mane and tail evident
240	Hair of poll, ears, chin, muzzle and throat evident
270	Whole of body covered with fine hair, longer mane and tail hair clearly seen
310	Allantoic sac volume 8.5 l
320	Testes may drop from this time onwards
320–340	Birth of fully developed fetus

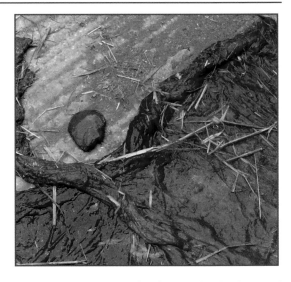

Fig. 3.34. The hippomane often found within the placenta of the mare. This example is 7 cm long.

production, from one or a number of CL, has to be maintained until at least day 75. If there is a failure of the functional CL during this time, the pregnancy will fail.

3.3.1.1. Maternal recognition of pregnancy

It may be argued that the first recognition of pregnancy occurs at day 5 as the conceptus controls its passage through the utero-tubular junction (Section 3.2.2). At this stage the conceptus produces PGE and PGF2α. It is this local secretion of PGs, rather than conceptus size or presence of the capsule, that then appears to drive rapid movement of the embryo to, and relaxation of, the utero-tubular junction sphincter and allow the conceptus to pass into the uterus (Weber *et al.*, 1991, 1995; Robinson *et al.*, 2000; Stout and Allen, 2001). However, day 15 is classically considered to be the time of maternal recognition of pregnancy. The importance of day 15, with regard to the recognition of pregnancy, has been demonstrated in experiments with early-pregnant mares. If the embryo is removed from a pregnant mare prior to day 15, she will return to oestrus at her normal time (21 days after the last). If, however, the embryo is removed at day 16 or later, the mare will not return to oestrus as expected and will show a prolonged dioestrus, due to the persistence of the CL. The length of the delay will depend to a certain extent on the age of the embryo at removal (Freeman *et al.*, 1991).

from the uterine hystotroph or secretions. No major changes from the non-pregnant cycle are evident as yet (Freeman *et al.*, 1991). However, by day 15, a message has to be received by the reproductive system of the mare if it is to continue in a pregnancy mode, blocking luteolysis (destruction of the corpus luteum, CL) so preventing the drop in progesterone, and allowing progesterone levels to remain elevated (Fig. 3.35). Elevated progesterone and/or related progestogenic compounds is essential for the initial maintenance of pregnancy. If the mare is pregnant then ovarian progesterone

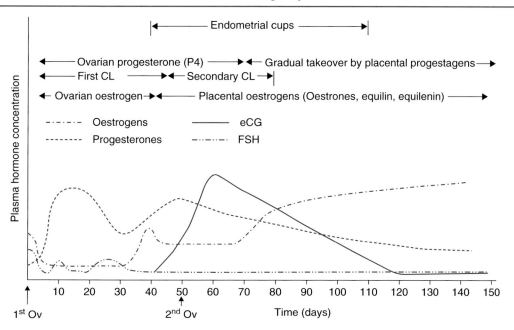

Fig. 3.35. A summary of the plasma hormone concentrations during early pregnancy in the mare (days 0–150). CL, corpus luteum; eCG, equine chorionic gonadotrophin; FSH, follicle-stimulating hormone; Ov, ovulation.

Although it is well established that, as far as the hormonal control of pregnancy is concerned, 'D-Day' is day 15, embryo transfer work suggests there may be some progressive recognition of pregnancy from day 8 onwards (Goff *et al.*, 1987). The exact nature of the message informing the mare of the presence of a conceptus is unclear, but there are several candidates. Oestrogens are known to be the signal of pregnancy in the sow (Bazer *et al.*, 1989); equine concepti are also capable of synthesizing oestrogens as early as day 10 (Sharp, 1993; Choi *et al.*, 1995; Klein and Troedsson, 2011). As such, oestrogens have been considered the likely candidates acting locally on the uterine epithelium to inform the mother of the presence of the fetus (Daels *et al.*, 1990; McDowell and Sharp, 2011). However, although some work indicates that oestrogens can prolong dioestrus and delay return to oestrus, this is now thought to be due to an inhibition of follicular development rather than luteotrophic activity (maintaining the CL); others dispute this role for oestrogens. For example, work by Goff *et al.* (1993) indicated that *in vivo* administration of oestrogens increased the release of PGs, as did the insertion of oestrogen-impregnated sialastic spheres into the uterus of mares. It is, therefore, suggested that oestrogen is not the message of pregnancy in the mare, but rather a means by which the conceptus drives and

controls endometrial gland secretion of histotroph and its uptake by the conceptus, so ensuring its own survival (Spencer and Bazer, 2004; McDowell and Sharp, 2011). It has been reported that the equine conceptus also produces three unknown proteins molecular weights of 400, 65 and 50 kDa around days 12–14 (Sissener *et al.*, 1996) and/or a single protein of molecular weight 6000 Da (Heap *et al.*, 1982), and most recently IFN-δ, a Type I interferon (Tayade *et al.*, 2008). Other species such as ruminants produce trophoblastic proteins (interferon tau) which act to inform the maternal system of a pregnancy; however, they are of a much higher molecular weight (17,000 Da; Hansen *et al.*, 1999; Bazer *et al.*, 2017). Other contenders suggested to be the message include an early pregnancy factor (EPF) (Takagi *et al.*, 1998) or a PIF (Paidas *et al.*, 2010; Stamatkin *et al.*, 2011) or heat shock protein 10 (Hsp10) (Bemis *et al.*, 2012). The more recent realization that inter-uterine marbles can be used to delay luteolysis (Rivera del Alamo *et al.*, 2008) have led some to reconsider the once rejected theory that conceptus size may play a role (Klein and Troedsson, 2011; Klein, 2016). Thus, in the mare, it is likely that proteins and/or early pregnancy factors produced by the conceptus are the messengers of pregnancy, with oestrogens driving uterine secretions that support conceptus development.

Regardless of the means by which the message is delivered, the result is the maintenance of the CL beyond day 15 (Ball *et al.*, 1991). In the non-pregnant mare the CL is destroyed at about day 15 by PGF2α, allowing the cyclical changes associated with oestrus and ovulation to begin (Chapter 2). Therefore, in the pregnant mare, this action of PGF2α must be blocked.

The exact mechanism for preventing the action of PGF2α is unknown, but there are several hypotheses. First, it has been suggested that PGF2α binding to the CL is reduced. However, doubt has been placed upon this hypothesis, as it appears that the CL concentration of PGF2α receptors is high during the period 16–18 days post-ovulation in both the pregnant and non-pregnant mare. The second hypothesis is that an alternative component is produced by the uterus that competitively binds with the PGF2α receptors on the CL. A suitable candidate would be PGE, which is very similar in structure to PGF2α but biologically inactive with regard to CL regression; however, there is little evidence to support this. The third hypothesis is that there is an alteration in the secretion pattern of PGF2α so it does not reach the CL. This is evident in the sow, where PGF2α secretion is redirected to the uterine lumen and away from the uterine vein and hence the ovary and CL (Bazer *et al.*, 1994), but there is no evidence for this in the mare. Finally the fourth, and currently favoured, option is that the secretion of PGF2α is reduced. This fourth hypothesis is supported by the reported reduction in the concentration of PGF2α in pregnant mare uterine washings, the reduction in PGFM in the mare's circulation (Kindahl *et al.*, 1982; Zavy *et al.*, 1984) and the ability of the conceptus at days 12–14 to suppress the endometrial production of PGF2α *in vitro* (Bazer *et al.*, 1994; Sissener *et al.*, 1996). The production of PGF2α in the non-pregnant mare is driven by oxytocin (Section 2.4.2.8) and appears to be a self-perpetuating cascade linking oxytocin and PG secretion until PG levels are adequate to cause luteolysis (Utt *et al.*, 2007). In the pregnant mare this cascade appears to be disrupted. It is known that the number of oxytocin receptors on the uterine endometrium is significantly reduced in the presence of a conceptus (Starbuck *et al.*, 1998); in addition, Aurich and Budik (2015) suggested there is a down-regulation of cyclooxygenase, which is required for PGF2α production. As a result, the endometrium response to oxytocin, in the form of PGF2α production, is significantly reduced. In turn this prevents the normal cascade of events in the non-pregnant mare, and so the CL and pregnancy are maintained

(Starbuck *et al.*, 1998; Stout *et al.*, 2000; Aurich and Budik, 2015). Although this is currently the favoured theory, not all work would support it (McDowell and Sharp, 2011).

The equine conceptus is unique in having a relatively long period of mobility (up to 18 days) (Section 3.2.3.1) and it is apparent that contact with much of the uterus by the moving of the conceptus is required to maintain pregnancy. Any restriction to that movement can be detrimental and the greater the restriction the greater the effect (McDowell *et al.*, 1988; McDowell and Sharp, 2011). Movement of the conceptus is due to localized uterine myometrial contraction driven by the conceptus secretion of PGF2α and PGE. On the face of it, it seems contradictory that the equine conceptus at the time of maternal recognition of pregnancy is actively producing its own PGs while also inhibiting endometrial secretion of PG. It has been suggested by Allen (2001b) that a failure to achieve a balance resulting in over-production of PG by the conceptus may be one of the reasons why early embryonic death is a significant problem in many mares.

From day 15 onwards maternal progesterone and embryonic oestrogens are the dominant hormones affecting the uterus, and are important in the production and composition of uterine hystotroph and pregnancy-specific proteins, collectively termed uterine milk. The composition of uterine milk is particularly important in the mare as the conceptus survives in a free-living form for a long period of time, no form of direct communication between the mare and the conceptus being evident until as late as day 40.

By considering the concentration of individual hormones a picture of how the mare maintains the conceptus can be developed.

3.3.1.2. Progesterone (primarily P4)

Maintenance of pregnancy in the mare relies on elevated levels of progesterone. Progesterone is often used as an umbrella term for a whole host of hormones that have similar, but sometimes subtly different, effects on the mare's reproductive system (Douglas, 2004). In the pregnant mare the prime progesterones are P4 and progestogens; often metabolites and derivatives of P4 such as pregnenolone (P5) and 5α-pregnane-3,20-dione (5 αDHP). All have similar biological functions, and inhibit PG release and hence uterine myometrial activity and maintenance of a closed cervix, providing a uterine environment conducive to conceptus survival (Ousey, 2011a). P4 is dominant during early pregnancy, with progestogens being first evident at day 60 and having a greater role in late pregnancy. Between days 6 and 14, the plasma concentration of P4 is 8–15 ng ml^{-1}, similar to that seen during dioestrus of the non-pregnant oestrous cycle. Day 15, decision time, heralds the divergence of P4 concentrations between the pregnant and non-pregnant mare. P4 levels in pregnant mares decline slightly after day 16 (but not to the extent seen in non-pregnant mares) to reach concentrations of approximately 6 ng ml^{-1} by day 30. Levels subsequently rise again to reach 8–10 ng ml^{-1} by days 45–55, and remain at this level, or possibly falling slightly, until day 150 (Holtan *et al.*, 1975b; Schwab, 1990, Ousey, 2011a). Experiments in the mare indicate that ovarian progesterone (P4), which is produced by CL, is essential for the maintenance of all pregnancies, at least until day 75 and in some cases up to day 150. During this period the placenta starts to produce progestogens. After day 150, placenta progestogens are adequate to take over and maintain pregnancy. All pregnant mares that are ovariectomized (the ovaries and hence the functional CL removed) before day 75 will abort. If mares are ovariectomized in the period between days 75 and 150, differing reports indicate differing abortion rates. After day 150, ovariectomy has no effect, and all mares successfully carry fetuses to full term (Holtan *et al.*, 1979). This demonstrates that ovarian P4 is essential prior to day 75 in all mares; in the period of days 75–150 placental progestogens gradually take over and, by day 150, ovarian P4 is not required. Indeed, at this time, the CL on the ovary can be seen to have regressed.

Ovarian P4 is not secreted continually by a single CL. In the mare, an increase in ovarian activity is evident between days 20 and 30 post-coitum: follicles develop, driven by FSH surges similar to those seen during dioestrus (Bergfeldt and Ginther, 1992; Chavatte *et al.*, 1997a). Dominant follicles become apparent and luteinize between days 40 and 60, forming several secondary CL (Figs 3.36 and 3.37; Chavatte *et al.*, 1997a). The cause of luteinization is unclear but is suggested to be increased eCG (Section 3.3.1.3). These secondary CL are unusual and largely unique to the mare. During the period of days 40–70 the secondary CL gradually take over the production of P4, although the primary CL does not necessarily regress (Conley, 2016).

These secondary CL are reported by most to be essential for pregnancy maintenance, although work by Allen *et al.* (1987) indicates that at least in donkey cross mare pregnancies they may not be essential. From day

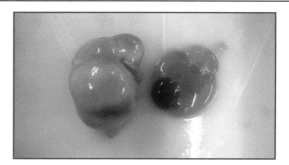

Fig. 3.36. Days 35-40 conceptus alongside the ovary taken from the dissected tract showing large follicles ready for luteinization to form secondary CL.

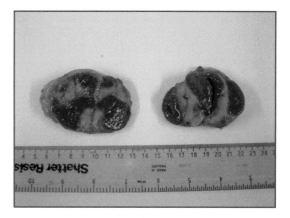

Fig. 3.37. A dissected ovary illustrating numerous secondary CL.

75 onwards, the placenta begins to produce progestogens, gradually taking over from the CLs by day 150 (Squires, 1993a; Ousey, 2011a; Conley, 2016). Placental progestogens are produced from steroid precursors that are transported from the mare to the fetus via the placenta. These are converted to pregnenolone (P5) in the fetal gonads which then passes back to the placenta for conversion to a range of progestogens; these then pass back into the maternal system where they take their effect (Rossdale *et al.*, 1992; Ousey, 2011a). The major placental progestogen is 5αDHP but others are also produced.

3.3.1.3. eCG

eCG (previously known as PMSG) is a glycoprotein hormone and is produced by the endometrial cups of the pregnant mare (Wooding *et al.*, 2001; De Mestre *et al.*, 2011) which, as discussed in Section 3.2.3.1, appear between days 35 and 40 of pregnancy. eCG is secreted into the mare's circulatory system from around day 40 and reaches a maximum concentration between days 50 and 70 post-coitum. It is secreted by the fetal tissue within the endometrial cups, and maximum concentrations achieved vary considerably, different reports giving levels of between 10 and 100 IU ml^{-1} (Wilsher and Allen 2011a; Antczak *et al.*, 2013). Levels are known to be affected by mare genotype, maximum levels reached and the duration of these levels being greater in mares mated to close relatives, e.g. brother-to-sister matings (Allen and Stewart, 1993; Wilsher and Allen, 2011a). The parous state of the mare also has an effect on eCG levels, multiparous (having had previous pregnancies) having lower levels than primiparous (first-time pregnant) mares (Wilsher and Allen, 2011a). Concentrations of eCG always decline and normally reach basal levels by days 100–120 (Steiner *et al.*, 2006; De Mestre *et al.*, 2011; Antczak *et al.*, 2013). The importance of eCG and why it is only secreted for a short period of pregnancy are unclear. However, several hypotheses have been suggested, including a role in the prevention of fetal immunological rejection by the mother; formation of secondary CL; maintenance of the secondary CL; and fetal gonad development (Daels *et al.*, 1995; Koets, 1995; Allen, 2001a; Flores-Flores *et al.*, 2014).

A direct involvement in immunological protection is now thought to be unlikely. However, it is interesting that the varying rates of decline in eCG are due to varying rates of maternal immunological rejection of endometrial cups. Slower decline in eCG is, for example, observed in sister-to-brother matings, where the relative genetic similarity of fetus and mother results in a delay in endometrial cup rejection, and so eCG is secreted longer than in non-related matings.

The most likely role for eCG is hormonal, as eCG is known to have FSH-like and LH-like biological properties and is used pharmacologically in other farm livestock to initiate follicle development and ovulation. It has been suggested, therefore, that eCG may be involved in follicular development in readiness for the formation of the secondary CL (Koets, 1995; De Mestre *et al.*, 2011). However, eCG is not secreted until around days 35–40, and follicular growth – in readiness for secondary CL – may start as early as day 20. It is, therefore, unlikely to have a major role in follicle development prior to secondary CL formation, but may act in connection with FSH pulses synonymous with those observed during dioestrus of the non-pregnant mare. The LH-like properties of eCG, however, may suggest a

role in luteinizing the developed follicles to form the secondary CL; additionally, a role in the maintenance of the primary CL has also been suggested (Daels *et al.*, 1991b; Allen and Stewart, 1993; Koets, 1995; De Mestre *et al.*, 2011; Conley, 2016). Finally, it has been suggested that the remarkable growth in fetal gonads between days 100 and 240 (Section 3.2.5.3) may be driven by eCG (De Mestre *et al.*, 2011), although its commencement at day 100 is somewhat late.

3.3.1.4. Maternal oestrogens

Like progesterone, more than one oestrogen is present in the pregnant mare: these include oestradiol 17β, oestrone, oestradiol 17α and their sulfoconjugates (e.g. oestrone sulfate) plus two oestrogens unique to the mare, equilin and equilenin. In the pregnant mare the major oestrogens are oestrone, equilin and equilenin. The plasma concentration of maternal oestrogens varies within pregnancy. Between days 0 and 35, levels remain very similar to those seen during the non-pregnant dioestrous period, despite oestrogen production by the conceptus, as conceptus production is very low and only has a localized effect. Around day 35 they rise sharply to reach 3–5 ng ml^{-1} around day 40. In the period of days 40–45 they decline slightly, and subsequently remain at this constant level until days 60–70, after which they slowly rise again and remain high until the last 2–3 months of pregnancy (LeBlanc, 1991; Stabenfeldt *et al.*, 1991; Ousey, 2011a; Conley, 2016).

These rising levels of maternal oestrogens between days 35 and 40 are thought to be secreted by the follicles developing prior to the formation of the secondary CL, in much the same way as oestrogens are produced by developing follicles prior to ovulation and oestrus in the normal oestrous cycle (Daels *et al.*, 1991a). These rising levels of oestrogens, however, do not result in normal oestrous behaviour although anecdotal reports indicate that some mares may show 'mareish' behaviour at this time. Evidence for the ovarian origin of these oestrogens is their absence in pregnant mares that have undergone ovariectomy prior to day 40, and the delayed decline in concentrations seen after fetal death not accompanied by immediate CL regression (Daels *et al.*, 1990, 1991b, 1995; Stabenfeldt *et al.*, 1991). However, the second rise in oestrogen at days 60–70 is unaffected by ovariectomy but is affected by induced or spontaneous fetal death (Darenius *et al.*, 1988) and can, therefore, be assumed to originate from the feto-placental unit. The precursors for these oestrogens originate in the fetal gonads that produce dehydroepiandrosterone (DHEA), which passes to the placenta where aromatase enzyme converts it to oestrone (Raeside *et al.*, 1982; Darenius *et al.*, 1988). By day 85, oestrogens in the mare's peripheral blood system are higher than those detected in non-pregnant mares, and are diagnostic of pregnancy. The continuing rise in oestrogens after day 80 is due to increased feto-placental production, initially of oestrone (peaking at 5–6 months), and then of equilin and equilenin (peaking at 7–8 months). The precursors for these increase significantly as fetal size increases (Raeside *et al.*, 1979; Ousey, 2011a, Conley, 2016; Section 3.2.4.3).

3.3.2. Late pregnancy

As far as the discussion on hormone control is concerned, late pregnancy can be classified as day 150 onwards (Fig. 3.38).

3.3.2.1. Progesterone (primarily progestogens)

In the later part of pregnancy progestogens, in particular 5α DHP, are primarily the progesterones produced. They originate from P5 produced by the fetal gonads from cholesterol from the maternal system. P5 then passes back across to the placenta where it is metabolized to 5αDHP and other progestogens, which then pass back to the maternal system where they take their effect (Chavatte *et al.*, 1997a). Hence progestogens are identified in the maternal circulation rather than P4 (Fig. 3.38). Progestogen levels which, prior to day 150,

were elevated and possibly slowly declining, remain at a steady 1–3 ng ml^{-1} until days 240–300. In the last few weeks they increase and then rapidly reach a peak 2–3 days prior to parturition and then dramatically decline in the last few hours (Allen *et al.*, 2002a; Ousey, 2011a). These high concentrations of progestogens pre-partum may be the result of an increase in fetal adrenal activity seen in the last few days of pregnancy (Allen *et al.*, 2002a; see Section 4.3.2). These elevated levels may then be responsible for maintaining a quiescent uterus despite increasing oestrogens, PGs and oxytocin. During the latter part of pregnancy, particularly day 150 onwards, P4 levels drop towards basal levels. Previous reports of changes in maternal progesterone concentrations may appear confusing (Barnes *et al.*, 1975; Holtan *et al.*, 1975a,b). This is due to the inability of early work to differentiate progesterones, particularly P4 and progestogens such as 5α pregnanes, due to cross-reactivity in the assays used (Hamon *et al.*, 1991; Houghton *et al.*, 1991; Squires, 1993a). Assay improvements now allow differentiation and the concentration of specific progesterones to be identified. It is now evident that, while numerous progesterones are produced, primarily P4 is produced in early pregnancy by the ovary; this gradually declines as progestogens from the placenta such as 5α-pregnanes are produced in later pregnancy.

3.3.2.2. Oestrogens

Oestrogen levels within the maternal system continue to rise in late pregnancy, reaching a peak, between days

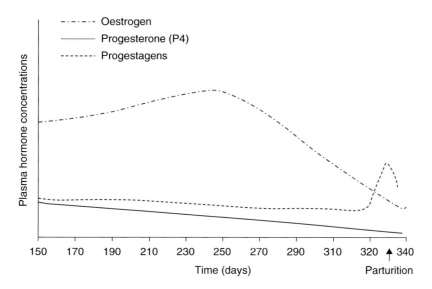

Fig. 3.38. A summary of the plasma hormone concentrations in the mare during late pregnancy (days 150–parturition).

210 and 280, of approximately 8 ng ml^{-1}. The three main oestrogens are oestrone and the equine-specific equilin and equilenin. The peak secretions of oestrones are reported to be somewhat earlier than that for equilin and equilenin (Cox, 1975). All oestrogen levels then decline as parturition approaches, reaching levels in the order of 2 ng ml^{-1} at parturition (Holtan and Silver, 1992; LeBlanc, 1997). This pattern reflects the development and regression of the fetal gonads (Section 3.2.5.3) that provide the precursors for placental oestrogen production, although it has also been suggested to play a role in changing photoperiod (Haluska and Currie, 1988). Oestrogen is thought to be responsible for increased placental blood flow (Bollwein *et al.*, 2002) and, therefore, fetal growth. Others, however, agree that oestrogen may be responsible for fetal growth but that this is not necessarily because of an oestrogen-induced increase in blood supply (Esteller-Vico *et al.*, 2017). Oestrogen also promotes uterine myometrial activity in the presence of PGs and oxytocin; however, in the presence of continued elevated progesterones, this role is negated (Leung *et al.*, 1999; Ousey, 2011a).

3.3.2.3. PGF2α

During the major part of late pregnancy, maternal PGF2α plasma concentrations remain at low levels, equivalent to those seen during early pregnancy (1–2 ng/ml). However, near to term, levels increase slightly in the form of short pulses; but significant elevations in concentration are not detected until parturition has started, when they play a major role in uterine myometrial contraction (Section 4.3.2 and 4.3.3 Daels *et al.*, 1996; Ousey, 2011a).

3.3.2.4. Relaxin

Little is known of the role of relaxin in pregnancy in the mare. However, it is evident that the maternal concentration of relaxin increases from around day 80, possibly declining somewhat after day 150 but then rising again from day 220, especially as parturition approaches. It is proposed that relaxin acts with progesterones to maintain a quiescent uterine environment throughout pregnancy, although the significant rise prior to parturition would seem to go against this hypothesis (Stewart *et al.*, 1992; Klonisch and Hombach-Klonisch, 2000).

3.4. Conclusion

Significant research has been carried out into many aspects of equine pregnancy. It is evident that pregnancy in the mare has a number of unique features – the period of mobility, the production of eCG and the reliance on two successive populations of CL – and so differs in several aspects from other farm livestock. Continuing development of our knowledge is essential if we are to understand and hence minimize embryo mortality, a significant cause of apparent infertility in the mare. When the factors affecting embryo survival are more fully understood, our management of the equine can be further directed towards minimizing losses.

Study Questions

Detail the means by which maternal recognition of pregnancy is achieved in the mare. How does this affect plasma hormone concentrations in order to ensure pregnancy is maintained?

Describe embryology in the mare (up to day 40).

Give an account of the various stages leading up to and including the establishment of the placenta in the mare (day 100) and evaluate their relative importance in the endocrine control of pregnancy and in the provision of nutrition to ensure the survival of the developing conceptus.

Give a detailed account of the development and structure of the placenta in the mare. How does the structure of the placenta affect the requirements of the new-born foal?

Detail the endocrine changes that occur in the mare during pregnancy. How do these ensure the continuation of pregnancy and survival of the conceptus?

'Progesterone is the hormone of pregnancy'. Discuss, with reference to the various roles progesterone plays in pregnancy and the site of production.

Suggested Reading

Ginther, O.J. (1992) *Reproductive Biology of the Mare, Basic and Applied Aspects*, 2nd edn. Equiservices, Cross Plains, Wisconsin, pp. 642.

Asbury, A.C. and LeBlanc, M.M. (1993) The placenta. In: McKinnon, A.O. and Voss, J.L. (eds) *Equine Reproduction*. Lea and Febiger, Philadelphia, Pennsylvania, pp. 509–516.

Flood, P.F. (1993) Fertilisation, early embryo development and establishment of the placenta. In: McKinnon, A.O. and Voss, J.L. (eds) *Equine Reproduction*. Lea and Febiger, Philadelphia, Pennsylvania, pp. 473–485.

Allen, W.R. and Stewart, F. (2001) Equine placentation. *Reproduction, Fertility and Development* 13, 623–634.

Betteridge, K.J. (2007) Equine embryology: an inventory of unanswered questions. *Theriogenology, 68 Supplement* 1, S9–S21.

Allen, W.R. and Wilsher, S. (2009) A review of implantation and early placentation in the mare. *Placenta* 30, 1005–1015.

Betteridge, K.J. (2011) Embryo morphology, growth and development. In: McKinnon, A.O., Squires, E.L., Vaala, E. and Varner, D.D. (eds) *Equine Reproduction*, 2nd edn. Wiley-Blackwell, Philadelphia, London, pp. 2168–2186.

Allen, W.R., Gower, S. and Wilsher, S. (2011) Fetal membrane differentiation, implantation and early placentation. In: McKinnon, A.O., Squires, E.L., Vaala, E. and Varner, D.D. (eds) *Equine Reproduction*, 2nd edn. Wiley-Blackwell, Philadelphia, London, pp. 2187–2199.

McDowell, K.J. and Sharp, D.C. (2011) Maternal recognition of pregnancy. In: McKinnon, A.O., Squires, E.L., Vaala, E. and Varner, D.D. (eds) *Equine Reproduction*, 2nd edn. Wiley-Blackwell, Philadelphia, London, pp. 2200–2210.

Bergfeldt, D.R. and Adams, G.P. (2011) Pregnancy. In: McKinnon, A.O., Squires, E.L., Vaala, E. and Varner, D.D. (eds) *Equine Reproduction*, 2nd edn. Wiley-Blackwell, Philadelphia, London, pp. 2065–2079.

4 Parturition

The Objectives of this Chapter are:

To detail the process and control of parturition in the mare.
To enable you to appreciate the risks to the mare and foal at parturition and so understand the possible preventions and treatments.
To provide you with the knowledge to understand subsequent chapters on neonatal adaptation and the application to breeding practice.

4.1. Introduction

Parturition is the active expulsion of the fetus, along with its associated fluid and placental membranes. Gestation length, and hence the timing of parturition, varies significantly in the mare but the average gestation (pregnancy) length is 320–335 days (Davies Morel *et al.*, 2002). This Chapter considers parturition (foaling) and, for ease of understanding, is divided into the physical process of parturition followed by the endocrine control of parturition.

4.2. The Anatomy and Physiology of Parturition

Parturition, as in most mammals, involves three distinct stages: stage 1, positioning of the foal and preparation of the internal structures for delivery; stage 2, the actual birth of the foal; and stage 3, the expulsion of the allantochorion (placental membranes). All three stages involve considerable myometrial activity, mainly within the uterus itself, but with some involvement of the abdominal muscles (Card and Hillman, 1993; Christensen, 2011b). In the mare it is expulsive, normally being very rapid compared to other mammals.

4.2.1. First stage of labour

Stage 1 involves uterine myometrial contractures, converting to stronger contractions, and positions the foal in the birth canal ready for birth (Nathanielsz *et al.*, 1997; Nathanielsz, 1998); it lasts between 1 and 4 h,

although exact timing is unclear as the mare may not show obvious signs of stage 1 labour immediately. In some cases, a mare may show signs of first-stage labour and then cool off, only to show further signs several hours later; this is particularly evident in Thoroughbred mares (McCue and Ferris, 2012). Figure 4.1 illustrates the forces involved in this stage (Ginther, 1993).

The uterine muscles contract in mild waves from the tip of the uterine horn towards the cervix. These contractions, helped by the movement of the mare and, to a certain extent, by those of the foal, result in the repositioning of the foal and its passage into the birth canal, the area of least resistance. Throughout late pregnancy the foal lies in a ventral-flexed position (its vertebrae lying along the line of the mother's abdomen) with its forelimbs flexed. In the approach to (and during) first-stage labour it rotates into an extended dorsal position, with its forelimbs, head and neck fully extended, and engaged in the birth canal (Fig. 4.2; Haluska *et al.*, 1987a,b; Ginther, 1993).

For successful parturition other changes, in addition to the engaging of the foal, must occur. The cervix gradually dilates; this is encouraged during the latter part of first-stage labour by the pressure of the allantochorionic membrane and the foal's forelimbs against the uterine side of the cervix. During the birth of a dead fetus, dilation of the cervix is less complete and slower, presumably as cervical dilation is actively encouraged by the movements of the foal (Volkmann *et al.*, 1995). The exact mechanism by which parturition is induced

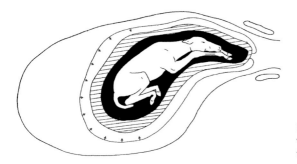

Fig. 4.1. The forces involved in the first stage of labour are provided by contractions of the uterine myometrium, as indicated by the arrows.

(A)

(B)

(C)

(D)

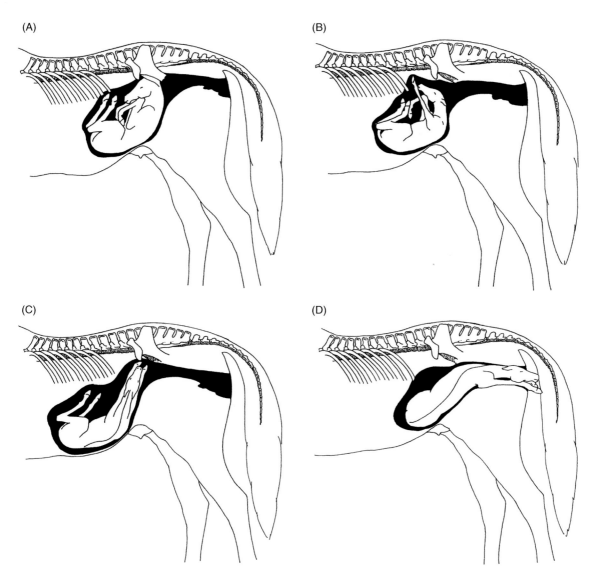

Fig. 4.2. (A–D) During the first stage of labour the foal is gradually rotated and positioned within the birth canal in readiness for expulsion during the contractions of second-stage labour.

and controlled is unclear (Section 4.3.2). However, active movement of the foal against the cervix and within the birth canal has been shown to increase prostaglandin F2α (PGF2α) and prostaglandin E (PGE) levels. Such a significant increase in prostaglandins, in particular PGE, is not seen during the birth of a dead foal. The cervix has a high concentration of collagen, the ratio of collagen to muscle fibres progressively increasing from the uterine horn through the uterus to the cervix. It is thought that PGE affects this collagen, causing it to change its configuration and so allow the cervix to relax (Rigby *et al.*, 1998). The hormone relaxin may also have a role (Bryant-Greenwood, 1982).

During this time the vulva continues to relax and secretions increasingly collect within the vagina. At the end of first-stage labour, the foal's forelegs and muzzle push their way through the dilating cervix, taking with them the allantochorion. At the cervix, this membrane is termed the cervical star and is one of the three sites devoid of microcotyledons and, therefore, there is no attachment to the maternal endometrium. The other two are at the entry to each Fallopian tube. The cervical star is the thinnest area of the placenta and hence it is this area that ruptures as the pressure of the myometrial contractions against the placental fluids increases, forcing them and the fetus through the cervix. The subsequent release of the allantoic fluid (breaking of the waters) is the trigger for the beginning of the second stage of labour (Wu and Nathanielsz, 1994; Nathanielsz *et al.*, 1997).

4.2.2. Second stage of labour

Stage two labour is the birth of the foal. Its start is heralded by the release of allantoic fluid that lubricates the vagina and is thought to trigger the stronger uterine contractions of the second stage. These strong contractions continue until the birth of the foal, normally within 20 min (acceptable range 5–60 min; Rossdale and Ricketts, 1980; McCue and Ferris, 2012). At the start of stage 2 the amniotic sack is often visible bulging through the vulva (Fig. 4.3), within which the foal's forelegs and muzzle can be felt (Figs 4.3, 4.4 and 4.5). Second-stage labour involves stronger contractions of the uterine myometrium, supplemented by abdominal muscle contractions (Fig. 4.6).

The supplementary force provided by the abdominal muscles is termed voluntary straining. During voluntary straining the mare inspires deeply, holding the rib cage and diaphragm at maximum inspiration, and increasing pressure on the abdomen. In addition the rib

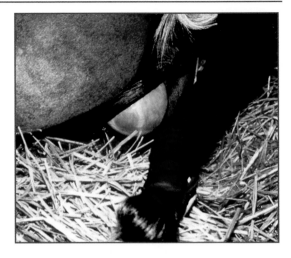

Fig. 4.3. The amniotic sack should be seen as a white membrane protruding from the mare's vulva. (Photo courtesy of Mr Steve Rufus.)

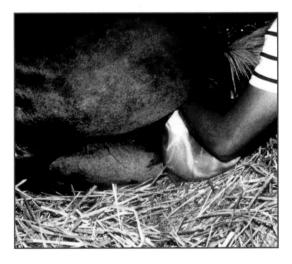

Fig. 4.4. At the start of second-stage labour, a brief internal examination may be made to ascertain whether the foal's feet and head are in the birth canal (meaning that the foal is correctly presented). (Photo courtesy of Mr Steve Rufus.)

cage and abdominal muscles react by contracting against the pressure; this further contraction force is transferred to the uterine contents, adding extra impetus to the expulsion of the uterine contents (Fig. 4.6). The area of least resistance is the cervix, and so the foal gets pushed forcefully further into the birth canal and out through the cervix and vagina.

At the end of first-stage labour, the foal lies in a dorsal-extended position. The soft tissue and surrounding

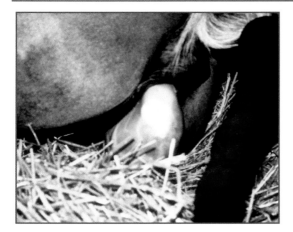

Fig. 4.5. The foal's forelegs should be seen within the amniotic sack. (Photo courtesy of Mr Steve Rufus.)

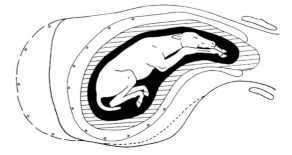

Fig. 4.6. Second-stage labour involves stronger contractions of the uterine myometrium, supplemented by contractions of the abdominal muscles, as indicated by the arrows.

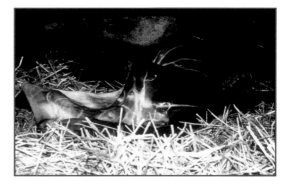

Fig. 4.7. The angle of the birth canal dictates that the foal is delivered in a curved manner, being expelled down towards the mare's hind legs. (Photo courtesy of Mr Steve Rufus.)

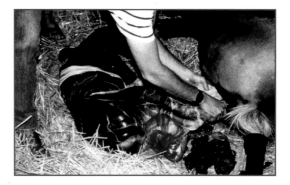

Fig. 4.8. The end of the second stage of labour is marked by the foal lying with its hind legs still within the vulva of the mare. (Photo courtesy of Mr Steve Rufus.)

bones govern the shape of the birth canal. The pelvis delineates the sides and ventral (bottom) part of the canal (ischium, pubis and ilium), and the sacral and coccygeal vertebrae delineate the dorsal (top, near the mare's vertebra) part. The diameter of the entry into the birth canal (20–24 cm) is slightly larger than the exit diameter (15–20 cm), and slightly more dorsal than the exit. Hence, the foal is funnelled through the birth canal in a curved manner, being expelled ventrally (down towards the mare's hind legs; Figs 4.7 and 4.8; Rossdale and Ricketts, 1980).

The foal is delivered forelegs first, followed by the head lying extended between the forelegs, parallel with the knees. The two forelegs are not delivered aligned: normally one leg is delivered slightly in advance of the other, the fetlock of one being in line with the hoof of the other (Fig. 4.9). This misalignment of the forelegs reduces the cross-sectional diameter of the foal's thorax, which is the widest part of the foal, so reducing trauma to both mare and foal at birth and easing foaling. Once the thorax and shoulders have passed through the birth canal, the remainder of the birth process is relatively easy. As the foal is forced through the birth canal the amnion that surrounds the fetus tears away, so the foal is born with the amnion pulled back away from its nostrils, allowing it to breathe immediately. At the end of stage 2 the foal lies with its head near the mare's hind legs, with its own hind limbs still within the mare's vagina and the umbilical cord attached (Fig. 4.8). The presence of the foal's legs within the mare's vagina has an apparent tranquilizing effect, most mares being reluctant to rise immediately post-stage 2 (Rossdale and

Ricketts, 1980). Soon the mare will stretch around to lick the foal while still recumbent, or she will rise and/or the foal will move, breaking the umbilical cord so separating the mare and foal.

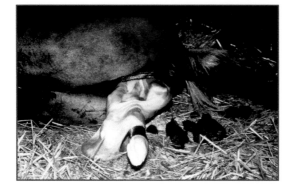

Fig. 4.9. In order to reduce the diameter of the foal's thorax passing through the birth canal the foal is delivered with one foot slightly in advance of the other. (Photo courtesy of Mr Steve Rufus.)

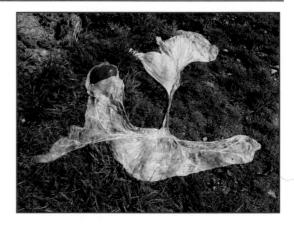

Fig. 4.10. The amniotic sack: the white membrane in the background and the allantochorion (placenta) in the foreground, after expulsion during the third stage of labour. As can be seen, the placenta is expelled inside out, with the red, velvety, outer allantochorion being inside and the white, smooth, inner allantochorion being outermost.

4.2.3. Third stage of labour

Stage 3 of labour is the birth of the placenta. Release of the placenta from the uterus begins at the later part of stage 2 and is normally completed within 4 h of the end of stage 2; an interval of longer than 8 h is of concern. Uterine contractions continue at a level similar to that evident during stage 1 labour, again originating at the uterine horns and passing down in waves to the cervix. At the same time, the allantochorion begins to shrink, as blood is drawn away from it towards the foal's pulmonary system (Section 19.2.2.2). The blood vessels constrict and draw the allantochorion away from the uterine endometrium. This releases the remaining attachments between the allantochorion and the uterine epithelium and forces the placenta to be expelled inside out. The placenta is delivered with its red, velvety outer allantochorion innermost and the white smooth, inner allantochorion outermost and should be examined as soon as possible (Figs 4.10 and 4.11). The contractions of third-stage labour also help to expel any remaining fluids and assist in uterine involution (recovery) (Christensen, 2011b; Schlafer, 2011a).

4.2.4. Hippomane

Passed out either during second-stage labour or along with the placenta during third-stage labour is a small, brown, leathery structure termed the hippomane (Fig. 3.34). It is found within the allantoic fluid and is an accumulation of waste salts and minerals collected throughout pregnancy. It has a high concentration of calcium, magnesium, nitrogen, phosphorus and potassium, and is first evident at around day 85 of pregnancy.

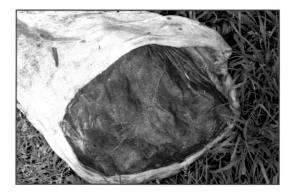

Fig. 4.11. A close-up of the placenta in its inside-out state, illustrating the innermost red allantochorion and the outermost smooth white allantochorion.

It has been associated with much folklore, including aphrodisiac properties and responsibility for keeping the foal's mouth open. There is, however, no evidence to support these claims (Morresey, 2011b; Schlafer, 2011a).

4.3. The Endocrine Control of Parturition

The endocrine control of the initiation of parturition and of parturition itself is still not fully understood in the mare. The following sections will outline current knowledge and hypotheses.

4.3.1. The timing of parturition

Parturition in the mare occurs at approximately 11 months (320–335 days), although ranges as large as 315–388 days have been reported to result in viable full-term foals (Davies Morel *et al.*, 2002; Perez *et al.*, 2003). The length of gestation in ponies tends to be shorter than in horses by 2 weeks, on average (Rossdale *et al.*, 1984; Satué *et al.*, 2011).

Within these averages, many factors may influence the exact timing of parturition including environmental, fetal and maternal factors. Environmental factors include the season of mating, with mares mated early in the season tending to have longer gestations than those mated later on. This is presumably nature's way of compensating for early and late matings, trying to ensure all mares foal at the optimum time of the year for foal survival – that is, during spring (Hodge *et al.*, 1982; Perez *et al.*, 2003; Rezac *et al.*, 2013; Talluri *et al.*, 2016). Climate (Astudillo *et al.*, 1960), year of breeding or foaling (Rophia *et al.*, 1969; Panchal *et al.*, 1995) and nutrition are also reported to have an effect (Hines *et al.*, 1987).

Fetal factors including the genotype of the offspring can affect gestation length. This can be demonstrated by comparing the gestation lengths of various crosses within the equine species. A stallion-cross-mare fetus has an average gestation of 340 days, a stallion-cross-jennet fetus 350 days, a jack-cross-mare fetus 355 days and a jack-cross-jennet 365 days (Rollins and Howell, 1951; Ginther, 1992). Breed of foal is also a reported factor (Aoki *et al.*, 2013), as is foal gender: colt foals have pregnancies on average 2.5 days longer than filly foals (Hevia *et al.*, 1994; Panchal *et al.*, 1995; Davies Morel *et al.*, 2002; Talluri *et al.*, 2016). Multiple births, although rare, also have shorter gestations than singles (Jeffcote and Whitwell, 1973).

Finally, maternal factors: the mare herself has some control over the exact time of delivery. It may be considered that the fetus determines the day of parturition and the mare dictates the hour. The majority of mares foal at night, when undisturbed (Fig. 4.12; Hines *et al.*, 1987; McCue and Ferris, 2012). There is evidence that this is linked to a circadian (daily) rhythm in oxytocin

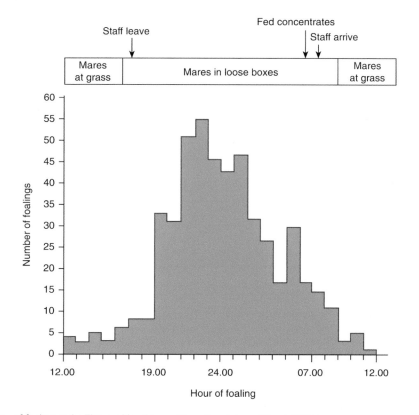

Fig. 4.12. The time of foaling in the Thoroughbred mare. (From Rossdale and Short, 1967.)

secretion around parturition (Nathanielsz *et al.*, 1997; McGlothlin *et al.*, 2004). This, in turn, may be related to stress such as the presence of staff. Work by Newcombe and Nout (1998) comparing two studs with different staff routines demonstrated that although most foaling occurred during the hours of darkness, the mares avoided foaling when staff were around. In addition, the mare's age (Bos and Van der May, 1980), parity (Panchal *et al.*, 1995), foaling-to-conception interval (Britton and Howell, 1943), genotype (Rophia *et al.*, 1969) and mating-to-ovulation interval (Ganowiczow and Ganowicz, 1966) have all been reported to affect gestation length, although many reports are inconclusive and often contradictory.

4.3.2. Initiation of parturition

Birth involves the rapid expulsion of the fetus, plus all associated placental membranes and fluid, and is achieved primarily by uterine myometrial activity (Section 4.2) which is inhibited by elevated progesterone/progestogens and depressed oestrogen concentrations, characteristics of pregnancy in most mammals. At full term, the ratio of progesterone/progestogens to oestrogen reverses, removing any inhibition and allowing myometrial activity to be facilitated by elevated oestrogens and driven by elevated PGF2α and oxytocin concentrations, all of which can be seen to rise at parturition (Chavatte *et al.*, 1997b; Ousey *et al.*, 2000). Efficient expulsion of the fetus and placental tissue is dependent upon sequential peristaltic contraction of the whole uterine myometrium (Macpherson and Paccamonti, 2011). There must, therefore, be immediate activation of muscle cells and efficient cell-to-cell excitation. This message transfer is affected by circulating hormone concentrations; elevated progesterone/progestogen concentrations reduce the spread of muscle cell excitation and contraction, whereas oestrogen, PGF2α and oxytocin actively facilitate and drive myometrial activity (Holtan *et al.*, 1991; Rossdale *et al.*, 1997). The exact mechanism for the initiation of this myometrial contraction for parturition in the horse or any other member of the Equidae is as yet unclear (Conley, 2016). However, in other mammals, two alternative mechanisms are apparent.

First, as seen in the ewe, goat, sow and cow, the fetus itself actively controls the initiation of its own parturition. Towards the end of gestation the fetus comes under increasing stress due to hypoxia (a shortage of oxygen), physical restriction within the uterus and an inability of the placenta to provide enough nutrients for growth and adequately remove waste products. These increasing stress levels activate the fetal hypothalamic–pituitary–adrenal axis, causing the production of adrenocorticotrophic hormone (ACTH) by the fetal anterior pituitary. ACTH activates the fetal adrenals to produce corticoids, so fetal cortisol levels increase (Ousey *et al.*, 1998). Cortisol passes to the placenta where it affects the metabolic pathways involved in conversion of progesterone to oestrogen. Under the influence of fetal cortisol, three enzymes in this pathway (17a hydroxylase, 17-20 desmolase, aromatase) are activated, and so increase the conversion of progesterone to oestrogen (Power and Challis, 1987; Nathanielsz, 1998). As a result the characteristic rise in oestrogens and fall in progesterone, as required for myometrial activity, is achieved (Fig. 4.13; LeBlanc, 1996; Ousey *et al.*, 2007, 2011a; Ousey and Fowden, 2012).

The second apparent method by which parturition is initiated is seen in primates. In such mammals the start of parturition is determined by a genetically controlled maturation signal linked closely to the time of gestation. It appears to be this maturation signal, and not fetal stress, that activates the fetal hypothalamic–pituitary–adrenal axis. In response, the adrenals produce increased levels of androgens, the precursor for placental oestrogens. Hence, elevated oestrogens are observed. In primates there is no involvement of the fetal adrenocorticoids. However, the result is the same, increasing oestrogen concentrations relative to progesterone/progestins (Nathanielsz *et al.*, 1997).

Regardless of the exact means of initiating parturition, the end result is the same: an increase in the ratio of oestrogen to progesterone/progestogens. The inhibitory effect of progesterones/progestogens on myometrial activity is removed, allowing the elevated oestrogen levels to drive activity by encouraging the synthesis of contractile proteins in the myometrial cells, in addition to being linked to increasing oxytocin production and increasing oxytocin receptors on the endometrium (Fuchs *et al.*, 1983; Wu and Nathanielsz, 1994; Challis *et al.*, 2002). This starts initial mild uterine myometrial activity, moving it from quiescence to activation (Fig. 4.14 phase 0 to phase 1); this initial mild activation is termed contractures and marks the start of stage 1 of parturition. Rising oestrogen levels facilitate myometrial activity (uterotrophin) and directly result in rising oxytocin levels and, as oxytocic is one of the two major inducers of uterine myometrial activity (uterotonic), it plays a central role in parturition. The second inducer

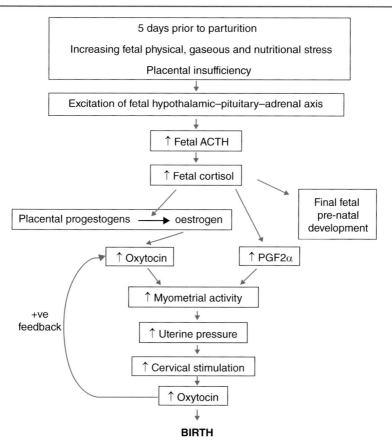

Fig. 4.13. The most likely model for the initiation of parturition in the mare. ACTH, adrenocorticotrophic hormone; PGF2α, prostaglandin F2α.

of myometrial contractions is PGF2α, which, as seen previously (Section 2.4.2.7) is produced by the uterine endometrium in response to rising oxytocin levels. PGE is also produced but is thought to be more concerned with cervical relaxation (Rigby *et al.*, 1998). So elevated oestrogen levels, characteristic of the end of pregnancy, drive the production of both oxytocin and PGF2α, both of which are major activators of uterine myometrial activity required during parturition. As PGF2α and oxytocin levels begin to rise, the contractures of the uterine myometrium are converted into full contractions, moving the myometrium from activation to stimulation (phase 1 to phase 2); the mare is now moving into stage 2 of parturition (Fig. 4.14; Ousey and Fowden, 2012). Initially it was thought that PGF2α played the major role, being involved in all three stages of parturition, particularly stages 1 and 2, whereas

oxytocin was thought to be primarily involved in stages 2 and 3. However, the importance of oxytocin is becoming increasingly evident, and it may indeed play more of a central role in driving the contractions of labour than previously thought (Nathanielsz *et al.*, 1997; Ousey and Fowden, 2012).

As the mare moves into stage 2 of parturition an additional neural stimulus supplements the existing hormonal activation. The increasing pressure from the allantoic fluid and fetus on the inside of the cervix, as it is pushed up into the birth canal, sends a neural message to the hypothalamus via the spinal cord. The hypothalamus activates the posterior pituitary, which in response produces oxytocin, so elevating circulating oxytocin concentrations. These elevated oxytocin levels then further drive the major uterine contractions (Wu and Nathanielsz, 1994; Nathanielsz *et al.*, 1997).

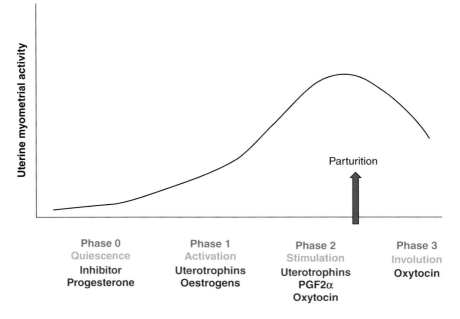

Fig. 4.14. The stages of activation of the mare's uterine myometrium during parturition. PGF2α, prostaglandin F2α.

The uterine myometrium is now in full stimulation (phase 2) and the mare in stage 2 of parturition (Fig. 4.14; Ousey and Fowden, 2012).There is also evidence of a circadian rhythm in oxytocin production. This rhythm is inherent but may be modulated by daylight, night-time being associated with increased oxytocin production (Fuchs *et al.*, 1992; Nathanielsz *et al.*, 1997; McGlothlin *et al.*, 2004; Roizen *et al.*, 2007; Murphy, 2019), so in part explaining the increased incidence of foaling during the hours of darkness (McCue and Ferris, 2012). The mare herself also appears to have some fine control over the exact timing of oxytocin release which can be inhibited, and so parturition temporarily suspended, by stress.

Once the foal has been born and the mare moves into stage 3 of parturition the levels of oxytocin and PGF2α decline, reducing myometrial activity although not eliminating it altogether, as mild contractions continue until the placenta has been passed and even into the first few days post-partum as uterine involution starts (phase 3; Fig. 4.14; Ousey and Fowden, 2012).

In summary, elevated oestrogen levels drive the production of oxytocin and PGF2α, which in turn (and provided progesterone levels are low) drive the uterine myometrial activity associated with the contractions of labour. In addition, the posterior pituitary produces additional oxytocin that provides the extra impetus required for second-stage labour.

Although there is no conclusive evidence of which mechanism initiates parturition in the mare, most of the evidence available indicates a system similar to that seen in the ewe (Silver, 1990; Silver and Fowden, 1994; Ousey *et al.*, 2004). Prolonged elevated corticosteroid levels in the later part of gestation, as seen in other mammals, have not been reported in the equine fetus, although this may be due to difficulties encountered in catheterizing such fetuses (Conley, 2016). However, significantly elevated corticosteroid levels have been reported in the equine fetus 72–96 h prior to parturition, reaching a peak 30–60 min post-partum (Silver and Fowden, 1994; Fowden *et al.*, 2008; Conley, 2016). Similarly, elevated cortisol levels have been reported in the mare prior to parturition and are correlated to a decline in progestins (Nagel *et al.*, 2012). It has been demonstrated that cortisol is essential in foals for final organ maturation, particularly that of the respiratory and digestive tracts. Pashan and Allen (1979) presented evidence that parturition in the equine is influenced by fetal stress, via an interaction between fetal and placental size, and that fetal constriction may be a trigger. This hypothesis is further supported by others

(Rossdale *et al.*, 1992; Ousey *et al.*, 2004, 2011) who demonstrated that treatment of fetuses in utero with ACTH resulted in an increase in corticosteroid production by the fetal adrenals, which caused premature parturition, as observed in ewes. It appears, therefore, that, as parturition approaches, foals become increasingly stressed owing to nutritional and physical restriction. As a result cortisol levels increase but, in the foal, cortisol levels increase more dramatically and over a shorter period of time prior to parturition than is evident in the ewe and cow (Silver and Fowden, 1994). The relatively short period of elevated cortisol levels apparently reflects the rapid maturation of the equine fetal adrenals, which is a necessity for post-partum survival and which occurs in the last 3–5 days of gestation (Chavatte *et al.*, 1997b; LeBlanc, 1997; Rossdale *et al.*, 1997).

4.3.3. Endocrine concentrations

The hormones involved in parturition will be considered in turn (Fig. 4.15).

4.3.3.1. Oestrogen

Average oestrogen concentrations in the maternal blood system continue to fall over the last 30 days of gestation and, as they originate from the fetal–placental unit, reach basal levels within hours of parturition (Haluska and Currie, 1988; Allen, 2001a). Concentrations are approximately 6 ng ml^{-1} at 30 days prior to parturition and fall to less than 2 ng ml^{-1} after parturition (Pashan, 1984). This appears to be opposite to that expected, as discussed in Section 4.3.2. However,

more recent detailed investigations demonstrate that, in fact, plasma oestrogen levels may not reach basal (undetectable) levels until after parturition. Hence, at foaling, oestrogens are still evident, possibly owing to pulsatile nocturnal release of oestrogens, which increases as parturition approaches (O'Donnell *et al.*, 2003), and this may be linked to increased nocturnal myometrial activity and the characteristic night-time foaling observed in mares. Oestrogens are uterotrophic in that they facilitate the activity of uterotonins such as oxytocin and PGF2α.

4.3.3.2. Progesterone/progestogens

As discussed in Section 3.3.1.2, several progesterones are produced in pregnancy, but in late pregnancy progestogen metabolites predominate, for example 5α pregnanes. P4 (the main progesterone in early pregnancy) concentrations have already declined to basal levels, but concentrations of progestogens such as P5 and 5α pregnanes peak at 10–15 ng ml^{-1} 2–3 days pre-partum and then decline to basal level at parturition (Hamon *et al.*, 1991; Holtan *et al.*, 1991; Schutzer and Holton, 1995; Conley, 2016). These increasing progestogen concentrations are not well understood, but may be due to fetal adrenals initially producing P5 rather than cortisol/corticosteroids, that pass to the placenta and on to the mare unchanged. The reason for these elevated progestogens is unclear, but they occur around the time of elevated prostaglandin and oxytocin, and so perhaps the increased suppression of myometrial activity by progesterone at this time is required to suspend parturition

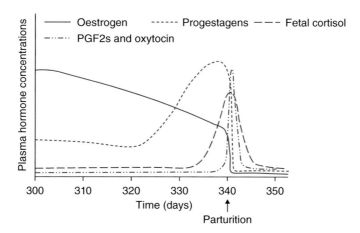

Fig. 4.15. A summary of the main changes in hormone concentration evident at parturition. PGF2α, prostaglandin F2α.

until the fetus is ready (Ousey *et al.*, 2005). Progestogens then fall, possibly as a result of the fetal adrenals now producing cortisol/corticosteroids, resulting in an alteration in placental metabolism driving the conversion of progestogens to oestrogens and so allowing parturition to commence (Rossdale *et al.*, 1991; Fowden *et al.*, 2008; Legacki *et al.*, 2016; Conley, 2016). It is evident, therefore, that despite previous reports to the contrary the endocrine changes in the mare at parturition are similar to those of other animals, albeit in a more truncated fashion, with relatively elevated oestrogen and low progestogen concentrations being evident in the last few hours prior to parturition.

4.3.3.3. Prostaglandins

Prostaglandins are primarily produced by the uterine endometrium and are uterotonic, actively driving uterine myometrial activity. Prostaglandin concentrations (both PGF2α and PGE) rise sharply in the plasma of the mare at term, mainly during the second stage of labour: 1–2 ng ml^{-1} in pregnancy, 20 ng ml^{-1} in first stage and 100 ng ml^{-1} in second stage, peaking 15 min or so before the foal is born (Silver *et al.*, 1979; Haluska and Currie, 1988; Fowden *et al.*, 1994; Vivrette *et al.*, 2000; Ousey, 2006). Fetal prostaglandin levels, as determined by catheterization, increase more gradually over the final weeks (40 days) of pregnancy (Silver *et al.*, 1979). Prostaglandin may also be detected in the allantoic fluid near to parturition. The major function of PGE is thought to be the induction of cervical dilation (Rigby *et al.*, 1998) and that of PF2α is to act as a strong inducer of uterine myometrial activity (Ousey, 2006). Prostaglandins were thought initially to be primarily associated with first- and second-stage labour; however, they are now thought to have a more encompassing role across all three stages (Ousey, 2006, 2011).

4.3.3.4. Oxytocin

Oxytocin is primarily produced by the posterior pituitary and (like PGF2α) is uterotonic, actively driving uterine myometrial activity. At parturition it is produced as part of the neuroendocrine response resulting from fetal stimulation of the cervix (the Ferguson reflex) (Christensen, 2011b). The actions of PGF2α and oxytocin are closely linked and they tend to show the same pattern of release, although oxytocin maybe a little delayed compared to PGF2α, as oxytocin levels remain low until the end of stage 1 when the

allantochorion breaks (Vivrette *et al.*, 2000). Oxytocin concentrations in the maternal system are low throughout pregnancy (<11 pg ml^{-1}) and then rise sharply to a peak at parturition, up to 6000 pg ml^{-1}, especially on the rupture of the allantochorion and release of the allantoic fluid and during the second stage (Haluska and Currie, 1988; Vivrette *et al.*, 2000). The central role of oxytocin is increasingly becoming evident and, like PGF2α, its primary role is in the induction of strong myometrial contractions, particularly important in second-stage labour, when it works in concert with PGF2α (Fuchs *et al.*, 1983; Haluska and Currie, 1988; Nagel *et al.*, 2014). Oxytocin appears to be the prime driver of the myometrial contractions of third-stage labour – the expulsion of the placenta – hence its use in cases of retained placenta (Hillman and Ganjam, 1979). The reported circadian rhythm to oxytocin release has been discussed previously (Section 4.3.2).

4.3.3.5. Cortisol

Cortisol concentrations do not change significantly in the maternal system during pregnancy although they rise, due to stress, at parturition (Chavatte *et al.*, 2000; Christensen, 2011b). Changes within the fetal system occur in late pregnancy with a sudden rise in cortisol evident 3–5 days prior to parturition (Silver *et al.*, 1984; Nathanielsz, 1998). As previously discussed (Section 4.3.2), this increase is shorter and sharper than the gradual increase observed in other species, and is thought to be associated with the maturation of the fetal adrenal cortex and its ability to react to increasing circulating ACTH (Silver and Fowden, 1994; Nathanielsz *et al.*, 1997, Fowden *et al.*, 2008). It may also be involved in final organ maturation, for example that of the respiratory system, in the equine fetus (Rossdale *et al.*, 1973).

4.3.3.6. Prolactin

Prolactin is produced by the anterior pituitary and is affected by day length, prolactin levels being generally elevated during long day length, the mare's breeding season. As far as parturition is concerned concentrations are reported to increase in the last 7–10 days of pregnancy (Heidler *et al.*, 2003). It is not apparent, however, that prolactin has a direct role in parturition, but its increase at this time may indicate a role in equine lactation, as seen in other mammals (Section 5.3; Forsyth *et al.*, 1975; Worthy *et al.*, 1986; Nett, 1993b).

4.3.3.7. Relaxin

Relaxin is produced by the placenta, and plasma concentrations are reported to be elevated in late pregnancy/parturition, when it is thought to maintain the quiescent nature of the uterine myometrium. Elevated levels at parturition seem paradoxical but perhaps at this stage relaxin is primarily involved in the relaxation and softening of pelvic ligaments and cervix as parturition approaches (Bryant-Greenwood, 1982; Stewart *et al.*, 1982; Christensen, 2011b). This is then overcome by the stronger uterotonin activation of oxytocin and PGF2α.

4.4. Conclusion

In the mare parturition occurs very rapidly and is driven by uterine myometrial activity. The mechanism for the initiation of this myometrial activity in the mare is unclear, but is likely, at least in part, to be due to fetal stress. Clarification of the hormonal control of equine parturition would be very beneficial as it would enable more accurate prediction of parturition and the successful artificial induction of parturition in the case of emergencies.

Study Questions

Evaluate the role that fetal stress may play in the timing of parturition in the mare.

Discuss the roles played by progesterone/progestogens and oestrogen in late pregnancy/parturition and how they affect the effectiveness of PGF2α and oxytocin.

Evaluate the role played by the uterine myometrium in parturition and the way in which its activity is controlled.

Explain how the endocrine changes that occur at the end of pregnancy result in parturition.

Detail the series of physiological events that culminate in the birth of the foal.

Suggested Reading

Ginther, O.J. (1993) Equine foal kinetics: allantoic fluid shifts and uterine horn closures. *Theriogenology* 40, 241–256.

Christensen, B.W. (2011) Parturition. In: McKinnon, A.O., Squires, E.L., Vaala, W.E. and Varner, D.D. (eds) *Equine Reproduction*, 2nd edn. Wiley-Blackwell, Philadelphia, London, pp. 2268–2276.

Macpherson, M.L. and Paccamonti, D.L. (2011) Induction of Parturition. In: McKinnon, A.O., Squires, E.L., Vaala, E. and Varner, D.D. (eds) *Equine Reproduction*, 2nd edn. Wiley-Blackwell, Philadelphia, London, pp. 2262–2267.

Conley, A.J. (2016) Review of reproductive endocrinology of the pregnant and parturient mare. *Theriogenology* 86, 355–365.

5 Lactation

The Objectives of this Chapter are:

To detail the anatomy of the mare's mammary glands so their role in lactation can be understood.
To describe the processes involved in the production of milk and how milk production is controlled.
To enable an understanding of the factors that might affect milk yield and so inform good breeding practice to ensure optimum milk production.

5.1. Introduction

The mammary glands are situated along the ventral midline in all mammals in a varying number of pairs. The mare normally has four glands (two pairs). Neither the anatomy and physiology of lactation, nor the control of lactation specific to the equine, have been widely studied. However, available evidence suggests that they are similar to those of other mammals, both in mammary gland structure and in control. Control is via both neural and hormonal pathways and can be divided into three stages: lactogenesis, galactopoiesis and milk ejection. Despite the lack of specific knowledge, an understanding of lactation is vital: optimum milk production is essential, both to provide vital immunoglobulins to the neonate and also for longer-term survival through the provision of vital nutrients up until weaning.

5.2. Anatomy and Physiology of Lactation

5.2.1. Anatomy

The mammary glands of the mare are situated in the inguinal region between the hind legs. They are covered and protected by skin and hair, except for the teats, which are devoid of hair. The whole of the skin surface is supplied with nerve endings, the concentrations of which are increased in the teat area, enhancing the response to touch. The mare normally has four glands –

two larger cranial ones and two smaller caudal ones – although six glands have been reported in the occasional mare. Each of the four mammary glands is completely independent and contained within, and supported by, a fibroelastic capsule, with no passage of milk from one quarter to another. The mammary gland halves are separated and supported by the medial suspensory ligament (fascial septum), running along the mare's midline. Further support is provided by the lateral suspensory ligaments running over the surface of the mammary gland under the skin, and by laminae, developing off the suspensory ligament and penetrating the mammary tissue in sheets (Fig. 5.1; Jacobson and McGillard, 1984; McCue, 1993; Knottenbelt, 2003; Dascanio, 2011a; McCue and Sitters, 2011).

Each udder half, on either side of the midline, is made up of two quarters; the openings from these two quarters exteriorize via a single teat (Fig. 5.2).

The mammary tissue itself is made up of millions of alveoli and connecting lactiferous ducts. This arrangement can be compared to a bunch of grapes, each alveolus being equated to a grape and the ducts to the branches (Fig. 5.3).

The alveoli are grouped together in lobules and then into lobes. These lobes join together via a branching duct system, which eventually leads to the gland cistern. Each quarter has its own gland cistern draining into a teat cistern and on to the streak canal, one from each quarter on that side (Dascanio, 2011a). At the end

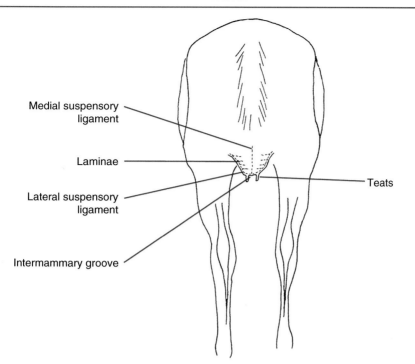

Fig. 5.1. A caudal (tail end) view of the mare's udder illustrating the suspensory apparatus of the mammary gland.

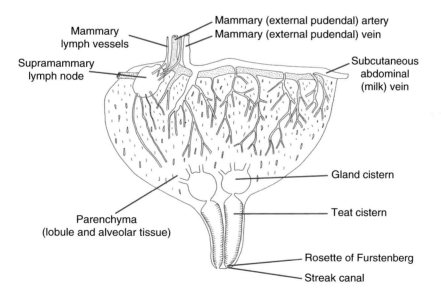

Fig. 5.2. A cross section through the mammary gland of the mare illustrating the exit of two quarters via a single teat.

of each teat is the rosette of Fustenburg, a tight sphincter that prevents the leakage of milk between sucklings. This sphincter can withstand a considerable build-up of milk pressure, though occasionally it may be breached, as in the case of mares that lose milk when parturition is imminent.

The alveoli, which are the milk-secreting structures, are lined by a single layer of lactating epithelial cells surrounding a central cavity or lumen. This alveolar lumen is continuous with the mammary duct system. Milk is secreted by the lactating cells into the alveolar lumen across the luminal or apical membrane. Surrounding each alveolus is a basket network of myoepithelial cells. These muscle cells also surround the smaller ducts, and their contraction is activated as part of the milk ejection reflex. Surrounding these myoepithelial cells is a capillary network supplying the alveoli with

milk precursors and providing hormonal control; there is also a series of lymph vessels. In addition, the alveoli have a nerve supply, which is responsible for the activation of the myoepithelial basket cells as well as for vasodilation and constriction of the capillary supply network (Fig. 5.4; Mepham, 1987).

The mammary gland as a whole is supplied with blood via two mammary or external pudendal arteries, one on each side of the midline, and entering the caudal end of the gland. Venous return from the mammary gland is via the venous plexus at the base of the gland and then on to the superficial vein of the thoracic wall (the subcutaneous abdominal milk vein) or via the external pudendal vein (Fig. 5.2). Both the external pudendal artery and vein enter and leave the body in the inguinal region. The subcutaneous abdominal vein, which runs along the abdomen of the mare, can be seen more clearly in lactating mares and is hence sometimes referred to as the milk vein. The mammary gland also has two supramammary lymph nodes, one on either side of the midline and at its base, and connecting the main circulatory lymph system to that of the mammary gland itself (Dascanio, 2011a).

5.2.2. Mammogenesis

Mammogenesis, or mammary development, is first evident in the embryo. Glands develop along either side of the midline in the inguinal region. Cells in this region proliferate to form nodules that develop to form

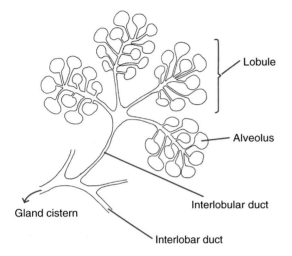

Fig. 5.3. A single lobe of the mammary gland made up of several lobules which in turn are made up of numerous alveoli.

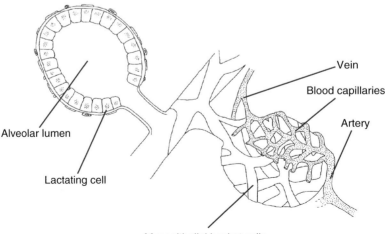

Fig. 5.4. The mammalian alveolus. On the left, a cross-sectional view illustrating the lactating cells surrounding the alveolar lumen, which is continuous with the mammary duct system. On the right, an alveolus illustrating the myoepithelial basket cells and alveolar blood supply.

mammary buds, evident from day 50 of gestation. Teats are present at birth, along with a few short branching ducts within the connective tissue associated with each teat (Mepham, 1987).

From birth to puberty mammary gland growth is isometric with (at the same rate as) body growth. Most of this prepubertal growth is an increase in fat and connective tissue, rather than in duct development. Puberty marks a change, as mammary development becomes allometric with (at a greater rate than) body growth. Beyond puberty, mammary growth increases and decreases with the oestrous cycle. The amount of mammary development within these cycles depends on the length of the dioestrous phase of the oestrous cycle, as elevated progesterone levels are responsible for mammary lobular–alveolar development. In the mare, the duration of dioestrus is such that just limited lobular–alveolar development takes place.

During pregnancy, elevated progesterone levels cause significant lobular–alveolar development, especially in the last trimester, but suppress milk production (lactogenesis). In the last 2–4 weeks of pregnancy progesterone declines; this removes the inhibition of lactogenesis and allows increasing prolactin, among other hormones, to begin to drive milk production (Section 5.3.1), so lactogenesis predominates (Leadon *et al.*, 1984; Ousey *et al.*, 1984; Mepham, 1987; McCue and Sitters, 2011). Elevated oestrogen levels,

characteristic of approaching parturition in many mammals, is also reported to induce the development of mammary ducts (Mepham, 1987; McCue and Sitters, 2011). During lactation mammogenesis continues, as cell division increases in line with milk production, to satisfy the increasing demands of the foal. Cell division then decreases after the maximum yield has been reached. At the same time, the size of the mammary gland slowly decreases until it returns to its normal non-lactating size post-weaning (Fig. 5.5).

5.2.3. Lactation curve and milk quality

There has been significantly less research conducted into the lactation of the mare compared with other livestock, especially the cow. Except in a very few cultures, mare's milk is of indirect rather than direct commercial importance, its value being assessed via the development of the foal reared, rather than directly by milk yield. As such, it is often not given the attention it warrants.

5.2.3.1. Lactation curve

There is much variation in the lactation curve demonstrated by different mares, largely due to man's interference and early weaning. As a general trend, milk yields in mares tend to increase during the first 2–3 months post-partum. Initial levels in the first 2 weeks are in the

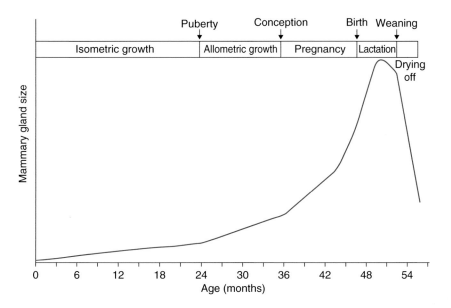

Fig. 5.5. Equine mammary development from birth to 4.5 years, including development during a mare's first pregnancy.

order of 3% of body weight, 4–8 l day^{-1} for Thorough-breds and 2–4 l day^{-1} for ponies (Fig. 5.6; Oftedal *et al.*, 1983; Oftedal and Jenness, 1988; Gibbs *et al.*, 1982; Santos and Silvestre, 2008).

Milk production reflects demand, which in turn reflects the size of the foal, and production therefore continues to rise as the foal grows until 2–3 months post-partum, when maximum levels of 10–18 l day^{-1} in Thoroughbreds, 14–17 l day^{-1} in draft mares and 8–12 l day^{-1} for ponies are reached (Tyznik, 1972; Oftedal *et al.*, 1983; Doreau *et al.*, 1990; McCue, 1993). In the first 3 months mares produce on average 2.1–5.4% of their body weight in milk day^{-1}. This corresponds to an average daily consumption by the healthy foal of 21–25% bwt day^{-1} in the first 2–3 months (Gibbs *et al.*, 1982). After 3 months, the foal's demand for nourishment from its mother decreases, as it starts to increasingly investigate grass or hay and its mother's hard feed. As the weaning process progresses towards full weaning, the lactational yield drops off further with decreasing demand (Jacobson and McGillard, 1984; Doreau and Boulet, 1989; Smolders *et al.*, 1990). As will be discussed later, milk quality also declines at this time, further encouraging the foal to seek nourishment elsewhere and to hasten the weaning process.

Lactation naturally lasts nearly a full year, the mare drying up completely a few weeks before she is due to deliver the following year's foal. However, in today's managed systems, humans normally dictate the length of lactation by weaning foals at about 6 months, at which time milk yield is less than that immediately post-partum (Fig. 5.6). At this stage the foal is obtaining little of its nourishment from its mother, deriving most from roughage and/or concentrate feeds, providing the foal is doing well. Weaning at 6 months, therefore, has little long-term effect on the foal's development.

The total milk yield of a Thoroughbred or one of the larger riding-type mares is 2000–3000 kg of milk per lactation. As a rough guide, in these larger horses, the natural daily milk yield averaged out over the whole lactation is 2–3 kg per 100 kg body weight. The corresponding equation for ponies is 5 kg per 100 kg body weight (Oftedal *et al.*, 1983). The foal normally suckles up to seven times per hour during the first week, consuming 70–100 g per suckle, then reducing to once an hour by week 10. Initial suckling ensures an intake of little but often; however, with age, the frequency of suckling declines and the intake per suckle increases up to 250 g or so at each suckling for larger riding-type horses (Frape, 1998). The number of suckles per day and the amount of milk taken per suckle reduce from peak lactation towards weaning.

5.2.3.2. Milk quality and composition

The composition of milk reflects the requirement of the young of that particular species, and provides the energy and the precursors needed for growth throughout lactation. In the case of some mammals, including the foal, milk additionally provides immunoglobulins during the initial stages of lactation (Table 5.1; Mepham,

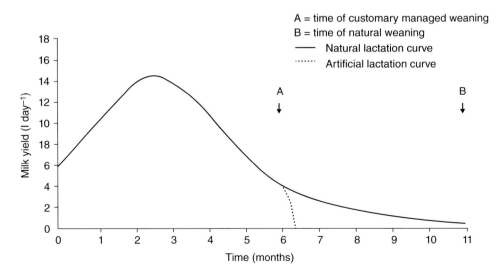

Fig. 5.6. The average lactation curve for a mare illustrating the natural extent of lactation along with that customarily imposed by man.

1987; Smolders *et al.*, 1990; Malacarne *et al.*, 2002, McCue and Sitters, 2011).

Colostrum

Colostrum is the first milk produced ready for the foal immediately after parturition; normally, 2–5 l is produced in total, at a rate of 300 ml h[-1] (Massey *et al.*, 1991; Knottenbelt and Holdstock, 2004a,b). In addition to being a source of nutrition, vitamins and lactoferrin (iron-carrying milk protein), for the neonate it is vitally important for the attainment of passive immunity via the provision of immunoglobulins, and as such contains a relatively high concentration of proteins (immunoglobulins). Protein concentration in colostrum is in the order of 13.5% compared to 2–4% in the main lactational milk. The main protein immunoglobulin in mare's colostrum is immunoglobulin G (IgG; 5000–11,000 mg dl[-1]); IgA (957 mg dl[-1]) and IgM (122 mg dl[-1]) are of less importance (Kohn *et al.*, 1989; Massey *et al.*, 1991; McCue, 1993; Erhard *et al.*, 2001). The levels of immunoglobulins reported varies considerably, and breed is thought to be at least one factor that affects IgG concentrations, being higher in draught than in light mares (10790 ± 4510 vs 7920 ± 1870 mg dl[-1], respectively). Age also seems to be a factor, older mares having lower colostrum IgG levels (LeBlanc and Tran, 1987; LeBlanc *et al.*, 1992; Chavatte-Palmer, 2002). This high protein concentration is at the expense of fats, which are present in relatively low concentrations. However, within 12–24 h colostrum production has ceased; protein levels fall dramatically, and fat levels rise. The relative concentrations within milk now stabilize, though both protein and lipid concentrations tend to decline gradually over time, as do mineral concentrations. However, lactose remains largely unchanged or even increases throughout the remainder of lactation, which is unusual in mammals (Table 5.2; Gibbs *et al.*, 1982; Smolders *et al.*, 1990). The digestive system of the foal is 'permeable' to complete protein molecules, such as immunoglobulins, for the first 24 h of life. This 'permeability' is due to enterocytes within the wall of the small intestine

Table 5.1. Comparative milk compositions of several species, expressed as percentages. (From Jennes and Sloane, 1970.)

Species	Total solids	Fat	Casein protein	Whey protein	Lactose
Human	12.4	3.8	0.4	0.6	7.0
Cow	12.7	3.7	2.8	0.6	4.8
Goat	13.2	4.5	2.5	0.4	4.1
Sheep	19.3	7.4	4.6	0.9	4.8
Horse	11.2	1.9	1.3	1.2	6.2

Table 5.2. The average composition of the milk during the main part of lactation in the mare. (From Oftedal *et al.*, 1983; Schryver *et al.*, 1986; Frape, 1989; Doreau *et al.*, 1990; Saastamoinen *et al.*, 1990; Martin *et al.*, 1991; Caspo *et al.*, 1995; Malacarne *et al.*, 2002; National Research Council, 2007.)

Component	Concentration
Water (%)	89.0
Protein (g kg[-1])(%)	19–40 (1.9–4)
Lactose (g kg[-1])(%)	51–69 (5.1–6.9)
Fat (g kg[-1])(%)	6–20 (0.6–2.0)
Energy (kcal 100 g[-1])	46–60
Ash (minerals, vitamins, etc.; g kg[-1])(%)	0.6–3.0 (0.06–0.3)
Ca (mg kg[-1])(%)	600–1200 (0.06–0.12)
P (mg kg[-1])(%)	230–800 (0.023–0.08)
Mg (mg kg[-1])(%)	30–100 (0.003–0.01)
K (mg kg[-1])(%)	400–700 (0.04–0.07)
Na (mg kg[-1])(%)	160–246 (0.016–0.025)
Cu (µg kg[-1])(%)	200–450 (2×10^{-5}–4.5×10^{-5})
Zn (µg kg[-1])(%)	1800–2500 (1.8×10^{-4}–2.5×10^{-4})

Ca, calcium; P, phosphorus; Mg, magnesium; K, potassium; Na, sodium; Cu, copper; Zn, zinc.

which absorb whole proteins via pinocytosis. After 24 h, this ability is irreversibly lost, as the enterocytes are replaced (McCue and Sitters, 2011). It is essential, therefore, that a newborn foal receives its colostrum well within 24 h of birth, as after this time it cannot take advantage of the immunoglobulins carried by colostrum: they will be broken down by intestinal proteolytic enzymes within the intestine into their component amino acids, and absorbed as such. The average composition of milk during the main part of lactation in the mare is given in Table 5.2.

Fat

The concentration of fats or lipids in mare's milk is reported to be relatively low when compared with other species (Table 5.1; Chavatte-Palmer, 2002; McCue and Sitters, 2011). However, there is some suggestion that this may be due to sampling error, as the highest concentration of fat is evident in the last milk milked out, which is not easily obtained. Fat is present in milk in the form of globules of saturated fat, cholesterol and unsaturated fats, as free fatty acids, phospholipids and triglycerides. The 8% concentration of triglycerides as a proportion of total fats is much lower than the 79% in cows. These fat globules exist as an emulsion within the milk and contain a high concentration of short-chain fatty acids, fewer than 16 carbons (C) in length (Oftedal and Jenness, 1988; National Research Council, 2007).

Proteins

Proteins during the main lactation are present in the form of near equal proportions of caseins (1.3%) and whey (1.2%; Doreau and Boulet, 1989). Caseins are unique to milk and have several functions. Under the influence of the stomach's acid pH, they form a clot with the enzyme rennin. This clot facilitates the digestion of proteins by the proteolytic enzymes of the digestive system. Caseins also contain essential amino acids and aid in the transport of minerals from the mare to the foal via milk. Caseins associate with calcium (Ca), phosphate (P) and magnesium (Mg) ions to form micelles, thus allowing a higher concentration of these minerals to be transported in milk than would be possible in a simple aqueous solution.

Two types of whey proteins are found in mare's milk and, unlike caseins, do not precipitate in acid pH. The whey proteins are divided into those that are specific to milk and those that can be found in both milk and blood. Those specific to milk can be further subdivided

into β lactoglobulin (28–60% of whey proteins) and α lactalbumin (26–50% of whey proteins; Gibbs et al., 1982). α lactalbumin is a good source of amino acids and is rich in essential amino acids such as tryptophan. It is also the B component which, along with an A component, make up the two halves of the enzyme lactase synthetase. Lactase synthetase is the terminal enzyme in the synthesis of lactose, the major sugar component of mare's milk. The second type of whey proteins found in mare's milk constitutes those also found in blood: serum albumin (2–15% of whey proteins) and serum globulin (11–21% of whey protein; Gibbs et al., 1982). Serum albumin is identical to blood serum albumin and is directly transferred unchanged from the blood through the lactating cell to the alveolar lumen. It is, therefore, only found in small concentrations, unless there has been cellular damage or haemorrhage within the mammary tissue. Serum globulin, on the other hand, is the immunological fraction of milk and, therefore, its concentration is very high in colostrum. Antibodies attach themselves to these globulins and it is via these that the foal attains its passive immunity (Zicker and Lonnerdal, 1994; McCue and Sitters, 2011).

Lactose

Lactose is the energy component of mare's milk (5.9–6.9%). Unique to mammals, each lactose molecule consists of a molecule of galactose and one of glucose. In the foal's intestine lactose is split into its two component parts: galactose which is then easily converted into glucose. Lactose is, therefore, in essence two molecules of glucose. The question then arises as to why lactose, not glucose, is present in milk, especially as there is an energy cost in converting glucose to lactose and vice versa. The answer lies in the effect of glucose on the osmotic pressure of milk relative to blood. The osmotic pressure of the two must be the same, and the component of milk that has the largest effect on osmotic pressure is the small molecule of lactose. However, if glucose were present, it would have an even greater effect on the difference in osmotic pressure. Additionally, one molecule of lactose gives rise to two molecules of glucose; that is, one molecule of lactose has twice the calorific value per molecule than glucose, and hence also per unit of osmotic pressure. It has also been suggested that lactose provides a more beneficial medium for intestinal activity, regulates bacterial flora and stabilizes pH, so aiding the absorption of minerals (Mepham, 1987; Smolders et al., 1990 ; McCue, 1993).

Mineral concentrations also vary with the stage of lactation. Potassium (K) and sodium (Na) concentrations in colostrum tend to be high, up to 1200 and 500 mg kg^{-1}, respectively, dropping to 700 and 225 mg kg^{-1} within 1 week and further dropping to 500 and 150 mg kg^{-1} in weeks 9–21. Ca tends to be raised in colostrum; it then falls slightly within hours, only to rise again to a peak of 1200 mg kg^{-1} at 3 weeks post-partum, but then drops as lactation progresses to 800 mg kg^{-1} at weeks 9–21. Mg levels are also elevated in colostrum, at 500 mg kg^{-1}, but fall off rapidly in the first 12 h and then continue to decline slowly throughout the rest of lactation to 45 mg kg^{-1} in weeks 9–21. Phosphorus (P) remains relatively steady at 400–700 mg kg^{-1} for the first 8 weeks of lactation and then concentration declines slightly; similarly, zinc (Zn) and copper (Cu) also decrease over lactation (Ullrey *et al.*, 1966; Oftedal *et al.*, 1983; Schryver *et al.*, 1986; Saastamoinen *et al.*, 1990; Martin *et al.*, 1991; National Research Council, 2007).

It is evident that there is a trend for the concentration of all the nutrient components of milk to decline as lactation proceeds. This is nature's way of encouraging the foal to obtain its nourishment elsewhere (Smolders *et al.*, 1990).

5.2.4. Milk synthesis

Milk is synthesized in the epithelial or lactating cells lining each alveolus. The precursors of, and components for, milk are obtained from the blood system supplying the udder. These components cross the basal membrane into the lactating cells. There is little information on how they pass across this membrane but, as the molecules are small, it seems likely that the majority pass by diffusion. The protein, fat and lactose components of milk are then built up within the lactating cells and pass across the cell membrane to the lumen of the alveolus (Mepham, 1987). Each of the major components of milk is discussed below.

5.2.4.1. Proteins

Proteins are built up from amino acids within the lactating cells. The total amount of nitrogen that crosses the basal membrane is equal to that within milk; however, there is a change in amino acids. Non-essential amino acids are synthesized within the cell and are built up into proteins along the mRNA within the ribosomes of the rough endoplasmic reticulum (RER). These proteins are then secreted into milk. Essential amino acids are passed unchanged across the basal membrane of the lactating cell, and are incorporated into proteins, along with the non-essential amino acids synthesized within the cell.

5.2.4.2. Lactose

Blood glucose is the primary precursor of lactose. However, glycerol, acetate and amino acids are also thought to contribute. The amount of glucose absorbed by the gland is much more than is needed solely for conversion to lactose. The difference is used as energy for general cell metabolism. The conversion of glucose to lactose involves five enzymes, the fifth being lactose synthetase, which is made up of two components, A and B. As discussed previously (Section 5.2.3.2), component B is the major milk protein α lactalbumin. The biochemical pathways involved in the conversion of glucose to lactose are summarized in Fig. 5.7.

5.2.4.3. Fat

The fat globules within milk are made up of esterified glycerol and free fatty acids, which aggregate to form a fat droplet emulsion within milk. There is much variation in the length of the free fatty acids making up the fat globules in the milk in females of varying species. The horse tends to have a higher concentration of short-chain fatty acids (less than 16 C atoms in length).

Fatty acids are derived mainly from three sources: glucose, triglycerides and free fatty acids. Glucose C is a significant precursor of free fatty acids in the non-ruminant, for example, the horse. Glucose is absorbed across the basal membrane and converted to acetyl coenzyme A (CoA) and on to malonyl CoA within the cytosol of the cell. Malonyl CoA is then built up, using a multi-enzyme complex, to free fatty acids which tend to be short chain (< 16 C). Blood triglycerides provide an

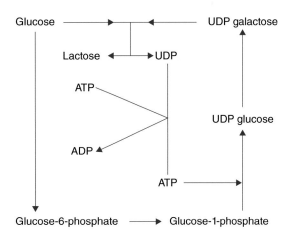

Fig. 5.7. A summary of the conversion of glucose to lactose within the lactating cell. UDP, uridine phosphate; ATP, adenosine triphosphate; ADP, adenosine diphosphate.

alternative source of free fatty acids for the lactating cell; these are broken down into glycerol plus free fatty acids within the cell. The free fatty acids obtained from triglycerides are longer-chain fatty acids, typically 16–18 C in length. Triglycerides, therefore, are not a very important source of fatty acids in the mare. The triglycerides are either broken down into amino acids and glycerol in the blood, similar to the way that proteins are broken down into amino acids and then absorbed into the cell, or they are absorbed directly (Mepham, 1987).

Glycerol that combines with the free fatty acids is derived again by three different methods: from the breakdown of triglycerides within the cell; by the absorption of free glycerol from the blood; or, finally, from the breakdown of glucose within the cell.

The free fatty acids and glycerol within the cell combine by esterification within the endoplasmic reticulum. These molecules then aggregate together to form the fat droplets within milk (Mepham, 1987).

5.2.5. Milk secretion

All the components of milk produced by the lactating cells have to pass across the apical membrane of the lactating cell into the alveolar lumen (Fig. 5.8). The different components of milk pass by different mechanisms.

5.2.5.1. Fat

The fat droplet size increases as the free fatty acids and glycerol continue to combine by esterification, and the resulting molecules aggregate into increasingly larger droplets as they migrate towards the apical membrane. In the vicinity of this membrane, strong London–Van der Waals forces attract these fat droplets and envelop

them in the membrane, forming a bulge in the apical membrane surrounding the droplet (Fig. 5.9).

The droplet and surrounding plasmalemma move away from the apical membrane into the lumen, forming a narrow bridge. This bulge then pinches off as the bridge gets narrower and releases the fat droplet plus surrounding plasmalemma into the alveolar lumen. The process is termed pinocytosis. Occasionally, part of the cell cytoplasm, sometimes including cell organelles, is enclosed in the bulge of the apical membrane along with the fat droplets, and then gets secreted into the alveolar lumen along with the milk fat. The formation of these structures, termed signets, occurs more commonly in the lower order of mammals, but they are evident in mare's milk (Mepham, 1987).

5.2.5.2. Protein

Proteins are built up from their constituent amino acids along the RER within the cell and then pass on to the Golgi apparatus. They accumulate as granules of proteins within the Golgi; this Golgi apparatus then migrates towards the apical membrane. The membrane of the Golgi apparatus fuses with the apical membrane and this releases the proteins into the alveolar lumen by reverse pinocytosis (Fig. 5.10).

By this reverse pinocytosis, plasmalemma lost during the secretion of milk fat is replaced during the secretion of milk proteins.

5.2.5.3. Lactose

The secretion of molecules of lactose, unlike that of milk fat and protein, is not visible using electron microscopy, and so the method of secretion is less clear. As discussed previously (Section 5.2.3.2), one of the mare's

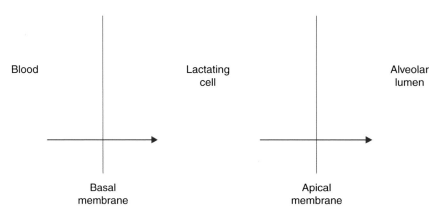

Blood

Lactating cell

Alveolar lumen

Basal membrane

Apical membrane

Fig. 5.8. The route of passage for all milk components from the mare's blood supply on the left through the lactating cell to the lumen of the alveolus.

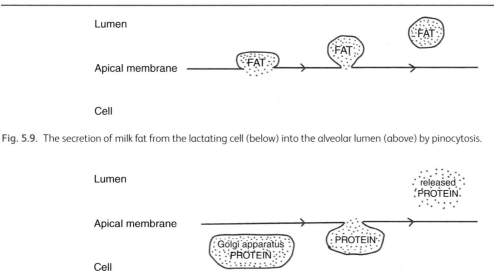

Fig. 5.9. The secretion of milk fat from the lactating cell (below) into the alveolar lumen (above) by pinocytosis.

Fig. 5.10. The secretion of milk protein from the lactating cell (below) into the alveolar lumen (above) by reverse pinocytosis.

milk proteins is α lactalbumin, and this protein is the B component of the fifth and last enzyme involved in lactose synthesis. It seems likely, therefore, that lactose secretion is closely linked to that of milk protein. The A protein of the enzyme lactase synthetase is known to be closely associated with the membrane of the Golgi apparatus. The B component (α lactalbumin) is synthesized, as are all other milk proteins, on the RER and then passed on to the Golgi apparatus. While the B component is in the Golgi apparatus, it becomes associated with the A component already there, and together they form active lactase synthetase. This enzyme catalyses the conversion of uridine diphosphate galactose (UDP galactose) and glucose to lactose. The lactose is then presumed to be secreted along with the milk proteins by reverse pinocytosis (Figs 5.10 and 5.11; Mepham, 1987).

5.2.5.4. Minerals

Milk has a relatively high concentration of K when compared to Na, and this is similar to the relative concentrations within the cytoplasm of the cell. Na and K in milk are derived from the intercellular fluid. The components within the lactating cell are derived from the blood system but the K/Na ratio in blood is the reverse of that within the cell and milk. Therefore, there must be an active transfer system across the basal membrane. This is via a Na pump, which pumps Na away from the cell cytoplasm and into the blood system and pumps K the opposite way towards the cell. This

maintains the high K/Na ratio within the cell. As the K/Na ratio in the milk is the same as that in the cell, Na and K are presumed to pass across the apical membrane to the alveolar lumen by simple diffusion (Mepham, 1987).

The concentrations of Ca, Mg and P are higher in milk than in the cell cytoplasm. Therefore, their passage must also be via an active transport system. The exact mechanism is unclear but all three ions are known to be closely associated with the milk protein casein. It is assumed, therefore, that this association occurs within the Golgi where the casein proteins are synthesized. These ions are then passed into the milk, along with proteins, via reverse pinocytosis (Mepham, 1987).

Iron is also secreted in association with proteins by reverse pinocytosis, as it is specifically bound to the milk protein, lactoferrin (Mepham, 1987).

5.2.5.5. Water

Water passes to the alveolar lumen from the cell cytoplasm by osmotic pressure. Fat and protein molecules in milk are in the form of large droplets, and so their effect on osmotic pressure is minimal. However, lactose and free ions are much smaller, and it is these that affect osmotic pressure and hence drive water diffusion from the cell into milk (Mepham, 1987).

5.2.5.6. Immunoglobulins

Colostrum, as discussed previously, has a high concentration of proteins; these proteins are immunoglobulins.

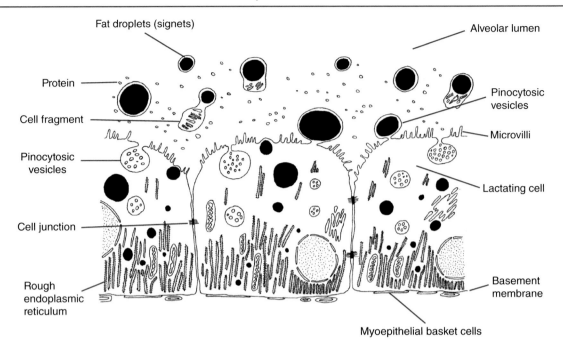

Fig. 5.11. Diagrammatic representation of a mammary secretory cell illustrating the build-up of protein and fat for release into the alveolar lumen.

These immunoglobulins are combined into large corpuscles termed bodies of Donne. The mechanism by which these are secreted is unclear. It is possible that engorgement of the lactating cell in late pregnancy results in the breakage of some of the junctions within the cell membranes, especially the basal cell membranes of the lactating cells. This allows the serum immunoglobulin proteins to pass into milk unchanged. There is also evidence suggesting an active transport system for these serum proteins, but the exact mechanism is unclear (Mepham, 1987).

5.3. Control of Lactation in the Mare

The control of lactation in most mammals, including the mare, is via both nervous and hormonal pathways. Unfortunately, information specific to the mare is very limited, though it is assumed that the control of lactation is similar to that evident in other mammals. Lactation may be divided into three stages as far as its control is concerned: lactogenesis, galactopoiesis and milk ejection.

5.3.1. Lactogenesis

Lactogenesis refers to the initial milk secretion that occurs in late pregnancy prior to parturition, resulting in a build-up of colostrum within the mammary glands. In the mare, lactogenesis is evident well before parturition occurs, as demonstrated by the presence of lactose, proteins and fat within the mammary secretions (Peaker *et al.*, 1979).

Control of lactogenesis is hormonal. High progesterone concentrations characteristic of pregnancy drive lobular–alveolar development, but inhibit milk secretion. Hence, with the decline of progesterone in late pregnancy, inhibition of milk production is removed (Mepham, 1987). Elevated oestrogen levels, also characteristic of approaching parturition, drive the development of the mammary ducts. Along with this elevated prolactin, growth hormone, insulin-like growth factor (IGF) and then thyroxine actively drive milk production (Heidler *et al.*, 2003). Evidence would suggest that elevated cortisol and insulin may also play a role, but more of a permissive or facilitating role, as opposed to actively driving mammary growth and milk production. It appears that, in the mare, prolactin may play a significant role as concentrations are observed to increase in the last 2 weeks of pregnancy and the first 2 months post-partum. Prolactin, in turn, is secreted by the anterior pituitary and is controlled via dopamine and is thought to work synergistically with oestrogens and progesterone to drive mammary gland development as well as to drive milk production (Neuschaefer *et al.*, 1991; Chavatte-Palmer, 2002; Heidler *et al.*, 2003). Elevated prolactin in the absence of previous exposure to elevated progesterone and oestrogens does not result in milk production (Nagy *et al.*, 2002). Lactogenesis, therefore, increases in late pregnancy and reaches a maximum immediately prior to parturition (Worthy *et al.*, 1986; Chavatte-Palmer, 2002).

In other mammals (for example, ruminants and humans) a placental lactogen has been identified and found to have an additional effect on lactogenesis. No such placental lactogen has been identified in equines, and it has been suggested that prolactin in the mare is responsible for the actions of placental lactogen in other mammals (McCue, 1993; Chavatte-Palmer, 2002).

5.3.2. Galactopoiesis

Galactopoiesis is the term given to the maintenance of milk production. Again, little information specific to the horse is available. However, it is assumed that control is similar to that in the sheep and the cow, and also that as with lactogenesis, prolactin, growth hormone, cortisol, insulin and thyroxine all act to drive galactopoiesis (Neuschaefer *et al.*, 1991). Interestingly, although prolactin seems essential for the establishment of milk production (lactogenesis and initial galactopoiesis), prolactin levels decline after the first few weeks but milk production remains high (Doreau and Boulet, 1989; Neuschaefer *et al.*, 1991). Galactopoiesis is also driven by, and mimics, the foal's demand for milk. This, in turn, dictates and governs the shape of the lactation curve and the quantity of milk produced. If the foal fails to suckle for a period of time, milk builds up within the mammary gland, causing back pressure that then inhibits galactopoiesis. If the foal fails to suck for a prolonged period this will have a permanent effect on galactopoiesis, milk production being reduced throughout that lactation. How this feedback is controlled is unclear but may involve the milk ejection reflex and/or oxytocin (Section 5.3.3).

5.3.3. Milk ejection reflex

Milk ejection, also termed milk let-down, differs from the other stages of lactation in that its control is both neural and hormonal. A nervous reflex acts as the stimulus or afferent pathway and hormones form the efferent path. Nerve receptors within the teats are stimulated by the action of suckling, and the nervous afferent pathway is activated, resulting first in a localized effect causing localized myometrial cell contraction. Second, this afferent nervous pathway acts via the central nervous system (CNS) to stimulate the paraventricular nucleus within the mare's hypothalamus. The hypothalamus then activates the posterior pituitary, which in response produces oxytocin. The efferent pathway of the milk ejection reflex is formed by this hormone oxytocin, which passes into the systemic blood system and hence to the mammary gland. The effectors that react to oxytocin are the myoepithelial basket cells surrounding each alveolus and the small ducts. It causes them to contract further and force milk out of the alveolus, along the ducts, to the gland cistern and on to the teat cistern, ready to be removed by the suckling action of the foal (Ellendorff and Schams, 1988; Nett, 1993b). Hence, at suckling, the milk initially available to the foal is that stored within the gland and teat cisterns, which is removed by the negative pressure exerted by the suckling action of the foal. This is then closely followed by the milk ejection reflex, which replenishes the milk within the gland and teat cisterns, making more available to the foal.

In addition to the above control mechanisms, the CNS has an overriding effect. For example, stress – especially as a result of fear or shock – reduces the effectiveness of the milk ejection reflex by increasing the levels of circulating adrenalin. Adrenalin causes vasoconstriction, so reducing the amount of oxytocin reaching the alveoli and hence the effectiveness of the reflex (Fig. 5.12). In instances of failed milk ejection, the teats become sore as the foal is only able to access the small volume of milk stored within the gland and teat cistern, necessitating frequent and relatively unsuccessful suckling attempts.

5.4. Conclusion

Our present knowledge specifically regarding equine lactation is still limited, largely due to the lack of direct commercial value for equine milk. However, by extrapolation from other species, a reasonable understanding can be achieved. Caution must be practised, however, in making definitive statements until these assumptions and extrapolations have been confirmed or refuted by more detailed research, specifically on equine lactation.

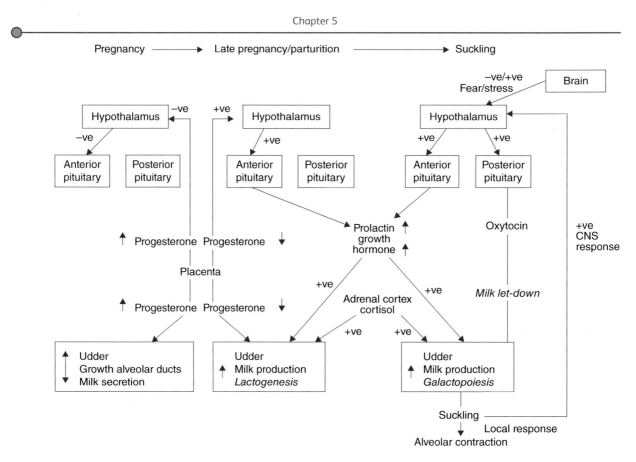

Fig. 5.12. Schematic representation of the control of lactation in the mare.

Study Questions

Detail the anatomy of the mammary gland and the role it plays in milk production.

The control of milk production can be divided into three stages. Name these stages and detail how they are controlled and how the foal itself may affect milk production.

Detail the components of milk, how these are produced, and how and why they change over the duration of lactation.

'Lactation quality is as important as lactation quantity'. Discuss the validity of this statement at all stages of lactation in the context of the well-being of the foal.

Suggested Reading

Mepham, B. (1987) *Physiology of Lactation*. Open University Press, Milton Keynes, UK, pp. 207.

Chavatte-Palmer, P. (2002) Lactation in the mare. *Equine Veterinary Education* 5, 88–93.

McCue, P.M. and Sitters, S. (2011) Lactation. In: McKinnon, A.O., Squires, E.L., Vaala, W.E. and Varner, D.D. (eds) *Equine Reproduction*, 2nd edn. Wiley-Blackwell, Philadelphia, London, pp. 2277–2290.

Dascanio, J. (2011) External reproductive anatomy. In: McKinnon, A.O., Squires, E.L., Vaala, W.E., Varner, D.D. (eds) *Equine Reproduction* 2nd edn. Wiley-Blackwell, Philadelphia, London, pp. 1577–1582.

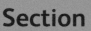

Section

B

Reproductive Anatomy and Physiology of the Stallion

Section B considers the biology of breeding the stallion, the anatomy of the stallion, the processes involved in sperm production and passage to the mare, and how reproductive activity is controlled in the stallion. This knowledge will then enable you to understand the following sections, which apply this knowledge to breeding practice.

6 Stallion Reproductive Anatomy

The Objectives of this Chapter are:

To detail the reproductive anatomy of the stallion.
To enable you to understand the process of spermatogenesis and the factors that might affect it.
To enable you to appreciate why infertility occurs and the possible treatments.
To provide you with the knowledge to understand subsequent chapters on endocrine control of stallion reproduction and the application to breeding practice.

6.1. Introduction

The reproductive system of the stallion, like that of the mare, may be considered to consist of extrinsic and intrinsic organs. The extrinsic organs are those associated with control (the hypothalamic–pituitary–gonadal axis) and will be considered in other chapters, plus the intrinsic organs, which are those that will be considered in this Chapter. The stallion's reproductive tract, similar to that of the mare, is a Y-shaped tubular system. The testes act as the manufacturing site for sperm, which are then matured and 'packaged' in the epididymis. After final maturation, through the addition of seminal plasma from the accessory glands, they are ready for delivery into the female tract via the penis. The reproductive tract of the stallion is illustrated diagrammatically in Fig. 6.1. Figures 6.2 and 6.3 provide a photograph and diagram of the reproductive system of the stallion after slaughter. Each of these structures will be discussed in turn in the following account.

6.2. The Penis

The penis of the stallion may be divided into the glans penis, the body or shaft and the roots or cura. In the resting position it lies retracted and hence protected within its sheath, or prepuce, out of sight; it is held in this position by muscles, including the retractor muscle which runs along the ventral side of the penis. The prepuce is a double-folded covering to the penis that folds back on itself to give a twofold protection. Within the inner fold lies the end of the penis, the glans penis (or rose), giving this sensitive area additional protection. Protruding by 5 mm from the centre of the glans penis lies the exit of the urethra (urethral process). Around this protrusion lies the urethral fossa and below it a dorsal diverticulum, both of which are often filled with smegma, a red-brown secretion of the prepubital glands lining the prepuce, plus epithelial cell debris (Fig. 6.4; Anamm, 2011a). These areas provide an ideal environment for bacteria, often harbouring venereal disease (VD) bacteria such as *Klebsiella pneumoniae*, *Taylorella equigenitalis* and *Pseudomonas aeruginosa*.

The penis of the stallion is attached by its two roots to the caudal part of the pelvis (ischium) by the ischiocavernosus muscles and to the lower part of the pelvis via the suspensory ligaments, one on either side. The urethra, running from the bladder, connects with the vas deferens and runs between the two roots before entering the body of the penis. The body of the stallion's penis contains a large percentage of erectile rather than fibrous tissue, which engorges as a result of increased blood pressure; as such the stallion's penis is termed a musculocarvenosus haemodynamic penis. Figures 6.5 and 6.6 illustrate a cross-sectional view through the stallion's penis (Chenier, 2008; Anamm, 2011a).

Figures 6.5a and 6.5b illustrate that the main body of the penis is divided into two sections: the lower

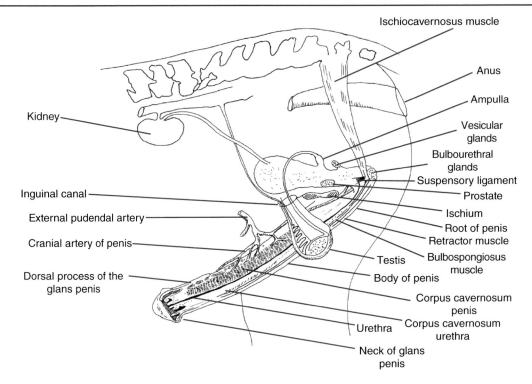

Fig. 6.1. A lateral (side) view of the stallion's reproductive system.

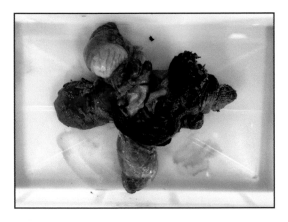

Fig. 6.2. The stallion's reproductive tract after slaughter and dissection; the accessory glands are not included.

corpus cavernosum urethra, sometimes called the corpus spongiosum penis, and the upper corpus cavernosum penis. Through the corpus cavernosum urethra runs the urethra, surrounded by a small area of trabeculae (sheets of connective tissue) enclosing small areas of erectile tissue, all enclosed within the bulbospongiosus muscle. The corpus cavernosum penis, the largest part of the penis, contains a dense network of trabeculae, associated muscle tissue and scattered cavities, and makes up the major erectile tissue of the penis. The corpus cavernosum penis is contained within the tunica albuginea, a fibro-elastic capsule or sheet, which maintains the integrity of the penis but still allows the doubling in size seen at erection. Finally, running along the bottom of the penis is a retractor muscle, contraction of which returns the penis to within the prepuce. The major erectile tissue of the glans penis is a continuation of the corpus cavernosum urethra, the corona glandis (Figs 6.6a and 6.6b). This erectile tissue, which is not confined by the fibro-elastic capsule of the corpus cavernosum penis, allows for the greater expansion (up to three times) of this area at ejaculation (Little and Holyoak, 1992; Chenier, 2008; Anamm, 2011a).

6.3. The Accessory Glands

The accessory glands are a series of four glands: bulbourethral, prostate, seminal vesicles and ampulla (some authors consider there to be three glands, excluding the ampulla), situated between the end of the vas deferens and the roots of the penis. Collectively these glands are

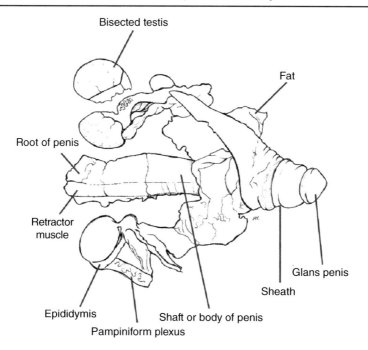

Bisected testis

Fat

Root of penis

Retractor muscle

Glans penis

Sheath

Epididymis

Shaft or body of penis

Pampiniform plexus

Fig. 6.3. A diagrammatic representation of the stallion's reproductive tract post dissection (as seen in the previous figure).

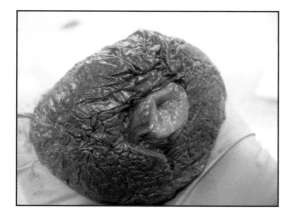

Fig. 6.4. The glans penis of the stallion, illustrating the protruding exit of the urethra and the surrounding urethral fossa and diverticulum.

responsible for the secretion of seminal plasma (Davies Morel, 1999).

6.3.1. Seminal plasma

Seminal plasma is the major fluid fraction of semen (the minor portion originating from the epididymis) and is testosterone dependent. Seminal plasma provides the substrate for conveying the sperm to the mare, and for ensuring final maturation. Other major functions are the provision of energy (glucose) and protection of the sperm from changes in osmotic pressure (citric acid, sorbitol), pH and from oxidization (ergothionine). It also contains a gel, which forms a partial clot in semen, the function of which is unclear, although it has been suggested that it might play a role as a paternity-protection mechanism (Davies Morel, 1999). Finally, seminal plasma is responsible for inducing motility in sperm. Sperm from the epididymis and the vas deferens are immotile, although their tails are functional, until they mix with seminal plasma.

Males of most species have this series of accessory glands, the relative size of which reflects the relative importance of their secretions within the seminal plasma. Owing to the difficulty of accessing the accessory glands, little information is available on their precise function and secretory products. However, composition does vary with species (Table 6.1); the most noteworthy as regards the stallion is the inclusion of glucose as the source of energy, rather than fructose as in most other mammals (Varner and Johnson, 2007).

6.3.2. The bulbourethral glands

The bulbourethral glands (formally known as the Cowper's glands) are the accessory glands situated nearest to

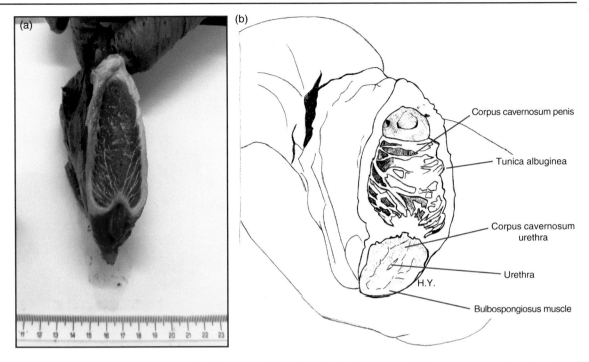

Fig. 6.5. Cross section through the main body of the penis of the stallion: (a) after dissection; and (b) a diagrammatic illustration of 6.5a.

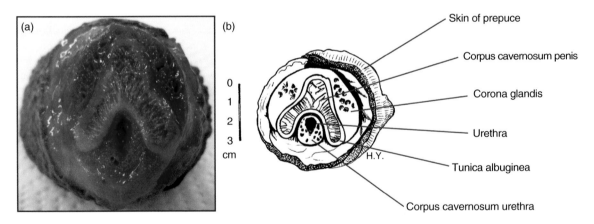

Fig. 6.6. Cross section through the glans penis of the stallion: (a) after dissection; and (b) a diagrammatic representation of Fig. 6.6a.

the roots of the penis on either side of the ischial arch. They are paired and oval in structure, approximately 3–6 cm in length and 1.5–4 cm wide, and lie on either side of the urethra. Their secretions are clear, thin and watery and form part of the main sperm-rich fraction and possibly also the pre-sperm fraction (Weber *et al.*, 1990; Setchell, 1991; Weber and Woods, 1993; Amann,

2011b; Paccamonti and De Vries, 2011; Varner and Schumacher, 2011).

6.3.3. The prostate

The prostate gland is a bilobed structure with a single exit to the urethra, situated between the bulbourethral glands and the ampulla; each lobe is 5–8 cm

Table 6.1. Composition of semen in stallions and bulls (Davies Morel, 1999).

Component	Stallion (mg ml⁻¹)	Bull (mg ml⁻¹)
Protein	1.2–12	3–80
Fructose	0.02–0.08	1.2–6.0
Glucose	0.82	–
Sorbitol	0.2–0.6	0.1–1.4
Citric acid	0.08–0.53	3.57–10
Inositol	0.19–0.47	0.25–0.46
Ascorbic acid	–	0.09
Ergothionine	0.03–1.1	< 0.01
Glycerylphosphorylcholine	0.4–3.8	1.1–5.0
Glutamic acid	–	0.35–0.41
Sodium	2.57	2.25
Potassium	1.03	1.55
Phosphorus	0.2–0.07	–
Calcium	0.26	0.4
Magnesium	0.09	0.08
Chloride	4.48	1.74–3.2
Bicarbonate	–	7.1

–, reliable results not available

long, 1.5–4 cm wide and 0.5–2 cm thick. Prostate secretions in the stallion are thin and watery, alkaline and high in proteins, citric acid and zinc. The significance of these is unclear, although it is known that proteins within seminal plasma attach to the sperm membrane; however, such attachment does not seem to affect fertility but may be responsible for conferring motility. Secretions of the prostate gland make a significant contribution to the pre-sperm fraction, helping to cleanse the urethra of urine and bacteria pre-ejaculation, as well as providing a lubricant for the passage of sperm. Prostate secretions also contribute significantly to the sperm-rich fraction (Weber *et al.*, 1990; Weber and Woods, 1993; Amann, 2011a,b; Paccamonti and De Vries, 2011; Varner and Schumacher, 2011).

6.3.4. The vesicular glands

The vesicular glands (formally known as the seminal vesicles) are again paired in structure and lie on either side of the bladder. Their size varies with season and sexual excitement but can be as large as 16–20 cm in length and 5 cm in diameter. They are lobed and can be compared with large walnuts in external appearance.

They secrete a major amount of seminal plasma, with a high concentration of potassium, citric acid and gel. Their secretions form part of both the sperm-rich and gel-like post-sperm fractions. Their function, and therefore their size and the volume of secretion, is particularly dependent upon circulating testosterone concentrations. As such, their contribution to seminal plasma declines significantly during the non-breeding season (Weber *et al.*, 1990; Amann, 2011a,b; Paccamonti and De Vries, 2011; Varner and Schumacher, 2011).

6.3.5. The ampulla

The ampulla glands are paired outfoldings of the vas deferens, where it meets the urethra, usually increasing the vas deferens lumen diameter from 0.5 cm to 1.5–2.0. The outfolding nature of the ampulla, as opposed to a discrete structure with connecting duct, is the reason why these glands are sometimes excluded as accessory glands. However, they make a considerable contribution to both the pre-sperm and sperm-rich fractions. Their secretions are high in ergothionine, an antioxidizing agent, which acts to 'mop up' toxic by-products of sperm metabolism (Weber *et al.*, 1990; Weber and Woods, 1993; Amann, 2011a; Paccamonti and De Vries, 2011).

6.4. The Vas Deferens

The vas deferens connects the epididymis of the testis to the urethra before passing the accessory glands and on into the penis. It has a diameter of 0.5–0.75 cm with a thick muscular wall, made up of three layers of muscle: inner oblique, middle circular and outer longitudinal (Fig. 6.7). These muscle layers actively propel the sperm plus surrounding fluid by peristalsis from the testis to the penis. The lumen of the duct is small and folded, especially near the epididymis, maximizing the surface

area and so aiding sperm storage and the reabsorption of testicular fluids.

The vas deferens, the testicular nerve supply, arterial and venous blood vessels, and the cremaster muscles pass out of the body cavity through the inguinal canal (Fig. 6.8). The cremaster muscle, which is divided into internal and external sections, is in part responsible for drawing the testis up towards the body in response to fear, cold, etc. (Section 6.6).

6.5. The Epididymis

The epididymis in the stallion lies over the top of the testis (Figs 6.9, 6.10 and 6.11) and is reported to be up

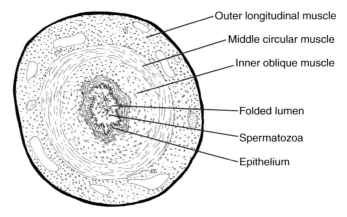

Fig. 6.7. Cross section through the vas deferens of the stallion.

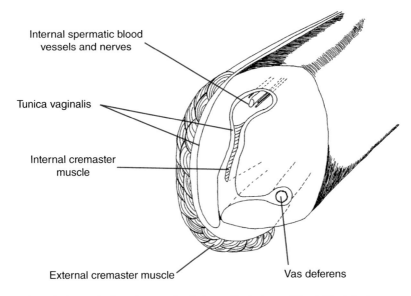

Fig. 6.8. Cross section through the inguinal canal connection between the testes and the stallion's body.

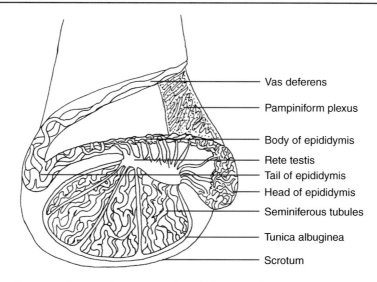

Vas deferens

Pampiniform plexus

Body of epididymis

Rete testis
Tail of epididymis
Head of epididymis

Seminiferous tubules

Tunica albuginea

Scrotum

Fig. 6.9. Diagrammatic illustration of a vertical cross section through the testes of the stallion.

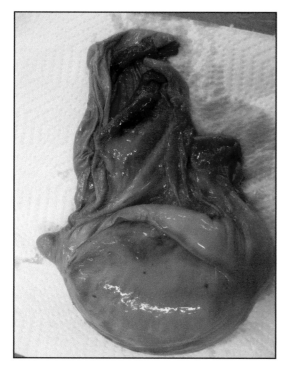

Fig. 6.10. The stallion's testis after slaughter and partial dissection.

to 45 m in length. It consists of convoluted ducts and is subdivided into three sections: the caput (head), the corpus (body) and the cauda (tail). The caput epididymis is connected by 12–14 highly convoluted ducts to the rete testis, a junctional area within the body of the testis, connecting the seminiferous tubules and the epididymis; as it continues into the corpus epididymis these 12–14 ducts merge and form a single duct which eventually emerges from the cauda epididymis as the vas deferens. The lining of these tubules is highly folded and is very similar to, and continuous with, the epididymal end of the vas deferens. These folds have additional microvilli, further increasing the surface area, and so facilitating the concentration, transportation, maturation and storage of sperm (Thompson, 1992; Amann, 2011a).

It is known that in order for sperm maturation to occur they must spend a period of time, maybe as long as 9–10 days, within the epididymis (24 h in the caput, 48 h in the corpus, 6 days in the caudal epididymis) (Senger, 2011). Such maturation is essential so that, once exposed to seminal plasma, released sperm are capable of movement via the beating of their tails and of further development (capacitation) within the female tract, enabling them to fertilize the waiting ova. The exact mechanisms involved in this maturation are unclear; however, they appear to be driven by the changing microenvironment, particularly within the corpus epididymis (Gatti *et al.*, 2004; Varner and Johnson, 2007). The three different parts of the epididymis have different functions, and the caput epididymis is primarily responsible for fluid absorption, resulting in a 10^5-fold increase in sperm concentration compared to the rete testis (Varner and Johnson, 2007). While in the

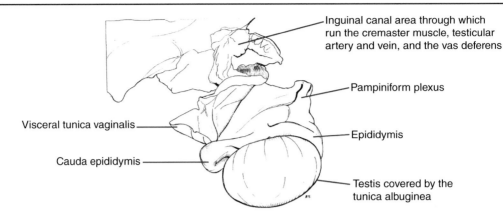

Inguinal canal area through which run the cremaster muscle, testicular artery and vein, and the vas deferens

Pampiniform plexus

Visceral tunica vaginalis

Epididymis

Cauda epididymis

Testis covered by the tunica albuginea

Fig. 6.11. A diagrammatic representation of the stallion testis shown in Fig. 6.10.

corpus epididymis the sperm mature, lose their cytoplasmic droplets and undergo biochemical changes, particularly to the acrosome region of the head (Yoshinaga and Toshimori, 2003). Sperm are then stored within the cauda epididymis in readiness for ejaculation. If they are not passed up to the vas deferens as a result of ejaculation they degenerate, and are reabsorbed over time, allowing a continual supply of fresh sperm to be available (Amann, 2011a). The cauda epididymis, along with the epididymal end of the vas deferens, acts as a storage site for sperm and also as a minor contributor to seminal fluid, in particular by secreting glycerylphosphorylcholine (GPC) (Samper, 1995a).

6.6. The Testes

The testes, like the ovaries, are gametogenic (the site of sperm production) and steroidogenic (site of endocrine/hormone production) in function. Figures 6.9, 6.11 and 6.12 illustrate the structure of the testis.

The testes hang outside the body of the stallion in order to maintain a temperature of approximately 3–5°C below that of body temperature (i.e. 35–36°C rather than 39°C). Sperm production is maximized at this lower temperature. Increases in testicular temperature due to disease or inflammation of the scrotum, testis or epididymis, even for just a few hours, result in a significant decrease in spermatogenesis (Amann, 2011b). This is transitory, as the duration of testicular dysfunction is related to the duration of temperature elevation, but may not be evident for 40–50 days owing to the 56-day duration of spermatogenesis. Testicular temperature is controlled primarily by means of the tunica dartos, and the arteriovenous countercurrent heat exchange mechanism provided by the pampiniform

plexus, plus the cremaster muscles and an abundance of scrotal sweat glands (Friedman *et al.*, 1991; Senger, 2011). In cold weather contraction of the tunica dartos muscle fibres lying in the scrotal wall draws the testes up closer to the abdomen, so reducing scrotal surface and hence heat loss; relaxation then allows them to drop lower and so cool down. The cremaster muscle was once thought to primarily control the proximity of the testis to the stallion's body and hence testis temperature. This is now not thought to be the case, although it may play a minor role, only causing a transitory raise in testes position. The pampiniform plexus (Figs 6.3 and 6.9–6.11) is formed by the dense capillary network where the testicular arterial and venous supplies come into close contact. In so doing, warm blood entering the testes via the artery loses heat to the cooler venous return and so forms an arteriovenous countercurrent heat exchange mechanism. Such an arrangement ensures that the testicular artery cools down prior to entry into the testes and the testicular vein warms up prior to its re-entry into the main body. The pampiniform plexus may also act as a pulse pressure eliminator. Arterial blood entering the pampiniform plexus does so at a pulse pressure of 40 mmHg but, as it passes through the pampiniform plexus, this reduces to 10 mmHg. The significance of this is as yet unclear (Senger, 2011).

The testes lie within a skin covering, termed the scrotum, under which lies the tunica dartos. This is followed by the tunica vaginalis, which is continuous with the peritoneal lining of the body cavity up through the inguinal canal (Fig. 6.12). In the fetus, the testes descend from a position high in the abdomen, near the kidney, through the inguinal canal and into the scrotum at (or soon after) birth (Fig. 6.13). The failure of one or both testes to descend fully results in a condition termed cryptorchidism, with the stallion often being referred to as a rig (Searle *et al.*, 1999, Arighi, 2011a; Pollark, 2017). In such stallions the retention of the testes within the body cavity results in elevated testicular temperature. This causes a reduction in sperm production, but has much less of an adverse effect on endocrine

function. Such stallions may, therefore, still be fertile (although sperm production from the retained testis is much reduced) and may exhibit near normal stallion-like behaviour owing to the continuing endocrine function. The condition may be further defined as unilateral, bilateral, inguinal or abdominal, depending on whether one or both testes have failed to descend, and how far descent has progressed (Section 18.3.4.1).

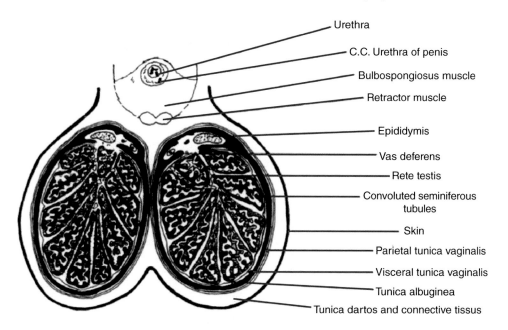

Urethra
C.C. Urethra of penis
Bulbospongiosus muscle
Retractor muscle
Epididymis
Vas deferens
Rete testis
Convoluted seminiferous tubules
Skin
Parietal tunica vaginalis
Visceral tunica vaginalis
Tunica albuginea
Tunica dartos and connective tissus

Fig. 6.12. Vertical cross section through the testes, epididymis and part of the penis of the stallion. cc, corpus cavernosum.

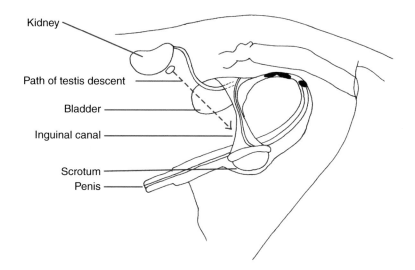

Kidney
Path of testis descent
Bladder
Inguinal canal
Scrotum
Penis

Fig. 6.13. The normal passage of descent of the testes in the stallion.

The testes of the stallion are ovoid and normally lie with their long axis horizontally, unless drawn up towards the body, when they may turn slightly. Their size varies considerably with stallion size or breed, and also season; their longitudinal axis is normally 6–12 cm with the height and width being 4–7 cm and 5–6 cm, respectively. On average the testes weigh 250–300 g each. Their size increases allometrically with (at the same rate as) general body growth until mature body size has been reached, at approximately 5 years of age.

Under the tunica vaginalis lies a fibrous capsule, the tunica albuginea, which surrounds each separate testis. Sheets of this fibrous tissue invade the body of the testis and divide it up into lobes. Each lobe is a mass of convoluted seminiferous tubules with intertubular areas (Figs 6.9, 6.12 and 6.14). Each area is largely responsible for one of two functions: gametogenic (seminiferous tubules and Sertoli cells) or steroidogenic (intertubular tissue and Leydig cells). The seminiferous tubules are U-shaped with the central convoluted area being responsible for spermatogenesis. They are lined by Sertoli cells that act as nurse cells, nourishing and aiding spermatozoa as they undergo spermatogenesis within the outer part of the tubules prior to their release as mature sperm into the lumen. Sertoli cells are also phagocytic, digesting degenerating germinal cells and residual bodies; they secrete luminal fluid and proteins, provide cell-to-cell communication and also form a blood–testis barrier, providing protection to the sperm from immunological rejection (Rode *et al.*, 2015). The two outer or straight ends of the seminiferous tubules are connected with the rete testis and on to the epididymis. The number of Sertoli cells is positively correlated with sperm production and varies with season, being significantly greater during the breeding season, hence the seasonal variation in sperm production (Johnson and Tatum, 1989). Sertoli cell number is also reported to be highly heritable (Hochereau-de Riviers *et al.*, 1987). Any condition or treatment that affects Sertoli cell numbers will, therefore, have an effect on sperm production. The lamina propria forms the walls of the seminiferous tubules and contains myoid cells (specialized muscle cells

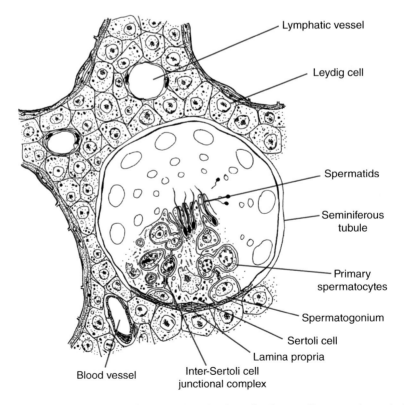

Fig. 6.14. A cross-sectional view through a seminiferous tubule within the stallion's testis, illustrating the gradual meiotic division of spermatogonia to spermatozoa.

that are thought to help propel sperm to the rete testis), fibroblasts and lamina (Varner and Johnson, 2007).

Outside the lamina propria, and so surrounding the seminiferous tubules, is the intertubular space in which is found the interstitial tissue. This is made up of the Leydig cells along with blood supply, nerves, lymphatic drainage and connective tissue. The Leydig cells are steroidogenic and so secrete hormones primarily responsible for sperm production and the development of general male bodily characteristics and behaviour (Section 7.3.2; Setchell, 1991; Amann, 2011a,b). As the stallion ages, the post-pubertal Leydig cells become more pigmented, and adult Leydig cells also produce more testosterone (Fig. 6.15; Amann, 2011a; Johnson et al., 2011). Additionally, the ratio of Sertoli to Leydig cells decreases with age, which may in part be responsible for the reported decline in sperm production in aged stallions (Pickett et al., 1989).

6.7. Sperm

Structurally sperm consist of five areas: the head, connected by the neck to the midpiece, then the principal piece and end piece (together often referred to as the tail) (Figs 6.16 and 6.17), with three distinct functions, all surrounded by a common plasma membrane (Davies Morel, 1999; Amann and Graham, 2011).

The head is mainly made up of nuclear material, containing the haploid number of chromosomes (half the normal number, 32, to allow fusion with the ova to give the normal diploid complement of 64). The head of the sperm is flat with a double membrane – the outer cell membrane and the inner nuclear membrane – except in the acrosome region at the top of the head, where there is an additional acrosome membrane. This membrane plays a vital role in fertilization (Section 3.2.1), as it is responsible for the breakdown of the cell membrane and the nuclear membrane at fertilization, allowing the fusion of the male and female nuclei. The midpiece of the sperm contains a high proportion of mitochondria – organelles within the cell that produce energy (ATP). The midpiece is, therefore, often termed the power plant of the sperm, providing the energy for metabolism and to drive the tail. The tail is made up of a series of muscle fibrils, equivalent to those found in the major muscle blocks of the body. Using the energy provided by the midpiece, the tail is whipped from side to side, driving the sperm movement in a wave-like motion (Davies Morel, 1999; Amann and Graham, 2011; Varner and Johnson, 2011). The average length of an equine sperm is 61–86 μm (Dott, 1975).

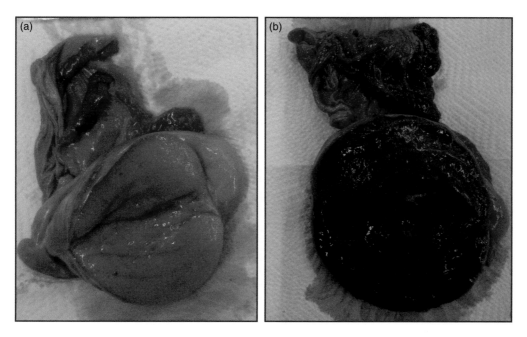

Fig. 6.15. Cross section of the testes from a young stallion (a) and older stallion (b), illustrating the increased pigmentation of the Leydig cells in the older stallion.

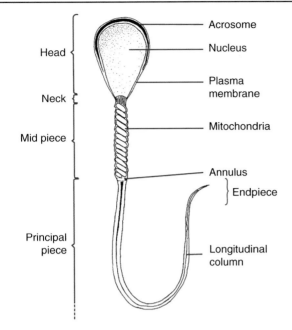

Head

Neck

Mid piece

Principal
piece

Acrosome

Nucleus

Plasma
membrane

Mitochondria

Annulus

Endpiece

Longitudinal
column

Fig. 6.16. A typical stallion sperm.

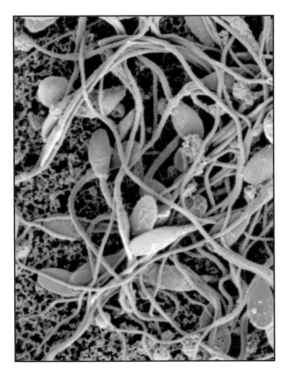

Fig. 6.17. Electron microscope image of fresh stallion spermatozoa, illustrating the flattened head, mid piece and tail.

6.7.1. Spermatogenesis

As discussed, sperm are produced within the seminiferous tubules and are supported, or nursed, by Sertoli
cells. They start as underdeveloped germinal cells or
spermatogonia, attached to the wall of the seminiferous
tubules (Fig. 6.14), and then by the process of spermatogenesis progressively develop into mature sperm
(Figs 6.14 and 6.18; Amann, 1981b; Amann and
Graham, 1993; Varner and Johnson, 2007). Spermatogenesis can be divided into spermatocytogenesis (19.4
days), meiosis (19.4 days) and spermiogenesis (18.6
days). The total time for spermatogenesis in the stallion
is 57.4 days (Fig. 6.18).

6.7.1.1. Spermatocytogenesis

Spermatocytogenesis is the first stage of spermatogenesis and in the stallion takes 19.4 days (Fig. 6.18).
Spermatocytogenesis starts with the development of
spermatogonia (stem cells) by spermatozoal division
from the underdeveloped germinal cells or gonocytes
in the base of the seminiferous tubule bordering the
lamina propria (tubule wall). The exact number of
spermatozoal divisions for the horse is unclear, but in
other mammals the number ranges from 1 to 14. This
is often referred to as the multiplication phase. At the
end of the spermatozoal divisions large numbers of A_1
spermatogonia are produced, which then enter the
spermatocytogenic phase and multiply further by mitosis. In the horse five different types of spermatogonia
are evident through the spermatocytogenic phase: A_1,
A_2, A_3, B_1 and B_2 (Johnson, 1991a; Johnson et al.,
2011).

The multiplication that results in the A_1 spermatogonia has two main functions: first, to produce more
stem cell spermatogonia (uncommitted A_1 spermatogonia) by mitosis which continue to replenish the supply of spermatogonia for future spermatozoa production; and, second, to produce committed A_1
spermatogonia which go on to produce and multiply
into A_2, A_3, B_1 and B_2 spermatogonia, and then primary
spermatocytes and eventually spermatozoa (Johnson
et al., 1997, 2011).

Those committed A_1 spermatogonia destined to
produce primary spermatocytes, once committed to
this line of development, divide by mitosis into four
stages to give initially a pair ($A_{1.2}$), then four ($A_{1.4}$), then
eight ($A_{1.8}$) and finally potentially 16 A_2 spermatogonia.
Throughout this division the groups of spermatogonia
originating from a single A_1 stay together, connected by
intercellular bridges (Johnson, 1991a). Each of these A_2

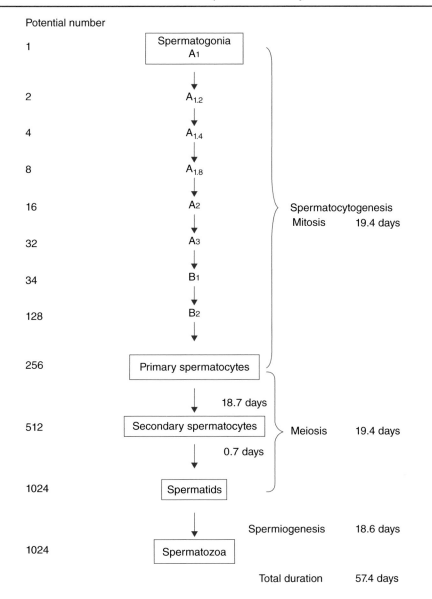

Fig. 6.18. The cell divisions within spermatogenesis in the stallion.

spermatogonia then, again by mitosis, divide to give two A_3; each of these then again give two B_1 and finally B_2 differentiated spermatogonia. Finally, each B_2 spermatogonia divide to form two primary spermatocytes, which enter the first division of meiosis. Therefore, in theory, one committed A_1 spermatogonia can give rise to 128 B_2 spermatogonia ready to become primary spermatocytes and to enter the next phase of spermatogenesis; however, this is not the case in practice, as many spermatogonia degenerate as they progress

through spermatocytogenesis. This rate of degeneration is particularly evident in seasonal breeders, such as the stallion, where it significantly increases in the non-breeding season, resulting in the characteristically lower sperm count (Hochereau-de Riviers *et al.*, 1990; Johnson, 1991a,b; Johnson *et al.*, 2011). Spermatocytogenesis does not cause any reduction in chromosome number, and hence the diploid (64 chromosome) A_1 spermatogonia give rise to diploid primary spermatocytes (Varner, *et al.*, 2015).

6.7.1.2. Meiosis

Meiosis is the means by which a single diploid cell divides to produce two haploid cells. This process only occurs in the gonads of the male and the female, allowing the production of spermatids and ova that are haploid in nature. This process also allows for the exchange of genetic material between chromosomes in the dividing cell. In the stallion meiosis follows spermatocytogenesis and takes 19.4 days; it starts with the primary spermatocytes (diploid), each of which results in the development of four round spermatids (haploid). Meiosis may be divided into two stages: the first and second meiotic divisions. The first meiotic division involves the multiplication and exchange of genetic material and results in two diploid secondary spermatocytes; it is by far the longest phase, taking 18.7 days. The second division results in the halving of the genetic material and the production of two haploid spermatids per single secondary spermatocyte and takes only 0.7 days (Johnson et al., 1997; 2011; Varner et al., 2015).

6.7.1.3. Spermiogenesis

Spermiogenesis is the final stage of spermatogenesis, lasting 18.6 days, and is the process by which spermatids are differentiated into spermatozoa (Johnson et al., 1997). Spermiogenesis is divided into four phases: the golgi, the cap, the acrosome and the maturation phases; the division of the phases is largely based on the development of the acrosome region. In addition, during this period the spermatids undergo dramatic changes to their nucleus, loss of cytoplasm and development of their tails (Holstein et al., 2003).

6.7.1.4. Spermiation

Although not strictly a stage within spermatogenesis, spermiation is important as the stage at which the fully formed spermatids, now called spermatozoa, are released into the lumen of the seminiferous tubules. From here they pass to the rete testes and on to the epididymis for final maturation.

As the sperm develop through spermatogenesis they migrate, attached to their Sertoli cells, away from the wall of the seminiferous tubules towards the open lumen. Once mature, they are then freed by their Sertoli cells, released into the lumen and, along with surrounding secretory fluid, are pushed along the seminiferous tubules by rhythmic contractions of the myoid cells within the lamina propria of the tubules. By this stage they have lost a considerable amount of cytoplasm and have developed tails, although the tails are not functional until epididymal maturation and contact with seminal plasma has occurred. The whole cycle of development takes 57.4 days and occurs in waves, ensuring a continual supply of mature sperm for ejaculation. The mean daily sperm production of a mature stallion is in the order of 7–8×10^9 sperm (60,000–70,000 sperm s^{-1}) and it may take up to 8–11 days for sperm to pass from the testes to the exterior (Johnson et al., 1997; Davies Morel, 1999; Varner and Johnson, 2007; Varner et al., 2015). Absolute sperm production is related to testis volume and Sertoli cell number.

6.7.2. Spermatogenic cycle

The spermatogenic cycle is the interval between connective release of spermatids. Spermatid release is determined by the timing of cohorts of committed A_1 spermatogonia entering into spermatogenesis, as cohorts of sperm develop together at the same rate. In the stallion this is 12 days and so within the 57 days that it takes for spermatogenesis to be completed there will be 4.75 (57/12) cohorts of sperm developing (Johnson et al., 2011).

6.8. Semen

Semen is the term applied to seminal plasma plus sperm, and in the stallion is a milky white gelatinous fluid. The sperm concentration of semen varies with the fraction examined. As previously mentioned, there are three identifiable fractions: pre-sperm, sperm-rich and post-sperm. The pre-sperm fraction is the initial fraction and contains no viable sperm. Its function is to lubricate and clean the urethra of degenerate sperm, stale urine and bacteria prior to ejaculation. The high concentration of bacteria in this fraction means that its collection should ideally be avoided when collecting semen for artificial insemination.

The sperm-rich fraction is the major deposit by the stallion and commences as soon as the glans penis swells to force entry into the cervix. This fraction is normally 40–80 ml in volume and contains 80–90% of the sperm and the biochemical components of semen.

The third fraction is the post-sperm or gel fraction. Its volume varies enormously from 0 to 80 ml, and is dependent on testosterone, and therefore is often related to libido: the higher the libido, the greater is the gel fraction. Season also affects the gel fraction (volume being lower in the non-breeding season), as does breed and previous use. If a stallion is used more than once per day, the second ejaculate frequently has half the gel fraction of the first.

At ejaculation the stallion secretes semen in a series of up to nine jets, the average volume of semen and the sperm concentration decreasing with successive jets (Fig. 6.19; Kosiniak, 1975; Love, 1992; Turner, 2011a).

6.9. Sperm Deposition, Erection, Ejaculation and Emission

Deposition of semen within the mare involves three stages: erection, emission and ejaculation. The control of these stages is discussed in detail in Section 7.3.2.8. Erection is the first reaction to a sexual stimulus and causes relaxation of the penile muscles and retractor muscle, allowing the penis to extrude from its sheath. This is followed by blood engorgement of the erectile tissue of the penis resulting in an initial turgid pressure. In order for intromission (entry into the mare) to be successful, penile blood pressure has to further increase to intromission pressure. This is essential before the stallion enters the mare; if not, permanent damage may be caused to the stallion or at least reduce his enthusiasm for future covering.

Emission (the passage of sperm and seminal plasma to the pelvic region) and ejaculation (the expulsion of semen through the penis) are the culmination of erection. Both are the result of contraction of the muscle walls of the epididymis, vas deferens, accessory glands, ischiocavernosus muscle and penile muscles, causing sperm to be forced from the epididymis up the vas deferens to be mixed with seminal plasma (emission) and passed out through the penis (ejaculation). Ejaculation

is marked by a series of pelvic thrusts at the end of which semen is released in the form of 6–9 jets over a period of 6–8 s. The semen jets can be divided into pre-sperm, sperm-rich and post-sperm (gel) fractions. The largest fraction and that containing the majority (70%) of biochemical components and sperm is the sperm-rich fraction; the pre-sperm and post-sperm fractions are smaller in volume and do not contain viable sperm (Weber and Woods, 1993; Davies Morel, 1999; Turner, 2011a).

At full erection, the penis doubles in size to 80–90 cm in length and up to 10 cm in width. At ejaculation, the glans penis triples in size, forcing open the cervix to allow sperm deposition directly into the uterus; it may also have a role in preventing initial leakage of semen from the mare. The glans penis has to return to near normal size (detumescence) before the stallion is able to leave the mare. Failure to allow time for detumescence can cause damage to the mare and/or stallion. Problems may be encountered in overzealous stallions that demonstrate enlargement of the glans penis prior to entry into the mare; in such cases, intromission is not safe until the glans penis has returned to its normal size. Such problems are especially evident in stallions of high libido and in young stallions, particularly if they have only a limited workload (Ginther, 1995; Turner, 1998; Davies Morel, 1999).

6.10. Conclusion

The male reproductive tract has specifically evolved for the efficient production, storage and subsequent deposition of sperm within the female tract. It also ensures that the sperm are deposited in a medium (seminal plasma) that is able to provide all the elements for their survival and final maturation, so maximizing the chances of fertilization.

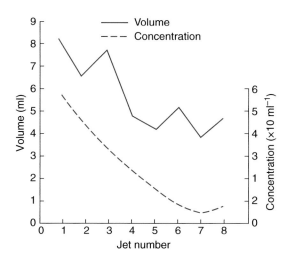

Fig. 6.19. Volume and sperm concentration of successive jets. (From Kosiniak, 1975.)

Study Questions

Detail how the testes of the stallion ensure a regular supply of sperm for release at ejaculation.

Describe the anatomical events that occur in the stallion during the deposition of sperm into the mare.

Discuss the means by which the stallion maintains a testicular temperature below body temperature and the consequences of this for reproduction.

Suggested Reading

Sack, W.O. (1991) Isolated male organs. *Rooney's Guide to the Dissection of the Horse*, 6th edn. Veterinary Textbooks, Ithaca, New York, pp. 75–78.

Samper, J.C. (1997) Reproductive anatomy and physiology of breeding stallion. In: Youngquist, R.S. (ed.) *Current Therapy in Large Animal Theriogenology*. W.B. Saunders, Philadelphia, Pennsylvania, pp. 3–12.

Bone, J.F. (1998) *Animal Anatomy and Physiology*, 3rd edn. Prentice-Hall, New Jersey.

Davies Morel, M.C.G. (1999) *Equine Artificial Insemination*. CAB International, Wallingford, UK, pp. 406.

Chenier, T.S. (2000) Anatomy and physical examination of the stallion. In: Samper, J.C. (ed.) *Equine Breeding Management and Artificial Insemination*. W.B. Saunders, Philadelphia, Pennsylvania, pp. 1–26.

Hafez, E.S.E. and Hafez, B. (2000) *Reproduction in Farm Animals*, 7th edn. Williams and Wilkins, Baltimore, Maryland, pp. 509.

Amann, R.P. (2011) Functional anatomy of the adult male. In: McKinnon, A.O., Squires, E.L., Vaala, E. and Varner, D.D. (eds) *Equine Reproduction*, 2nd edn. Wiley-Blackwell, Philadelphia, London, pp. 867–880.

Amann, R.P. and Graham, J.K. (2011) Spermatozoal function. In: McKinnon, A.O., Squires, E.L., Vaala, E. and Varner, D.D. (eds) *Equine Reproduction*, 2nd edn. Wiley-Blackwell, Philadelphia, London, pp. 1053–1084.

Control of Reproduction in the Stallion

7

7.1. Introduction

The stallion is a seasonal breeder, like the mare, but tends to show a less distinct season and, unlike her, if given enough encouragement is capable of breeding all year round. However, season does have an effect upon the efficiency of reproduction, with semen volume, sperm concentration, total sperm per ejaculate, the number of mounts per ejaculate and reaction time to the mare all being poorer during the non-breeding season (Pickett and Voss, 1972; Johnson, 1991b; Roser, 2008, 2011). Figures 7.1–7.5 demonstrate the effect of season on reproductive parameters. Additionally, the stallion's reproductive activity is continuous and is not constrained by cyclical events as seen with the mare's oestrous cycle. Hence the stallion is very often not the limiting factor to reproduction, and so less is known about the control of reproduction in the stallion than in the mare, with quite a lot of information being extrapolated from – and so presumed to be similar to – other species.

7.2. Puberty

Sperm production, like ova production, is governed by the hypothalamic–pituitary–gonadal axis and, as in the mare, commences at puberty. Sperm production then continues for the rest of a stallion's lifetime, although there has been a suggestion by some researchers that semen quality declines after 20 years of age (Fukuda *et al.*, 2001; Madill, 2002). The exact timing of puberty is unclear and varies with breed and stallion development, and is open to debate (Heninger, 2011). Various researchers have used histological changes within the testis, especially in association with the Leydig cells, to indicate the timing of puberty. Using such parameters, ages of 1–2.2 years have been suggested (Naden *et al.*, 1990; Clay and Clay, 1992; Heninger, 2011). However, other works using testicular weights, daily sperm production, testosterone concentrations and Leydig and Sertoli cell numbers and volumes (Berndston and Jones, 1989; Heninger, 2011) suggested that true puberty may occur nearer 2–3 years of age. However, it is generally accepted that stallions of 3 years of age are spermatogenically active and so capable of fertilizing a mare, although they have a limited sperm-producing capacity. By 5 years of age most are capable of producing adequate numbers of spermatozoa to cover a full complement (book) of mares (Johnson *et al.*, 1991). It was previously considered that stallions attain full adult reproductive ability at 5–6 years of age (when they reach mature body weight); however, other work suggests that, at least in slower-maturing draft breeds, full reproductive ability may not be reached until 10 years of age (Parlevliet *et al.*, 1994).

As with the mare, the reproductive activity of the stallion can be divided into physiological and behavioural changes, both of which are closely related, but for ease of understanding will be discussed separately.

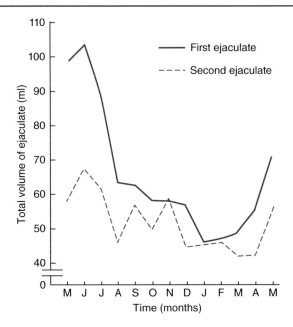

Fig. 7.1. Total semen volume produced throughout the year. (From Pickett and Voss, 1972.)

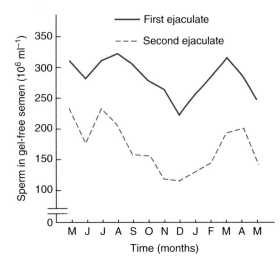

Fig. 7.2. Number of sperm in the gel-free fraction of semen throughout the year. (From Pickett and Voss, 1972.)

7.3. Physiological Changes

Hormone patterns are the major physiological events associated with stallion reproductive activity and indeed govern the remaining physiological and behavioural characteristics.

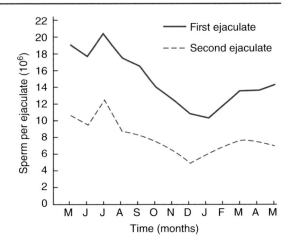

Fig. 7.3. Number of sperm per ejaculate throughout the year. (From Pickett and Voss, 1972.)

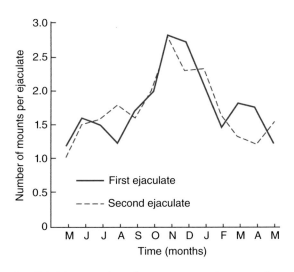

Fig. 7.4. Mean number of mounts required per ejaculate throughout the year. (From Pickett and Voss, 1972.)

7.3.1. Seasonality

As in the mare, environmental stimuli, in the form of day length, temperature and nutrition have an overriding effect on the hypothalamic–pituitary–testis axis (Figs 7.1–7.5). As discussed for the mare (Section 2.4.1), and so not repeated here, season is governed by the secretion of melatonin from the pineal gland in response to day length (see Section 2.4.1; Roser, 2011). Both melatonin and photoperiod can be manipulated, as in the mare, to alter the timing of the breeding season, but overstimulation with artificially long days for a

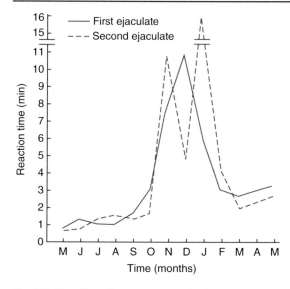

Fig. 7.5. The effect of season on sexual behaviour as measured by reaction time. (From Pickett and Voss, 1972.)

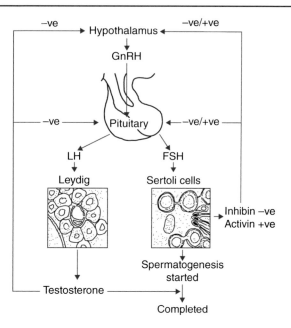

Fig. 7.6. The hypothalamic–pituitary–testis axis that governs reproduction in the stallion. GnRH, gonadotrophin-releasing hormone.

prolonged period of time results in refractoriness (failure to respond) to the photo stimulation (Argo *et al.*, 1991; Clay and Clay, 1992). This can be an issue when shuttling stallions from the Northern to the Southern hemisphere for all-year-round breeding (Roser, 2011).

Again, as discussed for the mare, prolactin concentrations are also affected by day length, increasing as day length increases; and that prolactin may be the means by which photoperiod controls non-reproductive activity such as coat growth, weight gain and food conversion efficiency. However, unlike the mare, there is as yet no definitive work that indicates a role for prolactin in reproductive seasonal activity in the stallion (Gerlach and Aurich, 2000; Aurich *et al.*, 2002).

7.3.2. The endocrinological control of stallion reproduction

Similarly evident in the mare, the control of stallion reproduction is governed by the hypothalamic–pituitary–gonad (Fig. 7.6); however, in the stallion the gonads are the testis (Nagata, 2000).

7.3.2.1. Gonadotrophin-releasing hormone

As discussed in the mare, gonadotrophin-releasing hormone (GnRH) is produced in a pulsatile fashion by the hypothalamus and acts on the anterior pituitary (adenohypophysis), driving the production of follicle-stimulating hormone (FSH) and luteinizing hormone

(LH) (Section 2.4.2.1; Nagata, 2000; Amann, 2011b) which in turn drive testosterone and sperm production. The importance of GnRH on reproductive activity, both libido and sperm quantity and quality, is demonstrated in GnRH immunization work (Malmgren *et al.*, 2001) and with the use of GnRH vaccines, agonists and antagonists to manipulate reproductive activity (Malmgren *et al.*, 2001; Stout and Colenbrander, 2004; Stout, 2005).

7.3.2.2. Luteinizing hormone and follicle-stimulating hormone

The anterior pituitary is stimulated via GnRH to produce FSH and LH, identical hormones to those produced in the mare (see Sections 2.4.2.2 and 2.4.2.5; Irvine, 1984). The release, and therefore the plasma concentrations, of LH and FSH are pulsatile in nature, again as seen in the mare. As suggested in the mare, the control of FSH appears to be less dependent on GnRH than LH secretion is (Cupps, 1991; Seamens *et al.*, 1991; Amann, 1993b; Kainer, 1993; Roser, 2011).

The testes, which are the target organs for LH and FSH, consist of two major cell types, Leydig and Sertoli cells. Leydig cells are found within the intertubular spaces or interstitial tissue of the testes and are responsible for the production of testosterone and oestrogens. These cells and, therefore, testosterone secretion are controlled by LH. Sertoli cells are found lining the seminiferous tubules and act as nurse cells for developing spermatids. These cells are controlled by FSH which, with testosterone, affects sperm production. The exact control of spermatogenesis is unclear in the stallion. It is possible that spermatogenesis in the stallion proceeds automatically and that hormones such as FSH act to modulate spermatogenesis. For example, under the influence of greater levels of FSH (and testosterone), less degeneration of spermatozoa occurs through the spermatogenesis process and so sperm production is increased. Based on evidence in other animals it has also been suggested that FSH and testosterone may act on different stages of spermatogenesis, FSH being responsible for driving the initial stages of spermatogenesis, (spermatocytogenesis and the first part of meiosis), developing spermatogonia to secondary spermatocytes; testosterone then completes spermatogenesis. Sertoli cells, however, also secrete inhibin, activin, androgen binding protein (ABP) and other growth factors such as transferrin and insulin-like growth factors (IGF), all of which are also likely to be involved in the control of spermatogenesis (Bidstrup *et al.*, 2002; Amann, 2011b; Roser, 2011).

7.3.2.3. Testosterone

Testosterone, a steroid hormone produced primarily by the Leydig cells, is driven by the pulsatile release of LH resulting in a pulsatile release of testosterone. The pulsatile nature of testosterone release means that analysis of a single blood sample for the hormone can give erroneous results; a hormone profile taken over a period of time and averaged is a much more accurate indication of true testosterone levels (Amann, 1993b).

Testosterone passes via attachment to ABP to the neighbouring Sertoli cells where it takes its effect. As discussed in Section 7.3.2.2., the exact control of spermatogenesis in the stallion is unclear, but testosterone may be specifically responsible for completing spermatogenesis (the second part of meiosis and spermogenesis) developing secondary spermatocytes to spermatozoa ready for passage to the epididymis for maturation (Davies Morel, 1999; Amann, 2011b; Roser, 2011).

Additionally, testosterone has a systemic role as it controls the development of male genitalia, testes descent in the fetus or neonate, pubertal changes and accelerated growth and muscular development, plus the maintenance and function of the accessory glands. It is also responsible for male libido and sexual behaviour by stimulation of the central nervous system (CNS), plus development of stallion personality and behaviour. It also affects the rate of germinal cell degeneration; elevated testosterone during the breeding season decreases germinal degeneration and hence increases sperm production. Finally, testosterone acts to feed back negatively on pituitary and possibly hypothalamic function to reduce the release of exclusively LH, and hence acts as a brake on its own production (Amann, 2011b). This is demonstrated in gelded stallions where, immediately post-removal of the testis (the major source of testosterone), LH increases significantly. It then takes 3–5 days for the system to adjust to the absence of testosterone and for LH to decrease (Collingsworth *et al.*, 2001). A derivative of testosterone, dihydrotestosterone, may also feed back negatively on the pituitary as well as having a limited additional effect on the other testosterone-driven stallion characteristics. Other work suggests that this feedback also involves oestrogens, elevated oestrogens having a positive effect on GnRH and LH release (Muyan *et al.*, 1993). These feedback mechanisms, which appear to work on both the hypothalamus and the anterior pituitary, ensure that the system does not overrun itself; for every driver there needs to be a brake. Testosterone may also be produced by a limited population of Leydig cells occasionally found in the wall of the vas deferens; this is evident in some geldings that have been successfully gelded but continue to demonstrate stallion-like characteristics. Testosterone is also produced by the adrenal glands in both the stallion and the gelding, and it is this testosterone that is responsible for the continued, but reduced, male characteristics of the gelding.

The production of testosterone is not only dependent upon season, but also a diurnal rhythm is suggested (Fig. 7.7). Testosterone concentrations have been reported by some to be elevated at 06.00 and 18.00 (Pickett *et al.*, 1989) and by others as just a morning peak at 08.00 (Kirkpatrick *et al.*, 1976). It has been postulated that, in the wild, this ensures that mating activity is greatest at dawn and dusk, times of least risk to stallions and mares from predators (Pickett *et al.*, 1989).

7.3.2.4. Inhibin and activin

Two other hormones are also involved in the control of male reproduction: inhibin and activin. Again, both are the same hormones as those secreted in mares (see Section 2.4.2.3). They are produced by the Sertoli cells in response to total sperm production and have additional

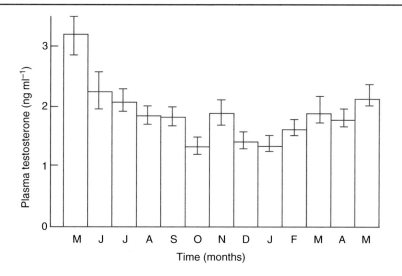

Fig. 7.7. Concentration (mean + standard error) of testosterone in the peripheral plasma of mature stallions over a 13-month period. (From Berndston *et al.*, 1974.)

feedback effects on hypothalamic and pituitary function, specifically on FSH production. As their name would suggest, inhibin acts as an inhibitor (negative feedback). Based on evidence in other animals, it is likely that activin acts as an activator (positive feedback) on pituitary activity, to ensure a steady secretion of FSH and, therefore, of sperm production. The precise mode of action of inhibin and activin in the horse is, as yet, largely unclear (Roser *et al.*, 1994; Roser, 1997; Nagata *et al.*, 1998; Amann, 2011b).

7.3.2.5. Prolactin

The role that prolactin may play in translating day length into non-reproductive seasonal physiological changes has already been discussed (Section 7.3.1 and Section 2.4.1.1). In addition, work in other farm livestock has suggested that prolactin may also have a role in enhancing the effect of LH on the activity of the Leydig cells by controlling the synthesis of LH receptors and on the functioning of the accessory glands; reduction in prolactin being associated with a reduction in seminal volume (Bachelot and Binart, 2007). Prolactin levels also increase with age and the breeding season, but it is unclear if this is a direct association or an indirect age and seasonal effect (Thomson *et al.*, 1987, 1996). The importance of prolactin specifically in the horse is, as yet, unclear.

7.3.2.6. Oestrogens

The stallion's testes are interesting in that they contain a high concentration of oestrogens and oestrones (150–200 pg ml^{-1}). This is surprising as these oestrogens are the same as those seen in the mare, and are specifically associated with female behaviour, and the levels in the stallion are much higher than in the testes of other mammals. The site of oestrogen production has been suggested to be the Leydig cells or the Sertoli cells (Seamens *et al.*, 1991; Amann, 1993b). The significance of testicular oestrogen is unclear; however, it has been suggested by some that oestrogens may act as a positive feedback on the pituitary and/or hypothalamus to increase the concentration of LH and decrease levels of FSH (Baldwin *et al.*, 1991; Muyan *et al.*, 1993; Tilbrook and Clarke, 2001). The elevated levels of oestrogen in the plasma of entire stallions serve as a useful way of determining if an apparent gelding is in fact a cryptorchid stallion (Sections 6.6 and 18.3.4.1).

7.3.2.7. Oxytocin

Oxytocin is reported to be elevated in the testes. It appears to be transported by the Sertoli cells into the lumen of the seminiferous tubules where it is postulated to drive the contraction of the seminiferous, rete testis and epididymis tubules, so facilitating sperm transport to the epididymis. It is unclear as to where oxytocin is produced but has been suggested by some to be the Leydig cells (Watson *et al.*, 1999; Thackare *et al.*, 2006; Amann, 2011b; Roser, 2011).

It is likely that the control of stallion reproduction is primarily by the hormones discussed above, but will also involve other hormones such as growth hormone

(GH) and thyroid hormone (TH) as well as growth factors such as testicular insulin-like growth factor-1 (IGF-1), transferrin, insulin-like peptides (INSL-3) and propiomelancortin, all acting at a more local level (Roser, 2011).

7.3.2.8. Control of semen deposition

There are three stages to semen deposition: erection, emission and ejaculation (Section 6.9), all of which can only occur in a system dominated by testosterone: that is, the stallion. Erection is initiated by a sexual stimulatory (erotogenic) signal, which may be visual (sight of a mare or facilities associated with mating or semen collection); olfactory (the presence of smells or pheromones associated with mating); or auditory (the sounds of a mare or other sounds associated with mating). This stimulatory signal is transmitted to the behavioural centres of the brain within the hypothalamus where neurons synapse with the parasympathetic and sympathetic efferent neurons that control vasoconstriction and vasodilation in the penis. Sexual excitation causes parasympathetic dominance which, via the splanchnic nerves, causes relaxation of the penis retractor muscle allowing the penis to extrude from its sheath. Additionally, the parasympathetic stimulation overrides the normal sympathetic stimulation and the parasympathetic nerve endings fire, releasing nitrous oxide (NO) from their terminals within the penis. NO activates the enzyme guanylate cyclase that is responsible for the conversion of guanylate triphosphate (GTP) to cyclic guanosine monophosphate (cGMP), which causes relaxation of the smooth muscle in the penis. This causes vasodilation and so increases blood flow, in particular to the erectile tissue of the corpus cavernosum penis, resulting in engorgement, which in turn causes turgid pressure to be achieved within the penis (Amann, 2011b; Senger, 2011).

However, in order for intromission (entry into the mare) to be successful, the blood pressure within the stallion's penis must be further increased to intromission pressure. This is achieved by further engorgement of the erectile tissue via two means. First, as blood flow increases to the penis, penile blood pressure continues to increase; this compresses the veins exiting from the penis against the ischium of the pelvis, restricting venous return of blood from the penis and so further increasing blood pressure. Second, CNS stimulation causes contraction of the muscles associated with the penis, in particular the ischiocavernosus muscle which draws the penis up against the ischium, further restricting venous

blood flow out of the penis and so further increasing blood pressure. This, along with an increase in heart rate and a general increase in circulatory blood pressure, causes intromission pressure to be reached within the penis in readiness for mating (Tischner et al., 1974; Amann, 2011b).

The second and third stages of semen deposition are emission, the passage of seminal plasma from the accessory glands and sperm from the epididymis to the urethral area of the penis; and ejaculation, the passage of this seminal plasma and sperm (semen) along the penis and into the mare after intromission. The control of these two stages is very similar and they occur as a continuum. Sensory stimulation, such as temperature or pressure, of the glans penis activates sensory afferent nerves which send impulses to the lumbosacral region of the spine. This results in a direct efferent neural return that activates the muscles associated with the reproductive tract. This activation causes wave-like, or peristaltic, contraction of the myometrial cells within the wall of the epididymis, vas deferens, accessory glands and penis, as well as contraction of the urethralis and bulbospongiosus muscle and further contraction of the ischiocavernosus muscle. This results in semen deposition into the mare in a series of jets (Tischner et al., 1974; Kosiniak, 1975; Weber and Woods, 1993).

Ejaculation follows shortly after entry into the mare and is signalled by the rhythmical flagging of the tail. Such mating behaviour is directly affected by circulating testosterone concentrations. At the beginning and the end of the breeding season reaction time to a mare lengthens and the number of mounts per ejaculate increases, these being direct indications that when testosterone levels are declining sexual enthusiasm or libido also wanes (Figs 7.4 and 7.5; Pickett and Voss, 1972; Weber and Woods, 1993).

7.4. Behavioural Changes

Testosterone is the prime driver of male behaviour especially that associated with reproduction. There is much variation between individuals, but in summary the following generalized behaviour is controlled by testosterone. On sight of a mare the frequency and amplitude of GnRH and hence LH and FSH release increase, driving testosterone production and hence driving stallion behaviour (libido) (Irvine and Alexander, 1991; Shand et al., 1995). In addition, 20% of GnRH released acts directly on higher behavioural brain centres (Pozor et al., 1991). In the feral situation, once a stallion has detected one of his harem mares as being in oestrus he will loiter in her vicinity, awaiting positive encouragement from the mare. It is invariably the mare that initiates the act of mating by approaching the stallion, reinforcing the message that she is receptive to mating. Once mating is imminent in both the feral and managed environment, the testosterone-driven behaviour of a stallion is similar and includes fixation on the mare, neck arching, stamping or pawing the ground and general elevated stallion stance. He will often show the characteristic flehmen behaviour of drawing back his top lip, drawing air into the nasal cavity and so detecting pheromones indicative of oestrus, reinforcing the erotogenic stimuli (Fig. 7.8; McDonnell, 2000a), accompanied by roaring. Intensively managed stallions tend to be more vocal than those breeding in a feral environment (McDonnell, 2011a). If the mare seems receptive he will approach her from the front, muzzle to muzzle, and in the absence of hostility will work his way over her neck, back and rump towards her perineum and vulva. If the mare still stands with no objection he will turn and approach her from behind and to one side. He will then mount her from that side, possibly after a few initial dummy mounts to test her reaction and confirm that she is willing to stand. In the feral environment a stallion may mate a mare in excess of 15 times in an oestrus, up to once per hour, depending on whether other harem mares are also in oestrus (McDonnell, 2011a).

It is known that social environment can affect behaviour via changes in testosterone; hence stallions housed in isolation have the lowest testosterone and therefore libido, as do stallions housed with other stallions, a situation that presumably emulates the natural

bachelor herd status. Stallions housed in close proximity to mares have the highest testosterone and, therefore, libido (McDonnell, 2000a; Christensen et al., 2002a, 2002b). However, more recent research suggests that mares closely related (major histocompatibility complex (MHC) similar) to the stallion are not beneficial as they induce lower testosterone concentrations and lower semen quality (Burger et al., 2015).

7.5. Conclusion

The control of reproduction in the stallion has evolved to ensure continual reproductive activity rather than cyclic activity, as in the mare. The only constraint on the stallion's reproductive activity is season, a limitation that only reduces the efficiency of, and does not eliminate, reproductive activity in the non-breeding season. This seasonal effect ensures that offspring are more likely to be born at a time of year most appropriate to their survival. In order to optimize reproductive success stallions should be housed with, or in near contact with, unrelated mares; not in traditional stallion yards; and not in isolation.

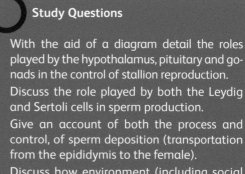

Study Questions

With the aid of a diagram detail the roles played by the hypothalamus, pituitary and gonads in the control of stallion reproduction.

Discuss the role played by both the Leydig and Sertoli cells in sperm production.

Give an account of both the process and control, of sperm deposition (transportation from the epididymis to the female).

Discuss how environment (including social environment) affects reproductive activity in the stallion and how this may inform management.

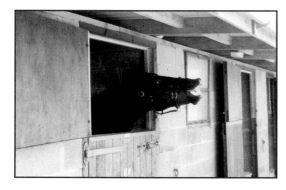

Fig. 7.8. Flehman behaviour typically shown by stallions in the presence of an oestrous mare. Such behaviour allows the stallion to detect pheromones in the air and so determine if the mare is in oestrus.

Suggested Reading

Gerlach, T. and Aurich, J.E. (2000) Regulation of seasonal reproductive activity in the stallion, ram and hamster. *Animal Reproduction Science* 58, 197–213.

Amann, R.P. (2011) Physiology and endocrinology. In: McKinnon, A.O., Squires, E.L., Vaala, E. and Varner, D.D. (eds) *Equine Reproduction*, 2nd edn. Wiley-Blackwell, Philadelphia, London, pp. 881–908.

Roser, J.F. (2011) Endocrin-Paracrine–Autocrine regulation of reproductive function in the stallion. In: McKinnon,

A.O., Squires, E.L., Vaala, E. and Varner, D.D. (eds) *Equine Reproduction*, 2nd edn. Wiley-Blackwell, Philadelphia, London, pp. 996–1014.

Senger, P.L. (2011) *Pathways to Pregnancy and Parturition*, 2nd edn. Current Conceptions Inc.

McDonnell, S.M. (2011) Normal sexual behavior. In: McKinnon, A.O., Squires, E.L., Vaala, E. and Varner, D.D. (eds) *Equine Reproduction*, 2nd edn. Wiley-Blackwell, Philadelphia, London, pp. 1385–1390.

Management of the Broodmare

Section C applies the mare anatomy and physiology considered in Section A to the management of the mare from preparation for covering through parturition to management at weaning. It also considers infertility and the reasons for reproductive failure. Various management options are discussed to enable you to make informed decisions with regard to managing a broodmare within a stud environment, ensuring optimum reproductive success, and also welfare.

Selection of the Mare for Breeding

8

The Objectives of this Chapter are:

To begin to apply the reproductive physiology knowledge you have gained from Section A to stud management.

To consider the criteria that need to be assessed when selecting a mare based on her reproductive competence in order to maximize the chance that she will breed a foal with minimal risk.

To evaluate the methods by which these criteria can be assessed and their appropriateness for different breeding establishments.

To introduce some of the causes of infertility in the mare and the methods by which they can be investigated; infertility will be developed further in Chapter 14.

8.1. Introduction

The choice of a mare for breeding can be a very time-consuming process. Often not enough importance is placed upon this selection, and the result is an oversupply of mediocre or poor stock and unnecessary difficulties with mares at covering, during pregnancy, at foaling and during lactation.

One of the most obvious selection criteria is that of performance or athletic ability, which is justified as the horse should be bred for a specific market or use. However, regardless of the performance criteria used for selection, stock should also be selected on reproductive competence. Unfortunately, all too often such criteria are not considered, with potentially serious consequences for the individual breeder and the equine breed as a whole. Regardless of the type of horse you intend to breed, reproductive competence, (the ability to produce healthy offspring with minimal danger to the life and well-being of the dam and foal) should also be of prime importance. Today's horse, unlike other farm livestock, has been selected primarily for performance ability, often at the expense of reproductive competence. As a result, there are many potential reproductive problems that the breeder should be aware of in selecting a brood mare.

The following sections will assume that the selection criteria for performance have been met and so will concentrate solely upon the criteria and techniques that can be used in the selection for reproductive competence. A wide range of techniques will be included in the following sections, many of which are costly in terms of time and money. Parts of this Chapter will overlap with infertility (Chapter 14), many of the more intrusive techniques not really being justified for use when selecting a mare and more suited to investigating infertility; however, they have been included here for completeness. Hence the extent to which these techniques are used when selecting a brood mare depends on personal choice, the value of the breeding stock concerned and the potential value of any offspring. Even if this information does not preclude the mare as a brood mare, much of this information can be used to inform her future breeding management. Further information specific to infertility and hence an expansion of some of the issues raised here is included in Chapter 14.

The selection criteria for reproductive competence in the mare can be listed as follows and are often referred to as breeding soundness evaluation (BSE):

- history;
- temperament;
- age;
- general conformation and condition;
- reproductive tract examination (external and internal);

- infections;
- blood sampling; and
- chromosomal abnormalities.

8.2. History

The history of the mare includes both her specific breeding and general history (Shideler, 1993a; Zent, 2011). At present many mares, especially those of any value, come with historical documentation. Such records are invaluable in assessing her ability to produce a foal, as well as in easing management. If there are no records available, contact should be made with her previous owners to find out as much information as possible.

8.2.1. Reproductive history

Details of her past breeding performance should ideally include answers to questions such as:

- Does she show regular oestrous cycles?
- What is the length of her normal oestrous cycle?
- When does her breeding season normally start?
- How long does her season normally last?
- Does she show oestrus well and are there any characteristic signs?
- How long is her typical oestrus?
- Does she demonstrate oestrus easily or under certain circumstances?

This information will indicate, among other things, whether or not she will be easy to detect in oestrus and to cover. Mares that do not demonstrate oestrus well tend to be hard to cover. This leads to frustration, due to missed oestruses and wasted journeys to the stallion, all increasing costs. In addition, mares that are habitually hard, or even dangerous, to cover may be refused by some studs, reducing the pool of potential stallions or necessitating the use of artificial insemination (AI). Other questions asked should include whether she has bred before. If so, has she had problems holding (conceiving) to the stallion? This will necessitate return journeys to the stud or a prolonged period of time away. Has she had problems during any of her pregnancies? Has she ever reabsorbed (suffered from early embryo mortality) or aborted? If a mare has a history of habitual reabsorption or abortion or the need for 'holding' injections (artificial progesterone supplementation) post-service, then she is really not a good candidate as a brood mare. Such problems may indicate an inherent inability to carry a pregnancy to term, due to hormonal imbalance, uterine incompetence and/or genetic abnormality.

Does she or her family throw twins? Repeated incidences of twins are a problem, in that the likelihood of one or both of the fetuses aborting, is very high. If only one of the twins aborts, the remaining one is often born weaker and smaller than would normally be expected. Spontaneous abortion of twins is not due to an inherent inability to carry a foal to term (Section 2.4.5), and such mares are perfectly capable of producing a foal provided a single pregnancy is conceived. They may, however, need to be checked routinely for twin pregnancies and intensively managed to eliminate one twin at an early stage or to induce abortion, and the mare returned to the stallion. The tendency to conceive twins is also an inherited trait.

It is important to find out whether there may have been any incidences of retained placenta or dystocia. Retained placenta can occur habitually in some mares and so necessitate intensive management. It is rare for abnormal fetal positions (fetal dystocia) to occur repeatedly, but past difficulties may have caused internal lacerations or damage, especially if a caesarean or manipulation of the fetal position was required. It is particularly important to know if the cervix has been affected. Limited damage to the uterus, vagina and vulva will repair quite effectively, although it may leave areas of weakness or adhesions. Damage to the cervix is more likely to cause cervical incompetence, allowing bacteria to enter the higher reproductive tract, and thus causing infection. Conversely, adhesions may hinder the passage of sperm at covering, making it less able to dilate during parturition, necessitating a caesarean delivery and preventing natural drainage after covering, so increasing the incidence of post-coital endometritis. Similarly, issues with the mare at foaling (maternal dystocia) such as placenta previa or uterine inertia may not necessarily repeat themselves, but may again have resulted in internal damage that would be of concern. Any reproductive surgeries should also be noted, such as perineal lacerations, Caslicks, removal of an ovary or caesarean section. The mare may have apparently recovered completely but there may be persistent internal damage or weakness.

Previous post-foaling problems may also be indicated, including rejection or even habitual attacking of foals. This could be a sign of a general temperament fault, or may not show up in subsequent pregnancies, particularly if such behaviour was associated with a first foaling. Records may show that the mare is not a good mother, producing ill-thrifty foals. It is, therefore, helpful to look at foal birth weight and subsequent development and growth rates. Such effects may be due to poor milk yield, which in turn may reflect faults in nutritional management rather than a specific mare problem, but if she has consistently produced foals that did not do well, it may be worth investigating further.

Records should also show any incidences of infections and the organism isolated, treatments given and success. The results of past cytology or biopsy samples should be noted, along with any abnormalities such as luminal fluid or uterine cysts identified at ultrasonic scanning. Minor infections may show no long-term effects. However, infections of the reproductive tract are largely responsible for the relatively high infertility rates in horses and are the single major cause of fertilization failure and abortion in mares (Ginther, 1992; McKinnon and Voss, 1993; Morris and Allen, 2002b). Previous mastitic infections, although rare, should be considered and such mares examined to make sure that their udders have not suffered permanent damage.

Detailed mare records not only prove invaluable as an aid to selection but also provide useful information for the stud to which you intend to send your mare. This is especially important if she is to stay at stud for a prolonged period of time, and if oestrus detection is to be carried out by staff at the stud (Zent, 2011).

8.2.2. General history

In addition to specific breeding records, information on the mare's general history is also very useful. This should indicate her vaccination and worming status, as well as operations and accidents, especially if these involved the pelvic area, abdominal muscles, internal injuries and damage to limbs or muscles. These may preclude natural covering, necessitating AI, and if not rectified in time may be exacerbated by pregnancy, especially in the later stages, and predispose the mare to problems and may prevent natural parturition.

Ongoing or past conditions should also be noted. Mares with a history of respiratory or circulatory disorders, recurrent airway obstruction (RAO), exercise-induced pulmonary haemorrhage (EIPH), umbilical hernias or vaginal/uterine prolapse would possibly not stand up to the strain of pregnancy. Such conditions may also be exacerbated by pregnancy itself (Turner and McIlwraith, 1982; Shideler, 1993a,b). Conditions such as severe laminitis, navicular disease and tendonitis may also have a bearing on the ability of a mare to carry a pregnancy to term. Mares with disorders that are potentially heritable may be able to carry a pregnancy to term, but it is debatable whether such

mares should be bred, and hence perpetuate the problem within the population.

8.3. Temperament

The temperament of the mare is obviously important for ease of management, especially at birth and with a young foal, when many mares tend to be antisocial. Her temperament also has a significant effect on the temperament of her foal. The temperament of any animal has both a genotypic (inherited) and phenotypic (environmental) component. Both parents have an equal genotypic effect on the temperament of the foal. However, the phenotypic component of temperament is affected much more by the mare, in whose company the foal spends much of its early life until weaning. The temperament of the mare could, therefore, be argued to be much more important than that of the stallion in determining the temperament of the foal.

A mare with a quiet and gentle disposition is much easier to handle and manage. Such mares tend to show oestrus more readily and are, therefore, easier to cover. Anxious and highly strung mares with poor temperaments may show signs of aggression towards a teaser or stallion even although she is in oestrus; stress may often mask the signs of oestrus in such mares. Such aggressive mares are obviously more difficult and dangerous to cover. Many need to be twitched and/or hobbled, which further increases stress and is not conducive to optimum fertilization rates or easy management. Such mares can, of course, be covered using AI but the problem of detecting oestrus/ovulation and optimizing the time of insemination remains. Highly strung and nervous mares may also suffer from higher embryo mortality and possibly abortion rates (Malschitzky *et al.*, 2015). Finally, a masculinized temperament may be indicative of hormonal abnormalities, for example granulosa cell tumours (Hinrichs and Hunt, 1990).

8.4. Age

The age of a mare at her first breeding influences the ease of her pregnancy and may have potential long-term effects, especially in mares under 5 or over 12 years of age. As mares reach puberty between 18 and 24 months of age, it is theoretically possible to breed a mare at 18 months to produce a foal at 27–28 months of age. Evidence would suggest that such young mares may not inherently be less fertile (Rose *et al.*, 2018) although the number of follicles on the ovaries does increase between puberty and mature size (Ginther *et al.*, 2004a). However, they may suffer detrimental long-term effects if nutrition is inadequate. A horse does not attain its mature body size until 5 years of age, on average, so for a mare under 5 years there are the additional demands of growth on top of those of pregnancy and maintenance. This should be reflected in her nutritional management. To breed a mare early in life is a decision not to be taken lightly. She must be well grown for her age and in a good, but not over-fat, physical condition. There must also be the money and other means to feed her additional good-quality food, especially in late pregnancy, and to provide good accommodation for her in order to minimize her body's maintenance requirement.

At the other end of the spectrum, maiden mares over the age of 12 may also find it difficult to carry a pregnancy and bring up a foal. There is considerable evidence to suggest that embryo survival rates, as well as fertilization rates, are reduced in old mares. This is due to an increase in the incidence of embryonic defects, a reduction in ova viability and an increase in age-related degenerative endometritis (Chapter 14; Ricketts and Alonso, 1991; Ball, 1993a; Allen et al., 2007b; Hanlon et al., 2012a,b; De Mestre et al., 2019). In addition, the mere fact that she has been alive longer also means that she has had a greater chance of exposure to reproductive tract infections which, if severe, may have permanently affected her ability to conceive. Older maiden mares may have also spent the majority of their lives as barren mares without the attention of the stallion; they tend, therefore, to reject or be antagonistic towards a stallion's approaches. They may also have problems associated with their previous life. Many such mares are ex-performance horses and, as such, they have been trained and kept in top athletic condition, which often disrupts reproductive activity. Prime athletic condition is associated with a variety of reproductive malfunctions such as delayed oestrus, prolonged dioestrus and complete reproductive failure (Malschitzky et al., 2015). These mares need a readjustment period before they are physically and psychologically capable of conceiving, bearing and rearing a foal. A prolonged period of rest of at least 6 months allows the mare's system to settle down into a non-athletic state; some mares may take as long as 18 months to adjust to their new way of life. If a mare has been treated with drugs, such as corticosteroids and/or anabolic steroids (illegally or legally), her system will require time to eliminate them, and in this period reproductive function may continue to be disrupted (Squires et al., 1985b; Zent, 2011). More recently gonadotrophin-releasing hormone (GnRH) antagonists have been used to suppress reproductive activity; the withdrawal time

for these is much longer than the more commonly used progestogen (Regumate®, DPT Laboratories, San Antonio, Texas, USA) (Farquhar et al., 2001; Stout and Colenbrander, 2004). A performance horse in top athletic condition develops musculature, especially in the abdominal and pelvic regions, that is not necessarily conducive to an easy pregnancy and parturition. Time should, therefore, be allowed for muscle tone to relax.

The ideal age to breed a maiden mare is at 5–6 years of age, at which time she will have reached her mature size. She will also not be old enough to have become set in her ways and will be less likely to have developed aggressive tendencies towards the stallion and to have contracted uterine infections. However, breeding at this age will not suit all systems. Most mares will not have proved their worth, so the decision to breed may not yet have been made. One increasingly popular way of overcoming this is the use of embryo transfer, discussed in detail in Chapter 22, which allows performance mares to breed but not at the expense of their performance careers.

Once a mare has borne one foal, she is more able to cope with the demands of subsequent pregnancies and, as such, is much more likely to breed successfully as an older mare well into her teens (Allen, 1992). If a mare has been a brood mare all her life, then age is less important. She may naturally be barren during the occasional year, and this has been suggested as nature's way of allowing recovery and regeneration. More care and attention is needed with older age, and it is not normally advisable to breed a mare over 20 years old, although this largely depends on the breed, type and condition of the individual mare. Mares of the native type tend to breed more successfully into later life than the hotblood/warmblood-type animals, although of course there are exceptions to every rule.

8.5. General Conformation and Condition

A mare's general conformation is of importance, not only to ensure that her offspring are well conformed, but also to ease her pregnancy. She needs to have a strong back and legs to enable her to carry the considerable extra weight of the fetus during late pregnancy. She should have correct pelvic conformation, with a pelvic opening adequate for a safe delivery. Ideally, she should also possess good heart and lung room across the chest, and have plenty of abdominal space. In general, rather fine, tucked-up mares tend to be poorer breeders and produce smaller foals, or have more problems during pregnancy and parturition.

A mare's general body condition is considered to have implications on reproductive activity, although evidence is conflicting (Gentry *et al.*, 2002a,b; Godoi *et al.*, 2002). There is evidence to suggest a link between leptin levels (which are related to body condition) and reproductive ability, especially in relation to seasonality (Fitzgerald and McManus, 2000; Fitzgerald *et al.*, 2002; Gamba and Pralong, 2006). The body condition of horses can be classified on a scale of 0–5, 0 being emaciated and 5 obese (Figs 8.1–8.4). The ideal condition score for a mare at mating is 3. Such mares have a good covering of flesh and the ribs may be felt with some pressure, as can the vertebrae of the backbone. It is widely believed that mares in condition score 3 have the highest fertilization rate and subsequent reproductive success (Fig. 8.3; Ridman and Keiper, 1991).

Thin mares (Fig. 8.2) may show prolonged anoestrus or very long/delayed oestrous cycles, along with suspension of all reproductive activity in cases of emaciation. At the other end of the spectrum, over-fat mares (Fig. 8.4) may suffer reproductive failure due to excess fat deposition on the reproductive tract, limiting its ability to move and expand with a developing pregnancy. Fat may also be deposited on the ovaries and around the Fallopian tubes, interfering with the process of ovulation.

It has been demonstrated that, in barren mares, an increasing plane of nutrition 5–6 weeks prior to mating, with an accompanying gradual improvement in body condition up to a score of 3, results in the best ovulation and fertilization rates (Van Niekerk and Van Heerden, 1972). This process is termed flushing and is a common practice in sheep and cattle management. It is discussed further in Section 9.2. Finally, body condition is reported to also affect the mare's response to hormonal treatment used in the manipulation of reproduction (Gentry *et al.*, 2002a).

8.6. External Examination of the Reproductive Tract

Poor external conformation of the mare's reproductive tract can have severe implications on reproductive performance (Section 1.3).

The perineal area forms the outer vulval seal of the tract (Section 1.3) and so should be examined (Fig. 8.5). First, the presence of features such as lacerations, damage,

puckers and scars should be noted, as they may be indicative of more extensive internal damage and will certainly affect the competence of the vulval seal (Fig. 8.6a and b). Second, the general conformation of the perineal area should be assessed. If the vulval seal is incompetent this allows bacteria and airborne pathogens to enter the vagina and challenge the upper reproductive system (Section 1.3; Figs 1.4, 1.7 and 1.9). This predisposes the mare to pneumovagina and urovagina. Both of these are common causes of reproductive tract infection and hence infertility. Such conditions are prevalent in lean athletic mares such as Thoroughbreds, mares in poor condition and mares with reduced vulval tone due to injury, damage, age, oestrus or foaling (Pascoe, 1979).

As discussed previously (Section 1.3), the height of the pelvic floor also has a bearing on bacterial contamination, and so should also be considered when selecting mares. It may be assessed by inserting a sterile probe into the vagina and resting it on the pelvic floor (Fig. 8.7).

In a normal conformation, at least 80% of the vulva should lie below the pelvic floor in order for the vaginal seal to be fully competent. In a mare with a low pelvic floor, the risk of contamination of the reproductive tract can be reduced if perineal conformation is correct and hence the vulval seal is competent.

The external perineal conformation and hence vulval seal competence can be assessed by eye, or a simple ruler and protractor can be used to allocate a Caslick index (Fig. 8.5; Section 1.3.1) and so indicate the likelihood of infection and the need for a Caslick vulvoplasty (Pascoe, 1979a). The competence of the vaginal seal can be assessed via the use of a sterile probe as indicated (Fig. 8.7) or may require a speculum. Speculum examination of the vagina and cervix is discussed in detail in the following section.

The selection of a mare with a Caslick vulvoplasty for breeding must be made with considerable caution. There are a finite number of times that the operation can be performed and, unless the more complicated Pouret operation (Pouret, 1982) or the more recent suggested adaptation of the Pouret (Bradecamp, 2011b; Papa *et al.*, 2014) is resorted to, there is – by implication – a limit to the mare's breeding career. An additional consideration is one of equine welfare and whether it is appropriate that a mare should go through such a procedure repeatedly. It may also be questioned whether such poorly conformed mares should be bred from at all as, in so doing, the trait is perpetuated within the equine population. However, a

CONDITION SCORE

	5	4	3	2	1	0
General	Obese	Fat	Good	Fair	Thin	Emaciated
Back/Pelvis/Croup	Ribs cannot be felt, buried in fat. Flat backbone with deep 'gutter' continuing over croup to base of dock. Pelvis buried in very firm fatty tissue and cannot be felt	Ribs well covered, only felt with firm pressure. Backbone well covered with slight 'gutter' continuing over croup. Pelvis buried in fatty tissue and only felt with firm pressure	Ribs, backbone and pelvis rounded and covered in fat but felt with light pressure. No 'gutter'	Ribs just visible. Backbone just covered in fat spinous processes easily felt but not visible. Croup well defined with some fat under skin. Pelvis easily felt. Slight depression under tail	Ribs and backbone easily seen, covered by slack skin. Pelvis and croup well defined with no fat under skin. Deep depression under tail	Ribs, backbone and pelvis very easily seen, prominent and sharp, covered by slack skin. Deep cavity under tail
Neck	Very wide and firm with excessive fatty tissue. Marked crest in mares and stallions	Wide and firm with folds of fat. Slight crest in mares and stallions	Firm with some fat. Crest only in stallions	Narrow but firm. No crest	Ewe neck, narrow and slack at base	Ewe neck, very narrow and slack at base

Fig. 8.1. Body condition scoring in the horse.

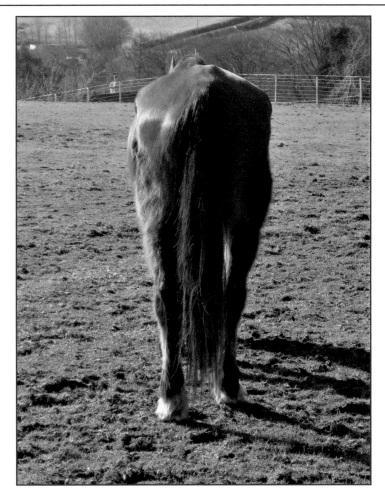

Fig. 8.2. Mare in poor condition, condition score 1.

Caslick vulvoplasty operation does effectively reduce the incidence of repeated uterine infection, which in itself may be considered a welfare issue (Hemberg *et al.*, 2005).

8.7. Internal Examination of the Reproductive Tract

Examination of the internal reproductive tract of the mare is the job of a skilled veterinary surgeon, necessitating the use of several examination techniques. Information given by these assessments can be indispensable in assessing the reproductive potential of a mare.

8.7.1. Vulva and vagina

Vaginal internal assessment can be carried out by means of a speculum (LeBlanc, 1993a; Zent and Steiner,

2011). The most commonly used is a Caslick's speculum (Figs 8.8–8.10).

The speculum consists of either an expandable or non-expandable hollow metal, glass, plastic or cardboard tube, sometimes with a light source attached. The sterilized and well-lubricated speculum is inserted into the mare's vagina. If an expandable speculum is used it is inserted in the closed position, and is expanded slowly, opening up the vagina. The integral light source or a separate pen torch is used to illuminate the mucous membrane lining and the cervix, allowing examination in detail. The use of a vaginal speculum must be accompanied by several precautions as, when in position, it opens up both the vulval and vaginal seals. The procedure should be carried out under conditions as sterile as possible, in a dust-free environment. The mare's tail

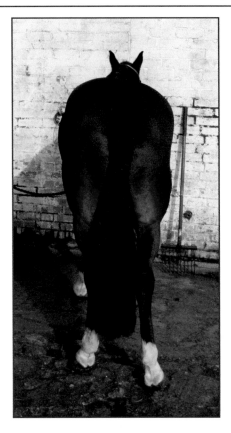

Fig. 8.3. Mare in the ideal condition for covering, condition score 3.

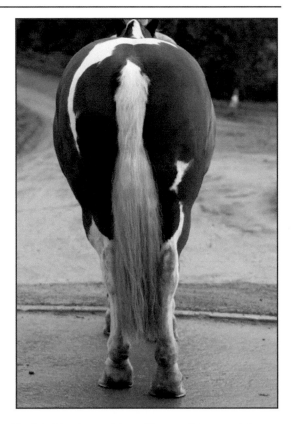

Fig. 8.4. Mare in over-fat condition, condition score 4.5.

should be bandaged and the perineal area thoroughly washed.

A more sophisticated technique – endoscopy or hysteroscopy – is often used today for viewing the mare's vagina and cervix before the endoscope is then passed up into, and used to view, the rest of the internal reproductive tract (Menzies-Gow, 2007; Card, 2011a; Assad and Pandey, 2015). Old endoscopes were rigid and, therefore, had limitations to their use. Today, fibre-optic endoscopes are flexible and so much more versatile, and can be used to view internal structures either through the body wall and into the body cavity; via the oral/nasal cavity into the digestive/respiratory system; via the rectum into the large intestine; or, finally, via the vagina into the reproductive tract.

The endoscope consists of a series of flexible carbon-fibre filaments with a light source and camera attached. The flexible carbon-fibre rod is passed through the vagina and up into the inner reproductive tract. One set of the carbon-fibre filaments allows the passage of light

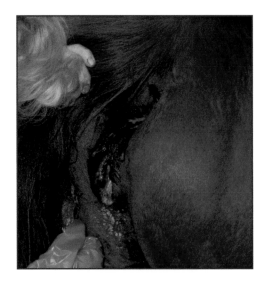

Fig. 8.5. Simple observation of the mare's vulva can be done by a lay person and can indicate mares with very poor perineal conformation, such as is evident in this mare.

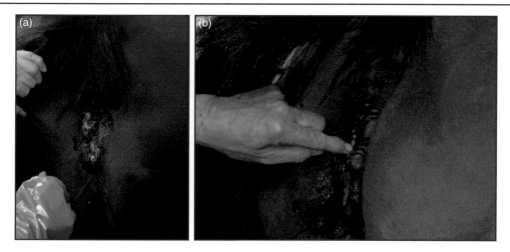

Fig. 8.6. Evidence of lacerations, puckers, abnormalities or repeated Caslick vulvoplasty on the vulva or perineal area will predispose the mare to a poor vulval seal, and may also indicate internal damage.

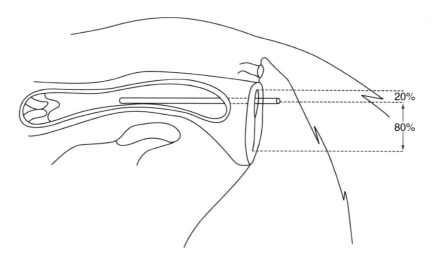

Fig 8.7. Assessment of the vaginal and vulval competence and hence the likelihood of pneumovagina.

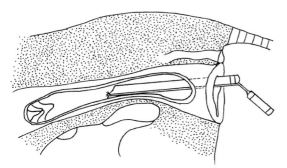

Fig. 8.8. Vaginal speculum examination of the mare's vagina. The attached light source allows the inside of the vagina and cervix to be illuminated and hence easily viewed.

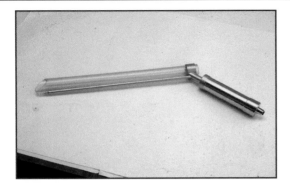

Fig. 8.9. A non-expandable Caslick vaginal speculum.

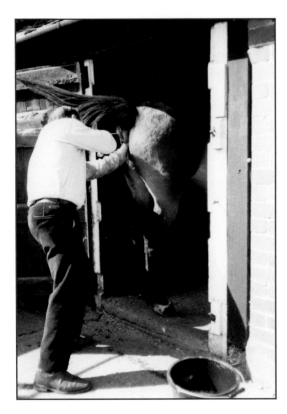

Fig. 8.10. Use of an expandable Caslick vaginal speculum.

from the external light source down the endoscope, illuminating the internal structures. The other set allows the transmission of the image back to the camera and on to a display unit. The positioning and angle of view of the endoscope can be controlled remotely from the exterior end of the endoscope. The use of the endoscope is expensive and is usually confined to examination of

the upper, less-accessible parts of the reproductive tract (Threlfall and Carleton, 1996; Card, 2011a; Assad and Pandey, 2015).

In the healthy mare, the mucous membranes lining the vulva and vagina should appear a healthy pink colour, whether viewed via a speculum or endoscope. Any mucus present should be clear and not cloudy or yellow-white in colour. An infected vagina appears red and inflamed and possibly covered in a cloudy mucus. Infections of the vagina are not uncommon and will be discussed in the following section on infections and also in Chapter 14. The vulva and inner vagina should also be free from bruising, irritation, scars and tears. They are susceptible to damage and injury at parturition and so should be carefully checked. Adhesions, if present, are caused by scar tissue and may render the mare unserviceable or cause her pain at mating and hence to reject the stallion. AI is a possible alternative but she is likely to still have problems at foaling (McCue, 2008).

Neoplasms of the vulva and vagina are relatively rare, although if present may cause problems at covering. Three kinds of neoplasms can be seen in horses: (i) melanomas, malignant growths of the melanin-containing pigment cells, particularly prevalent in grey mares and not necessarily confined to the vulva and vagina; (ii) carcinomas or malignant neoplasms of the epithelial cells; and (iii) papillomas or benign neoplasms. If a mare does show evidence of neoplasms, it is debatable whether she should be bred, as there is evidence to suggest that the tendency to develop some neoplasms is heritable.

Finally, urovagina (pooling of urine within the floor of the vagina) may be observed. Stagnant urine held within the vagina will increase the chance of infection. Urine pooling is evident in mares with poor perineal conformation, and in older multiparous mares in which vaginal tone has been lost, allowing urine to pass cranially towards the cervix rather than draining caudally towards the vulva. It may also result from past vaginal damage or injury.

8.7.2. Cervix

The cervix may be considered as the connection and final seal between the outer reproductive tract and the inner, more susceptible tract. As such, its competence as a seal is very important and anything that compromises this ability and/or the ability to dilate to accommodate the passage of the foal at parturition is of concern. This may also be assessed by means of a speculum or endoscope, as described above for vaginal examination. The cervix varies greatly with the stage of the oestrous cycle and pregnancy, and so can aid diagnosis. During oestrus the cervix is fairly relaxed, pink in colour, its tone flaccid and any secretions quite thin, and it appears to 'flower' (relax) into the vagina (Fig. 1.13) This is to ease the passage of the penis at copulation. During dioestrus and, to a greater extent, during anoestrus, the cervical tone increases, it appears whiter in colour, the seal becomes tighter and secretions thicker (Fig. 1.12). During pregnancy, the cervix is again tightly sealed and white in colour, with a mucus plug acting to enhance the effectiveness of the seal. The tone of the cervix may also be assessed via rectal palpation (Bowman, 2011). In general, the state of the cervix should correspond to ovarian activity and that of the rest of the tract. If not, infections or abnormalities should be suspected. Infection of the cervical mucosa, or cervicitis, will be discussed in detail later (Sections 14.3.4.5 and 14.3.5.4). Cervicitis is characterized by a red/purple swollen cervix, often protruding into the vagina and covered with mucus, clearly seen at speculum examination. In severe cases, cysts may be evident and may result in adhesions and long-term permanent damage, preventing correct closure of the cervical seal, with resultant infection. Adhesions as a result of cervical damage may not only close it completely, preventing entry of the penis, and so the passage of sperm to the upper tract, but also prevent the drainage of fluid from the uterus, resulting in serious uterine infections as well as preventing dilation at parturition. Minor cervical damage and/or adhesions can be helped by surgery (Sertich, 1993). Congenital abnormalities may occasionally be observed (Kelly and Newcombe, 2009).

8.7.3. Uterus

Examination of the mare's uterus is a more complicated procedure, as the uterus forms part of the inner and less-accessible reproductive tract. An appreciation of its gross structure can be obtained by rectal palpation and/or ultrasonic scanning. The colour and condition of the mucous membranes of the uterus may be inspected by means of an endoscope and further examined by uterine biopsy.

Rectal palpation is a commonly used and relatively effective way of obtaining a tactile impression of the inner reproductive tract and so identifying structural abnormalities (Figs 8.11 and 8.12). The procedure involves restraining the mare in stocks and inserting a well-lubricated, gloved hand and arm through the anus and into the rectum of the mare. The wall of the rectum

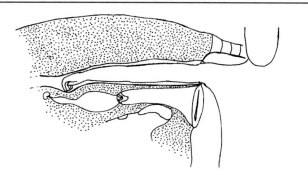

Fig. 8.11. Rectal palpation in the mare.

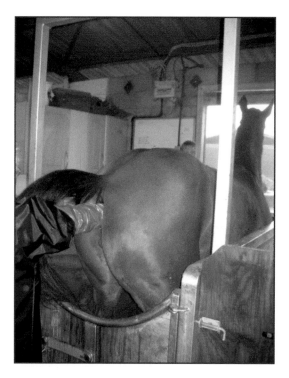

Fig. 8.12. Rectal palpation in the mare allows the practitioner to feel the reproductive tract through the relatively thin wall of the rectum.

is fairly thin, so the reproductive tract that lies immediately below it can be palpated with care through the rectum wall. The procedure, however, must only be carried out by an experienced operator, as rupturing the rectum is a risk. Rectal palpation can be used to assess the tone, size and texture of the uterus, uterine horns, Fallopian tubes and ovaries, and provides a tactile impression of the structures felt. It can be used to identify cysts, tumours, stretched broad ligaments, uterine endometritis, sacculations, adhesions, lacerations, scars and delayed involution (recovery after foaling). It is, therefore, a useful, cheap and immediate aid to selection of mares (Shideler, 1993c; McCue *et al.*, 2008b; Bowman, 2011b; Assad and Pandey, 2015).

Ultrasonic scanning is a newer and more expensive method of assessment, but gives an immediate, visual impression of the upper reproductive tract, rather than the tactile interpretation obtained with rectal palpation (Sertich, 1998; McCue, 2008; Assad and Pandey, 2015). The ultrasonic scanner is based on the Doppler principle. When high-frequency sound waves hit an object, they are absorbed or deflected back to a varying extent, depending on the density of that object. The reflected sound waves are transduced to appear as an image on a screen. Solid objects appear white and fluid appears black, with many variations of grey in between (Fig. 8.13; Pycock, 2011; McCue, 2008; Assad and Pandey, 2015; Pozor, 2017). In the case of ultrasonic scanners used in the assessment of a mare's reproductive status the transducer or ultrasonic emitting and receiving device is inserted into the rectum, or less commonly

placed on the mare's flank, and directed towards the reproductive tract (Fig. 8.14). The resultant image can be used to identify abnormalities similar to those assessed via rectal palpation, but is particularly useful in detecting cysts, intrauterine fluid, air, debris, neoplasms, etc. (McKinnon, 1998a; Assad and Pandey, 2015). The technique can also be used to assess the size and shape of the uterus and ovaries and so can be used to determine ovarian activity (Carnevale, 1998; McKinnon, 1998; Ginther and Utt, 2004). More recently colour Doppler ultrasonography has been suggested for use to assess uterine and ovarian blood flow, giving further information on function (Bollwein *et al.*, 2002, 2003, 2004; Ginther and Utt, 2004; Ginther, 2008).

When assessed via rectal palpation or ultrasonic scanning the healthy uterus should appear thin-walled and flaccid if the mare is in anoestrus; soft with little tone if she is in oestrus; firm and toned if she is in dioestrus; and more turgid with plenty of tone in early pregnancy. If the palpation is worked gradually from either uterine horn and across the uterine body, then local thickenings, cysts or fibrotic areas can be detected and

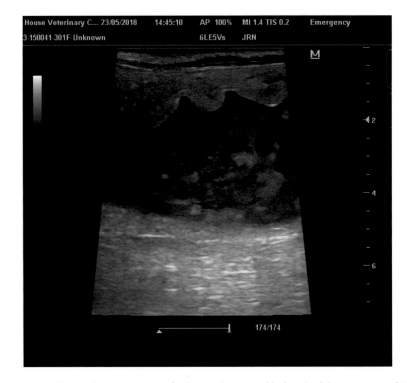

Fig. 8.13. The image produced by an ultrasonic scanner; fluid areas show up as black and solid structures as white, with variations in between. This image shows fluid within the uterus as dark grey with floating grey particles surrounded by the uterine wall as a lighter grey. (Photo courtesy of Professor John Newcombe.)

the diameter of each horn estimated and compared. The two horns should roughly match, although they are rarely identical in diameter in parous mares. Mares with a history of infections may show ventral outpushings of the uterus, especially at the junction between the uterine body and horns. These mares may well have difficulty in carrying another pregnancy to term as they often lose the fetus at the time of, or soon after, implantation. Incomplete involution of the uterus post-partum can also be detected, indicating infection, weakening or rupture of the uterine wall. In severe cases the uterus may never completely involute. This leaves a flaccid area of uterus with inadequate tone compared to the remainder. Again, such mares may well have difficulty carrying a pregnancy to term. Haemorrhages within the broad ligaments may be identified as local hard swellings. Stretched broad ligaments may also be detected, often due to excessive strain, accidents or damage. Again, such mares may be incapable of carrying a pregnancy to term, the broad ligaments being unable to support the weight of a full-term fetus. Luminal fluid, air or debris is not conducive to embryo survival, and uterine cysts not only reduce the uterine surface available for placental attachment, but impede embryo mobility and so compromise maternal recognition of pregnancy (Section 3.2.3.1).

An endoscope, as described earlier in this Chapter, may be used to examine the internal surfaces of the reproductive tract and to give a real-time image. Once the endoscope is inserted, sterile air or oxygen is passed into the uterus, separating the naturally apposed uterine walls and so easing the viewing of the mucous membranes and uterine epithelium. The normal healthy uterine epithelium is pale pink in colour and any mucus present is clear (Fig. 8.15). Any signs of redness or discoloration within the uterus, especially if it is associated with fluid (particularly cloudy or creamy mucus), are indicative of uterine infection, endometritis. Evidence of cysts, blood clots, thickening of the endometrium or scar tissue may indicate possible future problems in the mare's reproductive life (LeBlanc, 1993b; Card, 2012; Assad and Pandey, 2015).

The use of the endoscope, although very useful, is limited in routine mare selection owing to the cost of the instrument and to the skill required.

If any areas of concern within the mare's uterus are detected, a uterine biopsy may be performed to aid further investigation (Schlafer, 2007; Love, 2011b; Assad and Pandey, 2015). Uterine biopsies involve the removal of a small section of uterine endometrium with a small pair of forceps (Figs 8.16 and 8.17). The biopsy

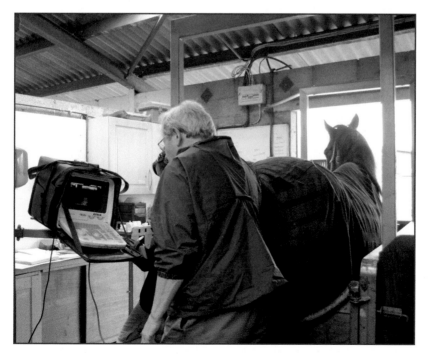

Fig. 8.14. The use of an ultrasonic scanning machine in the mare.

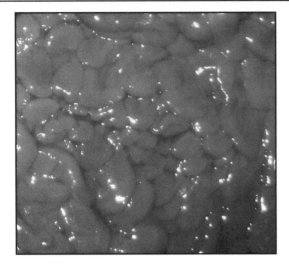

Fig. 8.15. The surface of the uterine endometrium should be pink in colour with obvious endometrial folds.

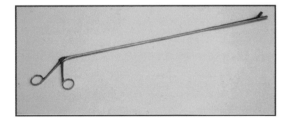

Fig. 8.16. Uterine biopsy forceps.

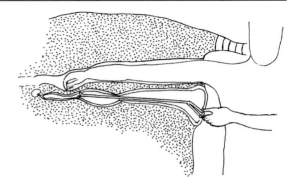

Fig. 8.17. The use of uterine biopsy forceps in the mare. The arm inserted via the rectum is used to ease the wall of the uterus into the jaws of the biopsy forceps.

forceps are passed into the vagina and guided up through the cervix by a well-lubricated gloved hand. The index finger guides the forceps through the cervix and into the uterus. The gloved hand is then removed and inserted into the rectum to guide the forceps to the section of the uterus that is to be biopsied. The jaws of the forceps are opened and the section of endometrium to be sampled is pushed between the jaws by this hand. The jaws are then shut and the forceps drawn back slowly until the pressure of the endometrium is felt. A sharp tug will then release the sample, which is immediately removed and fixed in readiness for histological examination (Fig. 8.17; Love, 2011b).

Samples taken from the mid-uterine horn have been shown to be representative of the uterine endometrium as a whole, so they are suitable for routine biopsies where no specific abnormality is being investigated (Kenney, 1978). In biopsies to further investigate suspected

abnormalities, samples should be taken from each suspected area and another sample from a seemingly normal area of endometrium. Biopsies can be taken at any time of the oestrous cycle but, normally, standard biopsies are taken in mid-dioestrus in order to standardize results (Kenney, 1978; Doig and Waelchi, 1993).

Such samples can allow identification of abnormalities and also indicate evidence of uterine degeneration. The evaluation of a histology sample is a skilled job but, in general, the examiner looks at a cross section of uterine wall to identify changes in cell structure, especially in luminal cells. These may be diagnostic of inflammation, presence of lymphocytes (indicating infection), fibrosis or necrosis, endometrial gland nests, etc. Mares are then classified as Grade I normal, Grade IIa or IIb (which show increasing evidence of infection and/or inflammation) and Grade III (which shows evidence of severe endometritis indicating a very poor prognosis for the mare as a breeding animal) (Fig. 8.18; Kenney, 1978; Doig et al., 1981; Doig and Waelchi, 1993). The process is reported not to disrupt the mare's reproductive cycle, although some people report a delay in the next oestrous period (Kenney, 1977).

Not all these methods discussed are necessarily used when selecting a mare; it largely depends on the value of the mare. Some techniques may be more appropriate to investigate specific abnormalities which have been indicated by the simpler and more routine procedures of rectal palpation and ultrasonic scanning.

8.7.4. Fallopian tubes

The competence of the Fallopian tubes (oviducts) is more difficult to assess. As mentioned previously, uniformity in size

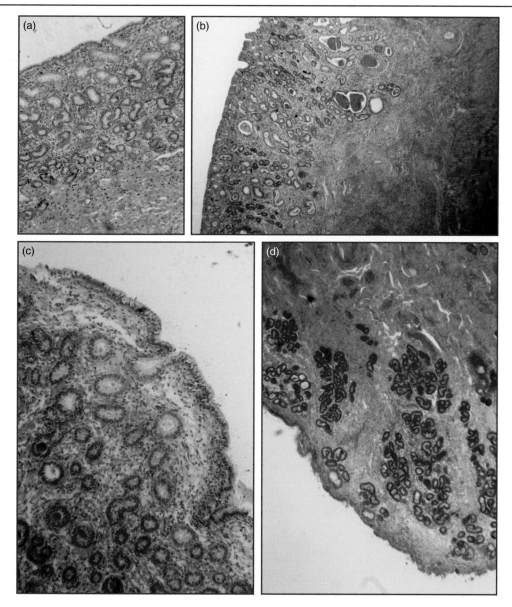

Fig. 8.18. Histological samples taken from mares via biopsy. (a) Grade I normal; (b) Grade IIa showing some lymphocytes (indicative of infection) in the endometrial stratum compactum; (c) Grade IIb showing separation of parts of the endometrial stratum compactum; and (d) Grade III showing endometrial glands bunched together (endometrial gland nests) indicating severe endometritis.

and shape can be assessed via rectal palpation, although this is not easy. In such an examination, the Fallopian tubes should feel wiry and uniform in consistency when rolled between the palpater's fingers. Severe abnormalities may be detected this way, especially adhesions connecting the infundibulum to the uterus or ovaries and scar tissue. However, salpingitis (inflammation of the Fallopian tubes) is hard to detect. Although it has been reported to be relatively uncommon in mares, any such inflammation is of importance, as it may hinder the passage of ova and/or sperm along the Fallopian tube and may even result in complete blockage of the Fallopian tubes.

Assessment of Fallopian tube blockage is very difficult. The traditional starch-grain test is relatively successful and relatively straightforward, but does not easily discriminate between left and right Fallopian tubes and, therefore, is of limited practical use (Allen, 1979). This technique involves injecting a starch-grain solution through the mare's back at the sub-luminal fossa, using a long needle. The ovary is manipulated, via rectal palpation, to lie immediately beneath the needle. Starch-grain solution (approximately 5 ml) is then injected onto the surface of the ovary. Washings are collected from the anterior vagina and cervix 24–48 h later. The presence of starch grains in the flushings indicates that the Fallopian tube associated with the ovary on to which the starch grains were injected is patent. A similar test used fluorescent microspheres deposited on the surface of the ovary via ultrasound-guided transvaginal needle and has been reported to be successful (Ley et al., 1998, Ley, 2011).

A more invasive form of investigation is the use of laparotomy/laparoscopy (Fig. 8.19) (Fischer, 1991; Hendrikson and Wilson, 2011; Köllmann et al., 2011) under sedation. Laparotomy involves the exteriorization and then examination of the Fallopian tubes through an incision in the abdominal wall. Laparoscopy involves the insertion of a rigid endoscope through a puncture hole in the abdominal wall, which allows the Fallopian tubes to be visualized in situ. Both these techniques allow the visualization of the uterine horns and Fallopian tubes, and their detailed examination, and allow for tissue biopsies to be taken. However, they are expensive and highly invasive, and so run the normal

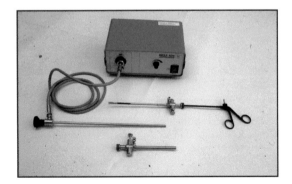

Fig. 8.19. A laparoscope, which may be used to view the internal structures of the mare's reproductive tract via the abdominal cavity. The trocars pictured in the foreground are inserted through puncture wounds in the mare's abdomen. The laparoscope is then passed through the larger one for viewing the internal organs, and the manipulating forceps through the smaller one for moving internal organs.

risks associated with puncturing into the abdominal cavity; they are, therefore, rarely used.

8.7.5. Ovaries

Ovarian activity can be assessed most simply by rectal palpation and more extensively by ultrasonic scanning. The appearance of the mare's ovaries varies considerably with season and reproductive activity. These changes are detailed and discussed in Section 1.9. Rectal palpation has traditionally been used to assess the stage of the mare's oestrous cycle and, therefore, to help in the timing of mating. It can be used in this context of selection for breeding to ensure that the mare is reproductively active and that follicles and corpora lutea (CLs) are being produced. It can also be used to ensure that the reproductive stage indicated by the ovaries is synchronized with developmental changes in the remainder of the mare's tract. Such techniques can also indicate the presence of adhesions and neoplasms, as well as cystic follicles, ova fossa cysts and other ovarian abnormalities, which may disrupt the mare's reproductive activity. Further detail on the assessment of the reproductive stage of the mare by ovarian examination is given in Section 10.2.2.2. Ultrasonic evaluation can be used to identify the same features as described for rectal palpation, but give a more detailed impression of the internal structures of the ovaries, including normal function as well as abnormalities.

Laparoscopy has been used experimentally to elucidate ovarian problems. It is not used in practical stud farm management owing to its cost and the need for sedation and puncturing of the abdominal cavity (Hendrikson and Wilson, 2011; Köllmann et al., 2011).

8.8. Infections

Mares are notoriously susceptible to reproductive tract infections, in particular endometritis (Ricketts and Mackintosh, 1987). For the last 100 years these have been known to be linked to temporary and possibly permanent infertility. Additionally, such infections can be transferred relatively easily to the stallion and hence on to other mares at mating (Ricketts, 2011). It is imperative, therefore, that infected mares are identified so that they can be discarded in the selection process and/or treated. One of the standard procedures used to detect such infections is swabbing followed by culturing for bacteriological examination and/or cytology examination (Davies Morel et al., 2013). Swabs may be taken from the uterus, cervix, urethral opening and/or clitoral area and assessed for pathogenic organisms, for example venereal disease (VD) bacteria such as *Klebsiella pneumoniae, Pseudomonas aeruginosa* and *Taylorella equigenitalis,* which are true sexually transmitted bacteria; or *Streptococcus zooepidemicus, Escherichia coli, Staphlococcus spp.* and less commonly *Enterobacteria cloaca* and *Corynebacterium* sp. which, although not strictly VD bacteria, may also be transferred at covering and cause uterine infections (LeBlanc *et al.*, 2007; LeBlanc and Causey, 2009; Nafis and Panday, 2012; Assad and Pandey, 2015).

Uterine swabs should only be taken during oestrus when the cervix is relaxed and moist, easing the swab's passage, and at the time when the mare's natural immunological response to accidentally introduced bacteria is heightened owing to the dominance of oestrogen. The swabs may be guided in through the cervix using a speculum or guided via a gloved, lubricated arm, as in the case of uterine biopsies. Once the swab is in the lumen of the uterus it is rotated against the endometrium to absorb uterine secretions and any bacteria. The risk of accidental contamination of the swab by either airborne pathogens or bacteria present in the cervix and/or vagina is minimized by careful washing of the mare and the use of a guarded swab. Such swabs are contained within two sterile tubes. The first tube is passed through the cervix and the second tube is telescoped into the uterus. The swab can then be pushed out through the second tube far enough to reach the endometrium. A reversal of this process will reduce the contamination on retraction of the swab (Figs 8.20–8.22; Blanchard *et al.*, 1981; Ricketts, 2011).

Cervical and urethral-opening swabs are easier to obtain (Fig. 8.21) and may be collected at any time of the cycle. The samples may be taken using a vaginascope by a similar process to that described for the uterus.

Clitoral swabs are taken from the clitoral sinus and the clitoral fossa. Gentle squeezing of the clitoris may produce smegma secretions for swabbing; care should be taken, however, as some mares object. The clitoral fossa is notorious for harbouring, among other pathogens, *T. equigenitalis*, the causal agent for contagious equine metritis (CEM).

Once the sample has been taken, the swab can be applied to a variety of growth mediums and incubated under various conditions (temperature, humidity,

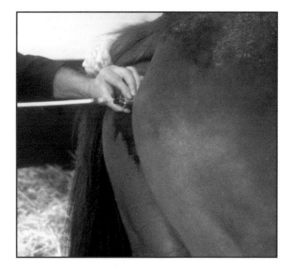

Fig. 8.21. Swabbing the mare.

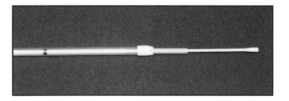

Fig. 8.22. A guarded swab used to collect samples from the mare's reproductive tract for bacterial assessment.

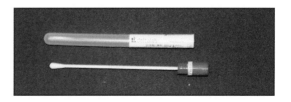

Fig 8.23. A standard swab used to swab the clitoral fossa and sinus of the mare.

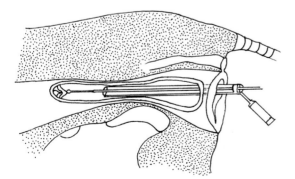

Fig. 8.20. Cervical swabbing in the mare.

atmospheric pressure, oxygen content – anaerobic, aerobic, etc.) in order to identify infective organisms (Mackintosh, 1981; Perry and Freydiere, 2007; Ricketts, 2011). Results are normally available within 48–72 h. More recently a polymerase chain reaction (PCR) test for *T. equigenitalis* has become available that allows much quicker turnaround times (24 h) and is reported to be nearly 100% accurate with respect to false positives (Ousey *et al.*, 2009). Finally, modern genomic technology now allows bacteria to be much more accurately identified, but at a much greater expense, and so is currently not widespread in its commercial use (Didelot *et al.*, 2012; Land *et al.*, 2015). Swabbing is a very effective method of assessing bacterial contamination of the mare's reproductive tract, but results must be treated with some caution. The presence of bacteria within the vagina and cervix does not necessarily indicate uterine infection, especially if the cervical seal is fully competent. The natural microflora of many mares contains pathogenic organisms. The actual process of taking a sample also increases the chance of reproductive tract contamination by airborne bacteria; hence the technique must be carried out under conditions that are as clean and sterile as possible. In general, and as indicated above, swabbing is best carried out during oestrus.

Samples of cells that line the reproductive tract can also be taken and assessed under the microscope (cytological examination) to identify any abnormal cell populations, in particular the presence of polymorphonuclear neutrophils (PMN) which, in high concentrations, indicate infection (Ricketts *et al.*, 1993; Ricketts, 2011). It is now good practice to perform uterine cytology alongside cultures in diagnosing endometritis (Davies Morel *et al.*, 2013). Sampling for cytology can be via swabs as well as with a cytology brush (Fig. 8.24) and is performed at similar times to swabbing, depending on the area to be swabbed. Cytology then allows the staining and rapid identification of cell types, results being available much more quickly than by culturing, which can take several days (Fig. 8.25; LeBlanc, 2011).

Swabbing also allows fungi to be identified, which although less common than bacteria can still be a cause of concern. The most common fungi are *Candida* spp. and *Aspergillus* spp., both of which can be identified by plating out on to appropriate plates (Dascanio *et al.*, 2001; Ricketts, 2011). Providing the possible drawbacks are borne in mind, swabbing is a simple procedure to carry out in the routine selection of mares for breeding. Indeed, as a result of the Thoroughbred Breeders Association Annual Code of Practice (1978 onwards) it is advised that all Thoroughbred mares, and increasingly many of those in other breed societies, should be swabbed prior to arrival at the stud and again at the oestrus of service, to ensure the absence of VD bacteria. Only mares with a negative certificate will be accepted at the stud and only those with a second negative certificate will be covered.

8.9. Blood sampling

If there are reasons to believe that a mare may have problems in carrying a foal to term, and no anatomical abnormalities have been detected using the previously

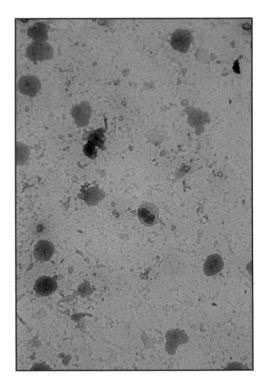

Fig. 8.25. Cytology image showing a binucleated polymorphonuclear neutrophil (PMN) in the centre of the image plus scattered endometrial cells.

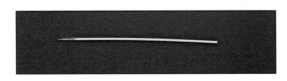

Fig. 8.24. A cytology brush used to collect cells from the lining of the reproductive tract for cytological examination.

discussed techniques, then the problem may lie in hormonal inadequacies. The endocrine profiles of mares can be determined by sequential blood sampling, and the most commonly tested is progesterone (Douglas, 2004; Fig. 8.26). Any deviations from the normal profile can be identified and the specific area of failure (i.e. follicle development, ovulation signal, oestrous behaviour or CL regression) can be determined. In the light of these results, appropriate hormone therapy may be possible to compensate for the natural deficiencies, or it can be decided that such a mare is not worth the risk or cost of such therapy. Details of the normal endocrine profiles for mares are given in Section 2.4.2.

Blood samples can also be used to indicate the general health status of a mare, bringing to light specific deficiencies related to diet, low-grade infections, blood loss, cancer and parasite burdens. Low red cell counts (i.e. below 10×10^6 ml^{-1}) indicate anaemia. Pack cell volume is a quick and easy assessment of red blood cell/fluid balance, and normal levels are 40–50%. Assessment of the

colour of the supernatant in the packed cell volume test is also a useful problem indicator. It is normally straw-like in colour, and discoloration can indicate problems: for example, red/pink indicates a breakdown of red cells and release of haemoglobin. Haemoglobin levels themselves are a well-established indicator of anaemia, and levels < 12–17 g l^{-1} indicate problems.

A high white blood cell count above 12,000–14,000 ml^{-1} indicates the presence of disease, in particular infection or cancer. A total protein index (protein content of serum after clotting) of < 15 g l^{-1} indicates blood loss, starvation or liver, kidney or gastrointestinal disease. Fibrinogen levels may also be indicative of abnormalities: high levels > 10 g l^{-1} suggest inflammatory, neoplastic or traumatic disease (Table 8.1; Varner *et al.*, 1991; Pickett, 1993c).

8.9.1. Chromosomal abnormalities

It is reported that 2–3% of the horse population have chromosomal abnormalities (Bugno *et al.*, 2007). Blood samples, or possibly a tissue sample, may be used for chromosomal analysis if genetic abnormalities are suspected (Bowling *et al.*, 1987; McCue, 2008). Genetic abnormalities are numerous and have not all been documented (Section 14.3.2). However, the majority involve the sex chromosomes and include a missing X chromosome, Turner's syndrome (63XO), chimerism or mosaic (63XO: 64XX), sex reversal (64XY) and extra X chromosome (65XXX; Halnan, 1985; Bowling, 1996; Lear and Villagomez, 2011).

8.9.2. Immunological infertility

Most recently blood samples have been used to detect infertility arising from humoral immunity such as anti-sperm antibodies, anti-zona pellucida antibodies, anti-ovarian stroma antibodies plus antibodies against seminal plasma and cauda epididymal extract (Risvanli, 2011). Infertility can also be the result of immunity against GnRH, equine chorionic gonadotrophin (eCG), etc., and can also be detected by a blood sample (Dalin *et al.*, 2002).

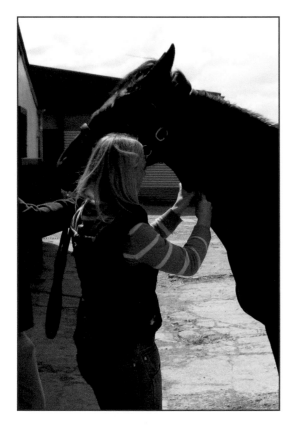

Fig. 8.26. Blood sampling can be a useful tool to assess general well-being as well as specific reproductive issues.

Table 8.1. Blood parameters indicative of disease.

Parameter	Value indicative of disease
Red blood cell count	< 10×10^6 ml^{-1}
Pack cell volume	< 40–50%
White blood cell count	> 12,000–14,000 ml^{-1}
Total protein index	< 15 g l^{-1}
Haemoglobin	< 12–17 g l^{-1}
Fibrinogen	> 10 g l^{-1}

8.10. Conclusion

If more attention were paid to assessment and selection of breeding stock on the basis of reproductive competence, significant amounts of money, time and effort would be saved in trying to breed from sub-fertile or infertile stock. Failure to select fertile stock leads not only to suffering for the mare and stallion, but also to frustration for all. Additionally, many problems are inherited and so will be perpetuated in subsequent generations, to the detriment of the equine population as a whole.

> **Study Questions**
>
> Evaluate the use of rectal palpation and ultrasound to assess the reproductive competence of the mare.
>
> Discuss the criteria that should be considered when selecting a mare based on reproductive competence. Include in your answer a critical evaluation of how reliable these criteria are in predicting the ease with which a mare may be bred.
>
> Critically evaluate the methods that could be used to assess the reproductive competence of a mare.
>
> Evaluate what can be done by a lay person/non-veterinary professional to assess the reproductive competence of a mare.

> Infections are a major cause of infertility in the mare. Critically evaluate what is likely to be observed at a breeding soundness evaluation that would indicate infections and how they may be specifically identified.

Suggested Reading

McCue, P.M. (2008) The Problem Mare: Management Philosophy, Diagnostic Procedures, and Therapeutic Options. *Journal of Equine Veterinary Science* 28(11), 619–626.

Bowman, T.R. (2011) Direct rectal palpation. In: McKinnon, A.O., Squires, E.L., Vaala, E. and Varner, D.D. (eds) *Equine Reproduction*, 2nd edn. Wiley-Blackwell, Philadelphia, London, pp. 1904–1913.

Card, C.E. (2011) Endoscopic examination. In: McKinnon, A.O., Squires, E.L., Vaala, E. and Varner, D.D. (eds) *Equine Reproduction*, 2nd edn. Wiley-Blackwell, Philadelphia, London, pp. 1940–1950.

Love, C.C. (2011) Endometrial biopsy. In: McKinnon, A.O., Squires, E.L., Vaala, E. and Varner, D.D. (eds) *Equine Reproduction*, 2nd edn. Wiley-Blackwell, Philadelphia, London, pp. 1929–1939.

Pycock, J.F. (2011) Ultrasonography. In: McKinnon, A.O., Squires, E.L., Vaala, E. and Varner, D.D. (eds) *Equine Reproduction*, 2nd edn. Wiley-Blackwell, Philadelphia, London, pp. 1914–1921.

Zent, W.W. (2011) History. In: McKinnon, A.O., Squires, E.L., Vaala, E. and Varner, D.D. (eds) *Equine Reproduction*, 2nd edn. Wiley-Blackwell, Philadelphia, London, pp. 1897–1899.

Assad, N.I. and Pandey, A.K. (2015) Different approaches to diagnose uterine pathology in mares : A review. *Theriogenology Insights* 5(3), 157–182.

9

Preparation of the Mare for Breeding

The Objectives of this Chapter are:

To detail the preparation of the mare in the months leading up to breeding.

To apply previous knowledge gained in Chapter 2 to understand how the mare's reproductive activity can be manipulated.

To evaluate the various methods by which the mare's oestrous cycle can be manipulated to ensure that she ovulates at a predetermined time.

To appreciate the various challenges presented when breeding maiden, barren and pregnant mares.

To understand how and why management of the mare prior to breeding can affect reproductive success.

9.1. Introduction

It is essential that preparation of the mare starts in plenty of time prior to covering. It is no use making a last-minute decision that you wish to put a mare in foal and then wondering why she does not conceive. A preparation time of at least 6 months is required to maximize the chance of conception. This Chapter will concentrate mainly on this period, with some reference to any earlier preparation that may be required. Brood mares may be classified as maiden (not previously had a foal), barren (previously had a foal but is currently not pregnant) or brood mare (currently pregnant, having been covered successfully last spring and may or may not currently have a foal at foot). There are some specific aspects of management for these three classes of mares which will be discussed first, followed by general management applicable to all mares.

9.2. Preparation of the Maiden and Barren Mare

If a mare is destined to be a brood mare, then she must be brought up with this aim in mind, with close monitoring of her general condition and growth. Horses normally reach puberty at 10–24 months of age, depending on the breed and their nutritional status in early life (Eilts, 2011). If you are considering breeding a mare at or near puberty, before she has reached her full mature size, then her stage of development and her general condition are of utmost importance. Breeding before attainment of mature body size places the additional burden of pregnancy on the mare as well as that of her own continued growth and development. Provided she is well grown and in good body condition, she should be able to cope with such additional demands, but this must be borne in mind when considering her management throughout pregnancy, especially that of nutrition.

Some maiden mares are bred for the first time relatively late in life, having already had a successful performance career, on the basis of which they have been chosen for breeding. This is to be commended but, in such cases, mares are older and so more set in their ways and have been managed to date as athletes and not as breeding stock. Performance mares must be allowed plenty of time to unwind, both physically and psychologically. This should start during the autumn prior to the planned covering, during which time workloads should be slowly reduced to a maintenance level. This is usually adequate for most horses, although much variation is evident between individuals, and some may take as long as 18 months to adjust. Intensive training is detrimental to reproduction in all mammals; this can be clearly demonstrated in women athletes who regularly fail to ovulate. Mares in peak athletic condition will characteristically demonstrate abnormal oestrous cycles, often showing delayed oestrus, silent heats and oestrous behaviour not accompanied by ovulation. However, given a long enough adjustment period, a mare should start showing regular oestrous cycles and can be mated successfully (Dobson and Smith, 2000; Berghold *et al.*, 2007; Malschitzky *et al.*, 2015).

Careful attention should also be given to the mare's nutrition and, related to that, her exercise (Lawrence, 2011). Mares should be in good, not fat, body condition at covering (Vick *et al.*, 2006; Miyakoshi *et al.*, 2012). The body condition score to aim for at mating is 3 (Section 8.5). In addition, it is generally believed that in maiden and barren mares better conception rates are obtained if they are on a rising plane of nutrition, in particular increasing energy, in the last 4–6 weeks prior to covering; this is termed flushing (Kubiak *et al.*, 1987; Morris *et al.*, 1987; Newcombe and Wilson, 2005; Morley and Murray, 2014). Flushing of barren mares has also been reported to advance the start of the breeding season by as many as 30 days (Newcombe and Wilson, 2005). The best regime is to ensure that the mare is in condition score 2–2.5 in the autumn prior to covering. As the season approaches, her energy intake can be increased gradually by turning her out onto lush grazing or by replacing some of her roughage intake

with concentrates in the last 4–6 weeks before planned covering (Fig. 9.1; Hintz, 1993a; Swinker *et al.*, 1993; Guerin and Wang, 1994; Frape, 1998).

If the mare is young, it may also be pertinent to supplement her diet during this period with protein, calcium, phosphorus and vitamin A. Requirements for these elements are higher in young maiden mares than in mature mares.

Exercise is also important, helping to maintain body condition and prevent obesity. Gentle riding or hacking provide a good form of exercise for maiden or barren mares during the preparation period (Fig. 9.2). All mares should be turned out daily and, ideally, mares (especially those not broken) should live out except in the most inclement weather or be turned out in to fields or specifically designed turnout or loafing areas, providing them with exercise ad libitum (Fig. 9.3).

A period of 6 months' preparation also allows time for a mare to be tested for infection, the appropriate treatment given and full recovery to occur. Any damage due to old infections can be investigated and either assisted in its repair or the mare discarded from the breeding scheme. If she is of sufficient genetic merit, the possibility of embryo transfer (ET) can be investigated, and necessary arrangements made. All barren mares, especially maidens, should be introduced to new handling systems, buildings and surroundings associated with breeding during this period. This is of particular

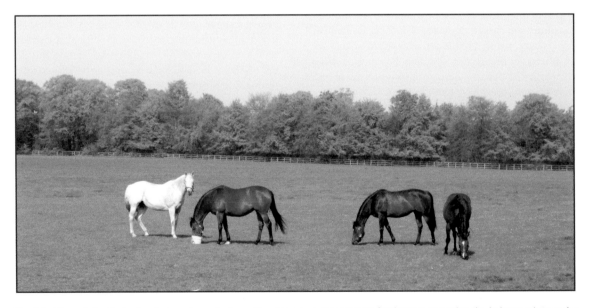

Fig. 9.1. Mares being flushed on lush pasture prior to mating, to encourage optimum fertilization rates; this also helps to advance the breeding season.

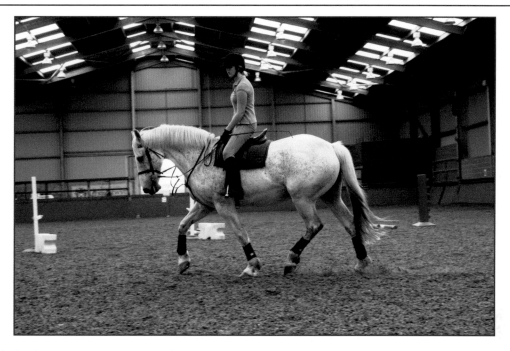

Fig. 9.2. Gentle riding provides ideal exercise for barren mares, to keep them fit for covering and any resultant pregnancy.

importance with ex-performance mares that are usually moved or sold in readiness for their new career. Familiarization with management practices associated with breeding, such as restraint in stocks, rectal palpation, ultrasonic scanning and teasing facilities should also be ensured prior to covering. Barren mares that have been covered several times before need only to be introduced to anything new a few weeks before the season starts. Any changes in diet must be introduced gradually; and also the introduction of new companions should be done early enough to allow a settling-down period and time for a hierarchy to be established (Kaseda *et al.*, 1995). Provided all changes are made gradually, and in good time, stress at covering can be minimized, so maximizing reproductive success.

9.3. Preparation of the Pregnant Mare

Care must also be taken in the preparation of the pregnant mare for re-covering the following spring. However, the presence of a pregnancy due to successful covering last spring limits to a large extent how she can be managed. One advantage with a pregnant mare is that she has seen it all before, at least in the previous year, and so no psychological or physiological adjustment

is required. However, a careful eye should be kept on her condition to prevent over or under condition. In particular, once a pregnant mare becomes overweight, it is very difficult to rectify (especially in late pregnancy) without endangering the fetus. Prevention is, therefore, much better than cure and it is essential that the mare is in a fit condition prior to initial covering and that a condition score of 3 is maintained throughout pregnancy and into her next covering. Flushing of pregnant mares while they are pregnant is not advised, and has no effect – or possibly a detrimental effect – on conception rates on the foal heat (Frape, 1998). If there is a reasonable period of time between foaling and re-covering, this can be used to flush mares and try to adjust body condition. Care must be taken, as alterations in nutrition can affect milk yield and hence the foal at foot. There is conflicting evidence with regard to the effect of nutrition during late pregnancy, and between parturition and foal heat on subsequent conception rates (Jordon, 1982; Henneke *et al.*, 1984; Newcombe and Wilson, 2005). However, it is generally accepted that a condition score of 3 is ideal during this period, and that mares should be fed well in lactation to maximize fertility, but with an eye to preventing obesity (Van Niekerk and Van Niekerk, 1997; Frape, 1998; Lawrence, 2011).

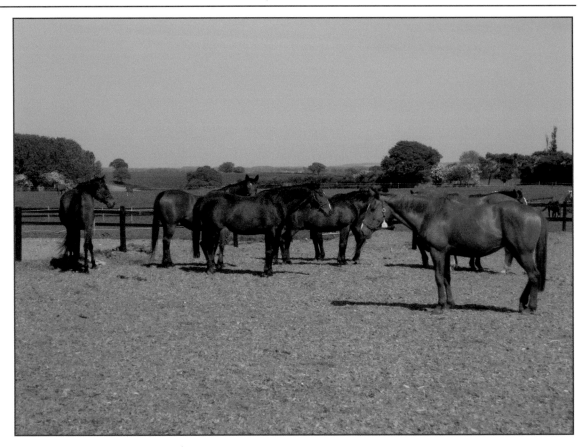

Fig. 9.3. If mares are not broken to ride, they must be turned out into fields or specially designed loafing areas, to provide enough exercise to maintain basic fitness.

Exercise is an important aid in maintaining a body condition score of 3 in the pregnant mare. Pregnant mares can normally be ridden safely up to the 6th month of pregnancy, but this depends on the individual. By the 6th month all strenuous work must be excluded. Mares that are not broken and those in late pregnancy should be turned out every day to help maintain fitness and blood circulation and to prevent boredom (Fig. 9.3). In an ideal world, mares would live out in established groups with plenty of opportunity to exercise; such systems are popular in temperate latitudes without the risk of adverse weather. Exercise not only helps to prevent obesity but also maintains the mare's fitness and muscle tone, both of which will be needed at and after parturition. In the absence of suitable fields, or in inclement weather, mares can be kept in open barns rather than in individual stables, as this allows for established groups to be maintained (Fig. 9.4).

9.4. General Aspects of Preparation for Breeding

In addition to management specific to the three different classes of mare there are a number of things that need to be considered for all mares.

9.4.1. Drugs

Many performance horses may have been on various drug regimes during their performance careers. Plenty of time must be allowed for the body to eliminate these drugs from the system. Corticosteroids, used as anti-inflammatory drugs to treat various injuries, can have seriously detrimental effects on reproductive performance in both stallions and mares (McCue and Ferris, 2011). They can also impair the body's ability to fight infection, which is of particular significance in the mare, hence such drugs are associated with a higher

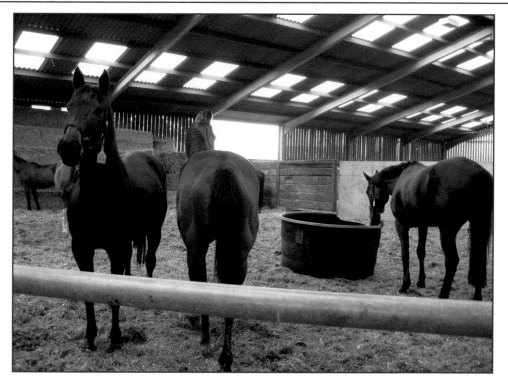

Fig. 9.4. If there are no suitable fields or turnout area, and/or the weather is inclement, then mares can be kept barned; this allows established groups to be maintained.

incidence of endometritis. Additionally, they are associated with a reduction in post-coital endometritis. This is a natural and ubiquitous response in the mare to mating and a means by which she eliminates dead sperm, seminal plasma, detritus, etc., from the uterus post-mating, so ensuring an appropriate uterine environment for the conceptus (Section 14.3.5.3; Ferris and McCue, 2010). The use of anabolic steroids to boost muscle development and hence performance also has severe detrimental effects on reproductive performance and should be eliminated from the animal's system well in advance of the breeding season (Squires *et al.*, 1985b; Maher *et al.*, 1983; Shoemaker *et al.*, 1989). Also, long-term use of progesterone/progestogens, often used to prevent oestrus (and so unpredictable behaviour) in performance mares, is associated with reduced immunological competence and so greater risk of endometritis.

9.4.2. Testing for infections

To prevent transfer of infections that will be detrimental to reproductive performance, testing for infections needs to be carried out.

Prior to covering, all mares – whether maiden, barren or pregnant – should be tested for reproductive tract infections. It is good practice for maiden and barren mares to have clitoral fossa swabs taken during their preparation. If done early enough and the results are positive, then there should be sufficient time for treatment, recovery and retesting before mating. It is the normal practice for many studs to require mares to be swabbed and proven to be clear of infection before being accepted for covering (Ricketts, 2011); indeed, the practice is contained within the Horse Race Betting Levy Board (HBLB) Codes of Practice for Thoroughbred breeders. Different swabbing practices are recommended for high-risk (mares that have been imported or have had previous positive results) and low-risk (all those not classified as high-risk) mares and for those boarding at studs and walking in. It is the responsibility of mare owners to make sure that they know and carry out the swabbing requirements before their mares go to stud. Requirements may change but they are published annually in the HBLB Codes of Practice (2019) and are increasingly being used as the basis for swabbing requirements by other studs and breeds societies. Normally, low-risk mares must have two clean swabs, one from the clitoral fossa before the oestrus of covering, and the second from the endometrium at the oestrus of covering. High-risk mares normally need three swabs: the two that low-risk mares have, with an additional clitoral swab taken before the mare arrives on the stud. All swabs must be sent to approved laboratories; the results are normally available within 48 h and so allow enough time for mares to be covered on the oestrus of testing (Ousey *et al.*, 2009). Swabs are tested primarily for *Taylorella equigenitalis*, the bacterium that causes contagious equine metritis (CEM; Timoney, 2011c), but they are also normally tested for *Klebsiella pneumoniae* and *Pseudomonas aeruginosa*, both venereal disease (VD) bacteria. Other bacteria such as *Escherichia coli*, *Streptococcus zooepidemicus* and *Staphylococcus aureus*, all present in the environment but which may still cause problems, may be also tested for. It must be remembered that, in the UK, CEM is a notifiable disease and, if isolated, must be reported by the testing laboratory to the Divisional Veterinary Manager of the Department for Environment, Food and Rural Affairs (DEFRA). Current codes of practice have largely eliminated the disease in the UK but sporadic incidences do occur (Jackson *et al.*, 2002). Although the other bacterial diseases are not notifiable, if they are identified, covering should immediately stop and advice/treatment sought. Most Thoroughbred studs require the completion of a mare certificate to indicate her previous coverings and any positive swab results. Whatever stud a mare is taken to (except many native pony studs), it is likely that they will require paperwork to confirm that the mare is free of infection. Native pony studs do not, as a rule, require swabbing to take place but this must be checked during stud selection.

Apart from bacterial infection, mares may also need to be tested for viral infections. The HBLB Codes of Practice now also include advice on equine herpes virus (EHV) 1 and 4, as well as on EHV 3 (equine exanthema) and equine viral arteritis (EVA) (Ricketts, 2011; Horse Race Betting Levy Board Codes of Practice, 2019). Since 1995, EVA has also been a notifiable disease. It is advised that all mares are blood-sampled twice at the beginning of the season, at least 14 days apart, to test for antibodies. If no antibodies are present or if the antibody levels are stable or declining, then the mare is free of active infection and is safe to be covered. However, if increasing antibody levels are identified, this means that the mare has an active infection and should not be covered. EHV and strangles (caused by *Streptococcus equi*) can also have disastrous consequences on breeding mares, being highly contagious, and in the case of EHV causing high abortion rates. Neither is notifiable but any mares suspected of having contact with EHV or strangles must be isolated, and certainly not sent to stud, and veterinary advice sought as to whether they can be covered at all that season (Metcalf, 2011). There is currently an effective vaccine for EHV although it is not advised for use in pregnant mares; newly developing vaccines may, however, be safer (MacLachlan *et al.*, 2007).

9.4.3. Nomination forms

Once a stud has been chosen, and during the preparation period for the mare, a nomination form (covering agreement) must be completed. This is a legal agreement between the mare and stallion owner, ensuring that the mare will be covered by that stallion the following spring. Nomination agreements are discussed further in Section 16.3.3.

9.4.4. General preparation

Immediately prior to sending the mare to stud she should at least have her hind shoes removed, be in good physical condition and have up-to-date tetanus and flu vaccination certificates. Some studs will also require that she is vaccinated against EVA, EHV etc., and/or blood tested for EVA, EIA, strangles, etc. She should also be wormed. Such requirements will be stipulated in the Nomination Agreement and it is up to the mare's owner to ensure that they conform to the stud's requirements, otherwise the cover will be refused. Most studs will not require the owner to bring any tack or equipment with the mare, preferring to use their own, to minimize the risk of losing other people's equipment. If the mare arrives at stud in good condition, then it is very likely that she will be returned to in a similar condition.

To have some control over the time of ovulation, and hence the time to cover a mare, many mares have their reproductive activity controlled with hormones. This is particularly the case with Thoroughbred mares where the start of the breeding season is advanced, and in mares covered by artificial insemination (AI). Problem breeders may also be put on hormone programmes under veterinary advice.

9.5. Manipulation of the Oestrous Cycle in the Mare

As the majority of equine matings are today influenced by humans we have, therefore, attempted to control the timing of covering to our advantage. There are several methods by which the timing of mating can be manipulated: first, by altering the beginning of the season; and second, by manipulating the timing of the mare's oestrus and ovulation within that season (Squires, 2008, 2009).

9.5.1. Advancing the breeding season

The horse is classified as a long-day breeder, with a breeding season extending on average from April to November in the northern hemisphere, and from October to May in the southern hemisphere (Section 2.4.1). The Thoroughbred industry, and increasingly other breed societies, registers the birth of all foals on 1 January (northern hemisphere) or 1 July (southern hemisphere), regardless of their actual birth date. It is desirable, therefore, to achieve perceived maximum advantage in the racing and young-stock sales, to ensure that mares foal as soon after 1 January as possible. As mares have an 11-month gestation, they need to be covered in February to achieve this. Hence, the arbitrary (or enforced) breeding season for Thoroughbreds in the northern hemisphere runs from 15 February to 1 July and in the southern hemisphere from 15 August to 1 January. This arbitrary breeding season, therefore, starts well before the natural season. Other breed societies also have similar arbitrary breeding seasons. Even in societies that do not stick to set foal birth dates, there is a desire to have foals born as early as possible in the year, to maximize their development during the showing and event season, and to enhance their chances of success and value at sales.

The existence of an arbitrary breeding season that does not correspond to the natural one is a major limiting factor in breeding mares. Manipulation of the mare's reproductive activity is required to advance the timing of oestrus and ovulation in order to accommodate these artificial limits. There are several means by which the breeding season in the mare may be advanced. These include the use of light or hormone therapy, or a combination of the two.

9.5.1.1. Light treatment

In a population of intensively managed mares only 10% will voluntarily show oestrus and ovulation during the non-breeding season. This figure is much lower for extensively managed feral populations. Artificial manipulation of light, along with nutrition, temperature and close association of mares and stallions, will significantly increase this percentage. Of these environmental factors, manipulation of light is the most successful (Meyers, 1997; Sharp, 2011c).

Light treatment of mares to advance the breeding season is well established and has been used for many years; hence a lot of the research work in the area is quite old. The use of light was pioneered by Burkhardt (1947) with later work by Kooistra and Ginther (1975), among others. Mares can be introduced to a 16 h light/8 h dark regime either suddenly or gradually. Light can be delivered by means of a 100 W light source (ordinary household light bulb) per 4 × 4 m loose box, or equivalent. A slightly lower-watt light source may be used if the stables are lined by reflective material or paint. Light treatment can be started any time from early November onwards; however, it is essential that the mare experiences an initial autumnal reduction in day length prior to light manipulation (Guillaume et al., 2000). Additionally, if light is started too early in the autumn (i.e. 1st October/1st November), it takes longer for the mare to show ovarian activity (100–120 days) compared to 1st December start (70 days), so in practice it is difficult to get mares to show ovarian activity before February (Professor John Newcombe, 2019, personal communication). Commencement of light treatment early in December will result in coat loss within 4 weeks, followed by ovarian activity normally 2–4 weeks later. The season may be advanced by up to 3 months, but there is considerable individual variation (Kooistra and Loy, 1968; Kooistra and Ginther, 1975; Oxender et al., 1977). In general, the earlier in the year light treatment begins, the longer the time interval to oestrus and ovulation. Light treatment from early December is often chosen, as it normally results in ovarian activity during early February. It has been reported that a photosensitive period exists around 01:00–03:00 and that a period of light for 1 h that occurs 8 h after dusk would suffice, resulting in the same effect as 16 continual hours of light (Palmer et al., 1982; Scraba and Ginther, 1985). However, in practice, as the timing of dusk varies it is easier to administer a 16 h block of light than continually move the period of 1 h of light. More recent work has reported good success with the use of short-wavelength blue light directly into the eye of the mare. Walsh et al. (2013) successfully used blue light from light-emitting diodes housed in blinkers on the mare's head, directed towards a single eye, to suppress plasma melatonin concentrations; this was reported to advance the breeding season (Fig. 9.5; Murphy et al., 2014). Further work by Murphy et al. (2014), plus others working on humans (Brainard et al., 2008), indicated

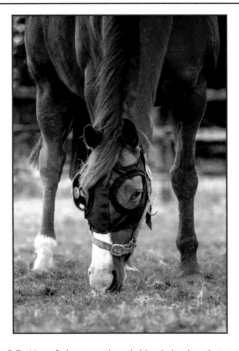

Fig. 9.5. Use of short-wavelength blue light directly into the mare's eye via blinkers to advance the breeding season. (Photo courtesy of Dr Barbara A. Murphy, Head of Equine Science, School of Agriculture and Food Science, University of Dublin, Ireland; Chairman and Founder, Equilume Ltd.)

that blue light is the most effective and that, in horses, low-intensity blue light directed into one eye successfully advances the breeding season. One of the major advantages of this system is that it allows mares to be turned out during this period, which is more natural than traditional housing.

The effects of light manipulation may be enhanced by increases in ambient temperature and nutritional levels, both of which are also associated with spring (Fitzgerald *et al.*, 2002; Gentry *et al.*, 2002b; Scaramuzzi and Martin, 2008). However, the relatively minor effect that temperature and nutrition have on advancing the season means that their use, beyond that of rugging up mares and increasing their energy intake, is not justified (Fig. 9.6; Meyers, 1997). Energy was considered to be the important nutritional component, but work by Van Niekerk and Van Niekerk (1997) suggested that protein is also of importance. Stallion effect, via pheromone and vocal stimuli, has also been reported to have an additional influence on advancing the season (Scaramuzzi and Martin, 2008). It is, therefore, advocated by some that stallions should be housed on the same yard

as, or near to, mares during January/February in order to enhance the effect of light treatment (Wespi *et al.*, 2014).

Despite the success of using lights to advance the breeding season, recent work has raised some concerns about how this may negatively impact on foal birth weight and development. Some workers report that mares under lights to advance their season have shorter gestation length, resulting in foals with lighter birth weights, and poorer subsequent growth rates (Kocher and Staniar, 2013; Beythien *et al.*, 2017; Nolan *et al.*, 2017). If such an association is evident this may make breeders rethink the long-held demand for early foals in the belief they will perform better and command higher prices at the sales.

Although light treatment is very successful in advancing the season, the timing of response within a group of mares is very variable. In an attempt to reduce this variation the use of hormone treatment has been investigated.

9.5.1.2. Exogenous hormonal treatment

The use of exogenous hormones to induce out-of-season breeding is very successful in anoestrous ewes and, as such, is a useful management tool (McCue *et al.*, 2007b). Unfortunately, the anoestrous mare's ovary appears relatively insensitive to exogenous hormone therapy. Treatment with equine chorionic gonadotrophin (eCG), human chorionic gonadotrophin (hCG) or follicle-stimulating hormone (FSH) by single or multiple injection, as used in other livestock, results in little if any response. However, natural crude equine pituitary extract (containing natural FSH and luteinizing hormone (LH)), if injected daily over a period of 2 weeks, does induce oestrus in the non-breeding season (Douglas *et al.*, 1974; Lapin and Ginther, 1977). Such a long period of treatment is required as the mare's ovary apparently requires a prolonged period of gonadotrophin stimulation in order to develop follicles adequately so that they can react to an ovulating agent (Section 2.4.2). Short-term treatments will not develop follicles to an adequate stage to allow them to react to any ovulation stimulus.

Gonadotrophin-Releasing Hormone

As some limited success had been achieved using natural pituitary extract, the use of gonadotrophin-releasing hormone (GnRH), naturally responsible for inducing

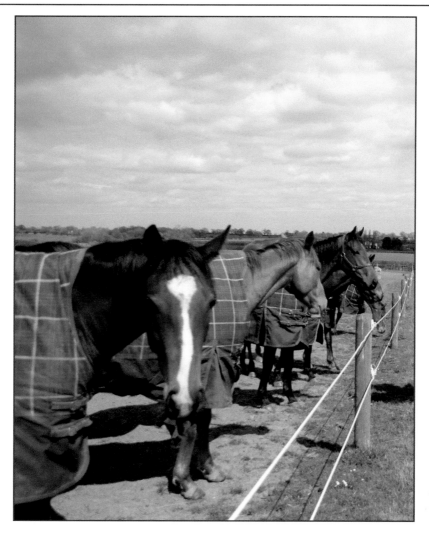

Fig. 9.6. Rugging up mares and increasing nutritional intake enhances the effect of light treatment in advancing the breeding season.

FSH and LH production by the pituitary, was investigated (Harrison *et al.*, 1990). As noted, prolonged stimulus of the pituitary is required, and so GnRH is administered as a series of injections or via infusion, mini pumps or subcutaneous (often vulval) implants, all of which have been reported to give some success (Ainsworth and Hyland, 1991; Harrison *et al.*, 1991; Mumford *et al.*, 1994; Camillo *et al.*, 2004). GnRH is now commercially available as an artificial analogue, most commonly as Deslorelin, but also as Buserelin and Histrelin. As with all artificial analogues, their potency is much greater than that of the natural hormone; in the case of GnRH the analogue Histrelin can be as much as 200 times more potent (although the most commonly

used analogue, Deslorelin, is only 114 times more potent, and this is reflected in the dose rates administered (Conn and Crowley, 1994). Licensed use of GnRH analogues varies with country (Lindholm *et al.*, 2012; Voge *et al.*, 2012). Despite this, GnRH analogues have been used with some success in commercial practice (Jochle and Trigg, 1994; Farquhar *et al.*, 2000; Morehead *et al.*, 2001; Briant *et al.*, 2004), especially in mares in the transition period from anoestrus to the breeding season (Hyland, 1993; Gentry *et al.*, 2002b; Raz *et al.*, 2009). The development of a longer-acting single injection of GnRH (Deslorelin) further enhanced the commercial use of artificial GnRH (Farquhar *et al.*, 2000).

Further development of the use of GnRH involved its inclusion in a hormone regime mimicking the natural concentrations of FSH, LH and progesterone in the normal oestrous cycle: a single injection of GnRH followed by daily injections of progesterone for 8 days. This regime is repeated twice more to give three artificial mini-oestrous cycles. This treatment, although not effective in mares in deep anoestrus, is reasonably successful in the transitional period (Farquhar *et al.*, 2000; Morehead *et al.*, 2001).

Progesterone

Progesterone has been used to induce oestrus and ovulation in anoestrous mares, but also seems only to be effective in the transition period (Alexander and Irvine, 1991; Handler *et al.*, 2006; Norman *et al.*, 2006). It is known that it is the decline in progesterone prior to ovulation that encourages LH and FSH release, which then drives final follicle maturation and ovulation. At the beginning of the season there is no such (or only limited) progesterone decline and the reaction, in terms of concentration of LH and FSH release, is limited. Ovulation, therefore, does not occur, or occurs in the absence of oestrus. The resulting corpus luteum (CL) of any such ovulations is often incompetent, and only at the second ovulation of the season are acceptable conception rates achieved. Therefore, if progesterone is artificially administered and then withdrawn, this mimics the natural decline in progesterone and helps induce the normal increase in LH and FSH required for ovulation and results in a competent CL (Cuervo-Arango and Clark, 2010). Ovulation accompanied by oestrus is then seen to occur within 7–10 days of cessation of a 10–12 days' progesterone treatment period; again, the best response is obtained in the transition period (Handler *et al.*, 2006; Norman *et al.*, 2006; Hanlon and Firth, 2012).

Progesterone is commonly used in the management of breeding mares; it is available in numerous forms and can be administered in various ways (Pinto, 2011). Traditionally, it was administered as an artificial progestogen (altrenogest) either orally (Regumate®, DPT Laboratories, San Antonio, Texas, USA) or via intramuscular injection, and in many countries altrenogest is the only approved progesterone drug for horses (Pinto, 2011). More recently it has been available for administration via a progesterone-releasing intravaginal device (PRID; Fig. 9.7; and PRID Delta; Newcombe 2002; Handler *et al.*, 2006; Crabtree *et al.*, 2018), controlled internal drug-releasing device (CIDR; Fig. 9.8a,b;

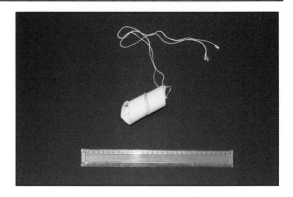

Fig. 9.7. A progesterone-releasing intravaginal device (PRID) can be placed in the mare's vagina for a set length of time as a method of administering progesterone.

Lubbeke *et al.*, 1994), sponges (Dinger *et al.*, 1981) or Cue-mare® (Bioniche Animal Health, Vetoquinol, Ontario, Canada; Grimmett *et al.*, 2002), all of which are impregnated with natural progesterone (rather than progestogen) and placed within the mare's vagina for the treatment period. Oestrus and ovulation post-progesterone treatment (PRID, CIDR and Cue-mare®) are reported to be quicker than post-progestogen treatment (Regumate® or injection), by virtue of the fact that natural progesterone allows some folliculogenesis to continue during treatment (Newcombe, 2002). Additionally, the elevated systemic progesterone levels resulting from treatment with PRID, CIDR or Cue-mare® decline over time, as the finite amount of progesterone within the devices is absorbed. This further ensures that significant follicle development can occur, especially towards the end of the treatment period, prior to their removal. The interval from the end of treatment to oestrus and ovulation is reported to be 5–10 days for PRID and CIDR compared with 8–10 days for Regumate® (Squires, 1993a,b; Arbeiter *et al.*, 1994; Newcombe and Wilson, 1997; Newcombe, 2002). In contrast, progestogen (Regumate® or injection) appears to depress follicular activity, which can only resume after the end of treatment, hence a longer interval to oestrus and ovulation. Intravaginal sponges, PRID and CIDR have the advantage of being labour-saving, and require only to be inserted and removed. They also ensure that a standard dose is administered. However, they can be lost and can cause vaginitis which, although of no real consequence to conception, looks unsightly. In common with these, the advantage of injection is that you can be assured that each mare has received her allotted dose.

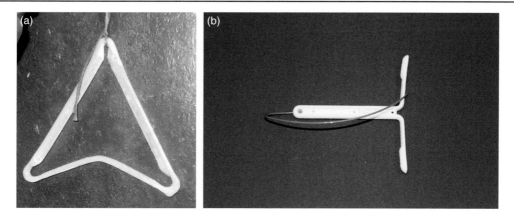

Fig. 9.8. A CIDR can similarly be used to administer progesterone to a mare by inserting into the vagina for a set period of time. Two different types of CIDR (a) and (b) are shown, both with the same function.

However, it is more expensive, especially when you consider the costs of the veterinary attendance, now required by law in the UK and many other countries, for the administration of injections to horses. Additionally, some horses do not tolerate repeat injections and there maybe problems with repeated injection sites. Oral administration (Regumate®) has the advantage that no vet is required, but some mares may refuse to take the feed in which it is mixed. If only part of the food is eaten, it is impossible to know how much progestogen has been ingested. Furthermore, all mares have to be dosed individually. While considering the use of progesterone, it is worth noting that its use has been associated with a decrease in neutrophil production in response to a bacterial challenge. This may well be of significance for mares with poor perineal conformation or a history of uterine infections and is a disadvantage of long-term use; hence, the recommended length of progesterone treatment is now much reduced (10 days rather than 15–20 days). Additionally, this presents a potential problem to animals such as in performance mares where it is used to suppress reproductive activity during competition periods (Pinto, 2011).

Prostaglandins

A further alternative investigated for use in late anoestrous mares is prostaglandin F2α (PGF2α), administered in a series of 2–3 injections at 48-h intervals. PGF2α is luteolytic in nature; that is, it destroys the CL and terminates the luteal phase of the cycle. In the natural cycle, in the absence of a pregnancy, prostaglandin is produced at a specific time (14 days) post-ovulation. As such, it both marks and causes the termination of the luteal phase and the commencement of the endogenous hormone changes associated with oestrus and ovulation (Section 2.4.2; Staempfli, 2011). It is this association with the termination of one cycle and commencement of the next which is exploited in this treatment. Ovulation has been reported in 73% of mares treated in this way in the transition period (Jochle *et al.*, 1987), but success is limited, and so PGF2α is not generally used on its own to advance the breeding season.

Prostaglandin is widely used in general mare breeding management and can be administered as natural prostaglandin (dinoprost) or prostaglandin analogue (cloprostenol); fluprostenol or the longer-acting fenprostalene are also prostaglandin analogues but are no longer commercially available (Staempfli, 2011). Prostaglandin, in particular prostaglandin analogue, does have some side effects including smooth muscle activation. Its use may, therefore, be linked to increased gastrointestinal activity, manifested as diarrhoea, sweating and possibly slight caudal ataxia (neurological uncoordination; LeBlanc, 1995; Nie *et al.*, 2001a; Coffman and Pinto, 2016). These side effects vary with the analogue used and the individual mare; however, provided the recommended dose rate is not exceeded, they are not serious. Additionally, more recent work would suggest that lower dose levels can be just as effective as higher traditional doses and have fewer side effects (Irvine *et al.*, 2002; Barker *et al.*, 2006; Coffman and Pinto, 2016).

Prolactin and Dopamine Antagonists

A link between prolactin and seasonal breeding activity is likely but the exact nature of this association is unclear.

It is thought by some to involve dopamine (a neuro-transmitter produced in the brain) which actively inhibits the secretion of prolactin and GnRH, both of which are involved in driving follicle development (Section 2.4.2; Melrose *et al.*, 1990; Bennett *et al.*, 1998; Tibary, 2011a). Elevated prolactin and suppressed dopamine concentrations are characteristic of the breeding season. Treating anoestrous mares with prolactin results in rapid follicle development. As prolactin receptors have been identified on large follicles it is likely that prolactin has an effect at the level of the ovary (Bennett *et al.*, 1998). If mares in the transition period (January time) are treated with a dopamine antagonist (which acts to remove dopamine from the system and so allows prolactin and GnRH to increase), such as sulfide or domperidone, many show advancement in their first ovulation of the year (Brendemuehl and Cross, 2000; Daels *et al.*, 2000; King *et al.*, 2008; Panzani *et al.*, 2011). However, not all mares respond and there is a significant variation in the timing of response. If light treatment (16 h day^{-1}) is introduced 2 weeks prior to dopamine antagonist treatment, a better and tighter response is obtained (Daels *et al.*, 2000). Neither of these treatment protocols is currently used in stud practice but may hold the key to future hormonal treatments.

Combination Hormone Treatments

In order to try and improve the success of hormone treatments, combinations of hormones have been used with some better success. For example Norman *et al.* (2006) reported good results with a combination of PRID, oestrogens and PGF2α, as did Newcombe *et al.* (2002) using PRIDs with hCG or GnRH. However, despite their reported better results, the increased costs of every additional hormone treatment mean that many of these hormone regimes are not commercially

viable as part of routine management, although they may be useful for individual mares. Although hormone treatment can time oestrus and ovulation more precisely than light treatment, it is only successful when the mare is in the transition period. The limitation of hormone treatment, therefore, is that it cannot be used with mares in deep anoestrus.

9.5.1.3. Combination light and hormone treatments

The use of light to advance the season is very successful but gives variability in timing of response. On the other hand, hormone therapy appears to work effectively and allow the relatively precise timing of oestrus and ovulation, but will only work in the transition period. A combination of the two may, therefore, be successful. Indeed, light therapy can advance mares into the transition period and then exogenous hormones can be used to time oestrus and ovulation more precisely. Progesterone alone, plus light treatment, can be successful. Light treatment (16 h light and 8 h dark) should be introduced during November/December in the northern hemisphere (May/June in the southern hemisphere), followed by progesterone for a period of 10–15 days from early to mid-January (July) onwards (Heeseman *et al.*, 1980; Scheffrahn *et al.*, 1980; Burns *et al.*, 2008; Squires, 2008, 2011b). There is individual variability in mares' responses, however. Table 9.1 gives an example of such a regime. The exact timing of the progesterone treatment depends on when covering is planned and when light treatment is commenced.

Some of the best and most consistent results have been obtained using a similar regime but with the addition of PGF2α: 16 h light and 8 h dark for 6–8 weeks, followed by 10 days' progesterone treatment; PGF2α is then administered on the last day of progesterone

Table 9.1. The advancement of oestrus and ovulation in the mare, using light treatment and progesterone supplementation (considerable variation in an individual mare's response may be observed).

Time	Drug to be administered/event
Day 0 (15 December)	Light treatment commenced 16 h light/8 h dark
Day 28 (12 January)	Coat loss in mare may be apparent
Day 42 (26 January)	Ovarian activity may be apparent
Day 43 (27 January)	Progesterone treatment started
Day 55 (8 February)	Progesterone treatment stopped
Day 60 + (13 February)	Oestrus commences
Day 63 + (15 February)	Ovulation may occur – covering/AI

treatment to induce luteolysis of any naturally occurring CL (Lopez-Bayghen *et al.*, 2008).

Although there are, in theory, very many ways of advancing the breeding season in the mare, most are too expensive and time-consuming to make them commercially viable and often achieve unreliable results. In practice, most commercial studs just use light treatment, possibly supplemented by rugging up mares, increasing nutritional intake and then possibly Regumate® (progestogen) treatment in the transition period.

9.5.2. Synchronization and timing of oestrus and ovulation

In addition to advancing the breeding season, there are many other reasons for manipulating the timing of oestrus, mainly related to easing mare management. In many countries, such as South America and the USA, mares are run in large herds that roam over vast tracts of land. In such systems, handling needs to be kept to a minimum. It would, therefore, be ideal if mares could all be treated in batches right through from conception to birth and foal rearing. For this to be successful a reliable and exact method of timing ovulation and oestrus is required. If this could be achieved it would also alleviate the need for teasing, rectal palpation, scanning, etc., and would be most useful in conjunction with AI. Such treatment would also allow the ovulation and oestrus of a single mare to be timed precisely, again to ease her management, but would be specifically useful for AI and ET. It also allows closer management of stallion workloads to both natural service and AI.

The methods used to time or synchronize oestrus and ovulation work on the principle of either artificially prolonging and then terminating the luteal phase (progesterone), or of prematurely terminating the natural luteal phase (PGF2α) of the oestrous cycle, or of variations on these two themes (Fig. 9.9).

9.5.2.1. Progesterone

Progesterone supplementation and subsequent withdrawal may be used to time oestrus and ovulation. The use of progesterone or one of its progestogen analogues works on the principle of imitating the mare's natural dioestrus or luteal phase. This is achieved by mimicking natural progesterone production through the administration of exogenous progesterone/progestogens. Termination of this artificial luteal state, achieved by the cessation of treatment, acts like the end of the natural luteal phase and so induces the changes in the mare's endogenous hormones responsible for oestrus and ovulation.

Within 2–3 days of progesterone supplementation, a mare will normally cease all oestrous activity, which will remain suppressed until treatment is terminated (Storer *et al.*, 2009; Bradecamp, 2011a). After 15 days' treatment, oestrous behaviour is apparent at 2–4 days and ovulation at 4–6 days post-progesterone withdrawal (Table 9.2). If progestogen analogues are used, the time intervals are longer: nearer 10–20 days (the interval to oestrous behaviour beginning) and 10–12 days (the interval to ovulation) (Newcombe and Wilson, 1997). As discussed in Section 9.5.1.2, there are various methods of administering progesterone. Generally, treatment is either with artificial progestogen (which tends to inhibit reproductive activity completely) or with natural progesterone (which, as in normal dioestrus, allows some follicular development to occur). Hence, the mare returns to oestrus and ovulation sooner after progesterone than after progestogen treatment. Conception rates post-progesterone/progestogen treatment are comparable to those associated with naturally occurring oestrus (Handler *et al.*, 2006). Traditionally, long periods of progesterone supplementation were used, up to 20 days, and although oestrus was suppressed, ovulation occasionally did occur during treatment. Hence, the timing of ovulation was not that successful. Additionally, it is known that prolonged progesterone treatment is associated with an increase in endometritis due to suppression in the neutrophil defence mechanism. For this reason, and particularly in mares prone to endometritis, shorter periods of progesterone supplementation (8–12 days) are now advocated. As such, the period of progesterone supplementation may not be long enough to ensure that the natural CL has regressed in all mares, and a combination of progesterone supplementation and prostaglandin treatment is, therefore, used.

9.5.2.2. Prostaglandins

Natural PGF2α or one of its analogues (Section 9.5.1.2) provides a successful means of timing oestrus and ovulation in the mare (LeBlanc, 1995; Staempfli, 2011). As discussed, PGF2α both marks and causes the termination of the luteal phase and the commencement of the endogenous hormone changes associated with oestrus and ovulation (see Section 2.4.2.7). Administration of exogenous prostaglandins, provided it is within certain time limits in the luteal phase, allows its termination to be controlled and with it the timing of oestrus and ovulation, normally 4–7 days and 8–11 days

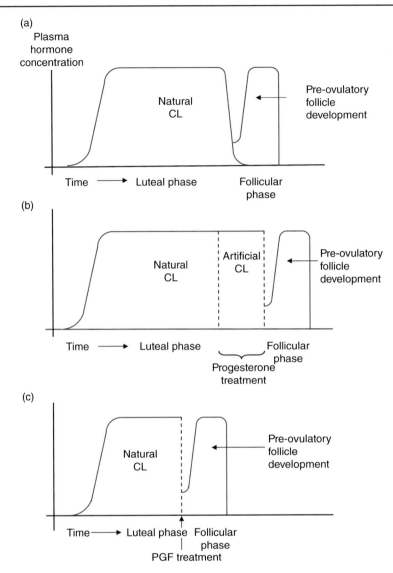

Fig. 9.9. Methods to synchronize or time oestrus and ovulation: (a) the natural cycle; (b) artificially prolonging and then terminating the luteal phase of the cycle (progesterone treatment); or (c) prematurely terminating the natural luteal phase (PGF2α). CL, corpus luteum; conc., concentration; PGF, prostaglandin F.

post-injection, respectively (Barker *et al.*, 2006; Samper, 2008; Staempfli, 2011).

The success of prostaglandin in timing oestrus in the mare is variable and depends upon the stage of the cycle. The CL of most mares is largely refractory to prostaglandin treatment prior to day 5 of the cycle. The best response is normally obtained when treatment is given between days 6 and 9 (Bergfeldt *et al.*, 2006), with oestrus and ovulation occurring at 5–7 and 8–11 days,

respectively (Bradecamp, 2011a). To be successful, the treatment must not only terminate the luteal phase but also induce ovulation. Considerable variation exists between the time of prostaglandin treatment and ovulation; a range of 24 h to 11 days has been reported (Staempfli, 2011). The time interval is determined by the stage of follicular development at treatment. Follicles 3–4 cm or greater in diameter ovulate, on average, within 4 days, although considerable variation is reported. If the follicle ovulates within 72 h it is often accompanied by an abbreviated oestrus or no oestrus at all. Occasionally, when a large follicle is present, prostaglandin treatment results in the regression of that follicle and the development and subsequent ovulation of another follicle from the next follicular wave; hence, there is a longer time interval between treatment and ovulation (longer than 8 days). The most consistent results are obtained when treating mares earlier in the cycle with small follicles (less than 3–4 cm in diameter), as less variation exists and the interval to oestrus followed by ovulation is on average 6 days (Table 9.3).

The previously described use of prostaglandin relies upon a single injection, the major disadvantage of which is that the stage of the mare's oestrous cycle must be known. In smaller intensive studs, where individual mares are monitored, this may present no problems. However, in large groups of mares kept in herd situations, or in mares whose stage of the oestrous cycle is unknown, a double injection of prostaglandin is required. These two prostaglandin injections need to be administered 14–15 days apart (Table 9.4). In this regime all mares between days 5 and 14 of the oestrous cycle will react to the first prostaglandin injection and will ovulate on average within the next 5–9 days. All

those mares between day 15 and ovulation will naturally ovulate anyway in the next 5 days. This leaves the remaining mares, those between days 0 and 5, which will not react to the prostaglandin injection as they do not have a fully functional CL. So, in 14–15 days' time when the second prostaglandin injection is given, the majority of mares are likely to then be between days 5 and 16 of the cycle and so the vast majority will react to the second prostaglandin injection (Bradecamp *et al.*, 2007; Staempfli, 2011).

The majority of mares are reported to commence oestrus 5–10 days after the second injection. However, the synchrony and timing of ovulation is still very variable, and ovulation may occur anywhere between 0 and 17 days after the second injection (Squires, 1993a,b; Bradecamp, 2007, 2011a). Hence, it is not advocated for use when tight synchrony or precise ovulation is required (e.g. AI or ET).

9.5.2.3. Human chorionic gonadotrophin

Further refinement of these protocols includes the use of hCG, a human placental gonadotrophin with LH- and FSH-like properties (Newcombe, 2011b). As such, it enhances and supplements the natural release of gonadotrophins, which drive follicular development and, more specifically, ovulation. Its addition has been advocated to hasten ovulation and reduce the duration of oestrus (Table 9.5; Harrison *et al.*, 1991; Vanderwall *et al.*, 2001).

Several timings for the injection of hCG have been advocated, most of them between 4 and 6 days after the second prostaglandin injection. Up to 90% of mares are reported to ovulate within 72 h of an hCG injection; however, there is much variation in response (Yurdaydin *et al.* 1993; Newcombe 2011a). It has been advocated that hCG be used twice, on day 7 (7 days after the first PGFα) and on day 21 (7 days after the second

Table 9.2. The timing of oestrus and ovulation in the mare, using progesterone supplementation (considerable variation in an individual mare's response may be observed).

Time	Drug to be administered/event
Days 0–14	Progesterone supplementation (intravaginal sponges or PRID)
Day 17 onwards	Oestrus
Day 19 onwards	Ovulation may occur – covering/AI

PRID, progesterone intravaginal device; AI, artificial insemination.

Table 9.3. The timing of oestrus and ovulation in the mare, using a single injection of prostaglandin (considerable variation in an individual mare's response may be observed).

Time	Drug to be administered/event
Day 0	Oestrus
Day 7	Prostaglandin
Day 12	Oestrus commences
Day 15	Ovulation may occur – covering/AI

AI, artificial insemination.

Table 9.4. The timing of oestrus and ovulation in the mare, using two injections of prostaglandin (considerable variation in an individual mare's response may be observed, particularly in the timing of ovulation).

Time	Drug to be administered/event
Day 0	Prostaglandin
Day 14	Prostaglandin
Day 20	Oestrus commences
Day 22	Ovulation may occur – covering/AI

AI, artificial insemination.

PGF2α injection; Table 9.6). The aim of this is to encourage the development of competent CL from the first prostaglandin injection, which would then react with less variation to the second prostaglandin injection. This regime is reported to result in up to 95% of mares ovulating on either day 22 or 23 but, again, variation in response is observed (Voss, 1993). The biggest challenge and likely cause of the reported variation in response is the inability of the follicle to react to hCG until it is mature enough to do so. The prior use of prostaglandin to eliminate the CL, and so time the start of final follicular development, certainly reduces the variability in the stage of follicle maturity when hCG is subsequently administered. It does not eliminate it, however, and so several follicles may not be mature enough to react to the hCG injection (Barbacini *et al.*, 2000; McCue *et al.*, 2004; Newcombe, 2011a).

Not only can hCG be used in combined hormone regimes to synchronize or time ovulation, but it is very often used alone in commercial practice, to control the

Table 9.5. The timing of oestrus and ovulation in the mare, using two injections of prostaglandin and a single injection of hCG (considerable variation in an individual mare's response may be observed).

Time	Drug to be administered/event
Day 0	Prostaglandin
Day 14	Prostaglandin
Day 20	Oestrus commences
Day 21	hCG
Day 23	Ovulation may occur – covering/AI

hGC, human chorionic gonadotrophin; AI, artificial insemination.

Table 9.6. The timing of oestrus and ovulation in the mare, using two injections of prostaglandin and two injections of hCG (considerable variation in an individual mare's response may be observed).

Time	Drug to be administered/event
Day 0	Prostaglandin
Day 7	hCG
Day 14	Prostaglandin
Day 20	Oestrus commences
Day 21	hCG
Day 23	Ovulation may occur – covering/AI

hCG, human chorionic gonadotrophin; AI, artificial insemination.

precise timing of ovulation in mares cycling naturally but which are monitored closely using ultrasonic scanning (Section 10.2.2.2). hCG is then administered once a large pre-ovulatory follicle (a follicle beginning to soften and with a diameter of 3.5 cm or greater) has been identified. As indicated previously, the ability of the follicle to react to hCG is determined by its maturity. While maturity is linked somewhat to follicle size there is considerable variation between breeds and mares in the correlation between follicle size and adequate maturity to react to hCG. Mature follicle size is normally reported to be around 3.5–4 cm in diameter but may range from 3 cm to 7 cm (Samper *et al.*, 2002; Newcombe, 2011a; Sauberli, 2013). Normal dose rates are 2000–2500 international units (IU) administered intravenously (IV) or intramuscularly (IM) (Barbacini *et al.*, 2000; Berezowski *et al.*, 2004) although dose rates as low as 750 IU are reported to be just as effective (Davies Morel and Newcombe, 2008). Up to 90% of mares treated with hCG are reported to ovulate in 24–48 h, allowing the timing of mating/AI (McKinnon *et al.*, 1997; Barbacini *et al.*, 2000; Samper *et al.*, 2002; Newcombe, 2011a; Newcombe and Cuervo-Arango, 2016; Phetudomsinsuk, 2017). The use of hCG is also reported to be associated with increased fertility rates (Vanderwall *et al.*, 2001); however, this is likely not to be an effect of hCG per se but due to the better synchronization of covering and ovulation that the treatment affords. As such, it is popular in studs with mares being covered by high-value stallions with high workloads, allowing these to be managed more efficiently. It is now also normal practice to 'walk mares in', having identified at home that they are oestrus. Treatment with hCG will then ensure better synchronization of arrival at the stud to ovulation and stallion availability, reducing the necessity for repeat visits, which are often over a long distance. Although successful in inducing ovulation, particularly when used in the presence of a mature follicle, there are two reported disadvantages of hCG: (i) an increase in multiple ovulation rates (Perkins and Grimmett, 2001; Veronesi *et al.*, 2003), although this is not supported by other workers (Davies Morel and Newcombe, 2008); and (ii) the reported association between repeated administration and the development of antibodies to hCG rendering the mare refractory to hCG (Wilson *et al.*, 1990; Green *et al.*, 2007). Although this effect is not reported to be a problem by others (Barbacini *et al.*, 2000; Evans *et al.*, 2006; Newcombe and Wilson, 2007), it is yet to be reported whether dose rates affect the antigenic response. In the light of these reported disadvantages, GnRH and its analogues have been suggested for use in its place.

9.5.2.4. Gonadotrophin-releasing hormone

GnRH acts to stimulate the natural release of LH and FSH from the anterior pituitary. As such, its administration as a series of multiple injections (four at 12-h intervals) or via a subcutaneous implant has been demonstrated to significantly advance the onset of ovulation in mares with follicles greater than 3.5 cm in diameter (Table 9.7).

Success rates of 88–100% of mares ovulating within 48 h of treatment (with Deslorelin) have been reported (Meinert *et al.*, 1993; Jochle and Trigg, 1994; Mumford *et al.*, 1995; Miki *et al.*, 2016; Dias *et al.*, 2018). It has been suggested that GnRH may be more successful than hCG in inducing ovulation in larger, thicker-walled follicles. Additionally, because of its smaller molecules, GnRH may also have the possible advantage of being less likely to induce refractoriness of response due to antibody formation (Mumford *et al.*, 1995). As seen with hCG (Section 9.5.2.3), GnRH can also be used with prostaglandin to time oestrus and ovulation. Results have been variable, but it is generally accepted that the timing of ovulation as a result of prostaglandin plus GnRH treatment is similar to that with hCG, and more precise than with the use of prostaglandin alone (McCue *et al.*, 2002; Newcombe and Cuervo-Arango, 2016; Dias *et al.*, 2018). The regime suggested in Table 9.7 is, therefore, another feasible alternative to time ovulation. When compared to hCG, however, the interval to ovulation is reported by some to be longer (McCue *et al.*, 2002).

Table 9.7. The timing of oestrus and ovulation in the mare, using two injections of prostaglandin and GnRH implant (considerable variation in individual mare's response may be observed).

Time	Drug to be administered/event
Day 0	Prostaglandin
Day 15	Prostaglandin
Day 19	Oestrus commences
Day 21	GnRH implant
Day 23	Ovulation may occur – covering/AI

GnRH, gonadotrophin-releasing hormone; AI, artificial insemination.

As with hCG, much of the current commercial use of GnRH is in mares during their natural oestrous period, to time ovulation in closely monitored mares, rather than within a synchronized oestrous regime. Use of GnRH alone to induce ovulation, as discussed for hCG, is reported to be successful. A single injection given to a mare with a follicle greater than 3.5 cm in diameter is reported to result in ovulation in up to 90% of mares in about 40 h (McKinnon *et al.*, 1997; McCue *et al.*, 2002; Newcombe and Cuervo-Arango, 2016; Dias *et al.*, 2018).

9.5.2.5. Recombinant equine LH

Recombinant LH (rLH) can be used in the same way as hCG and GnRH and the mare is reported to run a much lower risk of developing antibodies due to its smaller molecular weight. As with hCG and GnRH ovulation occurs, on average, at 48 h after injection (Yoon *et al.*, 2007). As yet rLH is not commercially available.

9.5.2.6. Combination treatments

Several combination treatments are used, some of which have already been mentioned. Two most commonly used and not previously discussed in detail are progesterone and prostaglandin, and progesterone and oestradiol.

Progesterone and Prostaglandin

Combination treatments of progesterone and prostaglandin are increasingly popular; they improve the timing of ovulation and may reduce the length of progesterone supplementation required. Administration of progesterone for 20 days is very likely to ensure that, on termination of progesterone treatment, any natural Cl will have already regressed and so post-progesterone treatment ovulation rate is acceptable. In the natural cycle PGF2α drives the demise of CL, so prostaglandin administration on the day progesterone treatment ceases ensures that any natural CL will be eliminated. This results in oestrus commencing 24–48 h later, followed by ovulation on days 3–6 post-PGF2α injection (Blanchard *et al.*, 1992). Today, owing to concern over the suspected side effects of long-term progesterone treatment, administration of progesterone is normally only for 8–10 days. This means that, for some mares, there is a risk that their natural CL will still be functioning when progesterone treatment is finished. Hence, using this protocol (Table 9.8), oestrus occurs 3–4 days earlier and with better synchrony than for progesterone treatment alone. However, these reported timings are average and disguise significant variability, ovulation being reported to occur up to 8–15 days after prostaglandin injection. This variation appears greater with shorter-term progesterone supplementation, especially during the early breeding season (Lofstedt and Patel, 1989; Bradecamp, 2011a).

Progesterone and Oestradiol

Used in combination, oestradiol and progesterone give a more profound negative feedback on LH and FSH release, and hence tighter synchrony at the end of treatment. Both hormones may be administered daily via intramuscular injection for 10 days; or, more commonly and easily, by using PRIDs containing progesterone plus 10 mg oestradiol (held within a gelatin capsule) inserted for 10 days. This may be followed, as in the previous protocols, with an injection of PGF2α at the end of the treatment (Table 9.9). It has proved to be successful, with more than 80% of treated mares ovulating 10–12 days post-PGF2α injection (Newcombe *et al.*, 2002; Card *et al.*, 2003; Norman *et al.*, 2006; Sudderth *et al.*, 2013). Normal

Table 9.8. The timing of oestrus and ovulation in the mare using progesterone supplementation, plus prostaglandin (considerable variation in an individual mare's response may be observed).

Time	Drug to be administered/event
Days 0–8	Progesterone supplementation (intravaginal sponges or PRID)
Day 8	Prostaglandin
Day 12	Oestrus
Day 16 onwards	Ovulation may occur – covering/AI

PRID, progesterone-releasing intravaginal device; AI, artificial insemination.

Table 9.9. The timing of oestrus and ovulation in the mare, using progesterone and oestradiol treatment followed by prostaglandin (considerable variation in an individual mare's response may be observed).

Time	Drug to be administered/event
Days 0–10	Progesterone and oestradiol treatment
Day 10	Prostaglandin
Day 14	Oestrus
Day 20	Ovulation may occur – AI

AI, artificial insemination.

pregnancy rates have been reported to AI after such treatment (Jasko *et al.*, 1993b). Further refinement of PRIDs, or the development of slow-release subcutaneous capsules, may further enhance the use of such combination treatments and remove the need for time-consuming daily injections. Some success has also been reported with a single injection of oestradiol at PRID insertion (Norman *et al.*, 2006). Although successful, the commercial availability of progesterone/oestradiol preparations is very limited and so it is rarely used in practice.

hCG or GnRH are also increasingly used with combination treatments, such as those discussed above, to further encourage and more precisely time ovulation (Newcombe *et al.*, 2002; Phetudomsinuk, 2017). As a broad generality the more hormones that are used to mimic the natural cycle the better the timing/synchrony, but this comes at a managerial and financial cost, and often precludes their use.

Follicle Ablation

Ultrasound-guided transvaginal follicle ablation of follicles, followed by prostaglandin and possibly hCG, has shown promise in reducing the length of treatment but does not seem to improve synchrony rates (Bergfeldt *et al.*, 2007).

9.5.3. Veterinary use

Many of the hormones discussed above may also be used to 'restart' the oestrus cycle in mares with ovarian inactivity, persistent CL, etc., during the breeding season. It is beyond the scope of this book to discuss these in detail; suffice to say that PGF2α is the first option to treat persistent CL (McCue, 1998; Staempfli, 2011) and progesterone with/without PGF2α plus hormone combinations such as GnRH plus PMSG/hCG have been successfully used to 'restart' ovarian inactivity in the breeding season (Medan, 2014). Further information on ovarian inactivity is included in Section 14.3.4.1.

9.5.4. Suppressing oestrous activity

Although not strictly part of stud management, oestrous suppression is important in many performing mares. Oestrous activity is often associated with poor concentration and attitude to work and, therefore, poor performance. The most drastic means of stopping reproductive activity is ovariectomy, which has the major disadvantage of being irreversible. Alternatively, hormone manipulation can be used. While progesterone concentrations are high, oestrous activity is suppressed. This occurs naturally during dioestrus; therefore, as mentioned previously, performance mares can be treated with exogenous progesterone (often Regumate®) to suppress oestrous activity. More recent work suggests that the addition of oestradiol treatment produces a better suppression of oestrus. It has also been reported that insertion of a small glass ball or marble (25–35 mm in diameter) into the uterus of the mare prolongs luteal function (Nie *et al.*, 2001b, 2003), and as a result also suppresses oestrous activity. The explanation for such a reaction is unclear, but it is possible that the marble simulates a pregnancy and, by its movement within and contact with the uterine endometrium, prevents the release of prostaglandin (as seen in early pregnancy), and so the CL is maintained (Rivera *et al.*, 2008). Although successful it has been reported to be associated with an increased incidence of chronic endometritis (De Amorim *et al.*, 2016). Further, more recent work by Stout and Colenbrander (2004) and Imboden *et al.* (2006) suggested that preventing the action of GnRH by blocking its action on the pituitary, via GnRH vaccines, antagonists and agonists, is a possible alternative for reversibly suspending a mare's reproductive activity. Additionally, GnRH overdose may also suppress reproductive activity by down-regulating pituitary receptiveness (Farquhar *et al.*, 2001). Finally, and most recently, it has been suggested that daily oxytocin injections on days 7–14 days post-ovulation will result in CL maintenance for up to 2–3 months and so can be used in place of progesterone treatment or marble insertion. It is hypothesized that oxytocin treatment before day 10 after ovulation has an 'antiluteolytic' effect as it inhibits the upregulation of cyclooxygenase 2 (COX-2) – the key enzyme necessary for PGF2a production – and hence prevents PGF2α release (Rebordao *et al.*, 2017; Sarnecky *et al.*, 2019).

It is evident that manipulation of the oestrous cycle results in variable success in advancing the breeding season and, when used to time ovulation in the mare during the breeding season, it reduces the random spread of ovulations within a population rather than allowing the exact timing to be predicted. Even so, manipulation of the cycle is routinely practised for AI and ET. In general mare management it also allows ovarian examination or teasing to be concentrated into a shorter period of time, so reducing labour costs and facilitating stallion workload management, etc. Manipulation of the oestrous cycle is, therefore, regularly practised and, with the additional use of ultrasonography, is regularly used to allow an accurate and precise prediction of ovulation to be made.

9.6. Conclusion

It is evident that the preparation of the mare for covering needs planning and thought, especially if the mare is maiden and/or has the added complication of an athletic career behind her. However, provided adequate time and forethought are invested, most mares that are anatomically and physiologically sound are capable of breeding and carrying a pregnancy to term, regardless of their previous careers. The manipulation of reproduction is widely practised and, especially if used in conjunction with rectal palpation or ultrasonic scanning, allows accurate prediction of the timing of ovulation; as such, it is a very useful stud management tool.

Suggested Questions

Evaluate the factors that need to be considered when planning to breed an ex-performance maiden mare in order to maximize the chances that she will conceive as easily as possible.

Discuss the uses of the following in stud farm practice when breeding mares:

- Progesterone
- hCG
- PGF2α
- GnRH

You have ordered semen from a stallion standing in France with the aim of having a foal born during the second week of April, hence the chilled semen has been booked to arrive with you in the UK on May 15th. Your mare is barren and both the mare and stallion are in their late teens, so it is particularly important that you do all you can to ensure the mare conceives successfully. Detail how you would manage the mare in the last month leading up to the arrival of the semen.

Given the requirement that a maiden mare needs to be covered as close to February 15th as possible, evaluate how would you choose to manage her prior to covering in order to achieve this aim.

Detail the preparations that need to be made from autumn onwards when considering breeding a barren mare in late May.

Suggested Reading

McCue, P.M., Logan, N.I. and Magee, C. (2007) Management of the transition period : hormone therapy. *Equine Veterinary Education* 19(4), 215–221.

Samper, J.C. (2008) Induction of estrus and ovulation: Why some mares respond and others do not. *Theriogenology* 70, 445–447.

Scaramuzzi, R.J. and Martin, G.B. (2008) The importance of interactions among nutrition, seasonality and socio-sexual. *Factors in the development of hormone-free methods for controlling Fertility Reproduction in Domestic Animals* 43 (Supplement 2), 129–136.

Squires, E.L. (2008) Hormone manipulation of the mare : A review. *Journal of Equine Veterinary Science* 28(11), 624–627.

Squires, E.L. (2009) Changes in equine reproduction : have they been good or bad for the horse industry? *Journal of Equine Veterinary Science* 29, 268–273.

Morley, S.A. and Murray, J. (2014) Effects and body condition on the reproductive physiology of the broodmare. A Review. *Journal of Equine Veterinary Science* 34(7), 842–853.

Horse Race Betting Levy Board (2019) Codes of Practice 2018–19 on Contagious Equine Metritis, *Klebsiella pneumoniae, Pseudomonas aeroginosa,* Equine Viral Arteritis and Equine Herpes Virus 1. Horse Race Betting Levy Board, London.

Management of the Mare at Mating

10.1. Introduction

Reproductive activity is governed by season and commences at puberty. The mare will only allow mating to occur when she is in her sexually receptive oestrous phase, which can be referred to as oestrus, season or heat. This period of sexual receptivity occurs on average every 21 days during the breeding season and lasts 2–10 days (average 5 days). Oestrus is synchronized with ovulation and so ensures that the mare is mated or covered at the optimum time for fertilization (Chapter 2).

Ovulation occurs normally about 24 h before the end of oestrus, so in an average mare it will be on day 4 of a 5-day oestrus (Ginther, 1992). There is, however, considerable variation between mares. Sperm are reported to survive for 24–72 h within the mare's reproductive tract, but the exact time remains in doubt, as most experiments on longevity have been carried out *in vitro* (Watson and Nikolakopoulos, 1996). Some reports have suggested that sperm longevity may be as long as 7 days (Newcombe, 1994b; Tarapour, 2014). The ovum, on the other hand, is thought to survive only 8–12 h, although longer times have been reported, again in *in vitro* work (Hunter, 1990). The timing of mating is, therefore, very important, and in practice most mares are covered every 48 h while oestrus lasts or until the mare has ovulated (Stone, 1994).

10.2. Mating Systems

The human desire to control the covering process has led to a wide variety of mating systems, varying from the two extremes of natural covering to intensive in-hand covering.

10.2.1. Natural mating

In the natural system, stallions run with their mares in a harem and detect those in oestrus at will, examining them often for signs of sexual receptivity. This process is ongoing, leisurely and unrushed, and the signals used by the stallion to detect oestrus are primarily smell and taste rather than sight (Stone, 1994; McDonnell, 2005). Natural courtship may occur over several days, as the mare slowly progresses from dioestrus into full oestrus, and takes place between a mare and stallion that are well known to each other. The stallion spends increasing lengths of time grazing in the vicinity of the mare. When she is fully in oestrus and receptive, the courtship culminates in mating. Courtship of a mare in full oestrus appears to follow a sequence of events, especially in intensively controlled mating systems that do not allow this natural prolonged interaction of mares and stallion. In such intensive systems the stallion is often particularly overt in his display of interest and may stand and fix his eyes upon a mare, arch his back and neck, vocalize and draw himself up to his full height; he becomes restless, pacing and perhaps pawing the ground and stamping his feet. However, in the natural mating scenario such displays are not so often seen, and mating activity may almost go unnoticed. In both systems the stallion is likely to show the typical facial grimace, termed flehmen, or tasting of the air (olfactory stimulation), possibly accompanied by roaring or vocalization, which for some mares appears to be particularly attractive (Fig. 10.1; Pickerel *et al.*, 1993). He will approach the mare and gauge her response to his attentions. The whole process takes some time, during which the mare, if she is truly receptive, will stand quietly and possibly nicker in response if interested. She may turn her head towards the stallion with one foreleg flexed; this appears to be particularly inviting to the stallion, and may be an additional message that she will not kick him (McDonnell, 2011a). Once the mare's interest has been ascertained, the stallion will have the confidence to approach her more closely, normally from the head, working his way slowly down her neck, nickering as he does so; he may nudge her slightly or lightly bite her neck (Fig. 10.2). He is watching for her response and for signs of rejection all the time. If he feels confident, he will then work his way down her flanks and to her hindquarters, and to her perineal area. At any time, he may pause to reassure himself that she is still interested. If she is still amicable, he will nudge her vulva and clitoral area. If the mare is in full oestrus she will stand still, relatively passive throughout the whole procedure, showing her interest by curling her tail to one side, urinating (often bright yellow urine with a characteristic odour), or she may just take up the urinating stance. She will expose her clitoris by inverting the lips of the labia around the ventral commissure, termed winking (Figs 10.2 and 10.3; Ginther, 1992; McDonnell, 1992, 2011a; Crowell-Davis, 2007).

If she is not in oestrus, she will show hostility to the stallion, which will be unable to get closer to her other than the initial advance. In nature, the stallion will then turn away, transferring his attentions elsewhere, and

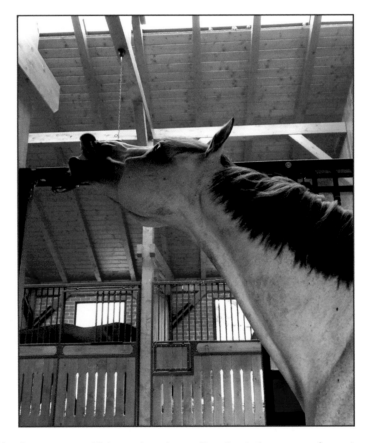

Fig. 10.1. The typical facial grimace, termed flehmen, shown by a stallion when in the presence of an oestrous mare. (Photo courtesy of Ms Ema Korak.)

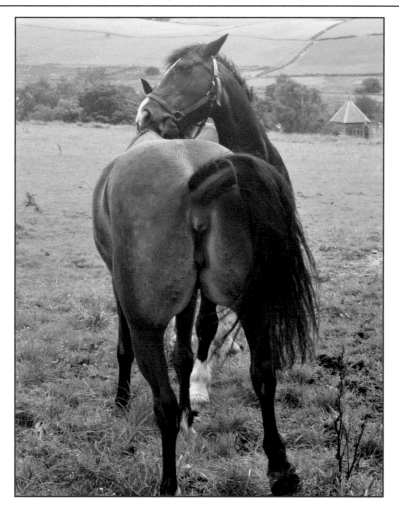

Fig. 10.2. Interaction between stallion and mare in the natural mating scenario, the stallion working his way down the mare towards her vulva and testing her reaction to his attentions. (Photo courtesy of Dr Ruth Wonfor.)

return to her later that day or on the next day (McDonnell, 2000a; Mills and McDonnell, 2005).

Once the stallion is sure that the mare is truly receptive he will mount her. His penis normally becomes erect as he approaches the mare and she shows interest. Mounting will only occur when his penis is fully erect (intromission pressure; Section 6.9). If the stallion is very sure of himself and the mare, he will often mount her directly and ejaculate immediately. A stallion with less confidence, or one not so sure of the mare, may nudge or push her forwards slightly prior to mounting, or half mount, to ascertain her reaction before he fully commits himself and runs the risk of injury. The number of mounts per ejaculate tends to be higher at the beginning and end of the season and in stallions with a low libido but, in stallions bred by natural breeding, the number of mounts per successful ejaculation is near to one and is much less than seen in controlled mating systems (McDonnell, 2011a). Ejaculation follows a varying number of pelvic oscillations, during which time the stallion may move on his hind feet. Successful ejaculation is signalled by rhythmic flagging of the tail. Ejaculation is followed by a terminal inactive phase when the stallion remains quiescent on the mare while penile erection subsides (detumescence). The stallion will not naturally dismount until his penile erection and the engorgement of the glans penis has completely subsided (Fig. 10.4; Section 6.9; Davies Morel, 1999).

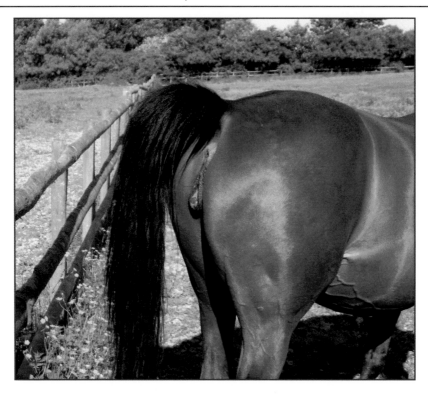

Fig. 10.3. A mare 'showing' she is in oestrus by lifting her tail to one side, winking her clitoral area.

The time taken to achieve ejaculation varies with stallion and circumstances. On average, a stallion will achieve erection within 2 min of contact with the mare; be ready to mount within 5–10 s of full erection; and achieve ejaculation within 5–20 s of mounting, with a final post-coital quiescent stage of up to 30 s (McDonnell, 2000b, 2011a).

It is of note that, in the natural system, the mare takes a very active part in courtship, often seeking out the stallion, soliciting his attentions from other mares and encouraging mating (McDonnell, 2011a).

In the natural system a stallion will cover a mare in oestrus many times, up to 8–10 matings in 24 h, sometimes even as frequent as hourly. Nature's system works extremely well, with high pregnancy rates (Ginther *et al.*, 1983; Bristol, 1987). It is a system, however, that is rarely practised today, although occasionally seen in pony studs, or with horses run on large expanses of land with minimal managerial input. For such a system to run completely naturally the stallion will only cover the mares within his harem, and no outside mares may be introduced solely for covering. The introduction of foreign mares causes a disruption in the hierarchy and can result in jealousy and hostility from other mares, and uncertainty between the stallion and the introduced mares (Ginther, 1983). The need to introduce outside mares to a natural mating system is accommodated in some native pony studs by running the stallion out with specific groups of mares (Davies Morel and Gunnarsson, 2000). Visiting mares can then be put in their own group, and home-bred mares in another, while the stallion is moved around between the groups and allowed to cover the mares at will when they come into oestrus.

Although conception rates are higher in natural breeding than in a controlled system (Bristol, 1987; Davies Morel and Gunnarsson, 2000), the natural breeding system has many disadvantages from the breeder's point of view, when maximum financial return from the stallion is required. The natural system limits the number of mares the stallion can cover in a season, as each mare gets covered numerous times per oestrus, whereas if mating is timed correctly, in theory only a single service is required. As a result, breeders feel the need to control events to protect the investment made, maximize the number of mares covered per season and hence financial return, and minimize the risk

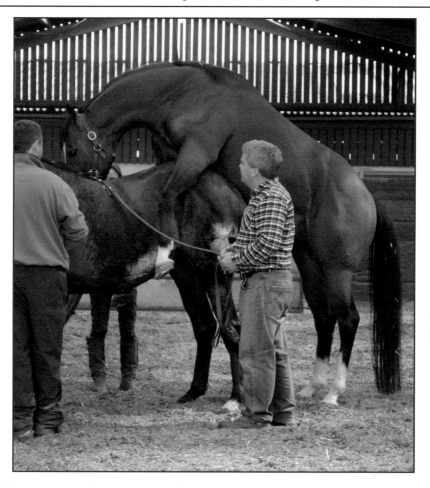

Fig. 10.4. The final stage after ejaculation, where the stallion remains inactive as detumescence occurs.

of injury to stock. This interference is at the root of many of the challenges associated with stud management today.

10.2.2. Mating in hand

Mating in hand is practised by the majority of studs today and involves complete control over the events surrounding covering. In general, humans now control the life of the horse, particularly with respect to mating, to such an extent that there is little similarity between the natural life and the one imposed.

It is common practice to segregate fillies and colts early on in their lives, sometimes from birth, and always at weaning. Naturally, colts and fillies would run together as part of a herd. Colts would be disciplined by other mares and the stallion, socially interact with fillies and learn respect at a young age, when the chance of

serious damage is reduced (Christensen *et al.*, 2002b; McDonnell, 2011a). In the present intensive systems, this social introduction of the young stallion to fillies and mares is removed. In addition, stallions are expected to cover mares that are unknown to them. The failure to develop social awareness and respect for mares results in stallions being inept at the interaction associated with covering (McDonnell, 2000b; Christensen *et al.*, 2002b). When this is coupled with the strangeness of any unknown mare and the sexual tension present, it is not surprising that the risk of mare rejection and injury to both parties is high. An additional consideration is the significant value of some stallions and the need to control events to protect the financial investment, the stallion and to minimize the number of coverings per pregnancy, so as to optimize his use and maximize financial return.

To overcome the potential danger to stallions and to optimize their use, most systems mate in hand. Humans, therefore, have total control over the number of mares covered by each stallion (Umphenour *et al.*, 1993). However, one of the major drawbacks of this system is that there is the need to interpret the mare's oestrous signals before the stallion is allowed near her. As discussed previously, the stallion uses the senses of smell and taste to detect mares in oestrus; the breeder, however, has to rely on the sense of sight only (Stone, 1994). This method leads to inaccuracies and can prove unreliable. Hence, a teaser stallion is often employed.

10.2.2.1. Teasing

Teasing is the use of a stallion, often not that chosen for mating, to encourage a mare to demonstrate oestrous behaviour under controlled conditions. The principle is that, as soon as the mare is thought to be in oestrus, she is brought in contact with the teaser, an entire male horse under controlled conditions, in an attempt to enhance the signs of oestrus and confirm the initial diagnosis. Once the mare is confirmed as being in true oestrus, she can then be prepared for covering by the chosen stallion. This system allows the stallion destined to cover the mare access to her only when she is in true oestrus and at the optimum time for fertilization, so minimizing the risk of injury and maximizing the chance of conception (Squires, 1993c). Apart from allowing oestrus to be detected, teasing is now known to play a role in enhancing reproductive activity. Prolonged teasing results in elevated gonadotrophin-releasing hormone (GnRH) concentrations, which in turn increase gonadotrophin (luteinizing hormone (LH) and follicle-stimulating hormone (FSH)) release in both the mare and stallion, thus advancing ovulation in the mare and enhancing libido in the stallion (Irvine and Alexander, 1991; Lieberman and Bowman, 1994; McDonnell and Murray, 1995). In addition, it is becoming increasingly evident that teasing plays an important role in uterine clearance and reduction in persistent post-coital endometritis. Teasing causes the release of oxytocin and possibly prostaglandin which, owing to their ability to activate the uterine myometrium, cause mild uterine contractions. These not only help transport sperm towards the waiting ova, but also help expel exudate and dead sperm from the tract (Nikolakopoulos *et al.*, 2000a,b; Stecco *et al.*, 2003; Campbell and England, 2004; Woodward and Troedsson, 2013). Various stimuli are known to affect uterine contractility. Work by Madill *et al.* (2000) suggested

that teasing with a stallion results in the greatest uterine contractility, followed by artificial insemination (AI), then the sight of a stallion and finally the sound or calling of a stallion. Such uterine contractility is particularly important in mares that habitually suffer from persistent post-coital endometritis (see Section 14.3.5.3). Prolonged teasing of such mares may well prove to be good practice (Stecco *et al.*, 2003).

The teaser stallion is often kept purely to detect mares in oestrus. He is often of low value. If he is injured or damaged by an objecting mare, then there is no significant loss. Often a pony stallion is used. In many native pony-breeding studs, the stallion to be used for covering also acts as the teaser for his mares. This allows the reproductive state of the mare to be confirmed under controlled conditions, but does not give the stallion the ultimate protection of using a separate teaser. However, such stallions tend to be less valuable, native mares show oestrus more readily and the mare is very likely to be teased initially over a teasing board or equivalent, providing some protection.

There are problems associated with in-hand covering, mainly because the courtship, which naturally takes place over a prolonged period between two individuals known to each other, is concentrated into a short space of time and forces the attentions of the stallion upon the mare. Some mares object to such forced attentions, even if they are in full oestrus, and such objection may mask the signs of oestrus. Mares with foals at foot are especially likely to object, occasionally violently, to the removal of the foal prior to teasing and covering, a practice often carried out to protect the foal. In the natural system the foal would still be in the close vicinity of the mare, but seems to know instinctively to keep its distance. Teasing some mares before feeding or turnout can also give erroneous results, and environmental conditions of extreme heat, cold, rain or wind may mask signs of oestrus. Some mares need a longer time of teasing before they can be coaxed into demonstrating oestrus and, in a busy stud working to a tight schedule, there is little time for extended teasing and hence she may never seem to be ready to cover. Again, some mares will only show oestrus under certain circumstances, for example only in the covering yard, when the perineum is being washed, the tail bandaged prior to service, or when a twitch is applied (Lieberman and Bowman, 1994). This is where the mare's records are invaluable in identifying any such idiosyncrasy. There is also evidence that mares may have a preference for certain stallions and this may be associated with vocalization. It has been suggested that the more vocal a stallion, the greater is his popularity (Pickerel *et al.*, 1993).

When a mare is in oestrus she will be docile; accept the attentions of the stallion; take up the urination stance; expose her clitoris (referred to as winking or showing); and demonstrate a general lack of hostility towards, and signs of acceptance of, the stallion (Figs 10.2, 10.3 and 10.5a–d; Crowell-Davis, 2007). There is a wide range of methods used to tease mares, depending on the stud, the value of the stock and the facilities available (McCue *et al.*, 2011a).

Trying Board

One of the most common methods of teasing is a trying or teasing board. The mare and stallion are introduced, one on either side of the board, and their reactions monitored. The board is designed to provide protection for both and should be high enough to allow just the horses' heads and necks to reach over. It is solid in construction, often made of wood and ideally twice the length of the horses. Its top should be covered by curved rubber or equivalent, to provide protection if the stallion or mare attempt to attack each other over the board (Fig. 10.6).

The approach of the teaser to the mare over the board should mimic that of the natural approach. Initially muzzle to muzzle, the teaser is then allowed to stretch his muzzle along the mare's neck, possibly gently nipping her. The attitude of the mare to this attention is closely observed: signs of hostility include laid-back ears, squealing, biting and kicking out, indicating that the mare is still in dioestrus. In contrast, leaning towards the stallion, raising of the tail and the other typical signs of oestrus indicate that she is ready to be covered. If the mare is interested, then her flank can be turned towards the trying board and the teaser allowed to work his way further down her body. It is, however, very important that direct contact with the mare's genital area is avoided, to prevent possible disease transfer to

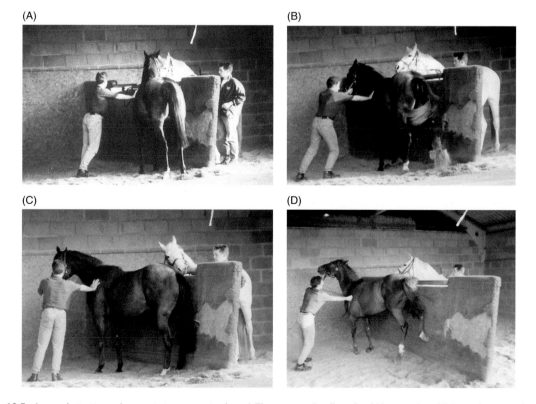

Fig. 10.5. A mare being teased over a trying or teasing board. The mare and stallion should be introduced (a) muzzle to muzzle; and (b), (c) the stallion allowed to work his way down to the mare's vulva. If she is in oestrus she will show little, if any, objection. A mare not in oestrus will usually object violently (d). (Photo courtesy of Ms Elizabeth Wood.)

other mares teased. After a few minutes of such attention, most mares will show definite signs of oestrus, although some mares (as discussed previously) may take longer.

Using the same principle, a stable door may act as an alternative to a purpose-built trying board, with the teaser in the stable and the mare introduced to him outside the door. This is a popular practice in the smaller, more native-type studs, but can be dangerous unless the teaser is well known and is unlikely to be overzealous (Fig. 10.7).

Teasing Over the Paddock Rail

Teasing over the paddock rail provides an alternative system, used in larger studs. The teaser is led in hand to the paddock rail of fields containing mares, which are

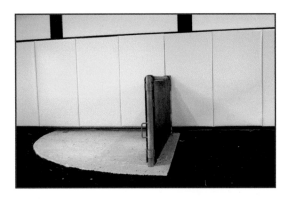

Fig. 10.6. A typical teasing board.

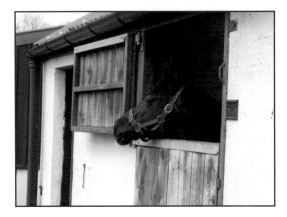

Fig. 10.7. Providing the stallion is of a known good temperament, then he may tease the mares over the stable door. This is a Section C Welsh Cob stallion who acts as a teaser for Thoroughbred mares that are presented to him outside his stable door for teasing.

running loose, normally in small groups. A permanent trying board is often built into the paddock rail or a movable trying board is placed there. The reaction of the mares to the teaser is noted. Most mares in oestrus will approach the teaser by the fence and show definite signs of oestrus; others may show hostility; and some may appear disinterested. Mares that show no reaction, often due to shyness or low social ranking, can be caught and brought up to the trying board to be tested individually. Those that show interest can also be tried individually for confirmation or brought in for covering immediately. This is an efficient method for use with mares that are turned out, as it greatly reduces time and labour. It is best to avoid teasing mares by this method immediately after turnout or just before feeding, as this can give erroneous results. Turning out a stallion or teaser into a neighbouring field or regularly walking past the paddock fence, a version of the above, can be practised, as long as the stallion or teaser has the appropriate temperament, alternatively a gelding can sometimes be used (Fig. 10.8). Taking a stallion or teaser past the paddock fence is of particular use if the teaser can be ridden or requires regular exercise in hand. The daily route can then be organized to pass appropriate paddocks and the general reaction of the mares observed. Those that show interest can be caught and taken to the covering yard.

This system does have potential problems when mares have foals at foot. There is conflicting opinion as to whether this presents a considerable danger to the foal, or that foals distance themselves as they do naturally; and that mares, especially in small groups, are very careful to avoid damage to their foals.

Not all mares react to these two forms of teasing. Those that are less demonstrative may well be missed, especially if they are low within the hierarchy (Curry *et al.*, 2007). It is essential in such systems, therefore, that a detailed record of the mare's normal oestrous behaviour is available.

Teasing in Chutes and Crates

In some parts of the world mares are run out in large herds, and are handled less frequently. In such enterprises, the mares may be run into chutes or crates and are held individually for a short period of time and teased from outside. This system reduces labour and enables large numbers of mares to be teased in as short a period of time as possible, with limited handling. The mares need to be accustomed to this system or errors may result.

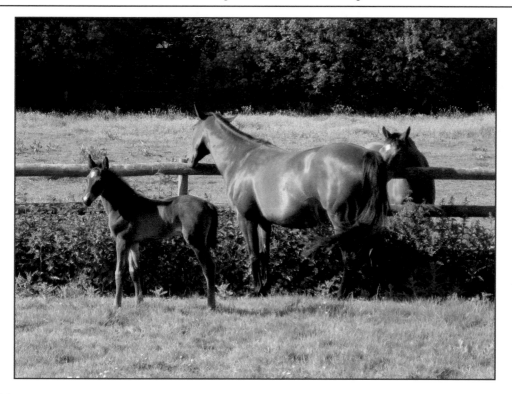

Fig. 10.8. Mare teased over a paddock rail. This mare is showing to a gelding who is in the neighbouring field. Stallions have to be well behaved to be turned out into fields next to mares but, as an alternative, a gelding can be used or the stallion can be led along the field fence to gauge the mare's reaction.

Teasing Pen

A further alternative system is to confine the teaser in a railed or boarded area in the corner of a paddock. The area confining the teaser normally has high boards with a grill or meshed fencing, possibly with a hole through which the teaser can put his muzzle (Fig. 10.9a,b). An alternative is the use of a small pony or miniature-breed stallion confined by a stout fence. If he escapes, it is not too disastrous, as his size limits his ability to cover the mares, although it is not impossible. These are again good systems for teasing a large number of mares, but they do require frequent observation of mares for signs of oestrus and, as with teasing over the paddock rail, it may be difficult to pick up shy mares. It must, of course, be remembered that the teaser can only be confined in the railed area for relatively short periods of time.

Along the same lines as the teasing pen or stable is a central teasing pen surrounded by a series of individual pens in which mares can be held.

A further variation on this theme is the use of two adjacent boxes, divided by a grill, one for the stallion and the other for the mare. Yet another involves the teaser being confined in a stable in the corner of a yard with the mare free within the yard to show to the stallion at will. Such an arrangement is used at the National Stud, Newmarket, UK, for maiden or shy mares that do not show oestrus well under more traditional methods (Fig. 10.10).

These last three systems are good for use with difficult mares, as they can be left alone to show in their own time without competition from other mares, and can be observed from a discreet distance.

Vasectomized Stallions

Vasectomized stallions may be used to run out with mares. This can be especially useful with maiden or difficult mares; those mounted can then be covered by the intended entire stallion. This system has the obvious danger of running unaccustomed mares and stallion out together and is therefore of limited use, especially with valuable stock. However, it is an extremely reliable method of detecting oestrus and has the reported

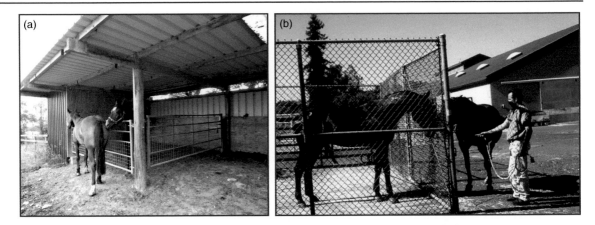

Fig. 10.9. A teasing pen or cage can be used to confine the stallion or teaser and allows observation of any mares, either (a) loose within the field; or (b) restrained. The reaction of the stallion to the mare, as well as the mare's reaction to the stallion, should be noted. (Photo a courtesy of Dr Ruth Wonfor; Photo b courtesy Dr Julie Baumber-Skaife.)

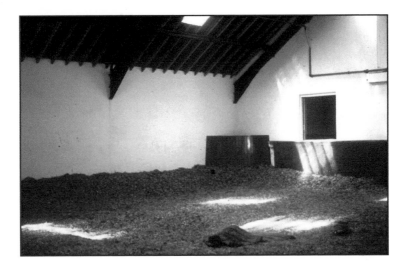

Fig. 10.10. An arrangement such as this can be used to tease shy or reluctant mares. The stable in the corner of a covering yard (open window in background) is used to confine the teaser; the yard (in the foreground) allows the mare to be free to exhibit oestrus at leisure.

advantage of increasing the number of mares showing regular 21-day cycles (Barnisco and Potes, 1987). The other major disadvantage is that this system allows intromission to occur, and so enables the transfer of venereal disease. Although this can be averted by surgical retroversion of the penis, causing it to extend caudally (between the hind legs) at erection and making intromission impossible (Belonje, 1965), the risk of venereal disease transmission via the stallion's muzzle is not eliminated and so the commercial use of vasectomized stallions is not seen.

Hermaphrodite Horses and Androgenized Mares

Hermaphrodite horses are very useful as teasers but are very rare and, therefore, not really a viable alternative. Androgenized mares (mares treated with testosterone) have been used successfully, but are not common practice (McDonnell *et al.*, 1986, 1988).

Teasing Mares with a Foal at Foot

A mare with a foal at foot may present problems. The foal often becomes agitated with the unaccustomed attention to its mother and so distracts her. To overcome this, the foal may be penned or held within reach or sight of its mother, or removed completely from sight and sound while teasing occurs (Fig. 10.11). Prior knowledge of a mare's normal behaviour in such circumstances is very useful. More recently in the Thoroughbred industry, because of the requirement for natural service and the increase in 'walk in' coverings, very young foals need to be transported long distances. This presents significant welfare concerns and so many foals are left behind while the mare is transported alone, especially if they are to be covered on the foal heat. Although this separation is only temporary, it has been suggested to increase the likelihood of stereotypical behaviour in the foal (which appears to be somewhat alleviated by human contact) and also increases mare stress, which is linked to reproductive success (McGee and Smith, 2004).

Conclusions on Teasing

Regardless of the teasing method, direct contact between the stallion's muzzle or penis and the mare's genitalia must, ideally, be avoided. Direct contact risks the transfer of disease to successive mares via the stallion. This is one of the major advantages of teasing over a trying board and a potential disadvantage of many of the other methods discussed.

As discussed, not all mares show under the above systems, and some require specific management, prolonged individual teasing, etc. The key to success is careful observation, as it must be remembered that all mares react individually and no system is 100% reliable. The physiological value of teasing and its role in advancing ovulation and uterine clearance is increasingly becoming evident. However, teasing only ever allows oestrous behaviour to be determined; it does not determine when the mare is due to ovulate. In the vast majority of mares the two occur concurrently, but the exact time of ovulation within oestrus is difficult to predict precisely. Hence further confirmation of a mare's reproductive activity is often required. This is achieved by veterinary examination.

10.2.2.2. Veterinary examination

Routine veterinary examination to confirm a mare's reproductive state is used in many studs, especially those running valuable stallions, with the aim of optimizing their use. Veterinary techniques allow the timing of ovulation to be estimated but do not detect oestrous behaviour. They may be used alone or to back up teasing, confirm diagnosis and optimize the timing of covering. There are three types of veterinary examination that may be used in this context: ultrasonic scanning; rectal palpation; and vaginal examination. All three techniques have already been described (Section 8.7). They are

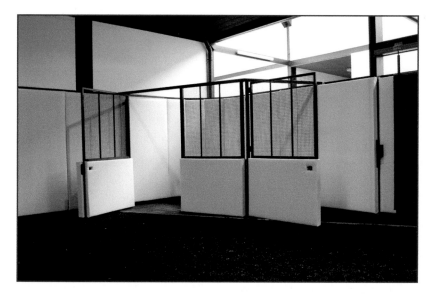

Fig. 10.11. Alternatively, when mares with foals at foot are teased or mated, a cage or padded area can be used to hold the foal, allowing reasonable access by the dam but ensuring the foal's safety during teasing and covering.

used primarily to assess ovarian activity, but uterine, cervical and vaginal activity can also be detected to aid diagnosis. This assessment can be used to confirm a mare's sexual state, correlate mating to ovulation and diagnose venereal infections. The mare should be restrained in stocks for all techniques (Fig. 10.12).

Ovarian Assessment

The main activity assessed in the context of covering management is ovarian activity. The techniques used are ultrasonic scanning and rectal palpation (Section 8.7). In particular, the presence of follicles and/or corpus luteum (CL), and their consistency, appearance and position are noted, so that the time of ovulation can be estimated and the most appropriate time for covering determined.

Follicles may develop on either ovary; often there are several follicles but many regress owing to an inability to react to hormonal stimulation (see Section 1.9.1). As oestrus and ovulation approach, normally one to two of these developing follicles can be identified as dominant (Gastal et al., 1997, 2006). The diameter of these follicles used to be advocated as a good predictor of the imminence of ovulation. However, although

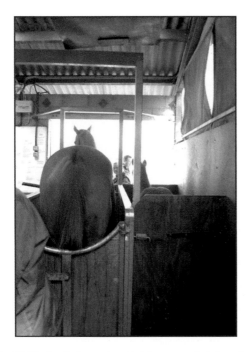

Fig. 10.12. Stocks for use in restraining mares for internal veterinary examination. Note the pen to the right to contain the foal during examination of the mare.

diameter may be used as a guide, pre-ovulatory follicular diameter varies considerably. Most mares ovulate follicles of 3.5–4.5 cm in diameter; others habitually ovulate follicles of up to 6.0–6.5 cm; and still other mares ovulate follicles as small as 2.0 cm (Fig. 10.13; Newcombe, 1994a; Samper et al., 2002; Newcombe, 2011a; Sauberli, 2013). Numerous factors affect follicle size at ovulation. These include breed, but also mares that are post-partum, transitional and aged tend to have smaller follicles (Ginther, 1992). Multiple ovulations are seen; double ovulations have been reported to occur in 23% of ovulations in the Thoroughbred (Davies Morel and O'Sullivan, 2001) but are rarer in other breeds, such as draught and Arab mares, and are very uncommon in native ponies (Newcombe, 1995). The incidence of multiple ovulations also appears to increase with mare age (Davies Morel et al., 2005). If multiple ovulations are present, they are likely to ovulate at a smaller size. The presence of multiple ovulations may well preclude a mare from covering. Despite the increasing success of managing twin conceptuses by pinching out (Section 11.3), studs may occasionally still prefer not to cover multiple-ovulating mares but rather to leave them and advance the next oestrus, which will, it is hoped, demonstrate only a single ovulation. Of further note with regard to multiple ovulations is that they may occur asynchronously but both may still be fertile. As such, scanning or rectal palpation may indicate a single dominant follicle, but examination up to 96 h later may indicate multiple CLs; and later examination may indicate a multiple pregnancy of very different conceptus sizes (Davies Morel et al., 2015). Close regular monitoring, especially of mares with a high risk of multiple ovulations (e.g. older Thoroughbred mares) is, therefore, essential. Ovulation occurs in two stages (Section 1.9.1). These two stages can be used as an additional guide to the imminence of ovulation (Professor J. Newcombe, Wales, 2019, personal communication). As ovulation becomes increasingly imminent, the follicular wall becomes thinner and the pressure of the follicular fluid contents decreases. On rectal palpation, this decline in follicular pressure can be felt and so the follicle feels softer. On scanning, the clear spherical shape of the follicle becomes less clear and the margins become thicker and more 'ragged' in appearance (Ginther, 1988; Sertich, 1998; McCue et al., 2011a). Such follicles would be expected to ovulate within 24 h and most studies advise that the mare should be covered immediately. Further detailed scanning work suggested that not only can the shape of the

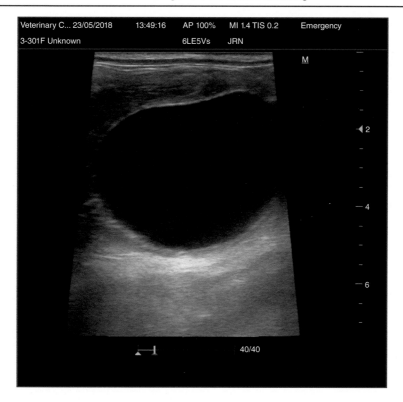

Fig. 10.13. An ultrasonic scanning photograph of a large (4-cm) pre-ovulatory follicle approximately 48 h before ovulation. Note the clear spherical shape. (Photo courtesy of Professor John Newcombe.)

follicle be used as a guide, but also that the echogenicity of the granulosa cells and the space between them and the theca cells lying below can be used to increase the accuracy of ovulation prediction (Fig. 10.14; Chan *et al.*, 2003). The best pregnancy rates are achieved by covering within the 48–72 h period prior to ovulation (Woods *et al.*, 1990; Katila *et al.*, 1996; Newcombe and Cuervo-Arango, 2008). If at re-examination 24–48 h later the mare has not ovulated, she should be re-covered immediately. In such a scenario human chorionic gonadotrophin (hCG) is often administered to advance ovulation (Section 9.5.2.3). The presence of a CL within the ovary indicates that the mare has ovulated and that, unless the ovulation is very recent (within 12 h) there is little point in covering the mare (Newcombe and Cuervo-Arango, 2008). Ova only remain viable for up to 12 h post-ovulation (Ginther, 1992), whereas sperm may remain viable for up to 7 days (Newcombe, 1994b; Tarapour, 2014). Coverings later than 12 h post-ovulation may result in fertilization but are associated with higher rates of early embryonic death, with

pregnancy rates for covering more than 24 h after ovulation at zero (Woods *et al.*, 1990; Newcombe and Cuervo-Arango, 2008). Recent CLs appear as semi-solid structures within the cavity of the old follicle. At scanning they are evident as a grey spherical shape (Fig. 10.15).

At rectal palpation a new CL can be detected as a soft spongy friable mass. At 24 h post-ovulation they feel firmer and a pit may be felt. Later on, when assessing via rectal palpation, they may be hard to distinguish from follicles.

Uterine Assessment

Uterine activity and appearance can be used as a further guide to reproductive activity (McCue *et al.*, 2011a). As with ovarian activity, this is assessed via scanning and rectal palpation. Striking changes occur within the uterus between oestrus and dioestrus. This is thought to be due to the presence or absence of progesterone, rather than oestrogens. Once the dominance of progesterone has been removed, as the mare goes into oestrus,

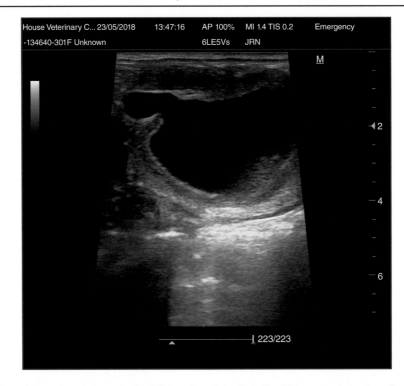

Fig. 10.14. An ultrasonic scanning photograph of a follicle as it ovulates. Note the thick, more echogenic wall and the loss of a clear spherical shape, as the follicular fluid begins to be released towards the ovulation fossa, in the top left-hand corner. (Photo courtesy of Professor John Newcombe.)

the uterine endometrial folds become oedematous (fluid collects within them) and can clearly be visualized at scanning (Ginther, 1992; Plata-Madrid *et al.*, 1994; Bergfeldt, 2000). The dense central portions of the folds appear echogenic (white/grey) and the oedematous portion non-echogenic (grey/black). Hence, when the uterine horn is viewed in cross section, it can resemble a sliced orange or cartwheel (Fig. 10.16; Samper and Pycock, 2007). This endometrial oedema can be scored and, as such, bears a close correlation to oestrogen concentrations and therefore behaviour scores indicative of oestrus (Pelehach *et al.*, 2002; Cuervo-Arango and Newcombe, 2008). However, other work by Plata-Madrid *et al.* (1994) indicated that oedema may peak up to 6 days prior to ovulation. Others have also questioned the correlation of oedema to the timing of ovulation and hence its usefulness (Watson *et al.*, 2003). Despite this, uterine oedema is used in practice as an additional useful indicator of imminent ovulation, and is a good indicator of basal progesterone levels and hence the likelihood of elevated oestrogens and so oestrus.

Rectal palpation may also be used to indicate uterine changes associated with reproductive activity. The tone, size and thickness of the uterus are assessed; these tend to increase under the dominance of progesterone, so during dioestrus the uterus appears larger and more toned, while during oestrus it appears smaller and more flaccid (Ginther, 1992; Bergfeldt, 2000).

Cervical and Vaginal Examination

Cervical and vaginal examination are less reliable determinants of reproductive activity; nevertheless, they can be useful tools in confirming a mare's sexual state. The cervix and vagina can be visualized via a vaginascope (Sections 8.7.1 and 8.7.2). During oestrus the cervix appears pink to glistening red in colour and is relaxed; it appears to 'flower' into the vagina; and its lining is oedematous (Fig. 1.13). Shortly after oestrus, the cervix begins to contract and becomes paler pink in colour, with a thicker secretion. By dioestrus, the cervix is closed, pale in colour, dry and retracted back against the cranial vaginal wall (Fig. 1.12; McCue *et al.*, 2011a). Pregnancy may be considered an extreme form of

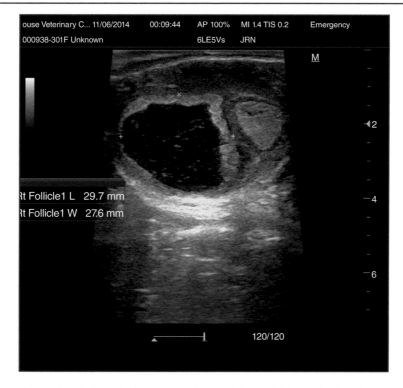

Fig. 10.15. An ultrasonic scanning photograph of a very recent corpus luteum (CL) (immediately post-ovulation) on the left. Note the thick wall as the follicle begins to luteinize and the fluid, blood-filled centre; and a mature CL with solid luteinized tissue throughout on the right. (Photo courtesy of Professor John Newcombe.)

dioestrus; as such, the cervix is very tightly closed and white in colour, with a central sticky mucus plug. Vaginal secretions largely originate from, and so mimic, cervical and uterine secretion. During oestrus the vagina appears red/pink in colour with fluid secretions; during dioestrus secretions appear more sticky and viscous, causing the vaginal walls to adhere together and make speculum examination more difficult. The vaginal secretion during pregnancy is thick, thickening even more as pregnancy progresses.

Ultrasound can also be used to assess cervical oedema, which follows much the same pattern as uterine oedema but is not as easy to assess; for this reason it is not diagnostic on its own and so is rarely used (Day *et al.*, 1995).

Hormone Profiles

It has been suggested that declining oestradiol plasma concentrations can be used as an indicator of imminent ovulation (Allen *et al.*, 1995) and also progesterone profiling (Nagy *et al.*, 2004). However, owing to individual variation, this is unlikely to be consistently diagnostic

in itself but may, like cervical and vaginal examination, be an additional aid in diagnosis.

10.2.2.3. Preparation for covering

Once it has been determined that the mare is in oestrus and ready for covering, and that she has the appropriate negative swab certificates (Horse Race Betting Levy Board, 2019), attention must be turned to the preparation of the mare and the stallion for actual covering (Umphenour *et al.*, 2011). Preparation depends entirely upon the system used for mating and varies, from the strict codes of practice within the Thoroughbred industry, to practically no preparation at all in the case of many native pony studs. The most cautionary preparation will be considered in the following account. Other studs dispense with some, if not all, of the preparation techniques. Exact management also depends on the size of the stud, labour available, stallion workload, etc. In larger studs there can be up to four breeding sessions per day, spaced at regular intervals (e.g. 06:00, 09:00, 14:00 and 19:00). Most mares are covered twice within an oestrus, at 24–48 h intervals or until ovulation

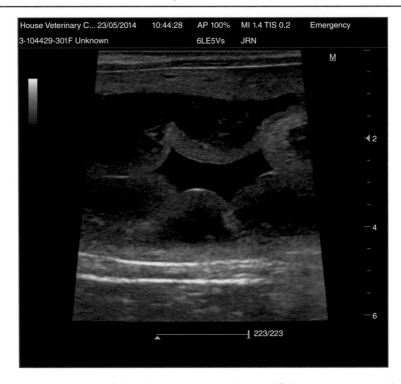

Fig. 10.16. The characteristic appearance of the oedematous uterine endometrial folds seen at scanning in the uterus of a mare in oestrus, particularly as oestrus commences. The oedema can be scored and the higher the score the closer oestrus/ovulation is; the oedema score for this image oedema was 3. (Photo courtesy of Professor John Newcombe.)

has been confirmed or oestrus has ended (Ginther, 1992; Newcombe, 1994b). The mare is prepared with all eventualities in mind. She is bridled and restrained, her tail bandaged and the perineal area washed thoroughly (Fig. 10.17). When washing the mare, gloves should be used and there should be a different swab of cotton wool for each swipe. Each swipe should be taken from the buttocks towards the perineum and the cotton wool discarded immediately to prevent contamination of the washing solution. If soap is used it should be mild, non-detergent soap, and the area thoroughly rinsed. Soap and disinfectants can act as spermicides and may also upset the natural microflora of the genital tract, opening up the opportunity for colonization by opportunistic bacteria and hence endometritis (Betsch *et al.*, 1991; Clement *et al.*, 1995). A hose may be used as an alternative to manual washing.

At this stage, the vulva of any mare with a Caslick vulvoplasty should have been opened (episiotomy). If any sutures remain from a recent Caslick vulvoplasty, these should also be removed to avoid damage to the stallion. Once the mare has been washed, she is led to

the covering area, where felt covering boots may be fitted to her back feet, which should have had their shoes removed prior to arrival at the stud (Fig. 10.18). She may also have a nose or ear twitch applied, depending on her temperament and past behaviour (Fig. 10.19). Some studs twitch as standard, believing that prevention is better than cure as far as damage to expensive stallions is concerned. If she has the reputation of being particularly bad-tempered she may need one of her forelegs held up in a carpal flexion, or hind leg hobbles may be fitted to prevent her lunging forwards and objecting when the stallion mounts. It is, however, questionable whether a mare requiring such drastic restraint is truly in oestrus. In such cases, conception rates are likely to be adversely affected, owing both to the incorrect timing of service and the stress of such treatment. Other articles used occasionally include blinkers, hood or blindfold, especially for highly strung maiden or difficult mares. A mare being covered by a stallion that tends to bite his mares can be protected by use of a neck guard (shoulder or wither pad), with or without a biting roll (Fig. 10.20).

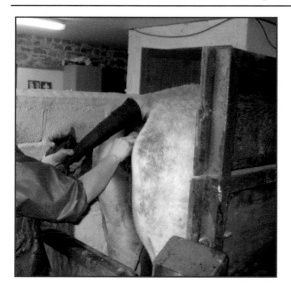

Fig. 10.17. In readiness for mating the mare's tail should be bandaged and the perineum washed.

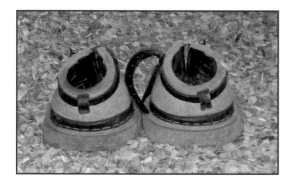

Fig. 10.18. Covering boots for a mare's hind feet to minimize damage to the stallion should she kick out.

On very rare occasions, tranquillizers may be administered 15–30 min prior to covering; this can be of use in particularly nervous or vicious mares. If such extreme restraint is necessary then the use of such a mare for breeding should be questioned, as there is a risk that such a temperament is heritable, and the stress associated with such management will negatively impact on conception rates (AboEl-Maaty, 2011; Malschitzky *et al.*, 2015).

This preparation of the mare, as described, represents the extreme of full precaution to avoid all possible transfer of bacterial infection and ensure stallion safety, and is referred to as the minimal contamination technique (Kenney *et al.*, 1975). In the Thoroughbred and sports horse industry, where the value of stock is high, such precautions are economically justifiable. In other studs, with progressively lower turnovers and less-valuable stock, preparation becomes less cautionary in nature. It is interesting to note that several of these procedures are gradually being introduced into the less-intensive studs. For example, many breed societies now require swabbing prior to covering, and some restrict the use of the yearly premium stallions to mares with negative swab certificates. The other extreme to that practised in the Thoroughbred industry is seen in many native studs, where no preparation of the mare or stallion is practised, except the possible bridling of the pair for restraint and removal of the mare's hind shoes. Such extensive systems run a high risk of disease transfer but are closer to the natural breeding scenario. One of the saving graces of native-type stock is that they appear to be less susceptible to genital infections, although of course they are not completely immune.

10.2.2.4. Covering

The management of the actual covering (mating) procedure varies considerably. In-hand covering is the norm within intensive breeding in most countries and, with the increasing value of stock, in-hand breeding is now widely practised.

During the covering process there should only need to be two handlers, one for each horse, ideally wearing stout footwear and a hard hat. The stallion handler should also carry a stick for reprimanding. In many traditional systems there may be up to two additional staff, an assistant to help the stallion gain intromission, if necessary, and to hold the mare's tail, plus a handler to hold the stallion steady on the mare and help to prevent the two tottering too far forwards. It is essential that all handlers know their exact roles and that an emergency procedure has been drawn up beforehand. Once prepared, the mare is normally taken into the covering area first, to await the arrival of the stallion. The stallion is then brought in to cover the mare immediately or, in some systems, the stallion may initially be introduced to the mare over a trying board positioned within the covering area. This provides him with protection during initial contact, and is required for some stallions to avoid a prolonged period with the mare in the covering area before full erection and mounting occurs, a potentially dangerous situation. The mare is then led away from the trying board ready for covering. At this stage she may be further restrained by means of a twitch or hobbles. Once the mare is ready, the stallion

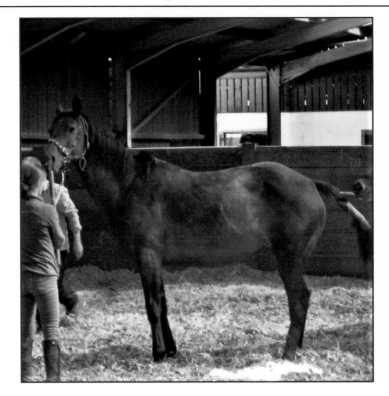

Fig. 10.19. Mare ready for covering: tail bandaged, perineum washed and with a twitch applied.

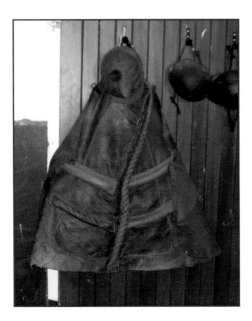

Fig. 10.20. A neck guard with built-in biting rolls to prevent a stallion savaging a mare's withers and neck.

is allowed to approach her, normally at an angle several feet from her nearside to avoid startling her and causing her to kick out.

Once the stallion's penis is fully erect he should be allowed to mount. Mounting before full erection should not be allowed. There are two blood pressures within the stallion's penis at erection: turgid and intromission pressure (Section 6.9). Attainment of intromission pressure is essential to avoid damage to the stallion on entry into the mare (Fig. 10.21).

As the stallion is allowed to mount the mare, all handlers should stand to one side of the animals, usually the left. If problems do occur, then both the stallion and the mare can be pulled towards their handlers, turning their hindquarters away from anyone likely to be kicked.

As the stallion mounts the mare she will probably totter forwards. This is to be allowed, within reason. Excessive tottering will put a strain on the stallion, which will rest more of his weight on her back and also cause her possible strain or injury. Tottering too far forwards can be prevented by placing the mare up against

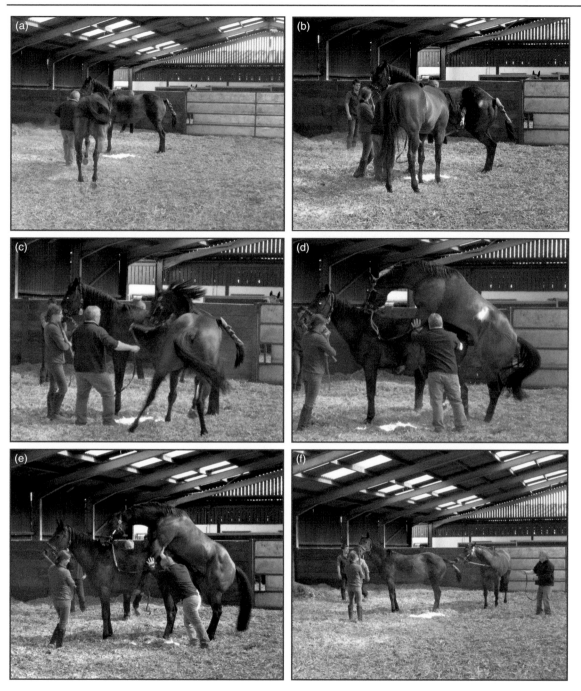

Fig. 10.21. The sequence of events associated with in-hand covering: (a) the stallion is bridled and brought into the covering area to meet the mare; (b) the stallion is then introduced to the mare and teases her immediately prior to covering; (c) the stallion is allowed to approach the mare from an angle. Ideally, the stallion should be calm and not over-enthusiastic; (d) the stallion is allowed to cover the mare; ejaculation is marked by flagging of the stallion's tail; (e) ejaculation is followed by a quiescent period prior to dismount; and (f) the stallion dismounts at will and is led away from the mare.

a protective barrier. This arrangement may also be used to protect handlers with mares that strike out. If a leg strap is being used to restrain the mare, it must be released at this stage. For this reason tight hobbles are not advocated, as they do not allow the mare to move in order to accommodate the weight of the mounting stallion.

As mentioned, many traditional studs still advocate the use of an assistant stallion handler to pull the mare's tail to one side and guide the penis into the vagina. However, this is no longer considered good practice, as any unexpected external stimuli may disrupt the normal sequence of events leading up to ejaculation, especially in young stallions.

Successful ejaculation is signalled by the rhythmic flagging of the stallion's tail (Fig. 10.21d). In most stallions this is clearly evident but, if in doubt, the urethral contractions can be felt by a hand placed along the ventral side of the penis. However, possible disruption of the natural sequence of events must again be considered.

After ejaculation, the stallion should be allowed to relax on the mare (Figs 10.4 and 10.21e). During this period of relaxation the glans penis, which has increased in size considerably at ejaculation, returns to normal, allowing the penis to be withdrawn. Early withdrawal can cause damage to the stallion and mare and the engorged glans penis may act to cause a vacuum, drawing semen out of the cervix/uterus. The stallion should then be allowed to dismount at will, which may take several minutes. The mare should then be turned towards her handler and walked slowly away, allowing the stallion to slide off and reducing the chance of him being hit should she lash out. The stallion should similarly be turned towards his handler after he has dismounted, again reducing the chance of injury to the mare or handlers. Some studs routinely collect a dismount semen sample from the drips on the penis at dismount, to confirm the presence of spermatozoa, and so confirm successful ejaculation; similarly, a dismount swab may also be taken from the urethral area, but these are not common practices. Increasingly, in studs running high-value stallions, the mating process is videoed to provide additional evidence that covering has taken place.

After covering, the stallion should be allowed to wind down and walked to the washing area. There his penis should be washed and his genitalia examined for abrasions. Many practitioners advocate walking the mare around slowly after covering to prevent her straining

and so losing semen. However, as the vast majority of the semen is deposited into the top of the cervix and uterus, beyond the cervical seal, it is very unlikely that there will be significant loss at post-coital straining. Any semen that is lost is likely to have been that deposited into the vagina and, as such, will have limited bearing on fertility.

Occasionally, the mare and stallion differ in size. If so, certain precautions should be taken. A very large stallion put on to a small mare should be considered carefully, as it may cause her problems in late pregnancy owing to potentially larger fetal size near term. The reverse situation poses no such problems. To assist in the mating of horses of unequal size, some covering yards have a dip in the floor or use a breeding platform to equalize the horses' heights (Fig. 10.22). Hydraulic breeding platforms are available and can be adjusted to the exact height required.

A breeding roll may also be used if there is concern that the stallion's penis is too long, or with maiden mares, to prevent vaginal rupture (Fig. 10.23). The breeding roll is placed between the mare's perineum and the belly of the stallion, preventing him from penetrating too far and so causing damage. The breeding roll is usually a padded leather roll of 15–20 cm in diameter and approximately 50 cm long. In an attempt to maintain sterile conditions, it can be covered with a disposable examination glove.

The Covering Yard

The covering yard can be any area that is quiet, dry and safe, with a non-slip surface and away from the melee of the general yard. A paddock, open yard or specially designed covered area (Figs 10.21 and 10.22) may be used. If large enough, this covering yard can double up as an exercise area.

If an area is to be specially designed, it should be at least 20 × 12 m, roofed and with two sets of wide doors to allow horses to enter and exit in different directions. It is very important that the floor of the covering yard is clean, non-slip and dust-free. Suitable surfaces include clay, chalk, peat moss and woodchip; rubber is now increasingly popular (Figs 10.21 and 10.22). The requirement for a non-slip surface makes floorings such as concrete not advisable, although they are occasionally used.

10.3. Management of the Foal at Covering

A perceived major problem when covering mares is the danger to any foals at foot (Figs 10.24a and b). The

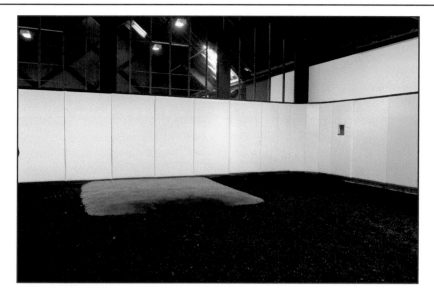

Fig. 10.22. Rubber is increasingly popular as a dust-free surface for a covering yard. Note also the raised matted area that can be used for mating horses of different heights.

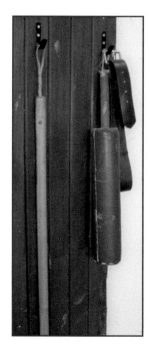

Fig. 10.23. A breeding roll (on the right) used to prevent large stallions penetrating mares too far and causing damage.

majority of mares either foal at the stud or, more commonly now, arrive with foals of a very young age. In nature, this presents no significant problems, as foals naturally move away from the mating activity but stay within the vicinity of the mare. If teasing and/or mating is to occur in a large open area, the foal may be let loose and will normally keep well away from the proceedings, or held within sight of its dam, reducing anxiety and stress (Fig. 10.24a and b). If mating is to occur in a small enclosed covering yard, or if the mare is difficult, the foal should be restrained for its own safety (Fig. 10.11). It may be removed and put in a loose box within sight of the mare and with a handler to watch it. However, some mares will become distracted by the antics of the foal. In such cases, more success may be achieved by removing the foal altogether, out of sight and earshot. The system used depends entirely on the character of the mare and foal, facilities available and personal preference. Further consideration of foal heat breeding is given in Section 13.2.2.

10.4. Management of Mares Susceptible to Post-coital Endometritis

All mares suffer from post-coital endometritis to some extent, but some mares appear to be more susceptible than others and, in such a situation, conception rates can be significantly depressed (Knutti *et al.*, 2000; Watson, 2000; Troedsson, 1999, 2006, 2011; Lui and Troedsson, 2008; Woodward and Troedsson, 2013). These mares can be managed in a number of ways to reduce excessive post-coital inflammatory response, including prolonged teasing, as mentioned previously; lavage; and/or treatment with oxytocin post-covering. Details of the management techniques that can be used are given in Section 14.3.5.3.

10.5. Variations in Mating Management

As mentioned previously, there are many variations on the above theme, many being more cost-effective and

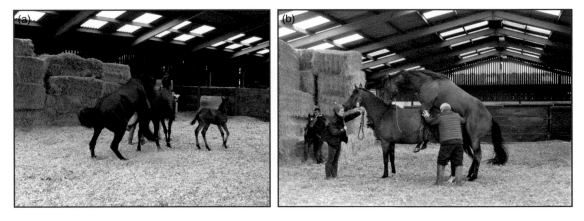

Fig. 10.24. Mares with foals at foot may prove difficult to tease and cover successfully. One method is to allow the foal to (a) move freely within a large covering area; or (b) be held close to the mare.

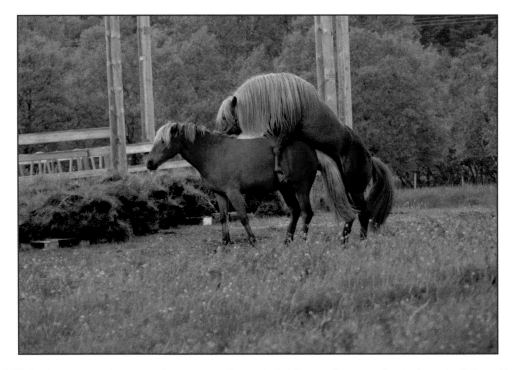

Fig. 10.25. In the most natural system stallions are turned out with their harem of mares and mate them at will. A good halfway house is to turn individual mares out with a stallion; this allows visiting mares to be accommodated in as natural a mating scenario as possible. (Photo courtesy of Ms Lillian Jensen, Norway.)

used on the smaller native studs. The alternatives include covering in a small open paddock, yard or railed area with a non-slip surface, possibly earth or grass. Many stallions, especially in the native pony industry, successfully cover mares in hand in a convenient field near to the main yard. This is how mares would have been covered historically, when stallions were walked around from farm to farm. If covering is to occur in a large field, then the stallion used must be well behaved and controlled, as his escape may incur considerable wasted time and disturbance to mares in adjacent fields.

The other extreme to in-hand breeding is pasture breeding, where the stallion is allowed to run free with his mares to cover them at will (Fig. 10.25). This system is the nearest to the natural situation but, as discussed at the beginning of this Chapter, presents problems with visiting mares. Pasture breeding is popular in semi-feral ponies such as the mountain ponies of Wales and Scotland, and in parts of Europe; it also takes place in South Africa and South America, where mares are run in large herds over wide expanses of land with stallions running out freely. Fertility rates in such systems are very good (Bristol, 1982; Davies Morel and Gunnarsson, 2000; McDonnell, 2000a).

A halfway house between in-hand breeding and pasture breeding is to allow the stallion to be loose in the field and to introduce the mares to him individually, either restrained or free. This system allows visiting mares to be successfully covered in a system that is quite near to the natural one. Stallions used in this system must, however, be of an appropriate temperament and their characteristics well known by the mare handler, so that any necessary avoiding action may be taken.

10.6. Conclusion

It is evident that there is a vast array of management practices for covering mares. The system ultimately chosen is up to the individual stud, its facilities, normal practices and labour available. Financial considerations also have a considerable bearing on management choices. Intensive breeding systems are commonly employed as they provide more protection for both handlers and horses, but often at the expense of natural equine behaviour and reproductive performance. More recently, alternative systems of mating mares are being considered, which address some of these concerns.

Study Questions

Discuss the use of teasing as a method to determine the most appropriate time to mate a mare.

Critically evaluate the effectiveness of methods, other than teasing, that are available to predict the timing of naturally occurring oestrus and ovulation in the mare.

Evaluate the various ways in which mares can be teased and the challenges these methods may present.

Evaluate the various methods that may be used to mate a mare. Include in your answer a discussion of the challenges these methods may present, both to stallion owners aiming to maximize their financial return, and to the safety and welfare of the mare. By which means can these challenges be overcome?

Detail how you would choose to manage a mare to be mated in hand for the period of time immediately before, during and immediately after mating.

Suggested Reading

Newcombe, J.R. (1994) A comparison of ovarian follicular diameter in Thoroughbred mares between Australia and the UK. *Journal of Equine Veterinary Science* 14, 653–654.

Bergfeldt, D.R. (2000) Anatomy and physiology of the mare. In: Samper, J.C. (ed.) *Equine Breeding Management and Artificial Insemination.* W.B. Saunders, Philadelphia, Pennsylvania, pp. 141–164.

McDonnell, S.M. (2000) Reproductive behaviour of stallion and mares: comparison of free-running and domestic in-hand breeding. *Animal Reproduction Science* 60–61, 211–219.

Mills, D. and McDonnell, S.M. (2005) *The Domestic Horse. The origins, development and management of its behaviour.* Cambridge University Press, Cambridge, UK, pp. 239.

McDonnell, S.M. (2011) Normal sexual behavior. In: McKinnon, A.O., Squires, E.L., Vaala, E. and Varner, D.D. (eds) *Equine Reproduction*, 2nd edn. Wiley-Blackwell, Philadelphia, London, pp. 1385–1390.

McCue, P.M., Scoggin, C.F. and Lindholm, A.R.G. (2011) Estrus. In: McKinnon, A.O., Squires, E.L, Vaala, W.E. and Varner, D.D. (eds) *Equine Reproduction*, 2nd edn. Wiley-Blackwell, pp. 1716–1727.

11 Management of the Pregnant Mare

The Objectives of this Chapter are:

To apply the knowledge of reproductive physiology and behaviour you have gained in Part A to the management of the pregnant mare.

To evaluate the various management options available, and so enable you to make informed decisions, when managing the pregnant mare.

To enable you to appreciate the various methods available for detecting pregnancy in the mare, and the appropriateness of their use at different stages of pregnancy.

To provide you with the information on and expectations of the normal pregnant mare, so you are aware when things are abnormal and know when to seek specialist help.

11.1. Introduction

Before the management of the pregnant mare is considered, it is essential to ascertain whether she is indeed pregnant. Once pregnancy has been confirmed the mare can be monitored and managed accordingly. The diagnosis of a twin pregnancy poses specific problems in the mare, and these will also be considered.

11.2. Pregnancy Diagnosis

Pregnancy detection may be carried out for a number of reasons. Ideally, it is conducted as soon as possible so that non-pregnant mares can be re-covered on their next oestrus, and twin pregnancies identified and appropriate action taken. It may also be necessary for sale or for insurance purposes, particularly relevant if the mare is in the last two-thirds of her gestation. Finally, if the agreement at covering is 'no foal, no fee', it establishes whether a fee is due. The customary date on which the buyer of a stallion nomination has to pay in the northern hemisphere is 1 October; the corresponding date in the southern hemisphere is 1 April.

The mnemonic 'AEIOU' describes the major requirements of an ideal pregnancy test:

A   Accurate.
E   Early.
I   Inexpensive.
O   Once only.
U   Uncomplicated.

There are problems with many tests in that some fail to indicate embryo viability, the presence of twin pregnancies, anticipate fetal death or differentiate between embryonic vesicles and uterine cysts. Numerous methods of detection are available; however, none (as yet) meet all the above criteria (Collins and Buckley, 1993; Lofstedt and Newcombe, 1997; Henderson *et al.*, 1998; McCue and McKinnon, 2011b).

11.2.1. Behaviour

The majority of mares that successfully conceive cease oestrous behaviour. However, it has been reported that 5–10% of pregnant mares display some oestrous-like behaviour, usually around days 35–40, as there is a peak in the oestrogen levels originating from the follicles destined to become secondary corpus luteums (CLs) (Section 3.3.1.4). It has also been suggested that this may be particularly evident in mares carrying filly foals (Hayes and Ginther, 1989). It might be assumed that the failure to return to oestrus in a mare that has been covered would indicate pregnancy; however, mares are known to fail to return to oestrus for other reasons, such as silent oestrus, prolonged oestrous cycle, early embryonic

© CAB International 2021. *Equine Reproductive Physiology, Breeding and Stud Management,* 5th Edition. (M. Davies Morel.)

death or even going out of the breeding season if bred late in the year. Hence, behaviour may be used only as an indicator of pregnancy, as it is far from 100% accurate.

11.2.2. External appearance

At 5–6 months of pregnancy the abdomen may take on a typical pear shape as the fetus appears to 'drop'. As pregnancy progresses, movement of the fetus may be seen through the musculature and tissue of the abdominal wall. This method of pregnancy diagnosis is of little use until late in pregnancy.

11.2.3. Manual tests

Manual methods of pregnancy detection are the oldest and cheapest, and still in use. A major advantage is that they give immediate results, although they can only be used accurately after day 20 post-coitum. Examination is carried out via rectal palpation or cervical/vaginal examination.

11.2.3.1. Rectal palpation

Rectal palpation, as described in Section 8.7.3, allows the uterus to be felt through the rectum wall. Initial work on this technique was carried out by Day (1940). This, and subsequent work, suggests that with experience an accurate diagnosis can be made from 20–30 days post-coitum. At this stage the embryonic vesicle can be felt as a discrete swelling on the ventral side of the uterus on either side of the midline, at the junction of the uterine horn and uterine body. Additionally, the uterus may feel turgid around the conceptus, rather than flaccid as in the non-pregnant state. Detection of pregnancy is reported to be possible at day 16 as an increase in uterine tone and thickening of the uterine wall, rather than identification of the embryonic vesicle itself, but poor accuracy precludes its regular use so early. Occasionally, with awkard mares, diagnosis is not possible until day 50. Normally, the accuracy of detection is very good and at its best at day 60, at which stage the age of the fetus can be estimated to within 1 week and the presence of twins detected (McKinnon, 1993; McCue and McKinnon, 2011b).

After day 60 the fetus appears to move towards the uterine body and, owing to its size, palpation of the margins of the fetal sack is difficult. In the case of twins, the fetal sacks merge, and their diagnosis becomes inaccurate. From this stage onwards, the whole uterus becomes progressively less turgid and more distended, with no discrete swellings detected (Fig. 11.1). Hence, the accuracy of pregnancy detection at these later stages

declines. However, as pregnancy progresses still further, it becomes possible to feel fetal structures, such as the head and ribs, through the uterine wall. After day 200, accuracy of detection returns to near 100%. At this stage, the fetus can be readily felt through the now much thinner uterine wall (McKinnon, 1993). Pregnancy will now become increasingly obvious from the mare's external appearance. Table 11.1 indicates the size of the embryonic vesicle at various stages throughout early pregnancy.

Pregnancy detection using rectal palpation is most commonly conducted between days 20 and 35 of gestation and is now considered accurate and safe, although some historical discussion with regard to a link with abortion has occurred (see Section 11.2.3.3).

The major disadvantage of rectal palpation is that it cannot accurately be used early enough to detect mares failing to conceive in time to allow them to be re-covered within one oestrous cycle, and is unreliable in the detection of twins. However, the technique is quick, simple and cheap, and gives immediate results.

11.2.3.2. Cervical/vaginal examination

Vaginoscopy, the examination of the mare's cervix and vagina via a speculum (Section 8.7.1), can be used as an aid to pregnancy detection, but is not accurate enough to be used in isolation (McCue and McKinnon, 2011b). By day 30 the pregnant cervix should appear white/light pink in colour, firm and with a sticky mucus. The vagina also contains sticky opaque mucus, making the insertion of the speculum difficult. However, there is significant variation in cervical/vaginal characteristics between mares, making the technique inaccurate when used in isolation (Asbury, 1991). Used in conjunction with rectal palpation, however, it can be a useful aid to diagnosis in awkward mares.

11.2.3.3. Abortion risk

Historically, there are conflicting reports associating manual manipulation of the mare's reproductive tract with an increased risk of abortion. Allen (1974) and Voss and Pickett (1975) produced no evidence of such an association in pony mares. In fact, they suggest that abortion of a twin by squeezing (pinching out) of the fetal sack through the uterine wall per rectum at day 40 requires considerably more relative force than ordinary rectal palpation, but is reported to carry only a minimal risk to the remaining fetus. However, Osborne (1975) demonstrated that uterine myometrial activity does

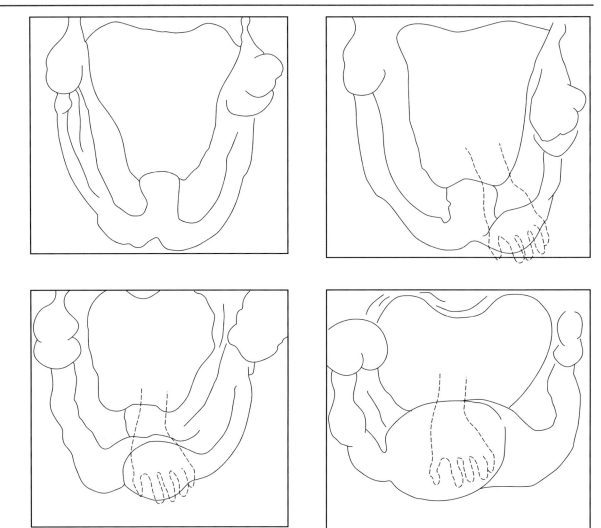

Fig. 11.1. The expected size of the fetal sack at various stages of pregnancy when undertaking rectal palpation. Top left: non-pregnant uterus; top right: 25-day pregnant uterus; bottom left: 45-day pregnant uterus; bottom right: 60-day pregnant uterus.

Table 11.1. The size of the embryonic vesicle at various stages during early pregnancy in the mare.

Age of pregnancy (days post-coitum)	Size of embryonic vesicle (diameter mm)	Comments
15	15–20	Feel for uterine tone
20	30–40	Embryonic vesicle first detected
30	40–50	–
40	60–70	–
50	80–90	–
60	100–130	Most accurate diagnosis

–, no comments applicable

increase at palpation, and that increased levels of such stress are associated with abortion. The current consensus of opinion is that any association between rectal palpation and abortion is due to the stress of unaccustomed handling, rather than by the technique per se. This association between stress and reproductive failure is increasingly evident (AboEl-Maaty, 2011; Malschitzky *et al.*, 2015) and underlines the need to ensure that mares are accustomed to their environment and breeding techniques. This link between stress and reproductive stress is of increasing concern now that mares are increasingly 'walked in' (arrive to be covered for the day, often with young foals at foot) rather than the traditional boarding at the stud (Baucus *et al.*, 1990).

11.2.4. Blood tests

Blood tests are of particular use in small ponies and mares with injuries or rectal/vaginal tears which render rectal palpation and ultrasonic pregnancy detection not feasible. Blood plasma concentrations of one or several hormones may be used to indicate pregnancy. These tests can be very accurate, but can be associated with false positive results, and also have the disadvantage of cost and a possible delay before the results are available.

11.2.4.1. Equine chorionic gonadotrophin

As discussed, in between days 35 and 100 of gestation, the endometrial cups produce equine chorionic gonadotrophin (eCG), also known as pregnant mare serum gonadotrophin (PMSG), which can be detected in plasma samples between days 35 and 100 post-coitum (Section 3.3.1.3; Allen *et al.*, 2002a; Antczak *et al.*, 2013). The presence of eCG is traditionally detected via the haemagglutination inhibition test, now more commonly known as the mare immunological pregnancy (MIP) test. This is still used, along with a range of more recent tests including immunological tests such as ELISA and radioimmunoassay (RIA) (Asbury, 1991; McCue and McKinnon, 2011b). During the period 45–100 days post-coitum, all three tests have an accuracy of 60–100%. The ELISA test, however, allows earlier detection at day 35 with 43% accuracy and is more accurate (100%) at day 40 than the MIP test (31–37% accuracy; De Coster *et al.*, 1980; Squires *et al.*, 1983). All three tests can be performed in less than 2 h.

Despite its accuracy, testing for eCG has two major disadvantages: variability in the time span in which the endometrial cups produce eCG, and an inability to determine whether the fetus is viable. eCG levels are typically raised from day 35; however, the rate at which they decline after the peak at around day 70 depends on individual mares (Section 3.3.1.3). Additionally, a mare carrying a twin pregnancy will have significantly greater eCG levels (McCue and McKinnon, 2011b). Most importantly, after spontaneous or induced abortion, the endometrial cups continue to secrete eCG for several days and, therefore, an erroneous positive result will be obtained. eCG is also, therefore, unable to inform if the pregnancy is viable or not (McKinnon, 1993; Steiner *et al.*, 2006).

11.2.4.2. Progesterone

Progesterone is the hormone responsible for the maintenance of pregnancy (see Section 3.3.1.2) and, as might be expected, elevated levels are indicative of the presence of a fetus. When testing very early in pregnancy at the time of the mare's possible return to oestrus, elevated levels (those greater than 1–5 ng ml^{-1}) on days 16–17 post-coitum are reported to be 71% accurate in indicating pregnancy (Villani *et al.*, 2000). In non-pregnant mares progesterone levels should be declining at this time. Hence progesterone levels below 1 ng ml^{-1} indicate no pregnancy or a failing pregnancy. However, it must be borne in mind that there are other reasons why a mare's progesterone levels may remain high at days 16–17, such as cycle variation, failure of CL regression or prolonged cycle (Hoffmann *et al.*, 1996; McCue and Squires, 2002). Use of progesterone to diagnose pregnancy after the placenta takes over progesterone production is less accurate, as the placenta produces a variety of progestins (Sections 3.3.1.2 and 3.3.2.1) which have varying cross-reactivity with assays used. Commercial kits are now available for the rapid testing of plasma progesterone concentrations.

11.2.4.3. Oestrogen

Oestrogens are present in a conjugated form such as oestrone sulfate or as unconjugated oestrogens (oestradiol 17β, oestrone, ostradiol 17). Various tests measure both conjugated and total (conjugated and unconjugated) oestrogens. Both can be identified in the mare's plasma during pregnancy and follow a similar pattern (McCue and McKinnon 2011b). Elevated levels are observed at days 35–60 (Section 3.3.1.4); however, at this stage they are ovarian in origin and so are of limited diagnostic value, but may be a preliminary indicator of pregnancy (Hyland and Langsford, 1990). However, the second rise in oestrogens (oestrones, equilin and equilenin) from day 60 onwards, and peaking around day 210, are feto-placental in origin (Section 3.3.2.2) and so post-day 80 provide an accurate, but late, diagnosis of a viable pregnancy (Henderson and Stewart, 2000). Schuler (1998) reported that plasma concentrations higher than 1.6 ng ml^{-1} are diagnostic of pregnancy and that concentrations lower than 0.8 ng ml^{-1} confirm a negative result. Concentrations between these two levels are inconclusive. Traditional biological tests and the chemical Cuboni test for oestrogens have been replaced by immunological (RIA and ELISA) tests. Most recently, the use of ELISA dipstick tests have been investigated (Henderson and Stewart, 2000, 2002). Oestrogen analysis has the major advantage of indicating fetal viability, as the fetal–placental unit is required for its production (Lasley *et al.*, 1990; Stabenfeldt *et al.*, 1991; McCue and McKinnon, 2011b). Despite this, the method is of no use for early diagnosis.

11.2.4.4. Early pregnancy factor

An early pregnancy factor (EPF) has been identified in the plasma of pregnant mares, using a rosette inhibition test in several animals as early as 6 h post-coitum (Shaw and Morton, 1980). An equine EPF has been identified from 2 days post-ovulation. After embryo transfer or embryonic death, EPF declines to non-pregnancy levels within 2 days; if pregnancy continues, EPF remains elevated. As such, this test has the potential to provide a useful tool not only for detecting pregnancy, but also for monitoring *in vivo* viability of equine embryos and for detecting embryonic death (Takagi *et al.*, 1998; Ohnuma *et al.*, 2000). More recently Barnea *et al.* (2012) and Paidas *et al.* (2010) have investigated the presence of preimplantation factor (PIF) in mares, as it has been identified in several other mammals. Whether this is the same as the previously identified EPF is unclear, but there has been limited success. Early detection of pregnancy failure would allow the mare to be prepared for covering on her next natural oestrus or at an artificially accelerated return to oestrus, but the test is not yet repeatable and hence not commercially available (Parker *et al.*, 2005). If diagnosis of fertilization ever becomes routinely possible as early as 6 h post-coitum, this will allow the mare to be re-covered at that same oestrus, giving her a second chance to conceive.

11.2.4.5. Relaxin

Plasma relaxin levels peak around days 180–200 and remain high until parturition (Klonisch and Hombach-Klonisch, 2000); as such they have been used with some success to detect pregnancy and inform on fetal viability (Ponthier *et al.*, 2008).

11.2.5. Urine tests

Urine tests, although not very popular, do have their uses in non-lactating mares where rectal palpation or blood sampling proves difficult. Oestrogens in the mare, being of a relatively small molecular weight, are capable of passing unaltered through the kidney's filtration system and can, therefore, be detected in the urine. As with plasma concentrations, pregnancy detection is possible from about day 90, although accuracy of diagnosis at this stage is low. By day 150, accuracy improves significantly (Daels *et al.*, 1991a; McCue and McKinnon, 2011b). Other hormones, such as eCG, have also been reported to be evident in urine and follow the same pattern of release as seen in plasma (Roser and Lofstedt, 1989).

11.2.6. Milk tests

Plasma hormone concentrations are most commonly used, but there may be occasions in lactating mares when obtaining a milk sample is easier and less stressful. Progesterone is the major hormone that can be isolated in milk for use as a pregnancy test. Milk progesterone concentrations increase in parallel with plasma concentrations. As with plasma progesterone, elevated levels are observed after oestrus; a subsequent decline after 10–15 days is indicative of no pregnancy, and continued elevated levels indicate pregnancy, but the same inaccuracies are evident. Conjugated oestrogens can also be identified in milk; again, the concentration pattern correlates closely to that observed in plasma and urine samples (Sist *et al.*, 1987; Raeside *et al.*, 1991).

11.2.7. Faeces tests

Unconjugated oestrogens have been isolated in the faeces of pregnant mares from day 120 and so may be used as a late pregnancy test. Such a test is particularly useful for feral mares and zoo equids (Sist, 1987; Raeside *et al.*, 1991; Linklater *et al.*, 2000; Celebi and Demirel, 2003).

11.2.8. Ultrasonic pregnancy detection

In recent years ultrasonic techniques have revolutionized the detection of pregnancy in many animals. Ultrasonic detectors are based on the principle that ultrasonic sound waves are absorbed or reflected by the objects they hit (Fig. 11.2; Section 8.7.3). This method has the advantage of giving an immediate result and of

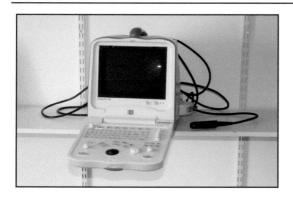

Fig. 11.2. The transducer probe (on the right) is placed in the rectum of the mare and angled down towards the uterus. The image produced is displayed on the monitor.

usually being done on the stud, as the equipment is fully portable (McKinnon, 1993; Sertich, 1998; Ginther, 2008; Bergfeldt and Adams, 2011b; McCue and McKinnon, 2011b). Ultrasonography provides accurate information on the status of the mare at scanning, but it is not able to predict the long-term outcome of any pregnancy, although there is a correlation between conceptus size and viability, small-for-age concepti having a much reduced chance of long-term survival (Newcombe, 2004).

Fraser *et al.* (1973) initially developed the use of the Doppler ultrasound. This machine enables movement, and hence fetal heartbeat, to be detected along with uterine arterial blood flow. The ultrasonic signal is emitted from, and received by, a transducer placed on the mare's abdomen or within her rectum via a rectal probe, and is transduced into an audible sound. The fetal heartbeat can be heard from day 42 of gestation onwards as a distinct beat, accelerated in comparison to the mare, although it is not consistently heard until day 120. The enhanced blood flow through the pregnant mare's uterine artery can also be heard at the same time. It is present as a distinct 'whooshing' noise at a slower beat than the fetal heart. This characteristic blood flow through the pregnant uterus is diagnostic in itself. This method is very accurate at day 120, but accuracy in early pregnancy is not guaranteed; thus, it cannot successfully be used within the timescale required for the mare to be returned to the stallion at her next oestrus. The timespan of use is similar to that of the test for eCG, but it has the obvious advantage of detecting a viable foal (Fraser *et al.*, 1973; Mitchell, 1973). This audio Doppler is not to be confused with the much

newer technology of visual Doppler (Ginther and Utt, 2004). The 1980s saw the development of visual echography, which allowed ultrasonic pregnancy detection by enabling the visualization of the embryonic vesicle within the uterus (McKinnon and Carnevale, 1993; McKinnon *et al.*, 1993; Ginther, 2008; Pycock, 2011). The embryonic vesicle can be detected from days 11–12 onwards as a discrete spherical sack (Ginther, 2008). This typical spherical nature of the equine trophoblast and its characteristic position (after day 17) at the junction of the uterine horn and body is fortunate and, as in the case of the human, allows detection at an early stage with an accuracy in excess of 98% (Ginther, 2008; McCue and McKinnon, 2011b). This method can also be used in the accurate detection of twins in early pregnancy, in addition to uterine cysts, fluid accumulation, sacculations, etc., or (at a later date) fetal viability.

The size of the embryonic vesicle (conceptus) at various stages of early pregnancy is given in Table 11.1. Pregnancy can be first detected at days 11–12, at which stage only the embryonic vesicle can be identified (Fig. 11.3a). At this stage the conceptus is mobile, and migrates within the uterus, making detection more difficult. In addition, there is a higher natural risk of embryo mortality in day 11 embryos than in older ones. By days 17–18 the conceptus has become 'fixed', normally at the junction of the uterine body and uterine horn, and so identification is easier (Allen, 2001a). By day 20 the embryo itself can be identified within the embryonic vesicle (Fig. 11.3b) (Bergfeldt and Adams, 2011b). Days 24–25 herald the first detection of the fetal heartbeat (Allen and Goddard, 1984; McCue and McKinnon, 2011b); by day 40 many of the features can be clearly seen (Fig. 11.3c,d); and, during two windows of time (days 55–90 and days 120–200) fetal gender may be determined (Mari *et al.*, 2002; Holder, 2011; Velde *et al.*, 2018). Most recently, transabdominal 3D tomographic ultrasound imaging (TUI) has been employed with additional success in determining fetal gender (Pricking *et al.*, 2019).

In practice most studs scan for pregnancy at day 18, which is the most accurate time, and early enough to allow arrangements to be made for re-covering. An additional scan at day 40, after the period of highest risk, may be considered. In the Thoroughbred industry, where there is a high incidence of twins, initial scanning is often carried out at days 11–12, to identify twins and manage the mare accordingly (Section 11.3). The mare is then re-scanned at days 18–20 and again at day 40. The period of greatest risk for pregnancy loss is prior to

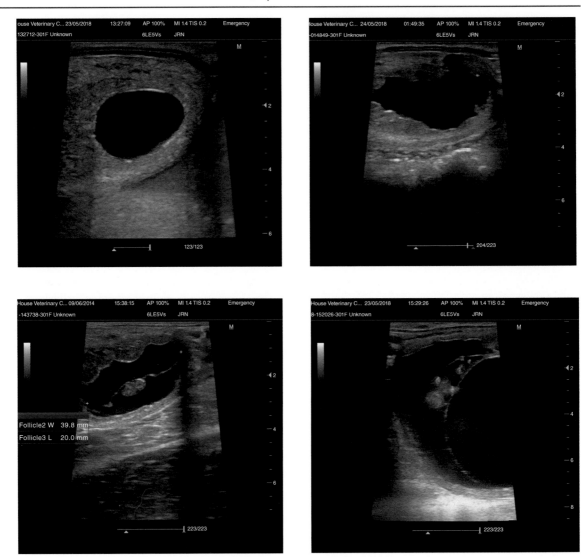

Fig. 11.3. A typical scanning photograph showing (a) a day-13 conceptus (note the clear spherical shape); (b) a day-20 conceptus (note the embryo at the bottom right of the black, and now somewhat collapsed, spherical conceptus); (c) a day-29 conceptus (note the embryo in the centre – you can just identify the head and forelimbs – and the clear demarcation between the growing allantoic sack and the shrinking blastocoel); and (d) a day-43 conceptus (note that the embryo's head and four limbs can be clearly seen). (Photos courtesy of Professor John Newcombe.)

day 40, so pregnancies present at this time are very likely to go to term (Section 11.4). Colour Doppler ultrasonography has been developed recently: this allows the movement of blood to be detected (Ginther and Utt, 2004; Ginther, 2008). The colours produced, usually red and blue, relate to the velocity and direction of blood flow (red towards the transducer, blue away from the transducer). As such, colour Doppler has been suggested as a tool to assess ovarian follicular development but, in the case of the pregnant mare, to assess uterine blood flow with the possibility of using it as a way to evaluate pregnancy viability (Bollwein *et al.*, 2004; Silva and Ginther, 2006; Ousey *et al.*, 2012; Freccero *et al.*, 2018). It has also been suggested to be a very accurate method of determining fetal sex (Rezende *et al.*, 2014).

11.2.9. Fetal electrocardiography

A fetal heart electrocardiogram may be obtained from electrodes strategically placed on the mare's body, which pick up the fetal electrical heart impulses. The electrocardiogram (ECG) readout given can be used to detect the presence of a fetal heartbeat and also any abnormalities (Adams-Brendemuehl and Pipers, 1987; Nagel *et al.*, 2010). Its popularity as a tool for diagnosing pregnancy is limited, due to the complication of setting it up, and it can only be used in late pregnancy. However, it does have its uses in detecting and monitoring fetal stress or cardiac abnormalities, especially near to parturition or during a difficult delivery. It can also confirm fetal viability and the presence of twins (Parkes and Colles, 1977; Buss *et al.*, 1980; Vera *et al.*, 2018).

11.3. Management of Twin Pregnancies

The conception of a multiple pregnancy (in the vast majority of cases, twin pregnancies) is a significant and increasing problem in pregnant mare management. As discussed previously (Section 3.2.4.2) the mare is monocotous, the uterus being unable to adequately support more than one pregnancy. Multiple pregnancies rarely survive to term, most commonly resulting in abortion in mid- to late pregnancy (9–10 months; Ball, 1993b; Card, 2000; McKinnon, 2011). Prior to the advent of ultrasonic scanning (Fig. 11.4) and the subsequent reduction of twins they were the most common cause of non-infectious abortion, accounting for 20–30% of all occurrences (Macpherson and Reimer, 2000). Of the twin pregnancies conceived it is reported that 64.5% result in two dead or aborted foals, 21% in one live foal and 14.5% result in two live foals (Fig. 11.5a,b; Ginther and Griffin, 1994; Card, 2000). Rates of twinning differ significantly between mares and breeds but, in the Thoroughbred, the incidence of twins has been reported to be as high as 16.2% (Newcombe, 1995; Davies Morel and O'Sullivan 2001; Davies Morel *et al.*, 2005). As such, it is advantageous to identify and manage twin pregnancies early on, so they can be managed appropriately. The advent of ultrasonic scanning has significantly helped the early identification and management of twins (Fig. 11.4).

There are four main management practices used to reduce the incidence of twins: monitor ovulation; wait and see; manually reduce; abort using prostaglandin F2α (PGF2α) (Card, 2000; Macpherson and Reimer, 2000; Hodder *et al.*, 2008; McKinnon, 2011). Historically, the incidence of twinning was reduced by monitoring ovarian activity using rectal palpation, and withholding mating from mares with more than one large follicle. The mare would then be mated on the next natural or the next artificially advanced oestrus. This successfully reduced twinning rates within a population, but with it conception rates declined and the time interval between parturition and successful covering increased (Pugh and Schumacher, 1990). To address these drawbacks, identification and treatment of actual twin pregnancies, rather than of potential twin pregnancies, is required. Naturally, in excess of 83% of twin pregnancies are spontaneously reduced to singles around the time of embryonic fixation (day 18; Ginther and Bergfeldt, 1988; Chavatte, 1997a). So, one option is to monitor the pregnancy and observe if natural reduction occurs. If it does not, induced abortion at a later stage may be advocated. The advent of scanning now allows such monitoring to take place easily. An alternative to natural reduction is to manually reduce. Manual reduction of twins to a single has been reported to be up to 96% successful between days 13 and 16 (Nath *et al.*, 2010). Manual reduction involves the manual squeezing of the smallest embryo, identified by ultrasound, either between the thumb and forefinger or by using the scanner probe to push the conceptus against the uterine wall and pelvis until the vesicle ruptures (McKinnon, 2011). This is best done prior to fixation (day 18) so is normally carried out at initial scanning, days 11–12 (Davies Morel *et al.*, 2012; McKinnon, 2011). However, asynchronous multiple ovulations are common and can be as far as 72 h apart, and so scanning at such an early stage runs the risk of missing the conceptus resulting from the later ovulation and so erroneously diagnosing the mare as not carrying a multiple pregnancy (Fig. 11.4a; Davies Morel *et al.*, 2015). It is common practice, therefore, to scan mares again at around the time of fixation (day 18). After fixation, and up to about day 30, the manual reduction of twins can still be successful, but reduction of unilateral twins (both in the same horn) is less successful than that of bilateral twins (one in each horn). In both cases there is a higher risk of losing the whole pregnancy than is seen with single pregnancies and with earlier reduction (Chavatte, 1997a; McKinnon, 2011). Other methods of manual reduction can be used, including transvaginal ultrasound-guided aspiration, which is reported to have a 70% success rate in eliminating just one embryo between days 16 and 35. Use after day 40 significantly increases the chance of both embryos dying (Macpherson

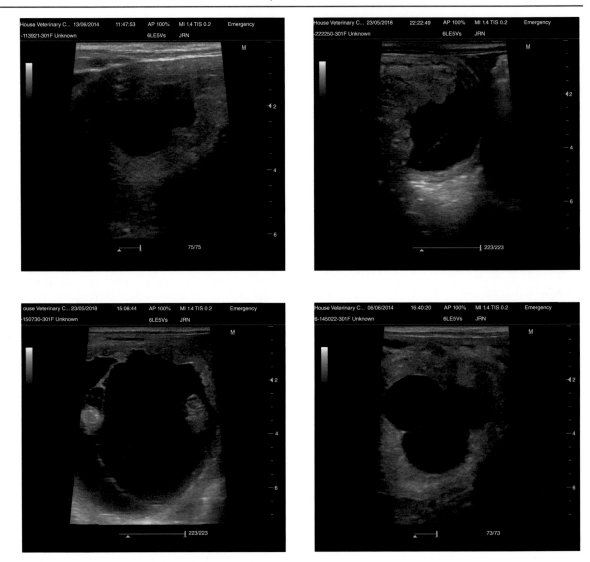

Fig. 11.4. Unilateral (in the same horn) twins: (a) asynchronous twins aged day 15 and day 13, conceived by ova that ovulated 48 h apart; (b) at day 17, the clear thin line separating the dark fluid into two demarks where the two concepti abut; (c) at day 40, the two embryos can clearly be seen within their individual allantoic sacks; and (d) day-14 unilateral triplet. (Photos courtesy of Professor John Newcombe.)

and Reimer, 2000; Mari *et al.*, 2005; Govaere *et al.*, 2008; Klewitz *et al.*, 2013). At a later stage of pregnancy (after day 40) ultrasound-guided allantocentesis (Macpherson *et al.*, 1995) and transabdominal fetal cardiac puncture have been used, but have not proved as successful as early manual reduction, and so are very rarely used commercially (Rantanen and Kinkaid, 1989; Chavatte, 1997a; Card, 2000; Dascanio, 2014a). Finally, and most recently, umbilical and fetal oscillation

between day 45 and day 50, which disrupts blood supply and therefore compromises fetal survival, has been reported to be successful (Beavers *et al.*, 2017). An alternative to manual reduction of one twin is to artificially induce abortion of the whole pregnancy and re-cover the mare at the next advanced oestrus. Abortion and subsequent return to oestrus and ovulation can be induced using a single injection of $PGF_{2\alpha}$, although multiple injections may be required later on in pregnancy.

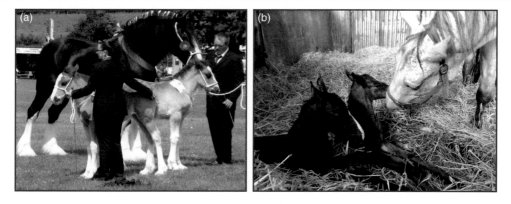

Fig. 11.5. Successful birth of twin foals is a very rare event. Owing to the size of the mare the chances of survival are greater in the Shire (a) than in a pony mare (Connemara) (b), but still very rare. (Photo (a) courtesy of Dr Debbie Nash; photo (b) courtesy of Ashley Middler on behalf of Craigmancie Stud.)

Abortion can be induced prior to the next expected oestrus; that is, before day 21 of pregnancy. This is often done at the time of first scanning, which may be as early as day 11, in which case the mare's return to pregnancy post-abortion may be within 8–10 days. However, with the success of ultrasonic-guided manual reduction of twins, abortion of the whole pregnancy at this stage is rarely an option chosen. Alternatively, the pregnancy may be allowed to progress longer in the hope that natural reduction may occur before $PGF_{2\alpha}$ is required. However, if a rapid return to oestrus is desired then $PGF_{2\alpha}$ must be administered prior to the development of the endometrial cups at day 40 (Chavatte, 1997a).

11.4. Embryonic Loss

Mares suffer from relatively high rates of early embryonic death (EED, prior to day 20) and embryo mortality (EM, prior to day 40). The times of highest risk are prior to day 20 and then prior to day 40. This further justifies the typical scanning routine discussed previously (Section 11.2.8) of scanning on days 12–14, then on days 18–20 and finally on days 35–40 of pregnancy, as they cover the periods of biggest risk. The reasons for, and causes of, embryonic loss and the subsequent failure to produce a foal are discussed in detail in Chapter 14. In an attempt to reduce embryonic loss, some studs routinely place their mares on daily progesterone supplementation therapy in the form of injections or oral treatment for the first 100–150 days of pregnancy. From day 100–150 onwards, placental progesterone alone should be adequate. The use of such routine progesterone supplementation is questioned by some, as there is little evidence that it prevents embryonic mortality in the

majority of pregnancies, and it prevents the expression of the warning signs of a return to oestrus should EM occur (Holtan, 1993; Canisso, 2013b). Having proven successful in cattle, gonadotrophin-releasing hormone (GnRH) administration on days 10–12 post-conception has also been advocated for use in mares, with a reported increase in pregnancy rates (Newcombe *et al.*, 2001; Newcombe and Peters, 2014).

11.5. Pregnant Mare Management

The general management of the pregnant mare is important to ensure that the fetus is given every advantage and that the mare's future reproductive capacity is maintained. A fit condition throughout pregnancy is advantageous, allowing a mare to foal with ease, and to be in optimum physical condition to embark on another pregnancy as soon as possible post-partum. An understanding of the developmental changes of both the mare and the fetus during gestation is essential in order to gear her management towards optimum reproductive performance. These developmental changes are detailed in Chapter 3.

There is little specific information on the environmental factors that affect fetal well-being. However, good management of the pregnant mare is clearly one of them, and can be reviewed under six main headings: exercise; nutrition; parasite control; vaccination; teeth care; and feet care. In addition, it is becoming increasingly evident that the stresses involved in much of the intensive management of mares, not least the ultimate control of the mating process, have a negative effect on reproductive success (Causey *et al.*, 2005; Malschitzky *et al.*, 2015).

11.5.1. Exercise

Exercise and nutrition are closely related and together are the major determining factors of body condition. As with most things, it is the extremes that can prove harmful, and so in the case of exercise a happy medium is to be aimed for. The absolute level of exercise depends on the individual mare and her history; ideally, mares should be turned out 24 h a day to allow them to exercise at will. Alternatively, a moderate exercise regime may be provided in the form of regular daily turnout or gentle ridden exercise in early pregnancy (Fig. 11.6a,b). Mares that are used to being ridden can be ridden with increasing gentleness up until 6 months of pregnancy. In the last trimester of pregnancy, forced exercise should cease, and ideally be replaced by group pasturing. Mares turned out in groups tend to exercise more effectively than those turned out alone (Kiley-Worthington and Wood-Gush, 1987).

Gentle exercise promotes and enhances the circulatory system. As discussed in Section 3.2.3.1, the fetus depends entirely upon its dam for its nutrient intake and waste output. This transport system is provided by the blood circulatory system, in particular the utero-ovarian artery and vein. Blood circulation through this system, and hence oxygen and nutrient supply to the fetus, is enhanced by exercise. Exercise reduces water retention (oedema), often associated with mares that are kept standing inside for prolonged periods of time, especially in late pregnancy. Exercise helps to maintain body condition and reduce obesity; hence the chance of

complications at parturition is reduced and the maintenance of muscle tone will enhance delivery.

Exercise must be consistent and not exhaustive, as this has been associated with high abortion rates. Excessive exercise may also cause stress, as may sudden movements, travelling, sale rings and even low-flying aircraft. Stress is known to increase abortion rates, especially in early pregnancy and around day 40, as well as during the last 6–8 weeks of pregnancy (Causey *et al.*, 2005; Malschitzky *et al.*, 2015).

11.5.2. Nutrition

The nutritional requirements of a pregnant mare vary according to whether she has a foal at foot and is lactating, or whether she was previously barren and so has only to satisfy the requirements for her own maintenance plus fetal growth (Hintz, 1993a). Lactation in the mare naturally lasts 10–11 months, although man normally dictates that foals are weaned at around 6 months. It is, therefore, during this time that the two groups of mares with or without foals at foot vary in their requirements. In an ideal system, and providing there are enough mares to justify it, these two classes of mares should be fed separately. During pregnancy, a mare's body condition and weight should be carefully monitored to ensure neither that excess weight is gained, nor that she has to mobilize her own body reserves to supplement inadequate nutrition. Her feeding management should vary accordingly. The use of a weigh pad (Fig. 11.7) is ideal to monitor weight on a regular basis, although a weigh band can still give an accurate indication of weight change up to about 6 months of pregnancy, after which it becomes increasingly less accurate. Assessment of body condition by eye and feel is also a

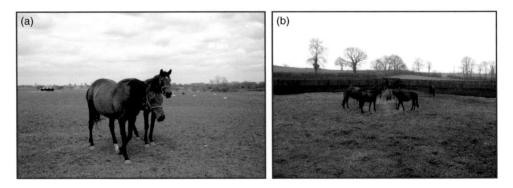

Fig. 11.6. Exercise is essential to maintain a mare's fitness – body condition score of 3 – and to prevent circulatory problems in the later stages of pregnancy. Ideally, mares should be turned out to grass (a) or, if not, then bark paddocks (b) provide a good alternative, allowing mares to exercise at will throughout their pregnancy.

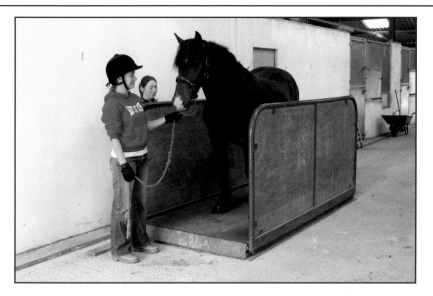

Fig. 11.7. A weigh pad is the ideal method of monitoring a mare's weight, especially when used in conjunction with assessment of body condition by eye and feel.

good way to assess whether nutrient requirements are being met, and not exceeded, and requires no expensive equipment (Figs 8.1–8.4); a condition score of 3 should be maintained throughout pregnancy.

The following discussion concentrates on the nutritional management of the non-lactating mare, as the management of the lactating mare is addressed more fully in Chapter 13. The general principles of nutrition apply to feeding the mare as they do to any formulation of a horse ration. The important nutrients are protein (Crude protein, CP), energy (Digestible Energy, DE), vitamins and minerals (Table 11.2), and they should all be balanced according to need. During pregnancy, requirements do not increase significantly until the last 3 months, when they should be adequate to allow a 14.5% increase in mare body weight at term. During early pregnancy the mare's weight gain should be minimal, although as she progresses into the last trimester (last 100 days), she should be expected to gain in the order of 0.25 kg day^{-1} (Frape, 1998; Card, 2000). This level of weight gain ensures that it is due to an increase in fetal weight and not to excessive deposition of internal body fat. At 7 months of pregnancy the fetus only weighs 20% of its birth weight (10 kg in a 500-kg mare expected give birth to a 50-kg foal) and less than 2% of the mare's weight. By full term the mare's body weight should have increased by 18–20%. Over-fat condition in mares during late pregnancy causes excessive pressure

on the internal organs at parturition, as well as limiting uterine size, and may reduce fetal birth weight and possibly post-natal viability. Others indicate that obesity may result in high foal birth weights and so an increased chance of dystocia (Smith *et al.*, 2015). Limited fat deposition in late pregnancy is desirable, to act as a temporary store for emergency mobilization during early lactation. Failure to gain the required weight may mean that the mare's limited fat reserves are already being mobilized, reducing the energy available to the fetus and hence its growth *in utero*. However, it has been reported that mares restricted to up to 55% of National Research Council requirements (Tables 11.3 and 11.4) give birth to normal birth-weight foals. This demonstrates that healthy mares will mobilize their own body reserves to compensate for low nutritional intake to ensure continuation of fetal growth (Van Niekerk and Van Niekerk, 1997; Frape, 1998).

As in the case of other animals, feed must be of good quality, with adequate roughage to aid digestion and prevent the development of vices through boredom (Winskill *et al.*, 1996). Any good stud will, as a matter of routine, have all batches of hay, haylage, etc., analysed to ascertain the dry matter (DM) content, protein, energy, vitamins and mineral concentrations. This allows accurate balancing of feeds available and identifies the appropriate supplements needed. The quality of feed is also important: conditions such as fungal contamination can cause abortion (Pugh and Schumacher, 1990).

Table 11.2. The average composition of feeds commonly used in horse diets. (From National Research Council, 2007.)

Feed	DM (%)	DE (Mcal/kg)	CP (%)	Lysine (%)	Fat (%)	Fibre (%)	Ca (%)	P (%)	Mg (%)	K (%)	Vitamin A(IU kg⁻¹)
Concentrates											
Barley (rolled)	91.0	3.67	12.4	0.45	2.2	20.8	0.06	0.39	0.14	0.56	817
Sugarbeet (molassed pulp)	88.0	2.84	10.0	0.42	1.1	44.4	0.89	0.09	0.23	1.11	88
Canola meal (mechanical extract)	90.3	2.94	37.8	2.12	5.4	29.8	0.75	1.10	0.53	1.41	–
Maize grain (cracked, dry)	88.1	3.88	9.4	0.27	4.2	9.5	0.04	0.3	0.12	0.42	–
Linseed (meal, solvent)	90.3	2.85	32.6	1.20	1.7	36.1	0.40	0.83	0.55	1.22	–
Oats (grain, rolled)	90.0	3.27	13.2	0.55	5.1	30.0	0.11	0.40	0.16	0.52	44
Sorghum (grain, dry rolled)	88.6	3.75	11.6	0.28	3.1	10.9	0.07	0.35	0.17	0.47	468
Soybean (meal, solvent 48% CP)	89.5	3.73	53.8	3.38	1.1	9.8	0.35	0.70	0.29	2.41	–
Wheat bran	89.1	3.22	17.3	0.70	4.3	42.5	0.13	1.18	0.53	1.32	1,048
Wheat grain (rolled)	89.4	3.83	14.2	0.40	2.3	13.4	0.05	0.43	0.15	0.50	–
Forages											
Lucerne	90.3	2.43	19.2	0.83	2.5	41.6	1.47	0.28	0.29	2.37	41,900
Grass (pasture)	20.1	2.39	26.5	0.92	2.7	45.8	0.56	0.44	0.20	3.36	–
Hay (grass, mature)	84.4	2.04	10.8	0.38	2.0	69.1	0.47	0.26	0.18	1.97	–
Hay (legume, mature)	83.8	2.21	17.8	0.89	1.6	50.9	1.22	0.28	0.27	2.38	–
Silage (grass, mature)	38.7	1.98	12.7	0.43	3.0	66.6	0.56	0.31	0.20	2.42	–
Silage (legume, mature)	42.6	2.19	20.3	0.87	2.1	50.0	1.30	0.33	0.26	2.87	–

DM, dry matter; DE, digestible energy; CP, crude protein; Ca, calcium; P, phosphorus; Mg, magnesium; K, potassium; IU, international unit; –, no/negligible amounts of Vitamin A

Table 11.3. The daily nutrient requirements of pregnant mares of varying weights. (From National Research Council, 2007.)

Stage of pregnancy	Non-pregnant (kg)	Daily gain (kg)	Actual-weight (kg)	DE (Mcal)	CP (g)	Lysine (g)	Ca (g)	P (g)	Mg (g)	K (g)	Vitamin A (mg)
< 5 months	200	–	200	6.7	252	10.8	8.0	5.6	3.0	10.0	8.0
	500	–	500	16.7	630	27.1	20.0	14.0	7.5	25.0	20.0
	900	–	900	30.0	1134	48.8	36.0	25.2	13.5	45.0	36.0
8 months	200	0.13	209	7.4	304	13.1	11.2	8.0	3.0	10.0	8.0
	500	0.32	523	18.5	759	32.7	28.0	20.0	7.6	25.0	20.0
	900	0.57	942	33.3	1367	58.8	50.4	36.0	13.7	45.0	36.0
11 months	200	0.26	226	8.6	357	15.4	14.4	10.5	3.1	10.3	8.0
	500	0.65	566	21.4	893	38.4	36.0	26.3	7.7	25.9	20.0
	900	1.17	1019	38.5	1607	69.1	64.8	47.3	13.8	46.5	36.0

DE, digestible energy; CP, crude protein; Ca, calcium; P, phosphorus; Mg, magnesium; K, potassium; –, not relevant

Table 11.4. The expected feed consumption of pregnant mares (percentage of body weight). (From National Research Council, 1989.)

Pregnant mares	Forage	Concentrate	Total
Maintenance	1.5–2.0	0–0.5	1.5–2.0
Mares in late gestation	1.0–1.5	0.5–1.0	1.5–2.0

General poor nutrition has been associated with prolonged gestation, developmental abnormalities and decreased birth weights. These problems are exacerbated if low nutrition levels are evident in late pregnancy. In particular, energy restriction is reported to increase the incidence of premature parturition and subsequent infertility after the foal is born. Protein restriction is reported to be associated with increased early fetal loss, as well as weight loss and slow return to reproductive activity post-foaling, and calcium (Ca) restriction retards fetal growth (Ousey *et al.*, 2008). Excess body weight has been associated with lower plasma concentrations of eCG (Wilsher and Allen, 2011a) and with uterine inertia and dystocia (Varner, 1983), although this is disputed by others (Henneke *et al.*, 1984; Kubiak *et al.*, 1988).

In late gestation gut restriction becomes a challenge to the mare as increased fetal size reduces the capacity of the gut, appetite decreasing from 2% to 1.4% of body weight, but the growing fetus continues to increase its nutritional demand. This necessitates an increase in quality but not quantity of feed, to ensure nutrient demands are satisfied. Hence, although for many mares good-quality forage will satisfy nutrient demands through most of pregnancy, in the last 2 months concentrate feed should be fed, up to a maximum of 35% of the diet.

11.5.2.1. Protein

For a horse weighing 500 kg or more, levels of crude protein (CP) in the order of 630 g CP day^{-1} are required in early pregnancy (Tables 11.3 and 11.4; Frape, 1998; National Research Council, 2007). However, as pregnancy progresses into the last 90 days, protein intake needs to increase in parallel with requirements. Levels of protein in the order of 759 g CP day^{-1} are required in the last 3 months of pregnancy, increasing to 850 g CP day^{-1} at term. This level may be achieved by feeding good fresh grasses, as dried grass or hay tends to lose protein in the drying process. Legume hay, for example lucerne, tends to have a higher protein content even after drying, and so may be adequate for the late-pregnant mare.

Protein can also be supplemented by the addition of animal products or plant products. Appropriate animal by-products include fishmeal and bone meal. Such products tend to be expensive and have now been banned in some countries, in the light of the bovine spongiform encephalitis scare in cattle. The other alternatives are plant products, such as soybean meal and linseed meal, which tend to be cheaper and more popular.

The total protein content of a diet is not the only important factor in satisfying the protein requirements; protein quality is also important. The component parts of all proteins are amino acids, some of which are essential; others can be manufactured by the body from other amino acids. The latter are termed non-essential amino acids. Certain protein-rich feeds may be lacking in specific essential amino acids, so that although the total protein content is high, its use to the body is limited. Barley, oats and linseed are all high in total protein content but are lacking in one or more essential amino acid. Soybean meal, on the other hand, contains all the essential amino acids required for the development of the fetus and is, therefore, a very useful protein supplement for use in late-pregnant mares. Lysine is the major limiting amino acid in the horse and is the one most lacking in horse diets (Table 11.2). Lysine intake of 27.1 g day^{-1} is required in the first 5 months, increasing to 38.4 g day^{-1} in the last month of pregnancy (Table 11.3; National Research Council, 2007).

11.5.2.2. Energy

Energy requirements increase significantly in late pregnancy, but are also important during early pregnancy, their deficiency being implicated as a cause of EM (Ousey *et al.*, 2008). Again, the energy demand of mares in good condition in early pregnancy may be met by good-quality forage. For a 500-kg horse, levels of 16.7 Mcal day^{-1} are required (Tables 11.2–11.4; National Research Council, 2007). However, if the mare is a poor doer, or being ridden, her energy intake may need to be supplemented. Her energy intake also needs to increase in the last trimester of pregnancy. This may be achieved, in theory, by an increase in hay intake. In late pregnancy, however, the increase in uterine size begins to limit the capacity of the digestive tract. Energy levels of 21.4 Mcal day^{-1} are required during this period. Good-quality feeds, low in bulk but high in nutrient value, are advised. In late pregnancy the mare's roughage intake should, therefore, be reduced and partly replaced by increasing levels of energy-rich concentrates. Care should be taken to ensure that the required protein intake is still maintained and adequate roughage for optimal gut function is still fed (Pugh and Schumacher, 1990; Frape, 1998; National Research Council, 2007).

11.5.2.3. Vitamins and minerals

Vitamins and minerals are classified as micronutrients. The specific effects of deficiencies in many micronutrients on the pregnant mare, and indeed on general equine welfare, are as yet unknown. However, the importance of Ca, phosphorus (P) and vitamins A and E is appreciated (Greiwe-Crandell *et al.*, 1997; Hoffman *et al.*, 1999). The Ca:P ratio is of special importance, and the involvement of both minerals in bone growth is well documented (Frape, 1998). In the pregnant mare, these micronutrients are important not only to the mare herself, but also to the fetus. Ca and P are normally stored within the bones, much of which act as a temporary store and can be mobilized to satisfy demands elsewhere. If the pregnant mare's dietary intake of Ca or P is inadequate, especially during late pregnancy, the mare will mobilize her own stores from within her bones to satisfy the fetal demand. If the dietary deficiency is great, then her bones will suffer, become brittle and possibly be unable to take the strain of the increased weight in late pregnancy or the stresses of parturition. The foals of such mares can also suffer from deformities in tissue and bone growth, and general ill thrift at birth (Estepa *et al.*, 2006a).

For a 500-kg mare, the levels of Ca and P required in the first 5 months of pregnancy are in the order of 20 and 14 g day^{-1}, respectively. During the last 3 months the demand increases from 28 g day^{-1} and 20 g day^{-1} in month 8 to 36 g day^{-1} and 26.3 g day^{-1} respectively, at term (Table 11.3). In the tenth month, 25.3 mg Ca kg^{-1} of the mare's body weight is deposited in the fetus daily (Frape, 1998; National Research Council, 2007).

Not only are the absolute levels of these two minerals important, but so are their relative amounts. Excess P interferes with Ca absorption and leads to an effect similar to Ca deficiency. A ratio of Ca:P of between 1:1 and 6:1 is considered acceptable. Legume hay is a good source of Ca and P, and supplementation of these minerals should not be required for mares fed legume hay *ad libitum* (Hintz, 1993a; National Research Council, 2007). It is important to know that straights, in the form of grains, tend to be relatively high in P; hence, feeding grains to late-pregnant mares, when concentrate intake is increased, may require Ca to be supplemented. Ca may be supplemented in the form of ground limestone flour, or as milk pellets, which are more readily available in today's market. The high concentration of P in bran largely precludes its use in late pregnancy, except perhaps in small quantities as a laxative.

As mentioned, Vitamin A is also important, especially as it is an essential component of epithelial cells. As such, it is important in reproductive function, cell regeneration and development. Vitamin E has been reported to be linked to immunoglobulin content of colostrum (Hoffman *et al.*, 1999). Adequate vitamin A and E levels are best ensured by feeding fresh green forage (Tables 11.2 and 11.3); mares with no access to fresh pasture must, therefore, be supplemented (Frape, 1998).

Cu deficiency has been linked to developmental orthopaedic disease, but more recent work did not support this (Gee *et al.*, 2005; Ytrehus *et al.*, 2007). Other minerals – for example, salt (NaCl), copper (Cu), potassium (K), magnesium (Mg), zinc (Zn), cobalt (Co), iodine (I) and manganese (Mn) – should also be supplemented, although their exact function is unclear (Ott, 2001; Kavazis *et al.*, 2002; Lawrence, 2011). These may easily be supplemented by one of the commercially available vitamin and mineral blocks, providing the mares with free access to (or controlled feeding of) pelleted or powder supplements.

Excess supplementation of – as well as deficiency in – minerals and vitamins has been implicated in abnormalities associated with bone growth, such as developmental orthopaedic disease, angular limb deformities and epiphysitis, so feeding the correct levels is important (Beard and Knight, 1992).

11.5.2.4. Water

As with all equine rationing, water is an essential but often forgotten component. The late-pregnant mare, kept at an ambient temperature of 20°C, requires large amounts of water, up to 50 l day^{-1} (7–8 l per 100 kg body weight per day), depending on the DM content of her ration (Huff *et al.*, 1985). This is about 10% more than a non-pregnant mare/horse at rest (45 l day^{-1}). This water must be clean, fresh and available at all times to allow consumption in small but frequent amounts.

11.5.3. Parasite control

Parasite control is of significant importance. A high parasite count is often the reason why some mares appear as poor doers, and parasites cause a large quantity of the food fed to be wasted. If a mare's internal worm burden is excessive, the damage caused may become permanent, condemning that mare to being a bad doer for the rest of her life or may even be a cause of death (Shideler, 1993d). *Strongylus vulgaris* (one of the three large strongyles) used to be biggest problem for adult horses including pregnant mares. The old-fashioned recommendation of frequent worming at 2–3-month intervals was designed to tackle *S. vulgaris* infection, as it takes 2–3 months for the *S. vulgaris* eggs to reappear after treatment (Kaplan and Nielsen, 2010). However, *S. vulgaris* is now rarely seen in managed horses and the parasite of biggest concern in adult horses is now cyathostomins (small strongyles), of which over 40 species have been identified in horses (Shideler, 1993d; Love *et al.*, 1999; Nielsen, 2016). Cyathostomins are found primarily in horses, but are relatively mild pathogens, not causing problems except in the case of high infestation. As such the previous high-frequency worming regimes are not justifiable and, owing to the differences in the life cycles of large and small strongyles, are not suitable for cyathostomin control. For this reason, and because of concerns over anthelmintic resistance, a more targeted approach needs to be employed including environmental management (Peregrine *et al.*, 2014; Leathwick *et al.*, 2019). As the cyathostome egg develops into the infective larvae within the faeces on the pasture, an effective control method is to remove all dung from pasture as quickly as possible. However, this is often not practicable. Eggs develop into larvae in warm, moist conditions; cold slows their development, as do high temperatures (which also kill the eggs) (Nielsen *et al.*, 2007; Gould *et al.*, 2012). Hence, in temperate climates, the use of anthelmintics can be more targeted in the autumn/winter (a time of low risk), with a second dose in the spring as the weather warms up and larvae begin to emerge. In tropical climates their use should be limited during the summer (the time of low risk), and used in the autumn as the weather cools and the larvae begin to emerge (Nielsen *et al.*, 2007). Most adult horses over 4 years of age will have developed a level of immunity to cyathostomins, but some will still harbour adult worms, and so be the main cause of pasture contamination. A further reduction in anthelmintic use, and so anthelmintic resistance, can therefore be achieved by periodic diagnostic testing. The most common test is faecal egg counts (FEC), plus the use of the more recent blood tests for cyathostomins and saliva test for tapeworms. This allows horses with high infestation to be identified and target wormed. Finally, rotational grazing of fields with ruminants (Fig. 11.8),

as equine cyathostomins are species specific, or leaving fields fallow or for hay are also successful ways of controlling parasites (Proudman and Matthews, 2000). As *S. vulgaris* has decreased in prevalence in horses, tapeworm (*Anoplocephala perfoliata*) has increased in prevalence (Gasser *et al.*, 2005) and has been reported by some to be the main cause of ileocaecal colic (Proudman and Trees, 1996; Osterman *et al.*, 2007), although others did not not agree (Abbott *et al.*, 2008). Hence, treatment for tapeworm is now also advocated by some. Pinworms and bots may be present but rarely result in life-threatening conditions (Card, 2000; Kaplan and Nielsen, 2010).

The development of resistance to wormers (anthelmintic treatments) can also be reduced by rotating the wormer types used (i.e. those based on the thiabendazole group followed by those based on the pyrantel embonate group). However, this is becoming more difficult as anthelmintic resistance increases, in particular in the case of cyathostomins. The industry has failed to develop new anthelmintics, and so resistance will become an increasing problem. To date, ivermectin remains the anthelmintic with least resistance but it is only a matter of time before parasitic resistance to ivermectin becomes evident (Pook *et al.*, 2002; Kaplan *et al.*, 2004; Traversa *et al.*, 2007; Osterman *et al.*, 2007). Care must be taken in worming pregnant mares, as not all wormers are suitable. Products based upon benzimidazoles, fenbendazole, pyrantel pamoate and ivermectin are considered safe (Card, 2000); others may not be suitable for very early pregnant mares (within the first 12 weeks) as their use has been associated with a risk of abortion. At the other end of pregnancy, organophosphate wormers used to control bot flies are not recommended, as they may disrupt and trigger smooth muscle contraction, and may induce late abortions due to uterine contractions. In general, it is recommended that no wormers be used in the last month of pregnancy, owing to the risk of inducing premature delivery (Varner, 1983). However, some have advocated worming immediately prior to parturition to ensure that the foal is not exposed to a high parasite burden at birth (Shideler, 1993d; Card, 2000). Regardless of anthelmintic use, the importance of clean grazing must not be overlooked, and a combination of worming treatment, routine diagnostics, clean grazing and rotational or co-grazing plus manure removal gives the best results (Kaplan and Nielsen, 2010).

Delousing powder may be administered to pregnant mares, but its use should be avoided in late

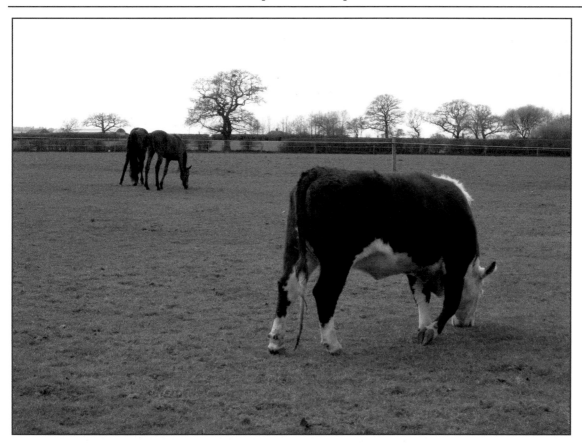

Fig. 11.8. Mixed and/or rotational grazing with cattle or sheep is a good aid to worm control.

pregnancy. Ideally, pregnant mares should not be allowed to get into such a condition that such treatment is required.

11.5.4. Immunizations

The vaccination programme required by a mare depends upon the endemic diseases prevalent and hence the country in which she lives (Wilson, 2011). In the UK, vaccination against tetanus and influenza is automatic and should be administered 4–6 weeks prior to parturition, to allow the mare's titre of antibodies to be raised adequately to ensure transfer to the colostrum, and hence provide protection to the foal immediately post-partum (Pugh and Schumacher, 1990; Robinson *et al.*, 1993).

Equine rhinopneumonitis (equine herpesvirus type 1, EHV 1) is a problem in the USA and is becoming increasingly so in the UK. This infection causes abortion, normally in the last trimester, in up to 70% of infected mares. If an outbreak is suspected, or routine protection is required, vaccination can be administered in months 5, 7 and 9 of pregnancy (Section 14.3.5.7; Mumford *et al.*, 1996; MacLachlan *et al.*, 2007; Wilson, 2011).

Equine viral arteritis (EVA) also causes abortion, and a modified live vaccine is now available. EVA has been a problem in parts of Europe and USA for a while and unfortunately is increasingly common in the UK. Vaccination is available and may be given to pregnant mares, but is not advised, especially in the last 2 months of pregnancy (Section 14.3.5.7; Timoney and McCollum, 1997).

Testing for, and confirmation of, disease-free status is often required by studs before a mare will be accepted for covering, in accordance with Horse Race Betting Levy Board Codes of Practice (see Section 14.3.5.3).

In other parts of the world, routine vaccination for eastern and western equine encephalomyelitis (essential in North America), West Nile virus, equine pneumonitis (EHV4), rotavirus, rabies and Potomac horse fever may be considered. All can be administered in the last 4 weeks of pregnancy to confer protection on the foal via colostrum (Sheoran *et al.*, 2000). Vaccination for strangles, botulism, anthrax, *Salmonella typhimurium* and leptospirosis is possible but only advised in areas of particular risk (Card, 2000; Chopin, 2011; Wilson, 2011).

11.5.5. Teeth care

The teeth of the pregnant mare should not be neglected. Regular teeth rasping ensures that all the plates are level and can efficiently grind food during mastication, enhancing digestion and maximizing the nutrient value of the food. This is of utmost importance when her system is under stress during late pregnancy.

11.5.6. Feet care

The majority of brood mares are unshod; even so, regular trimming should occur. Poor feet cause pain, and this pain can be exacerbated by the increased weight burden of late pregnancy. Such mares will be reluctant to exercise themselves, resulting in problems, as previously discussed. Some mares are turned to stud with musculo-skeletal problems and so may need orthopaedic shoeing, especially in late pregnancy. Even so, shod mares must have shoes removed prior to parturition, to prevent accidental damage to the foal.

11.5.7. Drugs

Not only should care be taken over what anthelmintics are used in pregnant mares, but care must also be taken in the use of non-steroidal anti-inflammatory drugs (NSAID). Recent work suggests that their use in early pregnancy may interfere with embryo mobility and, therefore, maternal recognition and pregnancy, and so pregnancy success (Okada *et al.*, 2019). This is of particular note, as it is not uncommon for mares to be sent to stud as the result of an injury obtained during their athletic career, for which NSAID were prescribed.

11.6. Conclusion

Accurate pregnancy detection is a major key to early pregnant mare management. Once pregnancy has been confirmed, mare management can be geared towards ensuring that pregnancy is stress-free, optimizing the chances of a healthy foal and a mare in the appropriate condition for lactation and subsequent re-covering.

Study Questions

Critically evaluate the various alternatives available for diagnosing pregnancy in the mare.

Critically discuss the methods that can be employed to control parasitic infections in the pregnant mare.

Your mare has been covered on 1st April and has been diagnosed as pregnant at 40 days on 10th May. Discuss how you would manage her from day 40 of pregnancy onwards to maximize the chance of producing a healthy foal.

Discuss the specialist veterinary, dental and farrier care a pregnant mare should receive throughout her pregnancy.

Suggested Reading

Collins, A.M. and Buckley, T.C. (1993) Comparison of methods for early pregnancy detection. *Journal of Equine Veterinary Science* 13, 627–630.

Lofstedt, R.M. and Newcombe, J.R. (1997) Pregnancy diagnosis and subsequent examinations in mares: when and why. *Equine Veterinary Education* 9(6), 293–294.

Kaplan, R.M. and Nielsen, M.K. (2010) An evidence-based approach to equine parasite control: It ain't the 60s anymore. *Equine Veterinary Education* 22, 306–316.

McKinnon, A.O. (2011) Orgin and outcome of twin pregnancies. In: McKinnon, A.O., Squires, E.L., Vaala, E. and Varner, D.D. (eds) *Equine Reproduction*, 2nd edn. Wiley-Blackwell, Philadelphia, London, pp. 2350–2358.

McCue, P.M. and McKinnon, A.O. (2011) Pregnancy Examination. In: McKinnon, A.O., Squires, E.L., Vaala, E. and Varner, D.D. (eds) *Equine Reproduction*, 2nd edn. Wiley-Blackwell, Philadelphia, London, pp. 2245–2261.

Bergfeldt, D.R. and Adams, G.P. (2011) Pregnancy In: McKinnon, A.O., Squires, E.L., Vaala, E. and Varner, D.D. (eds) *Equine Reproduction*, 2nd edn. Wiley-Blackwell, Philadelphia, London, pp. 2065–2079.

Proudman, C.J. and Matthews, J.B. (2000) Control of Intestinal Parasites in Horses. *In Practice* 22, 90–97.

National Research Council (2007) *Nutrient Requirements of Horses*, 6th edn. Revised. The National Academies Press, Washington, DC, pp. 315.

Lawrence, L.M. (2011) Nutrition for the broodmare. In: McKinnon, A.O., Squires, E.L., Vaala, E. and Varner, D.D. (eds) *Equine Reproduction*, 2nd edn. Wiley-Blackwell, Philadelphia, London, pp. 2760–2770.

Wilson, D.W. (2011) Vaccination of mares, foals and weanlings. In: McKinnon, A.O., Squires, E.L., Vaala, E. and Varner, D.D. (eds) *Equine Reproduction*, 2nd edn. Wiley-Blackwell, Philadelphia, London, pp. 302–330.

Management of the Mare at Parturition

> **The Objectives of this Chapter are:**
>
> To apply the reproductive physiology and behaviour knowledge that you have gained from Section A to the management of the mare at parturition.
>
> To enable you to evaluate the various ways in which the mare can be managed at parturition in order to make educated choices.
>
> To discuss the process of normal parturition to enable you to identify when things go wrong, and so to ensure speedy intervention.
>
> To give you the knowledge to make an informed decision about when to seek specialist help for the foaling mare, and to give you the theoretical knowledge to know what to do in the case of an emergency.

12.1. Introduction

Gestation in the mare lasts on average 330–336 days, although considerable variation is evident (Davies Morel *et al.*, 2002; Perez *et al.*, 2003). The physical process and endocrine control of parturition have already been detailed in Chapter 4. This Chapter will consider solely the management of the mare at parturition, including its artificial induction and dystocia.

12.2. Pre-partum Management

Approximately 6 weeks before the mare's estimated date of delivery, she should be introduced to the foaling unit or the yard at which she is to foal. This begins the gradual familiarization of the mare to the surroundings in which she will foal and be kept immediately postpartum, so reducing the stress of any sudden changes. Such familiarization allows her to become accustomed to particular management practices, especially if she is to foal away from home. Changes in feed, exercise, housing and routine can be introduced in plenty of time to allow a regular management system to be established prior to foaling.

If the mare is to foal away from home, a period of 6 weeks is also required to allow her immune system to raise the necessary antibodies against any challenges present in her new foaling environment. This will not only provide protection for the mare herself, but will also allow the antibodies to pass into the colostrum and so provide the foal with immediate protection at birth. Bearing this in mind, it is advised that all mares should be vaccinated with either their annual boosters or new vaccination programmes during this 6-week period. The vaccinations used depend upon the country of residence, prevalent diseases, and types and ages of mares, as discussed in Section 11.5.4 (Golnik, 1992; Card, 2000; Wilson, 2011).

Exercise is very important. Regular free exercise in a paddock or field will be adequate for most mares and will help maintain their fitness for foaling and reduce the chances of oedema (fluid retention) in the legs. A slightly laxative diet may be advised, as many mares suffer from constipation in late pregnancy, especially if exercise is limited. To this end, components such as bran or fresh carrots may be added in small quantities, but care must be taken not to upset the overall nutritional balance of the diet, especially the calcium:phosphorus (Ca:P) ratio, which is very important at this stage. Last, but by no means least, clean and fresh water must be available at all times. Many mares need large quantities of water (a 500-kg mare will need 27–35 l day^{-1}) in late pregnancy (National Research Council, 2007).

Throughout the preparation of the mare for foaling, she should be observed for the characteristic signs of imminent parturition: increase in mammary gland size; the secretion of milk; and general relaxation of the abdominal, pelvic and perineal area (Section 12.3).

By this time, except in the case of an emergency, it will have been decided whether the mare is to give birth naturally or if it is to be induced. If birth is to occur naturally then, as soon as any signs of imminent parturition are noticed, the mare must be put into her foaling box if she is to foal inside, or into a small quiet paddock if she is to foal outside. She should then be monitored closely.

If she is to foal inside, the box provided must be at least 5 × 5 m, with good ventilation but draught-free. Traditionally, the floor covering would have been a deep bed of straw, which provides a soft, warm, dust-free surface onto which the foal can be born (Fig. 12.1). Other alternatives, such as rubber matting, are increasingly popular, although expensive; they provide a clean, insulated and dust-free floor that can be easily washed and disinfected.

The foaling box should be free of any protrusions that may cause damage to the mare or foal. Ideally, it should have rounded corners to reduce the risk of the mare getting cast. Hay nets should not be used, as the foal can get itself caught up in anything left dangling. Hay should be fed off the ground. The use of high hay racks avoids the wastage of feeding off the floor, but does run the risk of the mare and foal getting seeds in their eyes and ears. In an ideal, purpose-built unit, each

box should have two doors: one to the outside for horse access and another facing into a central sitting area for human access and viewing. Closed-circuit television is also a good method of viewing mares with minimal disturbance. The provision of radiant-heat lamps in each box is an advantage for weak foals.

Once the mare has settled into her foaling quarters, it is a case of careful watching and patient waiting. Careful observation can minimize the time from the first signs of trouble to action and can, therefore, be crucial in saving lives.

More recently, with the increasing awareness of the stresses that can result from the intensively controlled breeding management systems, attempts have been made to accommodate a more natural environment for the mare. This can be done by keeping mares in established groups for much of the year. If keeping mares out or foaling out is not possible during the winter/early spring, they then can be housed in barns, rather than in individual stables (Fig. 12.2). Mares can then foal down in the barn and the closeness of the other mares and the freedom of movement in a much larger area appears to reduce stress and so ease parturition. Once the mare has foaled it may be prudent to remove her and the foal to a separate stable, until a bond is established, at which stage she can then be reintroduced to the group. This is eventually turned out together when the weather/facilities allow. This system is increasingly popular, and used successfully not only with native horses, but also with high-value horses.

12.3. Signs of Imminent Parturition

There are several signs that indicate parturition is approaching. These may become evident at any time in the last 3 weeks of pregnancy. It must be remembered that these signs (detailed below) should not be used in isolation, and that there is much variation between individuals and between successive pregnancies. Therefore, the mare should be assessed for a combination of the following signs (Wessel, 2005). It is also useful to have information on a mare's previous pregnancies, as general behavioural patterns may be characteristic to a particular mare.

Changes in the appearance of the udder are one of the first signs of imminent parturition. During the last month of gestation, as lactogenesis (milk production) commences, the udder increases in size as colostrum is produced and stored (Chavatte, 1997b; Christensen, 2011b).

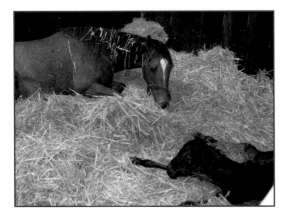

Fig. 12.1. The traditional floor covering for the foaling box is straw that provides a good, deep, soft bed for the foal to be born on to.

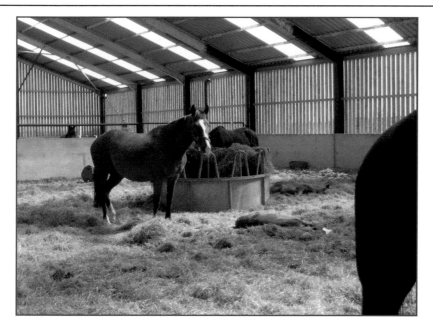

Fig. 12.2. To accommodate a more natural environment mares can be kept in a barn in established groups and allowed to foal down in their groups, reducing stress, and so easing parturition.

The udder may feel relatively warm to the touch as a result of the increased metabolic activity associated with milk production. At this time the udder may seem to increase in size at night, especially if the mare is kept in, and to decrease during the day when she is let out and able to exercise; exercise increases circulation and reduces udder oedema (fluid accumulation). When there is no such apparent change in udder size between exercise (day) and standing in (night), parturition is imminent. At this stage, the udder is so full of milk that exercise no longer affects its size. The extent to which udder size increases is dependent upon the size of the mare and her parity (number of previous foals; Rossdale and Ricketts, 1980; Macpherson and Paccamonti, 2011). Figure 12.3a shows the udder of a mare 5 days prior to parturition.

The teats also change, initially becoming shorter and fatter as the udder fills and the bases of the teats are stretched. As the time for parturition approaches the teats fill as milk production increases; they elongate and become tender to touch (Fig. 12.3a and 12.3b). Some mares may even start to lose milk, as production by the udder becomes too great for its storage capacity, and the sphincter at the end of the teat is breached. If a mare does start to lose milk, it is very important to minimize the loss. Milk at this stage is in fact colostrum, with a high concentration of immunoglobulins, and is vital for

the transfer of passive immunity to the foal. As there is a finite amount of colostrum produced, if a mare is seen to lose milk or habitually does so, it is a good idea to milk her out a little and store the collected colostrum for feeding to the foal immediately post-partum (foaling) (Chavatte, 1997b). Colostrum can be successfully frozen for more than 1 year for use at a later date. Many mares 'wax up', a term given to the clotting of colostrum at the end of the teat (Fig. 12.4). This is a good sign of imminent parturition. However, the lack of wax is not indicative that parturition is not imminent, as these colostrum plugs can easily be dislodged, especially in active mares.

The concentration of several minerals – sodium (Na), P, Ca and potassium (K) – within the mammary gland secretions as parturition approaches is also indicative of the imminence of parturition. These parameters are advocated for use when attempting to assess fetal maturity prior to the artificial induction of parturition (Section 12.4; Paccamonti, 2001; Ousey, 2002). In particular, Ca concentrations can be assessed via water hardness testing strips, and used to indicate the closeness of parturition (Ley *et al.*, 1993; Christensen, 2011b). Ca concentrations in excess of 4 mg/ml (10 mmol l^{-1}) or 200 parts per million (ppm) are reported to be indicative of parturition, as are a reversing of the relative relationship between Na and K. As parturition approaches, K becomes higher than Na (Ousey, 2002; Canisso *et al.*, 2013a). Linked to a change in mineral concentrations, a decrease in milk pH has also been reported to be an indicator of parturition (Canisso *et al.*, 2013a). Karouse (2013) suggested that lack of a pH drop indicates with 99% accuracy that the mare will not foal yet; however, pH drop, in itself, does not predict parturition with much accuracy because there are other reasons why this drop may occur.

Changes in the birth canal also become apparent as parturition approaches. Approximately 3 weeks prior to parturition, hollowness or softening may appear on either side of the mare's tail root, owing to relaxation of the muscles and ligaments, and particularly of the

sacrosciatic ligaments within the pelvic area (Fig. 12.5). The whole area may appear to sink with this relaxation and so allow expansion of the birth canal during the passage of the fetus. If the area on either side of the tail root is felt daily in the last 3–4 weeks of pregnancy, it may be possible to detect a change as the muscle tone relaxes (Christensen, 2011b).

Changes in the mare's abdomen may also be evident in late pregnancy. As the fetus increases in size, the abdomen expands correspondingly, becoming characteristically large and pendulous (Fig. 12.6). However, in the final stages of pregnancy, the abdomen appears to shrink as the fetus moves up out of the lower abdomen and into the birth canal ready for delivery.

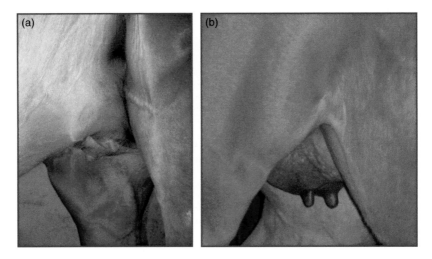

Fig. 12.3. As parturition approaches the udder of the mare enlarges: (a) 5 days away from parturition; and (b) at parturition.

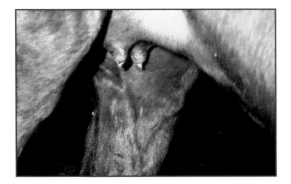

Fig. 12.4. One of the signs of imminent parturition is the accumulation of dried colostrum on the teats of the mare, termed 'waxing up'; dried colostrum may also be seen on the insides of the hind legs.

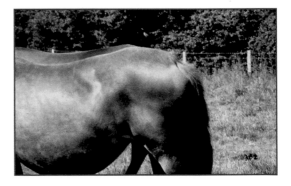

Fig. 12.5. A further sign of imminent parturition is a hollowing of the hindquarters either side of the tail root, above the pelvis, as a result of a relaxation of the birth canal.

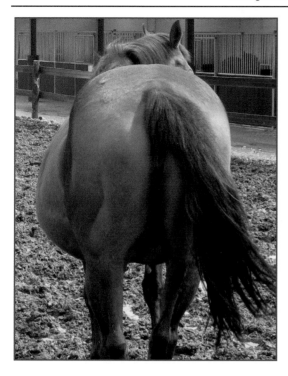

Fig. 12.6. One of the obvious signs of pregnancy is a large, pendulous abdomen. However, immediately prior to parturition, the size of the abdomen appears to shrink as the foal moves up into the birth canal.

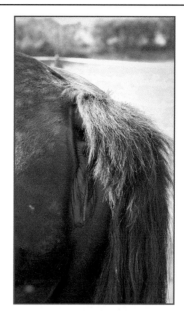

Fig. 12.7. As parturition approaches the vulva is seen to elongate and relax.

As parturition approaches closer still, the mare becomes restless and agitated, especially as she enters first-stage labour. Some restlessness may also be apparent in late gestation; in feral herds, at this stage, the mare would move away to the periphery of the group in readiness to move away completely once labour starts. As the mare moves into first-stage labour, her body temperature increases, and she may sweat profusely (Karouse, 2013). Internally, her cervix will dilate and the vulva may appear to relax and elongate, and secretions may be seen (Fig. 12.7; Volkmann *et al.*, 1995; Christensen, 2011b). During first-stage labour she may show signs very similar to those indicative of colic, such as walking in circles, swishing her tail, looking around at her sides and kicking her abdomen. If a mare does show signs of colic in late gestation, it is pertinent to consider that it may in fact be first-stage labour, and so her eating, drinking and defecating should be monitored.

As discussed, not all mares show all these symptoms, but a combination of one or two will give an accurate prediction that foaling is imminent. Ultrasound evaluation of fetal parameters such as eye length has also been used with varied success (Turner *et al.*, 2006). Additionally, commercial products have been produced in an attempt to aid in the diagnosis. These make use of some of the mare's natural signals, and the products include motion sensors attached to a head collar or strap around the mare's girth which attempt to detect when the mare lies down and/or stretches her head and neck out (detected by a device on a head collar or surcingle; Fig. 12.8a and b); an increase in body temperature or sweating (detected by humidity detectors on a neck strap); stretching of the vulval lips (detected by stretch receptors implanted into the vulval lips; Fig. 12.9); and accelerometers (detecting general increase in mare movement) (Karouse *et al.*, 2013; Hartmann *et al.*, 2018). Once triggered, they normally produce a signal transmitted to an audio and/or visual receiver or mobile phone. Closed-circuit television is also popular, allowing discreet observation.

12.4. Induction of Parturition

The mare shows a much wider variation in gestation length than other farm animals in which induction of parturition is practised. As discussed in Section 4.3.1, the natural length of gestation is very variable, and is affected by several factors. When considering artificially inducing parturition, it is essential that the date is as

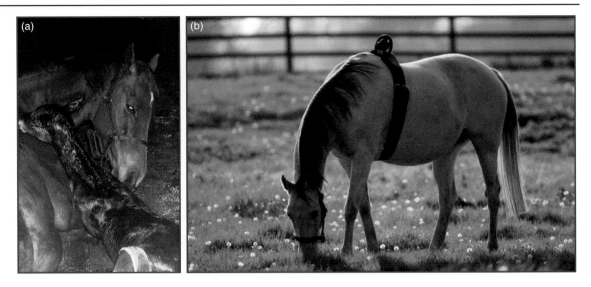

Fig. 12.8. Motion sensor attached to: (a) a head collar and (b) a surcingle around the mare's girth detects movement, in particular when she lies down. (Photo 12.8b courtesy of Inavata.)

close as possible to the estimated delivery date. In order to survive, the foal must have adequate energy reserves; a functional pulmonary and gastrointestinal system; and the ability to both suck and swallow and to maintain body temperature after birth (Paccamonti, 2001; Macpherson and Paccamonti, 2011). Premature induction will result in foals with all the classic symptoms of prematurity, including breathing difficulties, being late to stand and a delay in the normal post-partum adaptation mechanisms. Such foals may, if they survive, suffer long-term ill effects and there will be a dramatic increase in labour and veterinary expense. Induction of parturition in horses should, therefore, be carried out with great care in the case of medical emergency; its value as a routine management technique is very questionable.

Initially it was thought that induction would be useful as an aid to management, to ensure that all facilities and staff were available and ready when required, particularly if limited experienced labour was available and only a few mares were involved. However, high foal mortality rates mean that induction is now largely limited to emergencies, such as prolonged gestation, preparturient colic, pelvic injuries, ventral rupture, previous premature placental separation, pending rupture of the prepubic tendon, hydropic conditions, or painful skeletal or arthritic conditions which can be unbearable in late pregnancy. It may also be considered if the mare has a history of difficult foalings; premature placental

separation; uterine inertia; an inability to strain effectively; and if she has pelvic abnormalities or injuries. In all these cases induction of parturition is done under veterinary guidance and allows the organization of expert help to be on hand at parturition to assist both mare and foal.

12.4.1. Fetal maturity

As indicated, the timing of induction in relation to the expected natural delivery date and fetal maturity is crucial to maximize chances of fetal/foal survival. In horses, parturition is likely related to fetal development (Section 4.3.2; Ousey *et al.*, 2004), especially maturity of the adrenal cortex and its ability to secrete corticosteroids. In the 4–5 days preceding natural parturition, fetal cortisol levels are seen to increase significantly and are required for the final maturation of major organ systems (Rossdale *et al.*, 1997). For the fetus to survive parturition and early life it must have been exposed to these elevated cortisol levels; hence, induction of parturition prior to this runs increasingly higher risks of mortality (Chavatte *et al.*, 1997b). As gestation lengths are so variable in mares, it is not possible to use these as more than a rough guide to determine the expected parturition date; hence fetal maturity needs to be determined by an alternative means. The normal signs of parturition (Section 12.3) can give an indication, but are not accurate enough to use as a means to time artificial induction (LeBlanc, 1997). However, changes in

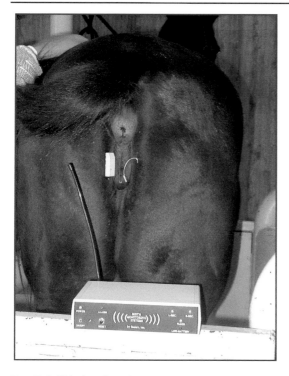

Fig. 12.9. Vulval implant that detects relaxation and stretching of the vulva as the mare goes into stage 2. (Photo courtesy of Foalert Inc.)

Table 12.1. Scoring system used to determine when the induction of parturition is safe. A total score of ≥ 35 suggests that safe induction of parturition is possible. (From Ousey *et al.*, 1984.)

Colostrum concentrations			
Ca(mg dl^{-1})	Na(mg dl^{-1})	K(mg dl^{-1})	Points for each electrolyte
≥ 40	≤ 69	≥ 136	15
≥ 28	≤ 115	≥ 117	10
≥ 20	≤ 184	≥ 78	5

secretions of the mammary gland are a good indicator. Ca concentrations increase significantly in the last 1–6 days pre-partum (Rook *et al.*, 1997; Macpherson and Paccamonti, 2011; Canisso *et al.*, 2013a). Hence concentrations ≥ 4.0 mg ml^{-1} have been reported to indicate a mature fetus, and concentrations ≤ 1.2 mg ml^{-1} to indicate an immature fetus (Ley *et al.*, 1993; Ousey, 2002). An inverse relationship between Na and K is also evident. As parturition approaches, Na concentration declines and K concentration increases. When Na < K, then the induction of parturition is reported to be successful. Based upon this, Ousey *et al.* (1984) devised a scoring system to determine when induction of parturition is safe (Table 12.1). These changes in electrolytes mainly occur at night. Water hardness indicator strips have been advocated to measure both Mg and Ca, but this results in false results as Mg rises earlier and more gradually in milk and so tests may prematurely indicate fetal maturity (Ousey, 2002). Further inaccuracies can occur in mares with placental problems, which often result in a premature increase in Ca (Rossdale *et al.*, 1991).

The extent of cervical softening has also been suggested to be associated with successful induction (Macpherson *et al.*, 1997; Rigby *et al.*, 1998), although this is not reported by others (Meyers *et al.*, 1991). Such an association is not surprising, as the closer the mare is to natural parturition the more successful induction is, and the closer the mare is to parturition the greater is the cervical dilation. However, Rigby *et al.* (1998) reported increased success by applying prostaglandin E (PGE) to the cervix, so encouraging softening.

Haematological assessment of the fetus has also been suggested as a means of determining the safety of induction (Jeffcote *et al.*, 1982), as well as rectal palpation, vaginal examination, amniocentesis, fetal electrocardiography, fetal eye diameter and length, and aortic diameter (determined by ultrasonography). When compared to Ousey's scoring system, however, they all have limitations (Reef *et al.*, 1995; LeBlanc, 1997; Turner *et al.*, 2006; Macpherson and Paccamonti, 2011).

12.4.2. Methods of induction

Once fetal maturity has been determined, there are several methods that may be employed to induce parturition (Macpherson and Paccamonti, 2011); these will be discussed in turn.

12.4.2.1. Corticosteroids

In ruminants, the most successful means of inducing parturition is the use of corticosteroids. Foaling can similarly be induced in large mares using 100 mg dexamethasone, a corticosteroid, administered daily for 3–4 days from day 321 of gestation. Parturition is reported to occur within 1 week and to result in live and healthy foals (Alm *et al.*, 1974, 1975). However other workers, using pony mares, report less success with slow, protracted, difficult labours, stillbirths and placental retention (First and Alm, 1977; Van Niekerk and Morgenthal,

1982). Interestingly, Ousey *et al.* (2006) demonstrated advanced fetal development but not necessarily parturition by administration of 100 mg dexamethasone for 3 days. Subsequently these foals were born naturally after a shorter gestation and were fully mature. Dexamethasone may, therefore, be useful in salvaging at-risk pregnancies.

12.4.2.2. Progesterone

Progesterone administration over a period of 4 days in late pregnancy, and its subsequent withdrawal, will induce parturition over approximately 1 week (Alm *et al.*, 1975). Such use of progesterone does not result in parturition in ruminants.

Both of these methods (corticosteroids and progesterone) are interesting as they are an indication of the possible differences in endocrine control of parturition when compared to ruminants (Section 4.3.2). However, they have the disadvantage of being relatively inaccurate in the timing of the reaction to their administration, which can be over a period of 1 week; in addition the number of stillbirths, and the need to administer the drugs over a period of time, make their use not commercially viable. A more accurate and more immediate induction agent is required.

12.4.2.3. Prostaglandins

The use of prostaglandins, both natural and synthetic, have been used with differing effects, but in general give a more immediate result than progesterone and corticosteroids. Natural prostaglandins are associated with a higher incidence of peripartum abnormalities (Ley *et al.*, 1989), hence prostaglandin analogues are normally used. For example, 250–1000 µg fluprostenol, administered intramuscularly, is sufficient to cause parturition within 2 h in a mare at full term. The mare will show the initial signs of parturition (stage 1) within 30 min. The foal is usually born within 2 h and the afterbirth appears 2 h later. Complications, such as insufficient cervical dilation and hence rupture and a decrease in foal viability, have been reported (Rossdale *et al.*, 1979; Ousey *et al.*, 1984; Ley, 1989; Knottenbelt *et al.*, 2004). In the natural course of events, the rise in prostaglandin coincides with the delivery of the foal, and fluprostenol presumably imitates this. Its use too early, therefore, has little effect, as elevated levels at this time are out of synchrony with other endocrine changes (Alm *et al.*, 1975). Currently fluprostenol is not commercially available; chloprostenol, the currently available prostaglandin, has not been widely used for induction.

12.4.2.4. Oxytocin

A further agent, and the one most commonly used today to induce parturition, is oxytocin. In the natural course of events oxytocin plays a central role in parturition, and concentrations rise markedly especially during second-stage labour, causing the rapid uterine myometrial contractions associated with birth. Initial research work used high levels of oxytocin (60–120 international units, IU) in a single injection, but these were associated with cervical rupture and reduced foal viability. These were a likely consequence of the sudden onset of myometrial contractions which bypassed the natural, more gradual, build-up of events. More recently, low levels of oxytocin (< 20 IU) have been used, administered intravenously over time (usually 3 h) either via multiple injections (every 15–20 min) or in an infusion over time in physiologic saline; this has been reported to result in parturition within 20 min (Camillo *et al.*, 2000; Chavatte-Palmer *et al.*, 2002). However, others using doses as low as 2 IU reported an increased incidence of retained placenta and decreased number of mares responding (Chavatte-Palmer *et al.*, 2002; Duggan *et al.*, 2007; Villani and Romano, 2008). The exact amount of oxytocin required depends on the endocrine balance within the mare at administration. It is known that, in many mammals, there is a synergistic relationship between oxytocin and prostaglandins, and that such an association does occur in mares. Oxytocin administration near term, therefore, results in an immediate release of prostaglandins, equivalent to the natural release. Oestrogen can be used in combination with oxytocin as part of an induction regime and presumably imitates the relatively high oestrogen levels at parturition. PGE topically applied to the cervix is reported to aid cervical dilation and hence ease the process and success of parturition (Hillman and Ganjam, 1979; Macpherson *et al.*, 1997; Rigby *et al.*, 1998; Witkowski and Pawłowski, 2014).

It cannot be emphasized enough that if induction of parturition is being considered then accurate records of the mare's date of service and expected delivery date are very important, along with close observation for signs of parturition, and a means of determining fetal maturity. Inappropriate use of induction agents has disastrous consequences. Most of the danger is to the fetus rather than to the dam, although the risk to both increases with the asynchrony between induction and the natural course of events. Induction of parturition in mares remains a risky business and must be used bearing this in mind.

12.5. Management of the Mare at Parturition

Whether the mare delivers naturally or is to be artificially induced, her management should be very similar (Riddle, 2003). The main difference is that the time of delivery with induction will be known and, therefore, preparation can be better timed and organized. The physiological process of parturition is discussed in Chapter 4. A mare may foal in a specifically built foaling unit or outside. Whichever system is chosen – and there are advantages in both – then the principles of the stages of labour and their management will be the same. Foaling mares outside is increasingly popular, as the risk of disease is lower, and the system is much nearer the natural situation. Foaling outside is normally restricted to pony or cob-type hardy mares or multiparous mares foaling later on in the season. Early foalers, maiden or difficult mares, and those of great value, are normally foaled inside and this allows closer observation.

12.5.1. Foaling kit

In readiness for foaling, the following equipment should be organized:

- veterinary telephone number (ideally, the vet should also be warned beforehand);
- mare halter and lead rope;
- towels;
- bucket;
- soap or antibacterial wash;
- cotton wool;
- access to warm water;
- obstetric lubricant;
- obstetric ropes;
- sharp knife or scalpel;
- radiant-heat lamp;
- antiseptic spray/navel dressing (e.g. 0.5% chlorohexidine);
- feeding bottles for milk/colostrum;
- gastrointestinal feeding tube; and
- access to colostrum (e.g. frozen colostrum).

12.5.2. First-stage labour

First-stage labour, the engaging of the fetus in the birth canal (Section 4.2.1), requires no special measures except close observation for the start of the second stage and for the identification of any potential problems. Once first-stage labour has been diagnosed, the mare's tail should be bandaged up and the perineal area thoroughly washed. Ideally, she should then be left alone, as excessive interference can cause a mare to suspend her labour (Frazer, 2011a). Some mares may lose milk prior to, or during, the first stage of delivery (Fig. 12.4). This milk is valuable colostrum, of which there is a finite amount. If a mare shows considerable milk loss prior to parturition, she should be milked lightly and the colostrum collected into a clean sterile container. As soon as the foal is born this can be bottle fed to it, or tubed if necessary, to ensure that valuable antibodies are received (Wessel, 2005; Frazer, 2011a).

At this stage an episiotomy (cutting of the vulva and perineal area) should be performed, if required. Unfortunately, today many mares routinely undergo Caslick's operation (Section 1.3.1; Fig. 1.10), owing to poor perineal conformation. Such mares, along with those that are naturally small, will need an episiotomy to allow passage of the fetus (Fig. 12.10).

During the first stages of labour the mare will seem restless and may repeatedly get up and lie down (Fig. 12.11). She may well lose her appetite, sweat profusely

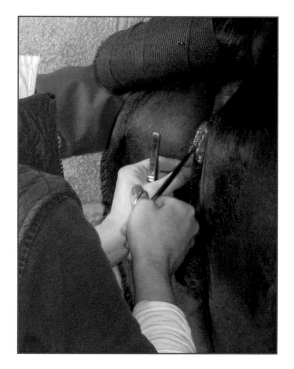

Fig. 12.10. An episiotomy should be performed by the beginning of stage 2 labour. This is routinely required in the case of mares having undergone a Caslick's operation.

and appear uneasy, glancing at her flanks and grimacing; she may also dig up her bedding, stretch as if she is going to urinate and pass small quantities of faeces (Frazer, 2011a).

This continual moving around is thought to help to position the fetus within the birth canal (Frazer, 2011a). The mare may well show signs of discomfort followed by quiet, and Thoroughbreds are reported to be notorious for this type of behaviour (Jeffcote and Rossdale, 1979). Her discomfort will increase with the frequency of contractions, culminating in the breaking of the waters (release of allantoic fluid) at the cervical star. Excessively prolonged first-stage labour may be a sign of problems, especially if the mare seems to be very distressed. It is very difficult to state how long first-stage labour should last, and at what stage you should call for assistance, as some mares will naturally show several false starts in the days preceding birth. However, as a general rule, first-stage labour is considered to last 20 min to 4 h (Christensen, 2011b). The assistance of a veterinary surgeon should be sought if the mare seems to be in prolonged discomfort, showing considerable agitation and profuse sweating, and before she is in any danger of becoming exhausted.

12.5.3. Second-stage labour

The management of second stage of labour, the delivery of the foal (Section 4.2.2) is more important and is marked by the breakage of the chorio-allantois (placenta) at the cervical star and the resultant release of allantoic fluid. In 90% of cases the mare will now take up a recumbent position, the most efficient for straining (Fig. 12.12; Wessel, 2005).

At this stage the amnion should be evident as a white membrane bulging through the mare's vulva (Fig. 12.13) and a brief internal examination may be made to ensure that the fetus is presented correctly (Fig. 4.4).

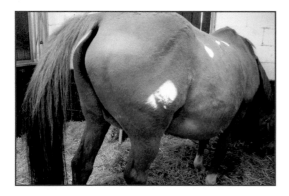

Fig. 12.11. During second-stage labour the mare will show signs of distress and may well stand up and lie down, look at her belly, pace around her stable, paw the ground, etc.

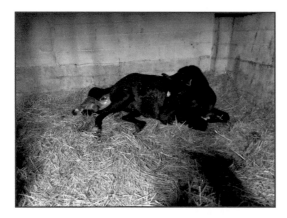

Fig 12.12. In the vast majority of cases, as the mare progresses into stage 2, she will take up a recumbent position (the most effective for straining). (Photo courtesy of Mrs Lienna Owen.)

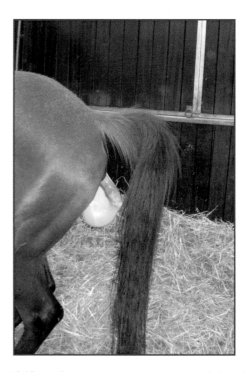

Fig 12.13. As the mare progresses into stage 2 the white amnion, possibly with a foot within it, may be seen.

If the forelegs of the fetus (one leg slightly in advance of the other, and behind that the muzzle) can be felt within the vagina, the mare should be left alone to deliver naturally (Fig. 12.14). If there are problems, assistance should now be called. Care should be taken not to rupture the amnion during this process; ideally, it should be left to break naturally. When it does, the colour of the amniotic fluid should be noted for evidence of meconium staining (dark brown/green coloration), which is indicative of fetal stress. If this is the case, then delivery of the foal should be speeded up by traction as soon as its head appears (Fig. 12.15).

If all is well, all attendants should now leave the box and allow the mare to foal unaided, but observed from a discreet distance. Most mares lie down during second-stage labour, as this is the most efficient position for voluntary straining (Section 4.2.2). Plenty of room is required to allow the mare to stretch out fully during straining.

The vast majority of foalings, up to 90%, require no outside interference (Vandeplassche, 1993). Things do go wrong occasionally, however, and it is as well to be prepared for – and have an understanding of – such eventualities. In such cases, prompt action can often save the life of both foal and mare. Foaling abnormalities are considered in Section 12.6.

Second-stage labour should last on average 15 min (range 5–30 min) (Christensen, 2011b). Mares foaling for the first time tend to have a longer second-stage labour and so do mares that have had a hard first-stage labour (Ginther and Williams, 1996).

12.5.4. Immediately post-delivery

After delivery the foal will undergo rapid adaptation to the extra-uterine environment (Section 19.2). It should be left with its hind legs still within its mother and the umbilical cord intact (Fig. 12.16); the umbilical cord must be allowed to break naturally to minimize blood loss (Section 19.2.1). The foal lying with its legs within the vulva of the dam appears to have a tranquillizing effect on the mare. As a result, most mares are reluctant to get up immediately, although they may turn to lick the foal. A mare may remain recumbent for up to 20 min post-partum. This should be encouraged, as it allows initial recovery of the tract and reduces the inspiration of air and, therefore, of bacteria passing in through the still-relaxed vulva (Fig. 12.17). Such contamination of

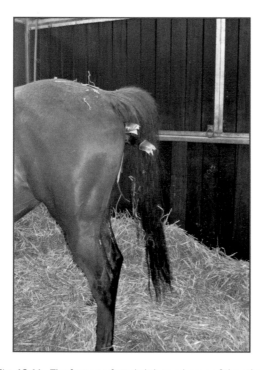

Fig. 12.14. The feet, one foot slightly in advance of the other, may be seen protruding from the vulva, often still within the amnion.

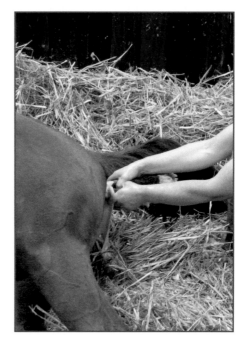

Fig 12.15. Gentle traction may be used to aid in the final stages of delivery, especially if the mare is showing signs of exhaustion.

the vagina increases the chance of post-partum endo-metritus or acute metritis, and delays uterine involution and any return to oestrus and covering success. Temporary Michel clips may be used after stage 3 to hold the dorsal (upper) vulval lips together and reduce air inspiration. These clips can easily be removed at the normal post-partum veterinary examination on day 2 or 3. They can then be replaced with a Caslick operation if required. This immediate post-partum period is very important and marks the beginning of mare–foal bonding and recognition. Minimal interference is required to maximize the chances of a good mare–foal bond developing. Interference, especially if the mare is stressed or a maiden, may cause her to get up and paw the ground, appear disorientated and confused, and present a danger to the foal.

If the foal has shown signs of distress and is limp or weak at delivery, the amnion should be broken immediately and the foal's head lifted to aid breathing (Fig. 12.18). Occasionally, the umbilical cord does not break after birth, despite drying up and constriction at the foal's abdomen. In such cases, it may be broken by a sharp pull, while placing the other hand on the foal's abdomen.

Immediately post-delivery the foal may be dried off, but this is not advocated unless the environment is particularly cold or the foal is compromised, as it removes allantoic fluid from the foal which is a trigger for the first mare–foal bonding. The severed umbilical cord must be dressed with an antiseptic agent such as 0.5% chlorohexidine or iodine to prevent infection (Fig. 12.19;

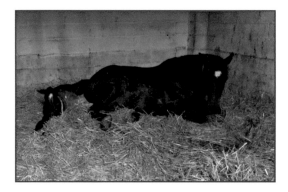

Fig. 12.16. Very soon after parturition, or often part way through, the healthy foal should be alert and struggle to sit up in a sternally recumbent position. (Photo courtesy of Lienna Owen.)

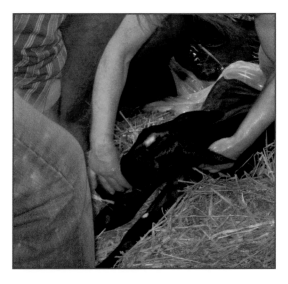

Fig. 12.18. The amnion may be removed from the foal's head and the nasal passages cleared to aid initial breathing.

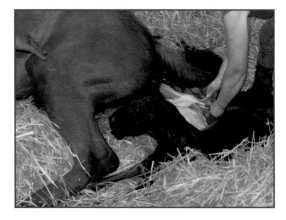

Fig. 12.17. The foal may remain for a while with its hind legs still within the vagina of the mare; the umbilical cord should be then left to break naturally.

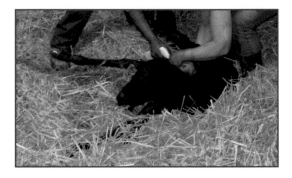

Fig. 12.19. The severed umbilical cord must be dressed with an antiseptic agent such as 0.5% chlorohexidine or iodine to prevent infection.

Section 19.2.1). At this stage the foal's heart rate may also be checked by placing a hand on the thorax or abdomen (Fig. 12.20). It may also be weighed; the birth weight of most normal foals is 10% of their expected mature weight. Details of management of the foal immediately after foaling, and the parameters required to be met by the foal at set stages in the first few hours of life, are given in Chapter 19.

12.5.5. Third-stage labour

During third-stage labour, the mare will appear restless again, similar to that during the first stage (Fig. 12.21). The average duration of this third stage is 60 min but there is wide variation. Occasionally the placenta may be expelled immediately after, or even with, the foal and still attached via the umbilical cord. At the other extreme, it may take several hours (Fig. 12.22). If the

placenta is not expelled before the mare stands, it may be tied up to prevent the mare standing on it and ripping it out prematurely. The extra weight provided by tying up also encourages its expulsion (Fig. 12.23). Third-stage labour in excess of 8–10 h is indicative of retained placenta (Section 12.6.3.1).

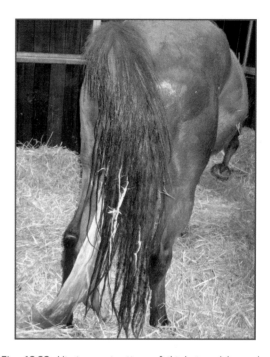

Fig. 12.22. Uterine contractions of third stage labour plus vasoconstriction of the placental blood vessels should result in expulsion of the placenta. Accidental tearing of the membranes can lead to partial placental retention, which must be treated immediately.

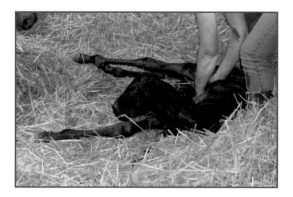

Fig. 12.20. The foal's heart rate may also be checked by placing a hand on the thorax or abdomen.

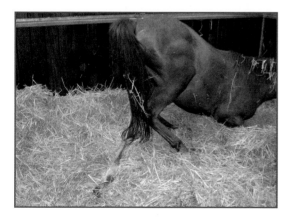

Fig. 12.21. During third-stage labour, the mare will appear restless again, similar to that seen during the first stage.

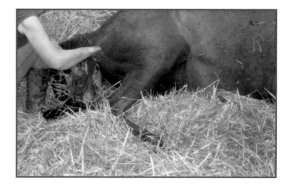

Fig. 12.23. If the placenta is not expelled before the mare strands, it may be tied up to prevent her standing on it, and ripping it out prematurely.

As soon as this third stage has been completed, and the placenta expelled, it should be removed from the box and examined for completeness (Figs 4.10, 4.11; Schlafer, 2004). An effective method of detecting holes and, therefore, any missing fragments, is to tie off both uterine horn ends of the placenta and fill the placenta with water through the cervical star. Leakage of water indicates a break, which should be examined to ensure that no membranes are missing. Tears in the placenta are of no consequence as long as there are no pieces missing. If this is suspected, then a veterinary surgeon should be called to ensure their complete removal. Placental retention of even just a fragment can lead to acute metritis, septicaemia and eventual death if not treated as a matter of urgency (Section 14.3.5.3). The temptation to pull the placenta to try and release it must be resisted, as this runs the risk of rupturing of the placental membranes and the danger of fragments being retained (Cuervo-Arango and Newcombe, 2009). Only a very small fraction is required to set up a septicaemic reaction.

During this period the bond between mare and foal starts to develop and can be irretrievably damaged by man's interference, however well intentioned. Damage to newborn foals by their mothers is very rare and, if it does occur, it is usually a result of her being disturbed or stressed by unwanted human interference. Occasionally, mares will nibble or gently bite their foals, to encourage them to move. Within reason this may be allowed but, if the dam is too aggressive, a muzzle may be used. Very occasionally, usually in maiden mares, real aggression towards the foal may be evident involving kicking and vicious attack. Such mares may be tranquillized for a short period of time. Tranquillizers may also be used on mares that will not stand still to allow the foal to suckle. After a while, most mares will get used to the foal and interference will not be required; some, however, never take the foal and it should be removed and put on a foster mare. Such behaviour can be seen in successive pregnancies. Occasionally mares will never accept their foals, which have to be removed and fostered at birth. It should then be considered whether the mare should be bred again. Use of the twitch should be avoided for the first 24 h post-partum as this is thought to increase the risk of internal haemorrhage.

Foals that appear to be weak and unable to get adequate colostrum from the mare may be bottle fed or tubed (Fig. 12.24). This ensures that they receive sufficient antibodies as soon as possible.

Enemas may be administered to foals if they show signs of meconium retention after 24 h. However, foals should be given the opportunity to suckle and pass meconium naturally, before the decision is made to use an enema (Section 19.2.1).

The mare should be given a feed about 1 h after the birth. A light, easily digested and slightly laxative feed is best, plus fresh hay and water. Water should be given only under supervision initially, unless automatic water feeders are installed, to minimize the risk of the foal drowning. The mare and foal should then be left in peace to bond (Fig. 12.25).

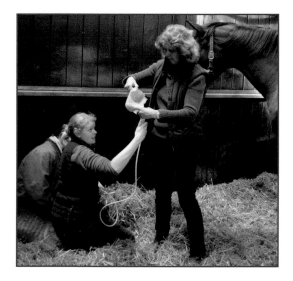

Fig. 12.24. Foals that appear weak and unable to suckle may be tube fed to ensure they get enough colostrum.

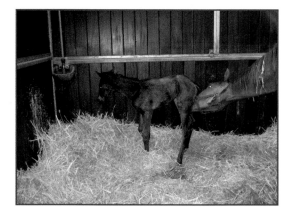

Fig. 12.25. The first few hours after foaling are critical for mare–foal bonding, which any interference at this stage can jeopardize.

12.6. Foaling Abnormalities

Foaling abnormalities or dystocia are relatively rare, especially in multiparous mares (mares having foaled before), although they increase with fetal size (Frazer, 2007; Langlois *et al.*, 2012; Squires *et al.*, 2013; Sabbagh *et al.*, 2014). Less than 4–10% mares experience problems (McCue and Ferris, 2012) and even lower incidences have been reported (Purohit, 2011). Dystocia can be classified as a condition or complication associated with parturition that prevents a natural birth. It can be divided into fetal dystocia (resulting from fetal complications) or maternal dystocia (resulting from maternal problems). Dystocia often causes a delay in parturition, which may result in a reduction in the oxygen intake by the fetus, due to partial placental breakdown or constriction of the umbilical blood supply. This may result in the birth of a weak, compromised foal requiring intensive post-natal care and/or more permanent problems, including brain damage and death in the more extreme cases (Frazer, 2011a). Delay in parturition due to dystocia may result in other complications, further hampering progress. The uterus may close around the fetus as it dries out and the lubricating effect of the allantoic fluid diminishes. As a result, manipulation of the fetus becomes increasingly difficult. Further drying out of the tract because of delay hinders passage through the birth canal, and thus makes any successful manipulation even harder (Pyn, 2014).

If dystocia does occur, fast action is essential. There are three main actions that can be taken: manipulation (manual correction of the fetal position) and traction (pulling the foal); caesarean; and fetotomy (Christensen, 2008). More recently mutation and traction have been subdivided into assisted vaginal delivery, when the mare is conscious and takes an active role in delivery; and controlled vaginal delivery, when the mare is anesthetized and hoisted to allow more significant mutation (Lu *et al.*, 2006; Frazer, 2007). Initially the least drastic option of manipulation (or mutation) of the fetus followed by traction, assisted and then controlled delivery, of the foal should be considered. This may or may not be accompanied by the use of relaxant drugs to reduce myometrial contraction (Frazer, 2011a). However, more drastic action may be required, such as a caesarean (Maaskant *et al.*, 2010; Freeman, 2011), especially in cases where extensive manipulation would be needed. A caesarean runs higher risk to both mare and foal and must be conducted under some form of anaesthetic or heavy sedation. Mortality rates for foals born by caesarean are approximately 70% (Embertson, 1992; Abernathy-Young *et al.*, 2014). The mortality rates for mares delivering by caesarean are lower than this, especially if they are operated upon before labour has progressed too far (Embertston 1992, 1999; Freeman *et al.*, 1999; Maaskant *et al.*, 2010; Abernathy-Young *et al.*, 2014). A caesarean involves either a ventral midline incision with the mare in a dorsal recumbent position (laid on her back) or, more commonly, a flank incision in the standing position and the foal born through the abdominal and uterine wall incision (Juzawiak *et al.*, 1990). Apart from the mortality risk, mares that have undergone caesareans have the added risk of developing adhesions and so lowered fertility in the future (Stashak and Vandeplassche, 1993). Adhesions form between internal structures that have become damaged, often by exposure to air, which then adhere (stick) to other internal structures. If the adhered structures include parts of the reproductive tract, there is a risk of interference with their function. Infection is also another potential problem, although with the advances in modern medicine this is nowhere near the risk that it used to be. A final alternative, in response to severe cases of dystocia, is fetotomy (Frazer, 2011b). This is performed on fetuses that have died *in utero* and involves the dividing up of the body of the fetus within the mare. A caesarean is a possibility in such cases but involves a higher mortality risk to the mare. Therefore, if the fetus is already known to be dead, fetotomy is often the preferred option.

12.6.1. Fetal dystocia

Fetal dystocia is caused almost exclusively by malpresentations *in utero*, making normal unaided birth impossible. Dystocia may be caused by the fetus being in one of many positions, and the ease of correction and likely outcome depends on its position and the skill of the manipulator (Vandeplassche, 1993; Blanchard, 1995; Frazer, 1999a,b, 2011a). Some of the more common positions and their treatment are given below.

12.6.1.1. Forward presentations

One or more forelegs may be flexed or folded under the fetus whose head is in the normal position within the birth canal. As discussed previously (Section 4.2.2), the widest cross section presented as the fetus passes through the pelvic cavity is the thorax area; therefore, in this position it includes the flexed forelegs, making passage impossible (Fig. 12.26).

The head of the fetus may be flexed back. In this position, its nose will not be felt in the birth canal. This again presents a much wider maximum cross section than the mare can deliver naturally (Fig. 12.27).

The legs of the fetus may be more misaligned than the normal hoof-to-fetlock alignment. One leg may become caught on the pelvic brim at the point of the elbow, preventing delivery (Fig. 12.28).

The forelegs of the fetus may lie over its head and be lodged behind its ears. This presents a cross section too large for natural passage and also runs the risk of rectal vaginal fissure if the hooves penetrate the roof of the vagina and into the rectum (Fig. 12.29).

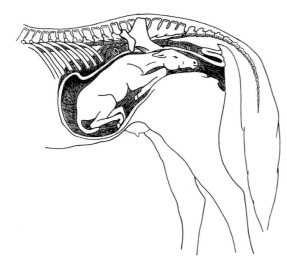

Fig. 12.26. Carpel flexion, which is flexion of one (unilateral) or both (bilateral) forelegs at delivery, significantly increases the cross section across the foal's thorax and, therefore, makes the passage of the foal very difficult.

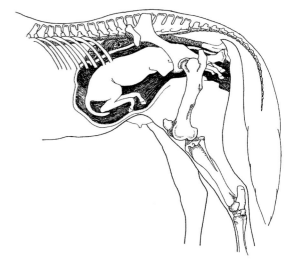

Fig. 12.28. A significant misalignment of the hoof of one leg and the fetlock of the other may be due to one elbow being flexed and becoming lodged at the pelvic brim.

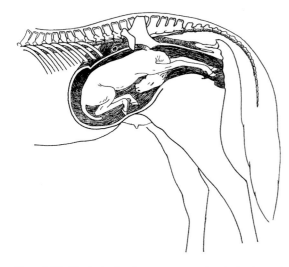

Fig. 12.27. If only the forefeet are presented in the birth canal the head may be flexed back, again presenting such a wide cross section of foal that it is very difficult for the mare to foal naturally.

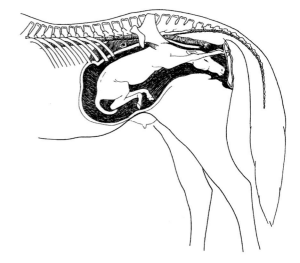

Fig. 12.29. The forelegs may be positioned over the foal's head. Not only does this increase the cross-sectional diameter of the foal but also creates the risk of a rectal vaginal fissure.

All four of these positions can, in theory, be corrected reasonably easily by pushing the fetus back into the uterus and manipulating it so it is presented in a normal position, followed by traction to aid the mare in her delivery. In practice, the strength of the uterine contractions can make this quite difficult, and to counter this muscle relaxants may be used. It must also be remembered that traction has to be applied in a curved manner (Section 4.2.2) to ease the fetus along the birth canal as dictated by the pelvic anatomy.

Other, more complicated positions, are seen; these require veterinary assistance, and in the worst scenario a caesarean may be required, especially if straining by the mare has caused damage to the cervix, vagina or uterus. The fetus may have both its head and neck turned back, presenting just two forelegs (a more extreme version of that shown in Fig. 12.27), or the presentation of the head and forelegs may be correct but the hind legs are also being presented at the same time (Fig. 12.30), putting four legs in the birth canal. Four legs may also be presented first, in a crosswise position (Fig. 12.31).

Finally, the fetus may be presented in a ventral position, in which case the arch of its vertebra does not allow expulsion in the required curved manner. This position must be corrected by rotation of the fetus before delivery is possible (Fig. 12.32).

12.6.1.2. Backward presentation

Backward positions may be evident with the back legs presented first, a position that need not be manipulated *in utero* but must be carefully watched and assisted during labour. In such cases, there is a danger that the umbilical cord may become trapped between the abdomen of the fetus and the pelvic brim, starving the fetus of oxygen. There is also the danger that the fetus may drown by inspiring allantoic fluid *in utero*. Fetuses in this position must, therefore, be pulled quickly and the amniotic sack removed from the muzzle immediately to allow extra-uterine breathing as soon as possible.

A more complicated backward position is indicated when no back legs are presented and only the tail can be felt. This position is known as a breech and veterinary assistance will be required to deliver such a fetus (Fig. 12.33).

Other positions, variations of the above, may be found; those discussed are those most commonly observed.

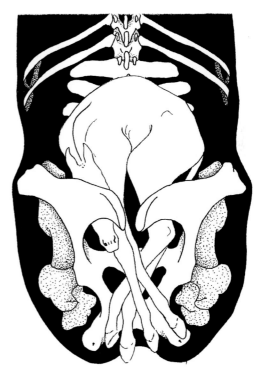

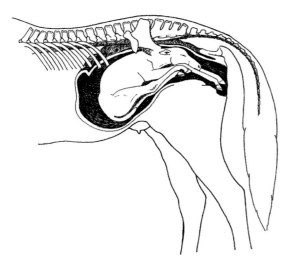

Fig. 12.30. If both forefeet and hind feet are felt within the birth canal, veterinary assistance should be called immediately, as this position can prove very difficult to correct, especially if the mare has progressed far into labour.

Fig. 12.31. A crosswise presentation also presents four feet first. This can, in theory, be corrected by pushing the hind legs back into the uterus.

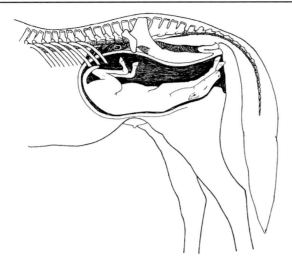

Fig. 12.32. Ventral position of the foal. The foal must be rotated into a normal position before delivery is possible.

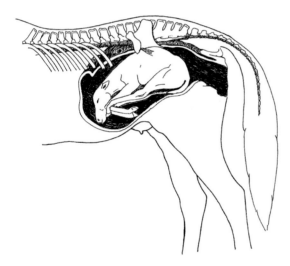

Fig. 12.33. If no legs can be felt within the birth canal, and only the tail and rump is presented, this is a true breech position and will require veterinary assistance.

12.6.2. Maternal dystocia

Maternal dystocia is the failure of natural delivery as a result of a maternal complication. These complications may be found in isolation or in combination (Blanchard, 1995; Purohit, 2011). Some of the more common ones will be discussed.

Placenta previa is evident as the protrusion of the intact red allantochorionic membrane through the mare's vulva, owing to its failure to rupture at the cervical star.

This may be due to extra-thick placental membranes, in which case manual breakage of the protruding allantochorion will allow parturition to progress normally. However, failure of the allantochorion to rupture at the cervical star may be due to rupture elsewhere, indicating placental weakness and/or premature separation of the placenta from the maternal epithelium, a much more serious condition. As this separation is one of the triggers for the foal's first breath there is a danger of suffocation and so the allantochorion must be cut immediately and the mare helped to foal (Higgins and Wright, 1999; Samper and Plough, 2012). The condition may also be indicative of placentitis (placental infection) which, if long-standing, is likely to have led to fetal brain damage or stress due to inadequate nutrition in late pregnancy (Asbury and LeBlanc, 1993; Vandeplassche, 1993).

Small pelvic openings or restriction to the birth canal may also cause problems. Restriction in this area may be the result of an accident or fracture or caused by malnutrition during the mare's early developmental stages of life. It may also be an issue with oversized foals (Vandeplassche, 1993) or partial/complete obstruction of the birth canal due to tumours, varicose veins, uterine torsion (Section 12.6.3), etc. (Jackson, 2004; Lopez and Carmona, 2010; Frazer, 2011a). Failure of the cervix to dilate is uncommon and can normally be rectified by manual manipulation. In such cases, a caesarean is often the only course of action that can be taken, and in the case of pelvic fractures it is questionable whether such mares should be used for breeding.

Uterine problems may also cause dystocia. Uterine inertia or failure to strain is a more common condition, and may often accompany fetal dystocia (Jackson, 2004). In such cases, the uterine myometrium becomes exhausted due to excessive straining, especially during second-stage labour. The condition can be accentuated by age, low body condition or previous uterine infections and may result in uterine rupture or placental retention. It may also result from abdominal hernia, rupture of the prepubic tendon, dropsical conditions, etc. (Section 12.6.3; Rose *et al.*, 2018; Rodgerson, 2011). Uterine inertia may not occur to the same extent across all the myometrium. In such cases, tight rings of muscle contraction may occur. As a result, there is a danger that the foal may be crushed or strangled. In most cases of uterine inertia, traction to aid the mare – along with an oxytocin injection to encourage myometrial contraction – is all that is required. Occasionally a caesarean may be advised (Vandeplassche, 1993; Lopate *et al.*, 2003). Rupture of the uterine wall occasionally may be seen and is most common due to mutation or traction; excessive straining, especially during second-stage labour; or significant intrauterine movement (Honnas *et al.*, 1988; Lofstedt, 2011b). In general many of these uterine problems are exacerbated in multiparous older mares in poor body condition.

12.6.3. Abnormal conditions

Abnormal conditions associated with parturition do not normally directly prevent normal delivery, but cause concern more indirectly (Lofstedt, 1993; Blanchard, 1995). These conditions include problems that become evident prior to labour, such as ruptured prepubic tendon, uterine prolapse and uterine torsion. The prepubic tendon is the tendon sheet attached to the abdominal muscles, and so it supports the entire abdominal contents, including the uterus. Its rupture results in loss of support for the abdominal organs, and death is the normal outcome for mare and fetus (Fig. 12.34; Jackson, 1982; Rodgerson, 2011), although some safe deliveries have been reported (Schutten, 2016).

Uterine prolapse results in the inversion of the vagina, and often part of the uterus, through the vulva due to incompetent uterine support, possibly associated with old age. It is relatively uncommon in mares compared to other farm livestock and normally occurs post-partum. In such cases, the uterus can be replaced manually after the administration of an anaesthetic or relaxant. This reduces the mare's straining and allows the uterus to be replaced and the vulva to be sutured to prevent a recurrence (Vandeplassche, 1975; Breen and Bowman, 1994; Spirito and Sprayberry, 2011).

A more rare condition is uterine torsion, where the uterus has become twisted, often as the result of a fall or

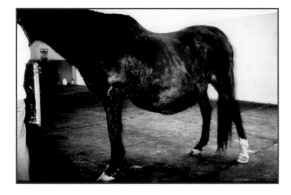

Fig. 12.34. Prepubic tendon rupture may occur in late pregnancy, resulting in the loss of all abdominal support. The prognosis is not good, and death normally results for both mare and fetus. (Photo courtesy of Dr Julie Baumber-Skaife.)

owing to weakened broad ligaments (Lopez and Carmona, 2010; Vasey and Russell, 2011; Yorke *et al.*, 2012; Saini *et al.*, 2013b). The twist, which is often towards the cervix end of the uterus, prevents any delivery through the birth canal. The prognosis for such cases is normally 50% chance of survival, but some success has been reported by enlisting the help of gravity and rolling the mare over rapidly, or by using manual surgical correction via a flank incision or via the rectum (Vasey, 1993; Lopate *et al.*, 2003; Chaney *et al.*, 2007; Jung *et al.*, 2008; Satoh *et al.*, 2017). Often a caesarean is required (Riggs, 2006; Lopez and Carmona, 2010).

Hydrops amnion and hydrops allantois are occasionally observed problems in the mare near parturition. Both cases involve excessive fluid accumulation in either the amnion or allantois and may occur separately or together. The reason for the condition is unclear, although it normally develops from 7 months of pregnancy onwards; treatment is via abortion or induction of parturition if the mare is approaching parturition. Prognosis for the mare is good, but foals are commonly significantly compromised and/or abnormal (Vandeplassche *et al.*, 1976; Christensen *et al.*, 2006; Lofstedt, 2011b; Waelchi, 2011).

Some conditions do occur during parturition itself, for example intestinal rupture, which is associated with the feeding of large, infrequent meals during late pregnancy (Littlejohn and Ritchie, 1975; Lopate *et al.*, 2003) putting the gastrointestinal tract under too much pressure as the mare strains during parturition. It may also be the result of a weakness arising from previous damage.

Finally, some conditions may not become evident until after parturition, but are a result of the forces of delivery. For example, haemorrhage, both internal (rupture of the uterine artery and often the cause of sudden death post-partum) and external (rupture of superficial blood vessels and so less drastic) may be a result of labour but not detected until after delivery (Lopate *et al.*, 2003; Byers and Divers, 2011). Rectal vaginal fistulas or perineal lacerations may be evident, resulting from the foal's hoof puncturing the roof of the vagina and passing through the floor of the rectum, opening up a cloaca as the foal is delivered (Fig. 12.35). Short fissures may be sutured, but longer ones cause significant problems, largely due to inaccessibility (Lopate *et al.*, 2003; Kay *et al.*, 2008; McKinnon and Jalim, 2011).

Delayed involution may be apparent after parturition. Under normal conditions, within 2 h the uterus should have shrunk to one-half of its fully expanded state, and continued low-grade myometrial contraction

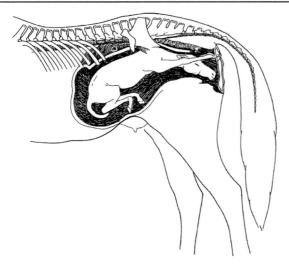

Fig. 12.35. During foaling, the foal's feet may pass through the vagina wall and up into the rectum, forming a rectal vaginal fissure.

will have expelled most of the fluid and bacteria remaining after parturition. By day 7 post-partum, it should be only 2–3 times the size evident in a barren mare, returning fully to its normal size by day 30 post-partum. Recovery of the uterine endometrium takes approximately 14 days (Section 13.2.2; Blanchard and Macpherson, 2011; Stanton, 2011a). Evidence of a dilated cervix or enlarged uterus at day 30 indicates problems, possibly associated with retention of placental membranes or dystocia. Uterine involution can be encouraged in such mares by daily infusion of oxytocin and antibiotics, plus gentle exercise (Blanchard and Varner, 1993a). Exogenous oxytocin may be used, not only to provide the extra impetus for placental expulsion, but also to help the following uterine involution (Threlfall, 1993; Haffner *et al.*, 1998).

Finally, hypocalcaemia, although not common in mares, if evident can be quite successfully treated by administration of calcium borogluconate post-partum. The incidence of hypocalcaemia is higher in mares suffering from dystocia and after caesarean section.

12.6.3.1. Retained placenta

Retention of the placental membranes may cause serious complications and is one of the more common complications post-partum (Threlfall, 2011). Normally the placenta reduces in size gradually as its blood flow reduces; it shrinks, therefore, and separates away from the endometrium and is delivered by the final contractions of the

uterus in third-stage labour. Retention of the placental membranes will result in infection that, if left untreated, will prove fatal (Hurtgen, 2006). Retention of the placenta for more than 10 h indicates problems. Retention is normally in the previously non-gravid uterine horn (the horn that did not contain the pregnancy), especially after dystocia or caesarean section. It may be due to a hormonal imbalance resulting in inadequate oxytocin or to exhaustion following a hard stage 1 and 2 and, therefore, reduced muscle activity. Selenium deficiency and an incorrect Ca:P imbalance have also been suggested as causes (Lopate *et al.*, 2003). Treatment can be in one of several ways, including manual removal and/or oxytocin treatment. Manual removal must be carried out with great care and, if attempted, you must be certain that the entire placenta is removed (Cuervo-Arango and Newcombe, 2009). After initial attempts, an antibiotic pessary can be inserted, and the rest of the membranes removed a few days later. It is imperative that the entire placenta is removed as soon as possible. If the whole of the placenta has been retained, then iodine solution can be pumped in through the cervical star to fill up the placenta. It may take 9–11 l for an effect to be obtained. After about 5 min the mare will be seen to strain against the filled placenta and so aid its expulsion, along with all the iodine solution. This method can be used in conjunction with oxytocin treatment, although the pressure on the uterus itself should induce an elevation in endogenous oxytocin (Threlfall, 1993). Other workers have reported success by injecting collagenase into the placenta via the umbilical cord in an attempt to speed up separation from the uterine endometrium (Haffner *et al.*, 1998). Placental retention is not only a potential problem in itself, but is linked to post-partum complications. Most notable of these is the significant reduction in conception rates to foal heat covering and potentially subsequent ovulations, and persistent post-coital endometritis (Blanchard and Macpherson, 2011). Such an association is not, however, supported by others, providing treatment is timely (Sevinga *et al.*, 2002).

12.7. Conclusion

Management of the foaling mare is of utmost importance in ensuring the birth of a healthy foal. Inappropriate management, or the failure to call in professional help when required, can have disastrous consequences. Induction is not appropriate as part of routine management of the foaling mare, but may be justified under veterinary advice, as inappropriate timing can have fatal consequences.

Study Questions

Gestation length in the mare is very variable and so cannot be used as an accurate predictor of the timing of parturition. Evaluate the various signs that may be used to predict parturition and discuss their relative effectiveness.

'Success in inducing parturition lies in the ability to accurately determine the maturity of the fetus'. Discuss this statement with reference to the methods that can be used to determine fetal maturity and the scenarios under which induction of parturition may be appropriate.

There is a range of facilities and conditions in which a mare may be foaled. Discuss how you would choose to manage a valuable mare foaling in February in the northern hemisphere, and justify your choices.

The breeding industry is increasingly aware of how different the intensively managed foaling environment is from the natural situation. Evaluate the management alterations that are being made to try and address this, with particular reference to the late pregnant mare and foaling.

Discuss the problems that may be encountered at parturition and how these may be managed.

As a stud hand you have been attending a foaling and the mare you are monitoring has shown signs of distress, possibly associated with first-stage labour, for 6 h. What should you do? If a problem is identified, evaluate the options that are available to maximize the chances of mare and foal survival.

Suggested Reading

Ousey, J. (2002) Induction of parturition in the healthy mare. *Equine Veterinary Education Manual* 5, 83–87.

Frazer, G. (2007) Dystocia and Fetotomy. In: Samper, J.C., Pycock, J.F. and McKinnon, A.O. (eds.) *Current Therapy in Equine Reproduction*. Saunders, Elsevier, St. Louis, Missouri, pp. 417–434.

Christensen, B. (2008) Managing dystocia in the mare. Proceedings of the Central Veterinary Conference, Baltimore p 1–5. Available at: https://www.dvm360.com/view/managing-dystocia-mare-proceedings (accessed 9 October 2020).

Macpherson, M.L. and Paccamonti, D.L. (2011) Induction of Parturition. In: McKinnon, A.O., Squires, E.L., Vaala, E. and Varner, D.D. (eds) *Equine Reproduction*, 2nd edn. Wiley-Blackwell, Philadelphia, London, pp. 2262–2267.

Christensen, B.W. (2011) Parturition. In: McKinnon, A.O., Squires, E.L, Vaala, W.E. and Varner, D.D. (eds) *Equine Reproduction*, 2nd edn. Wiley-Blackwell, Philadelphia, London, pp. 2268–2276.

Purohit, G.N. (2011) Intra-partum conditions and their management in the mare. *Journal of Livestock Science* 2, 20–37.

Pyn, O. (2014) Managing mare dystocia in the field. *In Practice* 36(7), 347–354.

Management of the Mare during Lactation and at Weaning

The Objectives of this Chapter are:

To apply the physiology of lactation knowledge gained from Section A to the management of the lactating mare and her foal.

To enable you to evaluate the various ways in which the lactating mare may be managed.

To understand the normal course of events through lactation and so enable you to be aware when things go wrong.

To provide you with the knowledge to make your own informed decisions when managing the lactating mare.

13.1. Introduction

After the birth, continued careful management of both the mare and foal is essential to ensure the foal is fit and well grown in preparation for weaning. This will also ensure that it reaches its genetic potential, whether in the athletic sphere or as a breeding animal. This Chapter specifically considers the management of the mare up to and including weaning. It should be read in conjunction with Chapters 19 and 20, which specifically consider the management of the foal at these times.

13.2. Mare Management in Early Lactation: the First 6 Weeks

The mare should be left in peace immediately post-partum, to bond with her foal (Fig. 13.1). The initial bond is the smell of the amniotic fluid, followed shortly by the smell of the mare's milk on the foal; the meconium; and then milk dung. She should have a good supply of hay or fresh grass plus clean water available to her. After 1 h or so she may be given a small nutritious feed, possibly laxative in nature, including bran or fresh apples/carrots, to address any continuing gut immobility from pregnancy. She should then have good-quality, nutritious feed, to provide for the increase in nutrient demand resulting from lactation. Her mammary gland can also be checked for milk production. She should then be observed discreetly from a distance (Asbury, 1993; Lawrence, 2011). Apart from being involved in the management practices applied to the foal, it is important that, during the first few weeks, she is watched carefully to ensure that she has not suffered any detrimental long-term effects from the birth (Asbury, 1993). In general, however, a lactating mare should be managed in much the same way as other stock: with common sense and an eye for potential problems.

13.2.1. Milk production

At about 72 h after delivery, the mammary gland predominantly produces milk rather than colostrum. Details of milk composition and quality, plus further details of the physiology of lactation, are given in Chapter 5. During the start of lactation it is important that the mare looks healthy and fit in herself, as any infections or disease will easily pass on to the foal. The general well-being of the foal should also be used as an indication of milk production. If the mare is not producing enough milk, the foal will appear tucked up; the mare's teats may be sore from continual unsuccessful suckling and she may begin to object to the foal suckling, risking the development of a perpetual situation making the condition worse. Low milk yields may be due to a physical inability, low nutritional intake, poor body

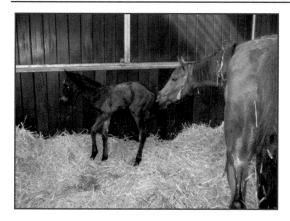

Fig. 13.1. Immediately post-partum the foal should be left in peace to bond with her foal.

condition or mastitis (McCue, 1993; McCue and Sitters, 2011).

Occasionally, immediately post-partum, the mare fails to produce any milk at all. This is usually due to either a failure in the milk ejection reflex or in the production of milk. Failure of milk ejection reflex is most common, and is thought to be due to high circulating adrenalin levels as a result of stress and anxiety. These cause vasoconstriction, hence reducing oxytocin reaching – and taking effect at – the udder. Injection of oxytocin and/or warm compresses applied to the udder, along with a quiet and calm atmosphere, will often rectify the situation. Failure of the udder to produce any milk (agalactia), the failure of galactopoiesis or lactogenesis, is a serious condition about which little can be done. The prime cause is the failure of any or adequate mammary gland development due to ingestion of ergot alkaloid from eating mouldy fescue grass, black oats or rye grass or due to a physical, often inherited, inability (Copetti *et al.*, 2001; Lezica *et al.*, 2009; Killian *et al.*, 2017). Many foals born to such mares have to be classified as orphan foals and brought up accordingly. Such mares should not be bred again, as the condition invariably repeats itself.

Teat abnormalities can also cause problems. Inverted nipples or conical nipples make it very hard for the foal to suckle, although the condition may not affect milk production itself. Supernumerary teats may also be present, but are rare, and do not seem to affect milk ejection from the normal teats. Oedema or fluid collection occasionally occurs within the udder of high-yielding mares and results in fluid accumulation around the udder and along the abdomen. As a result the udder becomes too painful to allow the foal to suckle and the condition predisposes the mammary gland to infections (mastitis) (Perkins and Threlfall, 1993).

In the relatively rare condition neonatal erythrolysis (Johnson, J.R, 2011) the mare becomes isoimmunized against the foal; that is, she has raised antibodies against the foal owing to previous exposure to specific non-compatible stallion antigens through blood transfusion, or by previous or current placental bleeding (Boyle *et al.*, 2005). This results in a fatal reaction within the foal if it ingests the mare's colostrum, as the colostral antibodies attack the foal's red blood cells (RBC). This can be identified prior to foaling via tests for blood incompatibilities or immediately after foaling by testing for agglutination between the mare's colostrum and foal blood. If a problem is identified the foal must be muzzled and alternative colostrum fed for at least 36 h post-partum until the gastrointestinal system loses the ability to absorb whole protein molecules. For the first 36 h the mare should also be stripped (or milked out) of colostrum. From 36–48 h onwards the foal can suckle normally.

Mastitis, an infection of the mammary gland, is relatively rare in the mare compared to the cow. It is characterized by a hot, swollen and painful udder, with oedematous swellings developing along the abdomen and up between the hind legs. Milk secreted tends to be thick and clotted and should not be fed to foals. If mastitis does occur, it is most often evident post-weaning, especially if the mare is still producing large amounts of milk, but is also seen in mares during the first 8 weeks of lactation and even in mares that are not lactating and have not lactated (McCue and Sitters, 2011). Mares that have had foals weaned prematurely are, therefore, at particular risk. Treatment is similar to that in cows, by the administration of antibiotics directly into the mammary gland via an intramammary tube inserted into the streak canal. This is repeated for several days. Alternatively, intramuscular injection of systemic antibiotics can be used, as many mares object violently to having a mastitic mammary gland touched (Perkins and Threlfall, 1993).

13.2.2. Uterine involution and breeding on the first oestrus post-partum (foal heat)

To prevent a drift of foaling dates later and later each year, it is desirable that mares are covered on their foal heat (the first oestrus post-partum), which normally occurs 4–10 days post-partum (Sharma *et al.*, 2010;

Blanchard and Macpherson, 2011). This provides little time for the reproductive system to recover from the last pregnancy, hence many studs perform a routine internal examination within 3 days of parturition and then again at 7 days to identify problems and check that uterine involution is progressing appropriately (Fig. 13.2). Any problems identified at this stage can be treated in time for either covering at the foal heat or, if not, by her next return to oestrus.

The rate of uterine contractility and involution to its pre-pregnancy state has a significant bearing on intra-uterine fluid, and hence on the conception rates at covering on the foal heat (Pycock and Newcombe, 1996; Stanton, 2011a). Although there is controversy regarding relative fertilization rates, it is generally accepted that foal heat conception rates may be as low as 50% of normal conception rates (Morris and Allen, 2002b; Blanchard et al., 2012). In fact fertilization rates may be unaffected, but embryo mortality at days 15–25 is reported to be doubled owing to an inappropriate uterine environment resulting from the failure of the uterus to recover post-partum (Meyers et al., 1991; Morris and Allen, 2002b). Within 7 days the uterus should have returned to two to three times its size in the barren mare and, by days 30–32, both the uterine body and horns should be back to their normal pre-gravid size (Blanchard and Varner, 1993a; Stanton, 2011a). In addition, recovery and return to pre-gravid state of the endometrium is required; this is normally completed by day 14 but can take up to 30 days (Blanchard and Varner, 1993a). Clearance of all uterine fluid discharge should also have occurred by day 15 (McKinnon et al., 1988a; Alghamdi et al., 2001;

Blanchard et al., 2012). The ability of the uterus to involute adequately has been linked to uterine blood perfusion which, in turn, can be linked to mare age and parity number (Lemes et al., 2017). In order for conception rates to be maximized, full uterine involution must have occurred. However, the mare invariably returns to oestrus and ovulation between 4 and 10 days post-partum and, as such, she will be covered before full uterine involution has occurred; as a result, conception rates are often poor. A correlation between uterine involution and conception rates is clearly documented, and mares that return to oestrus and ovulation 10 days post-partum, or later, have been reported to have significantly better conception rates to that oestrus, compared to those covered on the foal heat nearer to day 5 post-partum (Sharma et al., 2010; Blanchard et al., 2012). The time interval of 10 days prior to ovulation, plus 5 days for the embryo to reach the uterus, allows 15 days for the uterus to recover prior to receiving another embryo. As has been indicated, by day 15 uterine fluid clearance and endometrium recovery should be near complete. However, more recent work would suggest that the more appropriate cut-off date may be closer to 20 days (Blanchard et al., 2012).

Ideally, mares returning to oestrus prior to day 20 post-partum should not be covered, but left until their second oestrus post-partum. However, the industry demands foals that are born as early in the year as possible, and that a mare should produce one foal per year. The mare's 11-month gestation makes this difficult to achieve. In practice, there are several management techniques that can be used to help achieve these aims (Blanchard and Macpherson, 2011). The main aim is to encourage uterine involution, and potentially to manipulate the timing of the first or second ovulation and oestrus, to allow a 15–20 day recovery period prior to the arrival of the embryo in the uterus. The first thing is that all mares should have an internal examination 4–7 days post-partum, by either rectal palpation or ultrasonic scanning, and the extent of uterine involution, uterine inflammation or any luminal fluid retention can be ascertained (Reilas and Katila, 2002). At this stage it may then be decided that uterine involution is delayed and so not covering the mare at foal heat is the best option. Not only in such circumstances may covering of the mare at foal heat fail to result in pregnancy, but the effect on the already challenged uterus from the deposition of semen may increase the incidence of persistent post-coital endometritis, and so further decrease pregnancy rates. The mare's foal heat can be delayed using progesterone supplementation for 10–15 days post-partum, followed by

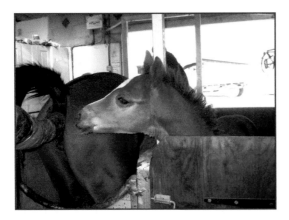

Fig. 13.2. Internal examination of the mare after foaling allows uterine involution to be assessed so that advice can be given on the appropriateness of foal heat covering.

withdrawal. It has been suggested that the addition of oestradiol to progesterone treatment helps to further suppress reproductive activity, and so delay oestrus and ovulation more effectively (Bristol *et al.*, 1983; Macpherson and Blanchard, 2005). This will induce a mare to ovulate within 3–4 days. Alternatively, the mare may be allowed to show her normal post-partum oestrus and ovulation, but her next ovulation is advanced by the use of prostaglandin F2α (PGF2α) 6–10 days after the foal heat ovulation, again ensuring at least a 15–20-day recovery period (Malschitzky *et al.*, 2002; Macpherson and Blanchard, 2005). Both these methods allow a longer time for uterine involution and hence result in better conception rates (Blanchard and Varner, 1993a). However the use of progesterone is suggested to run the risk of premature closure of the cervix, preventing natural drainage of luminal fluid, and a suppression of immune function compared to when oestrogen dominates the mare's system. Hence, some advocate allowing the mare to have her foal heat, and advancing the second oestrus, as being the best solution. In feral populations, conception and foaling rates to foal heat are in excess of 90%; this is thought to be owing to exercise, and so turning out mares as soon as possible post-partum is advised, to encourage uterine involution and especially uterine fluid clearance (Lowis and Hyland, 1991; McDonnell, 2000a; Blanchard *et al.*, 2004). Mares may also be lavaged post-partum, which removes any allantoic/amniotic fluid and associated bacteria, so promoting uterine involution (Mitchell *et al.*, 2019). Although this appears to be successful in mares with delayed uterine involution there is no evidence that it improves pregnancy rates in normal mares (Malschitzky *et al.*, 2002; Macpherson and Blanchard, 2005). Finally, evidence would suggest that close proximity to a stallion, as well as a warmer environmental temperature and an increasing plane of nutrition (Ishii *et al.*, 2001; Newcombe and Wilson, 2005), are associated with a reduced risk of persistent post-coital endometritis and better conception rates to foal heat covering.

Managing the foal when trying to detect oestrus by teasing or veterinary examination and at foal heat covering, or at any oestrus when the mare has a foal at foot, can be a challenge. There are various management practices, and these are discussed in Sections 10.2.2.1 and 10.3.

13.2.3. Nutrition

One of the specific areas to note in the management of the lactating mare is her nutrition. A lactating mare has higher nutritional requirements than any other equid, even one in heavy work (Doreau *et al.*, 1988; Harris,

2003) (Table 13.1). As parturition approaches, her nutritional demand increases to meet the demands of the growing fetus. After parturition, the mare continues to provide all the nutrients for that foal, but now the foal is extra-uterine and is larger. The supply of nutrients via milk is less efficient than nutrient transfer via the placenta. The efficiency of energy transfer in milk is only 60% (i.e. 40% of the energy intake does not appear as energy in the milk). After parturition the mare's nutrient requirements increase by 70–75% during early lactation, and by 50% in later lactation, to make up in part for this decrease in efficiency (McCue, 1993; Lawrence, 2011). Hence, even good grazing alone may not provide enough nutrients to meet demands (Fig. 13.3). At peak lactation, a mare may produce up to 3% of her body weight as milk, reducing to 2% during months 4–6. It is generally considered that it is beneficial for the mare to be in good body condition (condition score 2.5) and on an increasing plane of nutrition as she approaches post-partum covering; this is beneficial for conception rates and embryo survival (Van Niekerk and Van Niekerk, 1997; Newcombe and Wilson, 2005; Fradinho *et al.*, 2014).

13.2.3.1. Protein and energy

Protein and energy are important components of a lactating mare's ration. If her diet is nutritionally low in protein, she will not have enough to satisfy the demands of her milk production. Milk production will then decline (Martin *et al.*, 1991). Low dietary energy will result in mobilization of the mare's own body reserves in order to try and maintain production. If low dietary energy persists, milk yield will decline and the mare will lose body condition (Pagan and Hintz, 1986). Some weight loss, especially in mares that milk well, is to be expected, but should be minimized by appropriate feeding. It is reported that the mare's digestible energy (DE) requirements can increase by up 100% in lactation (Shepherd, 2015), hence significant weight loss is seen in mares that are deficient in energy. These may be accompanied by changes in endocrine profiles, resulting in poor reproductive success if they are returned to the stallion, especially on the foal heat (Cavinder *et al.*, 2007). Deficiency in dietary protein may also result in mare weight loss, but usually does not affect foal weight unless the deficiency is prolonged (Martin *et al.*, 1991). The protein and energy content of a lactating mare's ration are, therefore, important to her reproductive efficiency. For a 500-kg mare, DE intakes of 31.7 Mcal day^{-1} are required in the first month.

Table 13.1. Daily nutrient requirements of lactating mares of varying weights. (From National Research Council, 2007.)

Lactating mares	Weight (kg)	Milk production (kg day^{-1})	DE (Mcal)	CP (g)	Lysine (g)	Ca (g)	P (g)	Mg (g)	K (g)	Vitamin A (10^3 IU)
1 month	200	6.52	12.7	614	33.9	23.6	15.3	4.5	19.1	10.0
	500	16.3	31.7	1535	84.8	59.1	38.3	11.2	47.8	25.0
	900	29.34	54.4	2763	152.6	106.4	68.9	20.1	86.1	45.0
2 months	200	6.48	12.7	612	33.8	23.6	15.2	4.5	19.1	10.0
	500	16.2	31.7	1530	84.4	58.9	38.1	11.1	47.7	25.0
	900	29.16	54.3	2754	152.0	106.0	68.6	20.1	85.8	45.0
3 months	200	5.98	12.2	587	32.1	22.4	14.4	4.3	18.4	10.0
	500	14.95	30.6	1468	80.3	55.9	36.0	10.9	45.9	25.0
	900	26.91	52.4	2642	144.5	100.6	64.9	19.6	82.7	45.0
4 months	200	5.42	11.8	559	30.3	16.7	10.5	4.2	14.3	10.0
	500	13.55	29.4	1398	75.7	41.7	26.2	10.5	35.8	25.0
	900	24.39	50.3	2516	136.2	75.0	47.1	19.0	64.5	45.0
5 months	200	4.88	11.3	532	28.5	15.8	9.9	4.1	13.9	10.0
	500	12.2	28.3	1330	71.2	39.5	24.7	10.2	34.8	25.0
	900	21.96	48.3	2394	128.2	71.1	44.4	18.4	62.6	45.0
6 months	200	4.36	10.0	506	26.8	15.0	9.3	3.5	13.5	10.0
	500	10.9	27.2	1265	66.9	37.4	23.2	8.7	33.7	25.0
	900	19.62	46.3	2277	120.5	97.4	41.8	15.7	60.7	45.0

DE, digestible energy; CP, crude protein; Ca, calcium; P, phosphorus; Mg, magnesium; K, potassium; IU, international unit.

Similarly, crude protein intakes of 1535 g day^{-1} are required in the first month to ensure adequate nutrition for maximum milk production (Tables 13.1 and 13.2; Frape, 1998; National Research Council, 2007). In addition to protein quantity, quality is important, in particular the essential amino acid lysine, requirements for which are reported to increase by over 300% (National Research Council, 2007).

13.2.3.2. Calcium and phosphorus

In addition to protein and energy, calcium (Ca) and phosphorus (P) intakes are also very important and requirement increases by over 300%. For a 500-kg mare, average Ca intakes of 59.1 g day^{-1} in the first month of lactation are required to ensure that the foal obtains adequate Ca for bone and tendon growth and development. Deficiency in Ca and/or P has been reported to be associated with demineralization of the maternal skeletal system in order to satisfy the foal's demand (Glade, 1993). As previously discussed, the ratio of Ca to P is important; excess P causes a drain of Ca from the mare's bones in an attempt to redress the balance. P intakes of 38.3 g day^{-1} in the first month are required in early lactating mares of 500 kg.

To satisfy the demands for milk production the mare is likely to require concentrate feed in addition to good-quality forage. P and protein tend to be deficient with regard to lactating mares, even in very good-quality forage diets. The concentrate ration should address this but consist of no more than 50% of the total diet. Lysine is often a limiting essential amino acid in conventional grain and grass forage diets. This can be addressed by the inclusion of lucerne, or soybean meal (Frape, 1998).

As stressed in earlier discussions, it is imperative that all home-grown or bought-in straights and forages are analysed. An appropriate ration for a lactating mare can be ensured by using this information and the analysis of commercial concentrates (Tables 11.2, 13.1. and 13.2.).

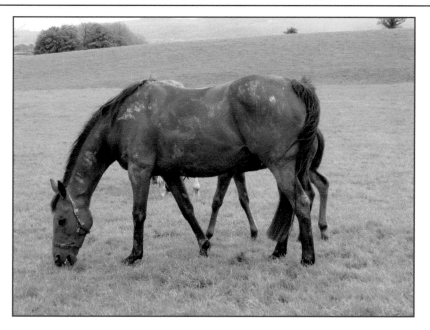

Fig. 13.3. A mare's nutrient requirements increase by 70–75% during early lactation, and so even good grazing alone may not provide enough nutrients to meet demands.

Table 13.2. The expected feed consumption by lactating mares (percentage of body weight). (From National Research Council, 1989.)

Mares	Forage	Concentrates	Total
Early lactation	1.0–2.0	1.0–2.0	2.0–3.0
Late lactation	1.0–2.0	0.5–1.5	2.0–2.5

13.2.3.3. Vitamins

Extra vitamins and minerals are also required during lactation. Deficiency will cause lacklustre and ill thrift in both the mare and foal, and inefficient use of other nutrients. Vitamins A and D are of particular importance. Vitamin A is available in fresh green forage, and Vitamin D from exposure to sunlight, underlining the importance of regular turnout (Frape, 1998; Duren and Crandell, 2001).

13.2.3.4. Water

Access to a clean, reliable water source is particularly important for the lactating mare, whose water requirement is as high as those of any other equine (Fig. 13.4). A 500-kg mare in mid-lactation in an ambient temperature of 20°C may require as much as 78 l day^{-1} (11–14 l per 100 kg body weight per day; National Research Council, 2007).

It is not appropriate to be too prescriptive about exactly what a lactating mare requires, as requirements will vary with individuals. Mares that produce more milk will probably require more feed and will probably require higher levels of concentrate to meet their demand. However, some mares seem to be better doers and more efficient as milk producers. In such mares, obesity may prove to be a problem and, therefore, limiting their concentrate intake should help. The yardstick to go by is the body condition of the mare; she should be fit, not fat, with a body condition score of 3. From 6 weeks of lactation onwards the foal, as far as nutrition is concerned, becomes increasingly independent. The mare's milk yield then decreases; her nutrition management must, therefore, reflect this change in demand.

13.2.4. Exercise

The importance of exercise in uterine recovery is not to be underestimated. Increasing exercise in the first few days post-partum is linked to accelerated uterine involution and hence better conception rates at the foal heat. It is interesting to note that conception rates to the foal heat in feral ponies are normal and in excess of 90% (Camillo *et al.*, 1997; McDonnell, 2000a). Confinement of domesticated mares may, therefore, be a contributory cause of decreasing foal heat conception

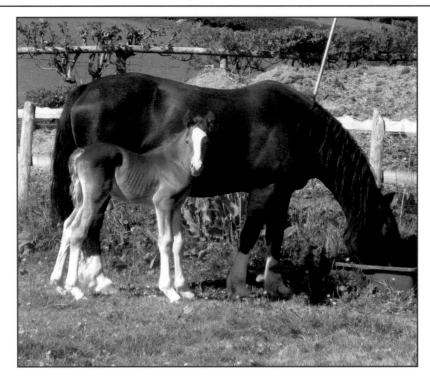

Fig. 13.4. A 500-kg lactating mare may drink up to 78 l of water day^{-1}, and so regular supply of fresh water is essential.

rates (Lowis and Hyland, 1991; Blanchard *et al.*, 2004). Outdoor exercise is also important to promote gastro-intestinal motility, improve appetite (which is particularly important at this time of high nutritional demand) and for Vitamin D production.

13.2.5. Immunization, parasite control, dentition and feet care

No specific immunization of mares that were appropriately vaccinated before parturition, apart from annual boosters, should be required at this stage. However, most mares are then mated and so pregnant again, and for them the vaccination advice given for pregnant mares will apply (Section 11.5.4). The parasite management for the pregnant mare has also been discussed previously (Section 11.5.3) and so will apply to many lactating mares. Worming can be carried out in the first week, especially against strongyles and ascarids, which are particularly significant in mares and young foals. Ideally, though, mares will be wormed in good time prior to foaling, and environmental control of parasites plus faecal egg count monitoring (FEC) will be practised. Teeth and feet care should not be neglected, and their care continued as normal.

13.3. Management of the Lactating Mare: 6 Weeks Post-partum Onwards

From 6 weeks post-partum, lactation yield decreases, along with the quality of milk produced. The mare's udder shrinks as milk demand reduces.

13.3.1. Nutrition

As the mare's milk yield decreases, so do her nutrient requirements. Concentrates should then be slowly reduced to ensure that she does not become obese. For a 500-kg mare protein intakes can be gradually reduced to 1468 g day^{-1} and DE to 30.6 Mcal day^{-1} by 3 months post-partum. Ca and P are still important and intakes of 55.9 and 36.0 g day^{-1}, respectively, are required (Tables 13.1 and 13.2). Particular attention should be paid to the mare's body condition, as mares often put on extra weight in the summer months as the demand for milk declines and before the demands of the fetus *in utero* become significant. It is not, however, appropriate to put a mare in foal on a strict reducing diet later on, in the autumn, in an attempt to lose excess weight gained during the summer months.

13.3.2. Exercise

At this stage exercise is essential to build up the mare's fitness again. Indeed, exercise, along with a decrease in nutrient intake, helps to dry up milk production. The mare and the foal should be turned out for as long as possible, ideally day and night; although, if the weather is too hot, it may be appropriate to bring them in during the day to avoid the flies and to be turned out at night.

13.3.3. Immunization, parasite control, teeth and feet care

Worming regime, immunization programmes, and attention to teeth and feet should be maintained as normal and not neglected, to ensure that the mare remains in optimum condition, especially if she is in foal again.

13.4. Post-weaning Care of the Mare

Weaning normally concentrates on the foal, but the mare should not be neglected (Section 20.2). If her foal has been abruptly removed (abrupt or sudden weaning; paddock or interval weaning) her udder may start to show signs of tenderness and discomfort due to the increase in milk pressure (Perkins and Threlfall, 1993). The milking out of a small amount of milk daily for the first few days is advocated by some, to reduce the pressure and hence the chance of mastitis. The amount of milk removed daily should only be small and should gradually be reduced over 5 days. The removal of too much milk will only serve to prolong the problem. If milk build-up within the udder leads to excessive pressure, infection and mastitis can result (McCue and Wilson, 1989; Gee and McCue, 2011). A post-weaning mare must, therefore, be watched for such problems, especially in the first few days. Mastitis in mares is relatively rare but, if it occurs, can prove fatal if not appropriately treated. Antibiotic treatment is usually successful, although there is always the danger of the infected half of the udder being lost. Using more gradual methods of weaning avoid the risk of weaning-induced mastitis. Additionally, turning a mare out onto into a paddock with limited grass cover and no supplementary feed helps to reduce the chances of mastitis (Fig. 13.5). This limits her nutritional intake and forces her to exercise in order to obtain what grass she eats. Exercise helps to relieve pressure within the udder and utilizes nutrients that would

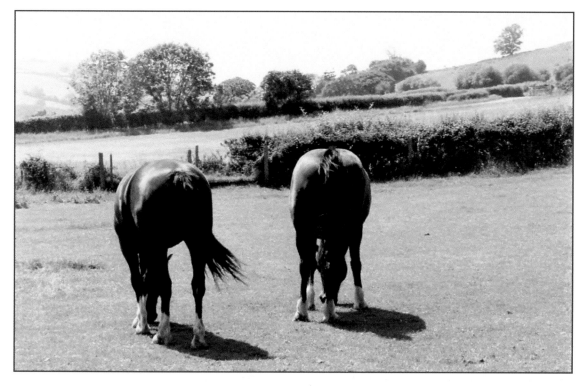

Fig. 13.5. After weaning mares can be turned out into a paddock with limited grass cover to help dry up their milk production.

otherwise be directed towards milk production. Her paddock should be secure and free of hazards, as some mares may be initially quite agitated owing to the absence of the foal. The mare usually recovers more quickly from the separation than does the foal and, in some cases, may even seem relieved to be free of the extra burden (Holland *et al.*, 1997; Siciliano, 2011).

Study Questions

Detail how lactation determines the nutritional management of the mare.

You own a mare that needs to be covered as soon as possible post-partum in order to ensure she foals early next year. Detail the management options to achieve this.

Suggested Reading

Chavatte-Palmer, P. (2002) Lactation in the mare. *Equine Veterinary Education* 5, 88–93.

Macpherson, M.L. and Blanchard, T.L. (2005) Breeding mares on the foal heat. *Equine Veterinary Education* 17(1), 44–52.

National Research Council (2007) *Nutrient Requirements of Horses*, 6th edn. Revised. The National Academies Press, Washington, DC, pp. 315.

Lawrence, L.M. (2011) Nutrition for the broodmare. In: McKinnon, A.O., Squires, E.L., Vaala, E. and Varner, D.D. (eds) *Equine Reproduction*, 2nd edn. Wiley-Blackwell, Philadelphia, London, pp. 2760–2770.

Blanchard, T.L. and Macpherson, M.L. (2011) Breeding mares on foal heat. In: McKinnon, A.O., Squires, E.L., Vaala, E. and Varner, D.D. (eds) *Equine Reproduction*, 2nd edn. Wiley-Blackwell, Philadelphia, London, pp. 2294–2301.

14 Infertility in the Mare

The Objectives of this Chapter are:

To use the anatomy and physiology knowledge gained from Section A to identify abnormalities and causes of infertility.

To gain an appreciation of why conception and/or pregnancy might fail.

To provide you with the knowledge to enable you to have an informed discussion with veterinarians when reproduction fails, and to make appropriate management choices.

14.1. Introduction

Infertility is a vast subject, and so this Chapter will only be an introduction to mare infertility, providing a basis from which further information can be sought. Infertility may have its root cause in either the stallion or the mare. This Chapter will discuss the mare, and a similar approach is taken regarding stallion infertility in Chapter 18.

Expected fertility rates vary enormously and are affected, among other things, by management. Per cycle covering rates are reported to be 60–85% for Thoroughbred/Thoroughbred-type mares bred by intensive management (Baker *et al.*, 1993; Morris and Allen, 2002b; Allen *et al.*, 2007b; Allen and Wilsher, 2018; Rose *et al.*, 2018). The definition of fertility is variable, however, and may be expressed in many ways including: percentage of mares pregnant per mating, percentage of mares pregnant per oestrous period or cycle, percentage of mares pregnant at the end of the season (often from coverings on numerous oestrous periods) or percentage of mares producing a live foal. It is, therefore, very difficult to make comparisons between reported fertility rates. Regardless of the precise definition of fertility, the ability of a mare to produce a live offspring the following year is the main consideration. Failure to do so can be from extrinsic or intrinsic factors, and this is the case with both the mare and the stallion. Extrinsic is the term given to external factors affecting reproductive performance, whereas intrinsic is the term given to internal, usually physiological, factors. As discussed above, reported fertility rates of 60–85% vary significantly with the definition of fertility, but also with the population of mares (Baker *et al.*, 1993; Pycock, 2000; Ball, 2011b; Lane, 2016; Allen and Wilsher, 2018). Of the 20,149 Thoroughbred mares bred in spring 2018 in the UK, 68.99% produced a live foal in spring 2019 (www.weatherbys.co.uk). Human interference in the reproduction of the horse has also had a significant effect on reproductive performance. Live foal rates for wild horses and ponies are in the region of 95% compared with 60% for in-hand-bred mares (Bristol, 1987). Early embryonic death (EED, prior to day 15) and embryo mortality (EM, prior to day 40) are held responsible for a significant amount of apparent infertility as opposed to abortion (after day 40) (Laugier *et al.*, 2011). EM rates of 5–20% have been reported for in-hand mating, compared to 1–2.5% for free mating, although higher rates of EED (up to 50% for normal mares and 70% for aged mares) have been reported by others (Baker *et al.*, 1993; Brinsko *et al.*, 1994; Bosh *et al.*, 2009a,b; Stout, 2012a; Rose *et al.*, 2018). As most loss is EED and so occurs prior to day 15 (Stout, 2012a) – indeed in aged mares prior to day 4 also appears to be a critical period (Ball, 2011b) – most measurements of infertility will also include EED. Unfortunately, despite recent better understanding, the causes of EED and EM are not completely understood, although they are still the biggest cause of pregnancy loss. Abortion is better understood and largely infective in nature (Laugier *et al.*, 2011).

Reproductive performance has been largely ignored in the improvement of the equine. This is in contrast with other farm livestock, where reproductive efficiency is of utmost importance. In addition, barrenness in a mare at the end of the season is not necessarily due to pathological infertility, but may also be a consequence of other environmental and managerial influences. Some mares are consistently barren in early life but breed successfully later on; others appear to take a year off breeding, especially as they age. Failure to produce an offspring in a particular year is, therefore, a complicated problem and is not to be confused with infertility and EM. Before the reasons for a mare failing to produce a foal are discussed in detail, the following glossary should be noted to prevent confusion in terms:

- Fertile – able to produce a live foal.
- Infertility – a temporary inability to reproduce.
- Barrenness – lack of a pregnancy at the end of the season, but perfectly capable of producing a foal, as demonstrated in previous years.
- Subfertility – inability to reproduce at full potential; this may be temporary or permanent.
- Sterility – a permanent inability to reproduce.
- EED – embryo loss prior to day 15.
- EM – embryo loss prior to day 40, often evident between scanning on days 15 and 40.
- Abortion – fetal death after day 40.
- Stillborn – fetal death after day 300.
- Fertilization rate – number of ova fertilized per ovulation.
- Pregnancy rate – number of mares pregnant on a specified day, expressed per oestrous cycle or per breeding season.
- Live foal rate – number of mares foaling per number of mares bred over the season. Arguably the best indicator of reproductive performance.

In the following account, the term 'reproductive performance' will be used, as it encompasses all the above definitions. In many texts the strict definitions of infertility, EED, EM and abortion are not adhered to, and this makes it very hard to distinguish precisely what is responsible for reported changes in reproductive performance. In the mare, reproductive performance does not just depend upon successful gamete production (as is the case with the stallion), but also upon an appropriate environment for fertilization, the free-living embryo, implantation, placentation and subsequent parturition. As such, the following sections will include consideration of fertilization failure, EED, EM and abortion, as appropriate. The failure of a mare to produce a foal at the end of a season may have numerous causes and can be divided into extrinsic and intrinsic factors.

14.2. Extrinsic Factors Affecting Reproductive Performance in the Mare

Extrinsic factors affecting reproductive performance in the mare may be considered to include lack of use; subfertile or infertile stallion; poor stallion management; poor mare management; and the artificially imposed breeding season.

14.2.1. Lack of use

A mare may not be covered in a particular season by design, or because of unavoidable circumstances. If she foals late in one season she may not be re-covered, to allow her to return to foaling earlier the following year. Disease or infection may preclude a mare from use, either because she herself is not in a fit condition to successfully carry a foal, or if there is a danger of systemic or venereal disease transfer. In the case of a performance horse she may not be bred in a particular year owing to work commitments. Advances in embryo transfer, however, now potentially allow such mares to foal via use of a recipient mare (Chapter 22).

14.2.2. Subfertile/infertile stallion

Half the responsibility for fertilization lies with the stallion. If a mare is covered by an infertile or subfertile stallion her chances of producing a foal are significantly reduced through no fault of her own. The causes of infertility in the stallion will be discussed in Chapter 18. Mares can only be expected to perform to their full reproductive potential if they are covered by a stallion whose semen meets minimum requirements. A stallion must also be physically capable of covering a mare effectively; a good semen evaluation in the absence of the ability or willingness to cover is of no use in the natural service of a mare. To a certain extent, this problem may be overcome by the use of artificial insemination (AI; Chapter 21), but, in such cases, it must be certain that the stallion's lack of libido or ability is not due to a potentially heritable fault.

14.2.3. Poor stallion management

Stallion management is considered in detail in Chapters 15–17. It is evident that, if any aspect of a stallion's management (especially his covering management) is not correct, then there is the potential for his fertility rates to be affected. Management in the earlier formative years also has a significant effect on a stallion's libido and hence reproductive performance.

The imposition of an artificial breeding season causes problems with reproductive performance. Even with the use of artificial lights, a stallion's performance during the months of December to February is lower than during his true breeding season. As a result, fertility rates for mares covered within this period cannot be expected to meet normal expectations.

Behavioural abnormalities often associated with inappropriate management (such as failure to obtain or maintain an erection, incomplete intromission and ejaculation failure) may cause apparently low fertilization rates, as can the incorrect detection of successful ejaculation.

14.2.4. Poor mare management

Mare management is discussed in detail in Chapters 8–13. Any deficiencies or inadequacies in brood mare management can lead to poor reproductive performance. Of specific significance is covering management, especially oestrus and ovulation detection. Better, more experienced management and the use of veterinary diagnosis and hormonal manipulation of the cycle are seen to significantly improve reproductive performance. This is suggested to be one of the reasons for the slightly improved conception rates reported over the last 20 years (Allen and Wilsher, 2018). Minimizing stress associated with handling and transportation is also important, as they are associated with EED and EM (Dobson and Smith, 2000; AboEl-Maaty, 2011), possibly via changes in plasma cortisol (Bacus et al., 1990; Alexander and Irvine, 1998; Breen and Karsch, 2006) and progesterone concentrations (Van Niekerk and Morgenthal, 1982). Finally, nutritional stress has also been reported to affect reproductive success (Ball, 1993a; Gentry et al., 2002a; Gastal et al., 2004).

14.2.5. Imposed breeding season

As detailed previously and in Section 9.5.1, there is considerable pressure for foals to be born as soon as possible after 1 January. The methods by which the mare's breeding season may be manipulated to achieve this are discussed in detail in Section 9.5.1. Regardless of the treatment used, pregnancy rates outside of the natural breeding season are not as high as those within the natural breeding season. As such, the continued imposition of an arbitrary breeding season places

unfair constraints upon a mare's potential reproductive performance.

14.3. Intrinsic Factors Affecting Reproductive Performance in the Mare

Intrinsic factors affecting reproductive performance in the mare include age; chromosomal, hormonal, pituitary, ovarian, Fallopian tube, uterine, cervical, vaginal and vulval abnormalities; and infections. All these will be discussed in turn; many, however, are closely interrelated.

14.3.1. Age

Age is reported to have the most significant bearing on reproductive performance (Barbacini et al., 1999; Allen et al., 2007b; Allen and Wilsher, 2018). In general, fertility decreases with age and EED increases (Carnevale et al., 1993; Hemberg et al., 2004; Bosh et al., 2009a; Hanlon et al., 2012a; Rose et al., 2018). It has been suggested that this decrease in fertility may, in part, be due to an increase in the transit time (greater than 4 h) for sperm to reach the oviduct (Scott et al., 2000), making the timing of covering in older mares more crucial. This would also in part explain the observation that significantly more cleaved ova can be collected at day 15 in 2–10-year-old mares compared to 20-year-old mares. It has also been reported that older mares produce less competent oocytes (Armstrong, 2001; Rambags et al., 2006) and possibly, as a result, yield more embryos with morphological abnormalities (Carnevale and Ginther, 1992; Carnevale et al., 1993; Cox et al., 2015; Rizzo et al., 2019) and demonstrate more multiple ovulations and so an increased likelihood of multiple pregnancies (Davies Morel and O'Sullivan, 2001). Embryos spend the first 5 days in the Fallopian tube and it is unclear whether poor reproductive performance is due to fertilization failure or EED in the Fallopian tube. In older mares in particular, embryo development during Fallopian tube transit is reported to be poorer (Brinsko et al., 1994; Ball, 2011b). Together, all of these factors suggest high apparent infertility rates in older mares. Evidence would also suggest that the occurrence of anovulatory oestrus is greater in mares over 20 years (Vanderwall et al., 1993). Rose et al. (2018) reported that 1.9% of young mares (2–4 years of age) suffered from EM between day 15 (1st scanning) and day 42 (2nd scanning) compared to 15.8% for mares over 19 years of age. This is because of an incompetent uterine environment.

Endometrial degeneration, and inflammatory changes in particular deteriorate with age, and have been held responsible for the high EM (days 15–40) rates reported in aged mares (Carnevale and Ginther, 1992; Carnevale et al., 2000c; Siemieniuch et al., 2017; Kabisch et al., 2019). Later in pregnancy the placental development, particularly blood supply to the microcotyledons, is reported to be adversely affected by old age and so leads to increased abortion rates (Bracher et al., 1996; Merkt et al., 2000; Allen, 2001a; Wilsher and Allen, 2012). Despite reducing reproductive performance, providing a mare is in good physical condition, she may breed successfully well into her 20s. However, welfare considerations may preclude breeding a mare of advanced age. In such cases, embryo transfer may prove a viable alternative to putting an older mare through the stresses of carrying a pregnancy to term (Chapter 22).

14.3.2. Chromosomal abnormalities

The normal chromosomal complement for the equine is 64 (32 pairs), the female complement being denoted as 64XX. Intersex conditions such as female pseudohermaphrodite have been reported where chromosomal complement is female (64XX) but the individual has male external genitalia or persistent infertility (Arighi, 2011b). Various variations of the normal complement of 64XX exist with a reported 2–3% incidence. These cause infertility, EED, EM and congenital abnormalities, and may remain undetected until the mare is put to stud (Lear and Villagomez, 2011). The most common abnormalities are to the sex chromosomes, which may or may not be inherited. These may be evident as changes in the reproductive tract and cyclicity such as 63XO (a female with a single X chromosome), termed Turners syndrome, the most common chromosomal abnormality (Gamo et al., 2019). Such individuals are characterized by small rudimentary ovaries; flaccid, poorly developed uterus; no ovarian activity; and, therefore, permanent anoestrus. Such mares tend also to be short in stature (Davies, 1995; Bowling, 1996). Mosaic chromosomal configuration may occur as 64XX complement in some cells, and 63XO in others; such individuals demonstrate erratic oestrous cycles with no ovulation (Kjöllerström et al., 2011; Lear and Villagomez, 2011; Neuhauser et al., 2018b), although successful breeding of a mosaic has been reported (Neuhauser et al., 2019b). Numerous other variations have been reported but are very rare (Dunn et al., 1981; Halnan, 1985; Kubien and Tischner, 2002; Lear and Villagomez, 2011; Anaya et al., 2014; Ghosh et al., 2016).

Other chromosomal abnormalities may not be evident as aberrations in the mare's reproductive tract or cyclicity, but result in EED and/or EM. Abnormalities like these involve a change in DNA organization, resulting in gametes with abnormal chromosome numbers incompatible with life (Lear and Villagomez, 2011). Such oocyte chromosomal abnormalities are reported to increase with mare age (Cox et al., 2015; Rizza et al., 2019). Additionally, embryo chromosomal abnormalities incompatible with life may also be a significant cause of EED, EM and/or abortion (Newcombe, 2000a; Lear and Layton, 2002; Rambags et al., 2005).

Positive diagnosis of chromosomal abnormalities is only possible by karyotyping (genetic mapping) via analysis of blood, hair or buccal swab samples, although the abnormalities may be indirectly indicated physiologically (Halnan, 1985; Bowling and Hughes, 1993; Lear and Villagomez, 2011; Anaya et al., 2014; Legrand and Bailly, 2019).

It is interesting to note that inbreeding, or what is often termed line breeding, is often practised within the equine industry in an attempt to fix traits within a population. Although it used to be considered that such levels of inbreeding did not result in the significant infertility and congenital problems seen in other mammals (Mahon and Cunningham, 1982), this is now not thought to be the case, and most recent work indicates that inbreeding may be becoming an issue in stud management.

14.3.3. Hormonal abnormalities

As discussed in Chapter 2, the control of the mare's reproduction is a finely balanced cascade and interrelationship of hormones involving the hypothalamic–pituitary–ovarian axis. Abnormalities/inefficiencies in any of these centres can cause imbalance throughout the whole axis. The majority of hormonal deficiencies are associated with pituitary abnormalities, for example Cushing's syndrome and insulin resistance, both of which may result in abnormal cycles (Van Der Kolk, 1997; Pycock, 2000; LeBlanc and McKinnon, 2011; Burns, 2016). Complete failure (or neoplasia) of the pituitary is relatively rare in the horse, but temporary malfunction may occur, especially in association with the transitional period at the beginning or end of the breeding season. During this transitional period mares tend to suffer from prolonged or persistent oestrus (nymphomania), prolonged dioestrus (persistent corpus luteum (CL)), silent ovulations (failure to exhibit oestrus despite ovulation), split oestrus (oestrus over a period of up to 3 weeks, possibly with a quiescent period in the middle), anovulatory follicles (follicles that luteinize but fail to ovulate), etc. Similar problems may be seen in post-partum mares owing to lactational anoestrus. In such cases, it is evident that a period of time is required to allow the mare's system to re-establish regular 21-day cycles.

Diagnosis of hormonal abnormality is initially via a mare's behaviour and the seeming inability to detect oestrus or, conversely, by apparent continual oestrus. Diagnosis of the cause is helped via scanning and rectal palpation, by which ovarian activity can be monitored. The incidence of hormonal deficiencies or abnormalities is particularly evident at the present time, as continued attempts are made to breed mares earlier in the season. The use of exogenous hormonal treatments and/or light treatment does successfully advance ovulation and oestrus within the year, but does not eliminate the transition period, which may still be associated with problems (discussed in Section 9.5.1).

Pituitary or hypothalamic tumours are rare in mares; they are associated with muscle wasting, hypoglycaemia, docility, alopecia, blindness and uncoordinated movement, in addition to prolonged anoestrus.

Hormonal deficiencies during pregnancy may also result in reproductive failure. In particular, progesterone insufficiency causes EED, EM or abortion, dependent upon when it occurs (Irvine *et al.*, 1990; Morgenthal and Van Niekerk, 1991; Allen, 2001b). Exogenous progesterone supplementation has been suggested to be successful in such mares, and it is routinely used in some stud practices as a safeguard, although such use is not normally justified with normal mares (Pycock, 2000; LeBlanc and McKinnon, 2011; Willmann *et al.*, 2011; Canisso *et al.*, 2013b).

Most recently anti-mullerian hormone (AMH) has been shown to correlate with antral follicle population in mares of different ages and possibly fertility (Claes *et al.*, 2015). Based on this and on work in other mammalian females, Scarlet *et al.* (2018) demonstrated a link between AMH in pre-pubertal fillies and future follicular reserves, and hence post-pubertal follicular development. As such the authors suggested that AMH in pre-pubertal fillies may be used as a biomarker to indicate gonadal function and so future fertility.

14.3.4. Physical abnormalities

There are a range of physical abnormalities, both genetic and due to accident/operation, which may be responsible for subfertility or infertility.

14.3.4.1. Ovarian abnormalities

Occasionally ovaries may be absent as a result of surgical intervention or chromosomal abnormality. Inactive ovaries and ovulation failure are often observed in mares and are exacerbated by the imposition of an arbitrary breeding season.

Follicular atresia

Follicular atresia is responsible for some incidences of ovulation failure. In such cases a group of follicles will develop normally, to about 3 cm in diameter, but there is a failure in the emergence of a dominant follicle (which would be expected to develop further). Conditions such as ovarian hypoplasia, granulosa cell tumours, ovarian cysts, uterine infections, malnutrition and season have all been implicated in follicular atresia (Pugh, 1985; Bosu and Smith, 1993; Ginther *et al.*, 2004a). The best cure appears to be time, especially in mares encountering problems during the transitional stage of the breeding season. Often, succeeding cycles will not demonstrate the same condition. Failure of follicular development may be due to ovarian senescence and has been suggested to be one of the reasons for poorer reproductive function in mares over 20 years. Older mares demonstrate longer follicular phase and interovulatory intervals. Complete ovarian senescence is rare but may be due to inadequate primordial follicle reserves (Carnevale *et al.*, 1994). Post-partum anoestrus is also evident as follicular atresia and is normally the combined effect of nutrition, lactation and season. The normal expectation is that mares will return to oestrus and ovulation (foal heat) 4–10 days post-partum. However, some mares, particularly those in poor body condition foaling early in the year, fail to come into foal heat and enter a period of prolonged anoestrus (Nagy *et al.*, 1998).

Corpus Luteum Persistence and Failure

CL persistence and, conversely, failure are also causes of reproductive failure in the mare, manifesting themselves as long or short oestrous cycles, respectively. Failure of the CL is less evident in the mare than persistence. However, CL failure is implicated in experiments using progesterone supplementation to prevent abortion (Pycock, 2000; Allen, 2001b; LeBlanc and McKinnon, 2011; Willmann *et al.*, 2011; Canisso *et al.*, 2013b). The effect of progesterone insufficiency has also been considered in Section 14.3.3. Premature luteolysis is often the result of bacterial endometritis causing the premature release of prostaglandin F2α (PGF2α). The presence of a persistent CL is more common in mares and is an important cause of anoestrus. The normal lifespan of a CL is 14 days, after which (in the absence of a pregnancy) the luteolytic hormone PGF2α, secreted by the uterine endometrium, takes effect. A persistent CL is presumably, therefore, a result of failure in the release of PGF2α, or in the ability of the CL to react appropriately. The presence of such conditions in a mare is implicated by the lack of oestrous behaviour, and confirmed by scanning or rectal palpation. The failure of the luteolytic message may be linked to chronic uterine infection, rendering the uterine endometrium unable to produce PGF2α. Dioestrus ovulation and EM after day 15, the time of maternal recognition of pregnancy, may also be causes. Treatment with exogenous PGF2α is normally successful (Pycock, 2000).

Anovulatory Follicles

Anovulatory follicles can be haemorrhagic, luteinized or persistent, and can be a cause of anoestrus (McCue and Squires, 2002; McCue and Ferris, 2017). They occur most commonly in the transition period into and out of the breeding season. Anovulatory follicles are characterized as large follicles that fail to rupture and ovulate. The majority will fill with blood and persist as haematomas (haemorrhagic anovulatory follicles) that then slowly luteinize (to become luteinized anovulatory follicles) and then persist as progesterone-secreting structures, possibly over a number of cycles. Occasionally an anovulatory follicle will not haemorrhage or luteinize, but will simply persist as a large follicle, slowly reducing in size over the season (persistent anovulatory follicle) (McCue and Squires, 2002; McCue and McKinnon, 2011a). Differentiation between haemorrhagic, luteinized and persistent anovulatory follicles is by means of scanning, when their content (blood, luteal tissue or follicular fluid, respectively) can be identified. Additionally, luteinized anovulatory follicles secrete progesterone, and so prolonged elevated plasma progesterone concentrations is indicative (Pycock, 2000; McCue and Ferris, 2017). Luteinized anovulatory follicles can be treated with prostaglandin, which destroys the luteal tissue, so allowing the mare to re-cycle. The majority of haemorrhagic anovulatory follicles convert into luteinized anovulatory follicles and so can be similarly treated with prostaglandin at that stage. Persistent anovulatory follicles, however, are harder to resolve, and so allowing time for them to degenerate is normally the solution (McCue and Ferris, 2017).

Ovulation Fossa Cysts

Ovulation fossa cysts are reported, especially in older mares. They appear to be associated with the epithelium of the fimbrae and may cause blockage of the ovulation fossa and, therefore, a disruption of ova release. They are often evident as a bundle of cysts, similar to a bunch of grapes, near the ovulation fossa. In the extreme, they may also interfere with the blood supply to the rectum (McKinnon, 1998b; Schlafer, 2011b; McCue and Ferris, 2017). Parovarian or paroophoron cysts are also reported, but rarely cause problems (McCue and McKinnon, 2011a).

Ovarian Tumours

There are a number of ovarian tumours, all of which are benign, and normally arise from epithelial cells, stroma cells or germ cells. They are all quite rare, however. The most common are granulosa cell (involving the granulosa cells) followed by theca cell (involving the theca cells) tumours (Figs 14.1 and 14.2). Both of these are an important cause of disrupted reproductive activity (Sundberg *et al.*, 1977; Rambags *et al.*, 2003; Nout-Lomas

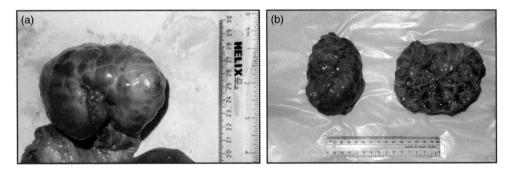

Fig. 14.1. Polycystic granulosa cell tumour in the mare, before (a) and after (b) dissection.

and Beacom, 2015; McCue and Ferris, 2017). They are usually unilateral (associated with a single ovary), but often affect the function of the other ovary through their hormone production, especially that of inhibin. The ovaries are either polycystic or large, solid structures and may weigh up to 8 kg (Figs 14.1 and 14.2; Norris *et al.*, 1968; McCue, 1992; McCue and Ferris, 2017).

The symptoms demonstrated by such mares depend on the hormones secreted by the tumours, and are largely behavioural. The main hormone produced is inhibin which inhibits pituitary function, so inhibiting the function of the contralateral ovary through negative feedback, resulting in anoestrus (Piquette *et al.*, 1990; Bailey *et al.*, 2002). The tumours may also secrete estrogen, in which case nymphomaniac behaviour (prolonged oestrus) in the absence of ovulation, is evident. Testosterone-producing cysts result in stallion-like behaviour and muscular development, and occasionally they may secrete progesterone, again resulting in delayed oestrus/suppression of reproductive activity. Removal of the affected ovary often allows the resumption of normal reproductive activity by the remaining ovary (Meager, 1978; McCue *et al.*, 2006).

Other ovarian tumours have been reported, such as cystadenomas, teratomas and dysgerminomas, but are very rare. They are also benign but not hormonally active and so do not cause behavioural changes or suppression of activity in the contralateral ovary (McKinnon, 1998a; McCue and Ferris, 2017). Ovarian teratomas arise from germ cells that undergo neoplastic transformation into endoderm, mesoderm and/or ectoderm tissue. They are therefore evident as containing hair, teeth, bone, muscular or nervous tissue, etc. (Fig. 14.3; Hughes, 1993; Schlafer, 2011b). They are also

unilateral but, owing to their non-secretory nature, they allow the other ovary to function normally; pregnancy rates may or may not be affected significantly.

Hypoplasia

Ovarian hypoplasia (underdevelopment) is a further cause of anoestrus. It is characterized by small, immature ovaries with no ovarian activity or increase in ovarian size within the breeding season. Hypoplasia is usually bilateral and is often associated with chromosomal or hormonal abnormalities, as previously discussed.

Cystic Ovaries

The term cystic ovary implies the presence of fluid-filled, hormonally active structures within the ovarian stroma. Such structures are reported in cattle, but are reported not to occur in mares, and are sometimes confused with granulosa cell tumours (Pycock, 2000).

Other Abnormalities

Several other abnormalities have been reported, but occur rarely, such as dysgerminomas (malignant tumours of cells resembling primordial cells), abscesses and haematomas (overfilling of the follicular cavity with blood post-ovulation) (Meuten and Rendano, 1978; Bosu *et al.*, 1982; Neely, 1983; Bosu and Smith, 1993; Card, 2011b; McCue and McKinnon, 2011a; Schlafer, 2011b).

Multiple Ovulation

Multiple ovulations, and the resulting multiple pregnancies, have been considered in Sections 2.4.5 and 11.3. However, they warrant mentioning here as a major cause of EED and abortion, hence reproductive failure. The

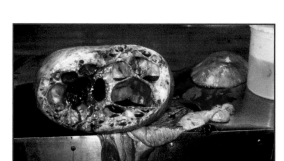

Fig. 14.2. A large solid theca cell tumour in the mare. (Photo courtesy of Dr Julie Baumber-Skaife.)

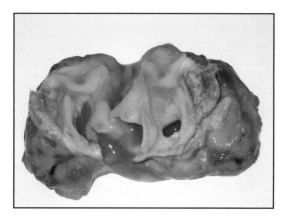

Fig. 14.3. An ovarian teratoma containing hair and cartilaginous tissue.

mare is monocotous and, as such, she is unable to satisfactorily support more than one fetus *in utero*. Fetal restriction results, causing either spontaneous abortion of one or both fetuses or the mummification of the smaller twin (McKinnon, 2011). Twins are, therefore, not desirable, and management in general is geared towards avoiding them (Section 11.3). Twinning is an inherited trait and can be avoided, and an awareness of its possibility can be gained by studying a mare's breeding history and any previous incidents of twinning.

14.3.4.3. Fallopian tube abnormalities

The extent of follicular tube abnormality is unclear (Ley *et al.*, 1998; Ley, 2011; Liu, 2011; Lyman and Sertich, 2019). However, if present, they are normally associated with adhesion of the infundibulum to other parts of the reproductive tract. Collagenous masses that may occlude the lumen of the Fallopian tube have also been documented (Lui *et al.*, 1990). Rarely, an ovarian cyst may be seen to block the entry to the Fallopian tube at the infundibulum. Tumours of the Fallopian tube are extremely rare. Treatment via the topical application of prostaglandin E (PGE) has been suggested (Allen *et al.*, 2006).

14.3.4.4. Uterine abnormalities

Uterine abnormalities due to congenital defects or infections are relatively well understood in the mare, compared to abnormalities of the remainder of the tract. The development of techniques such as ultrasonic scanning, endoscopy and uterine biopsy has significantly advanced our understanding of uterine physiology and pathology (Brook, 1993).

Endometriosis, Or Chronic Non-Infective Degenerative Endometritis

Endometriosis is caused by degeneration of the endometrium, rather than by infection, and may be classified as infiltrative or degenerative (Fig. 14.4). Infiltrative endometriosis may be a result of changes within the uterus owing to a busy breeding career, and is associated with a natural post-coital increase in leucocyte response to the normal bacterial challenge of mating (Ricketts and Alonso, 1991; Hoffmann *et al.*, 2009). Degenerative endometriosis is a degeneration of the endometrial glands that renders the uterus incapable of supporting a pregnancy. It is associated with EM (days 15–40) and is often the result of repeated gestations, especially in mares with a history of uterine infections (Bracher *et al.*, 1996). Degeneration of the endometrial glands

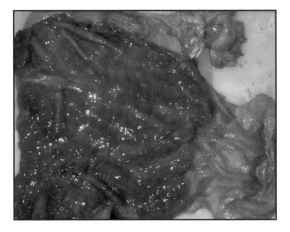

Fig. 14.4. Endometriosis is caused by degeneration of the endometrium, rather than by infection. This is evident in this uterus by the complete lack of endometrial folds. Note the uterine luminal cysts just inside the cervix.

results in a failure to return to normal, post-partum, leaving lymph-filled lesions (Walter *et al.*, 2001; Aresu *et al.*, 2012), but this does not necessarily affect the ability of the uterus to react to a bacterial challenge (the phagocytic activity of polymorphonuclear neutrophil (PMN) granulocytes; Zerbe *et al.*, 2004). Treatment may be attempted by the stimulation of growth of new healthy endometrium using mechanical or chemical curettage (see later in this section). However, such treatment is not very successful and runs the risk of further uterine damage. The prognosis for such mares is poor (Asbury and Lyle, 1993; Hoffmann *et al.*, 2009; Ball, 2011b).

Hyperplasia

Uterine hyperplasia (overdevelopment) is characterized by an overdevelopment of the uterus for the reproductive stage of the mare, or a failure to recover from a previous event such as pregnancy. Again, the endometrial glands are most significantly affected. As indicated, the condition is often a result of delayed involution post-partum, the uterine endometrium failing to return to normal within the time expected (see Section 13.2.2). Hyperplasia may also be a result of EM or abortion, or as a consequence of hormonal imbalance, often resulting from hormone-secreting tumours. Hyperplasia is normally a temporary condition that can be reversed by reproductive rest or hormonal treatment (Van Camp, 1993; Murphy *et al.*, 2005; Witkowski *et al.*, 2017).

Hypoplasia

Uterine hypoplasia (underdevelopment) is characterized by an inability to develop adequately in order to maintain a pregnancy. The endometrial glands are most significantly affected, tending to be very small and so incapable of adaptation to support a pregnancy. As a result, even if fertilization does occur, the EED rate is high. Covering mares too close to puberty is associated with high rates of EED due to hypoplasia, simply because the uterine development to date is inadequate. The actual age at which the uterus is fully mature depends very largely on the individual mare: 2–4 years is considered acceptable. Hypoplasia is most common, therefore, in young mares. If it persists beyond around 4 years old it is indicative of a problem that is likely to be permanent, and may be associated with chromosomal or hormonal abnormalities (Davies, 1995; Ricketts and Barrelet, 1997; Witkowski *et al.*, 2017).

Uterine Atrophy

Mares with uterine atrophy or senility are normally characterized as repeat breeders with high rates of EED and EM (Bracher *et al.*, 1992; Van Camp, 1993). Uterine atrophy is caused by a decrease in the number of endometrial glands due to atrophy or an inability to regenerate themselves. It is often associated with chromosomal intersex conditions; ovarian incompetence; or progressive wear and tear in multiparous mares (Hanada *et al.*, 2014; Kabisch *et al.*, 2019). It is also reported to have a greater occurrence late in the breeding season, presumably due to a decline in oestrus and ovarian activity. Generally, such late-season atrophy is of little concern, but evidence of it occurring early in the season may be indicative of a permanent problem and effect on reproductive performance. This condition is normally irreversible.

Uterine Fibrosis

Uterine fibrosis (periglandular fibrosis) is a degenerative uterine change, most commonly found in old multiparous mares, but has also been reported as the result of lavage with enrofloxacin antibacterial agent (Kiviniemi-Moore *et al.*, 2017); it is characterized by fibrotic changes around the endometrial glands forming glandular nests. As a result, the secretions of the endometrial glands decrease, the glands dilate, increasing the incidence of uterine cysts and resulting in increasing EED owing to a disruption of embryo mobility, or abortion in late pregnancy due to restricted placental size (Van Camp, 1993).

Uterine Luminal Cysts

Uterine luminal or endometrial cysts are the most common form of uterine lesion (Eilts *et al.*, 1995; Stanton *et al.*, 2004; De Mestre *et al.*, 2019). They are generally thin-walled, greater than 3 cm in diameter, filled with lymph and may occur singularly or in multiples (Fig. 14.5).

They are particularly evident in mares of 10 years old or over (Stanton, 2011b). Their effect on reproductive performance is disputed. They tend to be found at the base of the uterine horns and so, if present in any number, they are likely to interfere with embryonic mobility increasing EED and EM through interrupting conceptus mobility and, therefore, maternal recognition of pregnancy. They may also reduce the uterine surface area available for placental attachment, increasing abortion rates (Curnow, 1991) and are reported to be associated with reduced uterine blood flow (Ferreira *et al.*, 2008). Treatment may be attempted by puncturing the cysts via curettage, endoscopic manipulation and rupture or thermocautery, as well as laser therapy, although they may subsequently recur (Pycock, 2000; Rambags and Stout, 2005; Stanton, 2011b; Miller and Ferrer, 2014). More recently success has been reported using ethanol sclerotherapy (Carluccio *et al.*, 2018).

Uterine Curettage

Uterine curettage was traditionally used as a treatment for a whole range of conditions that resulted in damage to the uterine endometrium. It works on the principle of mechanical or chemical irritation of the endometrium, the rationale being that irritation stimulates and initiates a cleansing and regeneration process within the uterine endometrium and a mobilization of neutrophils

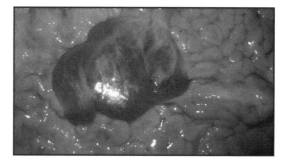

Fig. 14.5. A luminal cyst within the uterus. Luminal cysts do not necessarily cause excessive problems unless evident in large numbers, when they may interfere with embryo mobility and subsequent implantation.

to the affected site. Mechanical curettage involves physically scraping the entire surface of the endometrium, using a cutting edge mounted upon a long shaft that is passed through the cervix into the uterus. Chemical curettage involves the infusion of a chemical irritant such as povidone-iodine, or kerosene, which is reported to have a similar effect (Bracher, 1992). Curettage was once very popular but has largely been discredited as ineffective, with the potential to cause excessive scar tissue, haemorrhage and uterine adhesions.

Ventral Uterine Dilation

Ventral uterine dilation or sacculation is caused by uterine myometrial atrophy, normally in the base of one uterine horn, forming an outfolding or sacculation, which often collects fluid (Fig. 14.6). This is again more common in older multiparous mares, due to a weakening of the myometrium. It often occurs at the implantation site, and may be caused by a gradual weakening of the wall in an area of repeated excessive stretching. Treatment is relatively unsuccessful, unfortunately, but some beneficial results have been reported using oxytocin, or oxytocin in combination with warm saline lavage. The fluid accumulation is normally of greatest concern, making such mares susceptible to chronic endometritis and pyometra (Section 14.3.5.3; Brinsko *et al.*, 1990).

Uterine Adhesions

Uterine adhesions are present as single or multiple bands or sheets of tissue within or across the lumen of

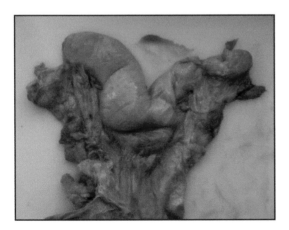

Fig. 14.6. Uterine dilation is often characterized by excess mucus or fluid within the uterus; and endometritis can be identified at rectal palpation when part or all the uterus feels enlarged, flaccid and doughy.

the uterus, and are the result of uterine trauma from dystocia, intrauterine infusion, severe endometritis or after treatment with caustic solutions. Their effect upon fertility depends upon their extent, but they may disrupt embryo mobility and restrict placental attachment, as well as causing fluid retention, leading to endometritis. As such, they may be associated with EED or abortion. Attempts may be made to remove or break adhesions manually via an endoscope and biopsy forceps, or via electrocautery (Van Camp, 1993; Hurtgen, 2011a).

Uterine Neoplasia

Neoplasia or tumours within the uterus are very rare. Leiomyoma are the most common and can be evident as single or multiple nodules; they can cause persistent haemorrhage (Quinn and Woodford, 2005). Treatment may be attempted with some success by surgery or endoscopy (Bradecamp *et al.*, 2017).

Lymphatic Lacunae

Poor uterine lymphatic drainage may result in oedema within the uterine wall, causing continuation of the normal ultrasonic 'cartwheel' appearance of the uterus beyond ovulation. Normally such oedema disappears soon after ovulation via absorption into the lymphatic system. Lymph is pumped along the lymph vessels by mild rhythmic contractions of the uterine myometrium but sometimes, especially in older multiparous mares, uterine myometrial contractility is impaired and so uterine oedema is not dissipated. This leads to a doughy, thick-walled uterus that is unable to sustain a pregnancy; pregnancy normally fails at 12–20 weeks (LeBlanc *et al.*, 1994, 2004; Kabisch *et al.*, 2019).

Foreign Bodies

Very occasionally foreign bodies such as a mummified fetus, fetal bone, tips of uterine swabs, straws used with frozen semen, etc., are found within the uterus, potentially resulting in chronic endometritis. Their removal, followed by treatment and recovery time, normally restores reproductive performance (Pycock, 2000; Hurtgen, 2011a).

14.3.4.5. Cervical abnormalities

Cervical abnormalities normally arise from damage at parturition. Lacerations or injuries to the cervix often do not heal properly, severely affecting the dynamic properties of the cervix, which allows it to vary from a tight seal to wide dilation at parturition. Damage often causes adhesions, which may block the entrance to the uterus through the cervix, or cause cervical incompetence. This will inhibit sperm deposition, allow infection to enter the uterus and prevent natural uterine drainage (Sertich, 1993; Katila, 2012). As discussed in some detail in Sections 1.3.1 and 1.5, the cervix naturally forms the final seal protecting the upper reproductive tract from infection, and so such mares are predisposed to uterine infection, fertilization failure and EED. Minor adhesions may be treated by physically cutting or electrocauterizing the scar tissue and inserting a plastic tube to prevent reoccurrence, and lacerations can be surgically corrected (Brown *et al.*, 1984; Aanes, 1993). Excess adhesions and interruption of the normal cervical relaxation at oestrus can prevent the natural drainage of uterine secretion, increasing the chance of endometritis. The prognosis in most cases, however, is not good (Hurtgen, 2011b). Occasionally cervical dilation failure might be evident. This can have an obvious effect on parturition but also at breeding, leading to reproductive failure due to failure of uterine clearance (Tibary, 2011b). Neoplasms of the cervix are very rare (Sertich, 1993). Inherited or congenital cervical incompetence, though, has been reported in pony mares (Lieux, 1972; Brown, 1984; Card, 2012).

14.3.4.6. Vaginal abnormalities

Vaginal abnormalities have several causes. Among these is damage at parturition, often a result of fetal malpresentations. Superficial damage will correct and heal naturally, although there is the risk of adhesions. Severe adhesions may cause the mare pain at subsequent coverings. Vaginal and vulval lacerations can occur at parturition; in the extreme, rectal vaginal fissures may be opened up by the foal's foot passing through the top of the vagina and into the rectum during parturition. The prognosis in such cases depends on the length of the opening formed, but can be very poor when substantial rectal vaginal fissures occur (Section 12.6.3; Fig. 12.35; Spensley and Markel, 1993; Saini *et al.*, 2013a; Anand and Singh, 2015; Elkasapy and Ibrahim, 2015).

Two of the most common vaginal abnormalities are associated with poor perineal conformation: pneumovagina (inspiration of air and bacteria into the vagina) and urovagina (urine pooling in the cranial vagina). Pneumovagina predisposes the mare to endometritis and so is a common cause of infertility, especially in Thoroughbred mares, and is due to the incompetence of the vestibular and vulval seals and associated poor perineal conformation. This can be alleviated quite successfully by a Caslick's vulvoplasty operation (Section 1.3).

Urovagina results from weakness within the vaginal walls and/or inward sloping of the reproductive tract causing collection of urine often around the vaginal fornix (posterior vagina), and so urine can easily pass through the cervix into the uterus. As such, it is associated with infection (endometritis, cervicitis and vaginitis) and hence adversely affects reproductive performance. The condition is normally observed in older, multiparous mares with pendulous reproductive tracts because of continual stretching and weakening with successive pregnancies. Occasionally it may also be seen as a temporary phenomenon at foal heat, but in most circumstances it will have rectified itself by the second heat post-partum. If it is evident, it is essential that the mare is not covered, as there is an increased chance of post-coital endometritis. Treatment using oxytocin has proved reasonably successful, as has surgical intervention (Jalim and McKinnon, 2010; McKinnon and Jalim, 2011).

Persistent Hymen

Occasionally, a persistent hymen may be evident. The hymen divides the anterior and posterior vagina and occasionally does not break in early life before first service, and so may be evident in maiden mares as a white/blue membrane possibly pushing through the vulva. A persistent hymen will impede natural drainage and, as such, when fillies reach puberty the secretions of the reproductive tract associated with oestrous cycles will build up behind the hymen causing it to bulge through the vulva. Simply manually breaking the hymen will allow the fluids to drain and the mare's subsequent fertility should be unaffected. If the hymen is not broken prior to the first service it may tear, causing the development of scar tissue (Hurtgen, 2011b; Dascanio, 2014b).

14.3.4.7. Vulval and perineal abnormalities

Vulval abnormalities most commonly involve inappropriate perineal conformation, as discussed in detail in Section 1.3, predisposing the mare to pneumovagina and urovagina. The resulting vulval-seal incompetence increases the chance of infection entering the reproductive tract. Lacerations of the vulva occurring at parturition or due to accidental injury can also compromise vulval-seal competence, owing to incorrect healing and adhesion formation (Saini *et al.*, 2013b; Anand and Singh, 2015). Vaginal lacerations can be surgically repaired with some success (Sang Kyu *et al.*, 2009; Elkasapy and Ibrahim, 2015). Failure to cut a Caslick's vulvoplasty prior to covering or parturition will also cause tearing and will predispose to adhesion formation, fibrosis and inappropriate vulval healing (Aanes, 1993).

Haemorrhage of the vulval lips may be evident, caused by the bursting of varicose veins. This has minimal direct effect on reproductive ability but may cause discomfort at breeding. Neoplasms of the vulva are reported, most commonly melanomas, originating in the pigment-producing cells of the skin, especially prevalent in grey mares. These tumours can spread from the perineal area around the anus and eventually throughout the whole of the body. Squamous cell carcinoma, normally associated with the penis, may also be seen on the vulval lips. Finally, enlarged clitorises (sometimes in the form of a vestigial penis) may be observed, and are associated with chromosomal abnormalities; such animals are sterile.

14.3.5. Infectious infertility

Infection, particularly of the uterus (endometritis) – whether bacterial, fungal or viral – is a major cause of subfertility or infertility in the mare.

14.3.5.1. Ovarian infections

As far as infection or disease is concerned, the ovary is essentially unaffected and the vast majority of ovarian abnormalities, and hence ovarian infertility, are not the result of pathogenic agents.

14.3.5.2. Fallopian tube infections (salpingitis)

Salpingitis, inflammation of the Fallopian tubes or saplings, is rarely seen; however, it may occur as a consequence of endometritis. Complete blockage of the Fallopian tubes is rare, but inflammation can interrupt the process of fertilization, the passage of ova towards the utero-tubular junction and sperm movement towards the ampulla. Infertility or subfertility may result. Occasionally, infection may cause inflammation of the utero-tubular junction, affecting the passage of sperm and/or fertilized ova (Ley, 2011; Lyman and Sertich 2019).

14.3.5.3. Uterine infections

One of the major causes of infertility and EED and EM in the mare is endometritis (inflammation of the uterine endometrium) (Card, 2005; Causey, 2006; LeBlanc 2008; Liu and Troedsson, 2008; Troedsson, 2011; Pasolini et al., 2016). Endometritis is primarily caused by infection by venereal and/or opportunistic bacteria, but may also be due to non-infectious degenerative endometritis and/or persistent post-coital endometritis

(Section 14.3.4.4). It is reported to be evident in 25–60% of barren mares (Traub-Dargatz et al., 1991; Christoffersen et al., 2015). The main consequence of endometritis is a uterine environment hostile to embryo survival and implantation, resulting primarily in EED and EM, but may also cause abortion. Endometritis is evident in four forms: acute endometritis; chronic endometritis; acute metritis; and pyometra. These will be discussed in turn later in the Chapter.

Several factors predispose the mare's tract to infections, including immunological, physiological or endocrinal deficiencies; these may be inherited, leading to a predisposition to endometritis.

Unfortunately, the mare's reproductive tract is horizontal or even declined inwards towards the ventral abdomen and, as such, is not well conformed for the natural drainage of infective organisms or the resulting exudate. Infections are difficult for the mare's system to eliminate naturally, therefore, and can easily develop into chronic infections. Chronic infections can cause serious problems to the mare if not treated in good time (Hoffmann et al., 2009). Temporary infertility is nearly always evident with endometritis, and, if the infection/damage is great, permanent reduction in reproductive performance will result. Bacterial infection is largely introduced at covering, or by inadequate hygiene precautions during internal examination or immediately post-partum, although an incompetent vulval seal is increasingly responsible for allowing bacterial invasion in some breeds. It is, therefore, most important that strict hygiene precautions are adhered to during covering, and in manipulation or examination of the mare's tract.

One of the major problems with uterine infections is that they may remain undetected for prolonged periods of time, thus not only reducing the mare's reproductive performance, but also risking transfer to the stallion and hence to other mares (LeBlanc and Causey, 2009). Regular swabbing is not only compulsory in many studs, but is good practice to ensure that all chronic endometritis infections and latent asymptomatic infections are identified and treated immediately.

Endometritis is often characterized by excess mucus which may be seen exuding from the vulva, high leucocyte counts and increased uterine blood flow. Uterine oedema (fluid accumulation) can be identified at scanning, and the uterus at rectal palpation can be felt as large, flaccid and doughy (Fig. 14.6). Uterine luminal fluid may also be evident (Fig. 8.13). The mare may also show shortened oestrous cycles, owing to the irritation of the uterine wall resulting in premature CL regression.

Potential Endometritis-Causing Bacteria

As indicated, endometritis is primarily caused by bacterial infection. There are six major bacteria causal to endometritis, with up to 15 different bacteria identified in some cases (Pycock, 2000; Causey, 2006). Bacteria may exist not only as isolates but also as biofilms (an aggregation of microorganisms with complex community interactions) (Ferris *et al.*, 2017). As such they are increasingly resistant to antibacterial agents and so have been suggested to be particularly associated with chronic endometritis. The six major bacteria will be considered and can be classified as opportunistic or venereal (Ricketts, 2011).

Opportunistic Bacteria

Opportunistic bacteria are those that are common within the environment. They often have no effect, living as commensals (interacting with each other within a stable micro-climate) but can rapidly invade a micro-environment once the opportunity arises. In the mare this often occurs after a disruption to the natural microfloral balance due to antibiotic treatment, stress, excessive use of soaps or antiseptics, etc. Disruption to the natural balance leaves a space into which opportunistic bacteria invade and then populate. Opportunistic bacteria are generally present within the environment and so can be introduced quite easily at covering, internal examination, AI, foaling, etc. (Samper and Tibary, 2006). As such, they are potential causers of acute endometritis, especially in compromised or susceptible mares (LeBlanc *et al.*, 1991; Ricketts, 2011). Numerous opportunistic bacteria have been associated with endometritis but there are three main opportunistic bacteria of concern (Riddle *et al.*, 2007; Barbary *et al.*, 2016).

Streptococcus zooepidemicus is a Gram-positive spherical aerobic bacterium and is implicated in 75–80% of acute endometritis cases, particularly during the initial stages (Christoffersen *et al.*, 2015). *S. zooepidemicus* is spherical and found normally in chain formation, often in the intestine and mucous membranes (Rasmussen *et al.*, 2013). *Streptococcus* is classified into two subgroups: alpha and beta. *S. zooepidemicus* is a beta *Streptococcus* and causes the destruction of red blood cells; it also has a major role in initiating infection of the mare's cervix and uterus. It may also promote the proliferation of other bacteria within the tract (LeBlanc *et al.*, 1991; Asbury and Lyle, 1993).

Haemolytic *Escherichia coli* is a Gram-negative rod-shaped aerobic bacterium that is found either alone or in short chains. It is the second most common cause of uterine infection. It is naturally found in the intestine and particularly associated with faecal contamination. It can cause not only acute endometritis, but also severe systemic infection, which can prove fatal (Asbury and Lyle, 1993; Tibary *et al.*, 2014).

Staphylococcus aureus is a Gram-positive spherical or oval anaerobic bacterium and is a less common cause of endometritis. It is a spherical or oval bacterium, normally evident in clusters, and found associated with skin and mucous membranes. Under suitable conditions, such as the disruption of the natural microflora, ill health or stress, it will invade the reproductive tract of the mare (Asbury and Lyle, 1993).

Venereal Disease Bacteria

Venereal disease bacteria are those that are transferred solely via the venereal route; that is, they are present within the semen and the reproductive tract of the mare and stallion, and are capable of producing endometritis in both the normal and susceptible mare. They may also be present in apparently asymptomatic animals, in particular the stallion, which rarely shows symptoms. There are three main venereal disease bacteria of concern (Ricketts, 2011; Pasolini *et al.*, 2016).

Taylorella equigenitalis is a Gram-negative rod or spherical bacterium. It is extremely contagious and the causal agent of contagious equine metritis (CEM). It was first isolated in Newmarket, UK, where it spread rapidly and widely owing to the reluctance of infected-mare owners not to present their mares for service (Crowhurst, 1977; Crowhurst *et al.*, 1979). The stallion is seemingly not affected by the bacterium, but is the prime means by which it is spread from mare to mare. In the mare, the typical symptoms of acute endometritis are characterized by uterine, cervical and vaginal inflammation along with copious grey discharge within 2–5 days of infection; she may then appear to recover but remains a carrier. In rarer instances, the mare may not show any clinical symptoms, but can still be a carrier capable of infecting a stallion. At the other extreme, the infection may develop to give chronic endometritis (Timoney, 2011c,e; Kristula, 2014).

Klebsiella pneumoniae is a Gram-negative encapsulated rod-shaped anaerobic bacterium associated with acute and chronic endometritis (Ozgur *et al.*, 2003; Tibary *et al.*, 2014). The bacteria of particular concern are capsular types 1, 2 and 5 (Pycock, 2000). These are endemic and widespread, but diagnosis is reasonably accurate via cervical–uterine swabbing. Unfortunately the bacteria are relatively insensitive to antibiotics and antiseptic washing agents.

Pseudomonas aeruginosa is a Gram-negative slender, rod-shaped anaerobic bacterium with rounded ends and flagellae, and is found widely within the environment. However, some strains of *P. aeruginosa* are causal to endometritis and may be isolated in a stallion's semen or in swabs taken from the urethral fossa, but clinical symptoms are rarely evident. In the mare, *P. aeruginosa* causes a greenish-blue or yellowish-green exudate, which appears to be more prevalent in older mares. It is relatively resistant to antibiotics and antiseptics, so early diagnosis and cessation of natural cover is the best course of action (Troedsson, 2011; Ferris *et al.*, 2017).

Diagnosis

Because of the highly contagious nature of venereal disease endometritis, diagnosis and prevention are very important. Many diagnostic techniques can be used, and a summary follows. Diagnosis of endometritis may be implicated owing to the mare's history of failure to conceive. If acute it may be obvious due to exudates; if more subtle, it may only be identified via scanning, rectal palpation, endoscopy, biopsy or through routine swabbing. Once inflammation has been diagnosed, the causal agent – whether infective or not – needs to be identified (Overbeck *et al.*, 2011; Walter *et al.*, 2012; Cadario, 2014).

Traditionally, bacterial infections were identified by swabbing of the reproductive tract. It is normal and recommended practice (Horse Race Betting Levy Board, 2019) that swabs are taken from the uterus, cervix, clitoris and urethra opening (Cocchia *et al.*, 2012; Riddle *et al.*, 2007; Walter *et al.*, 2012). Uterine swabbing should be carried out, using a guarded swab to prevent contamination en route and through an open cervix during oestrus (Section 8.8; Figs 8.20, 8.21 and 14.7; Ricketts, 2011). The other swabs may be taken throughout the mare's oestrous cycle. The resultant swabs can be plated out and incubated under varying conditions (anaerobic, aerobic, microphilic, etc.), or undergo genotyping to identify the bacterium (Section 8.8; Ricketts *et al.*, 1993; Walter *et al.*, 2012). Fungal infections may also be identified in a similar manner. The use of swabbing is a widespread and often compulsory practice. Some breed societies have successfully used it to eradicate specific causes of infection in many areas worldwide. In particular, within the UK the Horse Race Betting Levy Board publishes Annual Codes of Practice; these are used worldwide and have resulted in a near eradication of

T. equigenitalis (CEM) from the UK as well as significantly reducing the incidence of venereal diseases caused by *K. pneumoniae* and *P. aeruginosa*. The Horse Race Betting Levy Board also produces guidelines on equine herpes virus (EHV) and equine viral arteritis (EVA; Horse Race Betting Levy Board, 2019). These Codes of Practice are reviewed annually and detail the number and type of swabs and diagnostic techniques that need to be used for different classes of mare. CEM is now a notifiable disease in the UK, and Codes of Practice have been laid down for exportation and importation of stock and, in cases of suspected CEM, abortion, etc.

Uterine aspirations and washings may also be collected (Fig 14.10), especially if purulent material and fluid are present. Culturing of the washings allows bacteria to be identified (Freeman and Johnston, 1987; LeBlanc *et al.*, 2007).

Uterine cytology is increasingly used as a diagnostic aid (Riddle *et al.*, 2007; Cocchia *et al.*, 2012; Davies Morel *et al.*, 2013). Cytology samples are taken via swabs, cytology brush (Fig. 14.8) or low-volume lavage, and are examined for the ratio of epithelial cells to polymorphonuclear neutrophils (PMNs) which are characteristic of inflammation response (Section 8.8; Fig. 8.25). Various definitions have been proposed but, commonly, 1% PMN is indicative of endometritis (Troedsson, 2011; Davies Morel *et al.*, 2013).

Biopsy is another accurate method of diagnosing inflammatory response indicative of endometritis, and is particularly useful for identifying chronic endometritis (Section 8.8; Figs 8.16 and 8.17; Schoon and Schoon, 2003; Neilsen *et al.*, 2010; Woodward *et al.*, 2012). Mares can then be graded I (best) to III (worst),

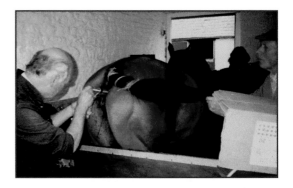

Fig. 14.7. Many studs require all mares to be swabbed prior to service. The swabs can be taken from clitoral sinuses and fossa along with the urethral opening, endometrium and cervix. (Photograph courtesy of Elm Stud, Ms Victoria Kingston.)

which correlates well with conception rates (Fig. 8.18; Section 8.7.3). Although these last two methods (cytology and biopsy) are very accurate in diagnosing endometritis, they are not accurate in identifying the causal agent. Swabs may also be used to identify the rarer incidence of fungi and yeast infections (Hartman and Bliss, 2011).

Finally, with the advent of genome sequencing, the identification of infective agents can be much more precise (but at a cost rendering it currently not commercially viable). However, as costs decline, this will become a commercially viable technique.

Acute Endometritis

Acute endometritis is a result of either significant bacterial challenge by venereal or opportunistic bacteria, or by a persistent acute reaction to covering. If infective, acute endometritis develops rapidly, giving immediate symptoms of exudate or pus, and irregular oestrous cycles. Internally, it causes deep haemorrhage and degeneration of epithelial cells of the endometrium and, in severe cases, degeneration of the deeper stroma cells, leading to areas of missing endometrium. This may lead to hypertrophy and abscessed uterine glands.

Acute Infective Endometritis

Acute infective endometritis is a major cause of infertility in the mare, providing a hostile environment for both sperm and embryo survival. Bacteria are potentially introduced into the system at covering, both natural or AI, or at veterinary inspection. It is now known that some degree of acute endometritis is always evident after all coverings regardless of the extent of bacterial invasion (post-coital endometritis); however, introduction of additional bacteria, or inability of the mare to deal with bacterial invasion, causes a significant uncharacteristic inflammatory reaction (persistent post-coital endometritis).

Treatment for general acute endometritis begins with identification of the infective agent and targeted use of local antibiotics, systemic antibiotics and/or uterine lavage (Dascanio, 2011b). Local antibiotics can be applied by placing them directly into the uterus via infusion, using an indwelling catheter passed through the cervix and placed into the uterus. The end of the catheter is looped into two ramshorn shapes, which help keep the catheter in place, and allow repeated infusions without the need to change and reintroduce the catheter (Fig. 14.9). This reduces the risk of introducing more opportunistic bacteria via the technique itself into what is already a compromised system (Dascanio, 2011b). Such antibiotic treatment must be used with care, as some antibiotics may cause necrosis or erosion of the endometrium. Bacterial resistance is increasingly a problem, so identification of the causal bacterium and use of a specific targeted antibiotic are very important. Excessive antibiotic use may allow fungal infections to develop, which will themselves require treatment

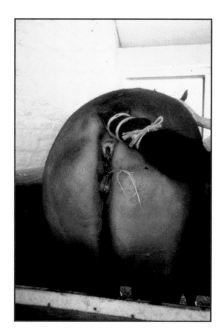

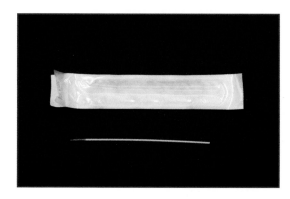

Fig. 14.8. A cytology brush may be used to obtain a sample of cells from within the mare's reproductive tract for evidence of inflammatory cells.

Fig. 14.9. An infusion catheter in situ allowing repeated treatment of mares with antibiotics in cases of endometritis. (Photo courtesy of Elm Stud, Ms Victoria Kingston.)

(Asbury and Lyle, 1993). Systemic antibiotics have been used, but evidence for their success is inconclusive. They have been advocated for use in conjunction with local antibiotics (Dascanio, 2011b).

Uterine lavage, using 1–2 l of saline, is increasingly popular (Fig. 14.10). Lavage has been demonstrated not only to remove debris and exudate but also to encourage neutrophil release to the infection site. The washings may also be used to identify causal agents. The extent and regularity of lavage again depends upon the severity of the condition (Asbury, 1990; LeBlanc and Causey, 2009). Uterine infusion or lavage with chemical irritants such as kerosene or disinfectants, as a form of chemical curettage, have been advocated. However, results are variable and such treatments should be used with great care. Povidone-iodine has been used with some success (Bracher *et al.*, 1991; Asbury and Lyle, 1993), as has plasma infusion (Asbury, 1984; Pascoe, 1995). In addition to treating the infection, any physical abnormalities that may be predisposing the mare to infection should be corrected through Caslick's vulvoplasty, a Pouret operation, removal of adhesions, etc. (Caslick, 1937; Pouret, 1982).

In the treatment of endometritis, topical treatment of vaginal or clitoral infections should be considered. This involves cleansing the whole area with a non-antiseptic soap for *K. pneumoniae* and *P. aeruginosa*, or chlorohex-idine for *T. equigenitalis*, followed by topical application of antibiotic creams. Unfortunately, *K. pneumoniae* and *P. aeruginosa* are particularly difficult to eliminate, in which case clitorectomy may be considered (Pycock, 2000). Clitorectomy – removal of the clitoris – is more widely practised in the USA than in the UK and Europe.

More recently the use of immunostimulatory agents, and intrauterine treatment with blood plasma and leucocytes, have been reported to improve pregnancy rates in mares with chronic endometritis (Rohrbach *et al.*, 2006; Neves *et al.*, 2007; Reghini *et al.*, 2016). Mycolytic agents such as N-acetylcysteine (NAC), used to remove excessive mucus and/or exudate, have also been reported to be successful (Witte *et al.*, 2012; Gores-Lindholm *et al.*, 2013). Chelating agents that affect the permeability of the bacterial wall have also been suggested for use (LeBlanc, 2010), as have immune modulators such as glucocorticoids (Wolf *et al.*, 2012; Meyers, 2018).

Persistent Post-Coital Acute Endometritis

Post-coital acute endometritis is the specific term given to acute uterine inflammation resulting from covering. This inflammatory response is characterized by an influx of polymorphonuclear neutrophils (PMN), resulting in uterine luminal fluid and endometrial secretion of PGF2α, which, if they persist, are incompatible with pregnancy

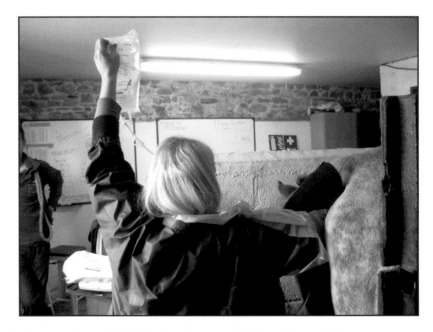

Fig. 14.10. Uterine lavage can be used to flush the uterus to remove debris, exudates and fluid.

(Troedsson, 1999; Maischberger *et al.*, 2008; Christoffersen and Troedsson, 2017). This response is seen in all mares to a varying extent but will usually resolve within 48 h. However, in susceptible mares, rapid resolution does not occur. The persistence of post-coital endometritis may be encouraged by several factors including general stress; a decline in the mare's general well-being; and cervical, vaginal or vulval abnormalities. However, even in the absence of these predisposing factors, acute endometritis may still persist, and it is evident that some mares are inherently more susceptible than others. At mating the stallion deposits semen directly into the top of the cervix/start of the uterus along with bacteria cell debris, etc. Sperm move rapidly up through the uterus towards the Fallopian tube, leaving a considerable amount of fluid and non-viable sperm (plus any bacteria, etc.), within the uterus. This causes transitory inflammation of the uterine endometrium, a ubiquitous and necessary reaction to mating. This excess fluid, bacteria, etc., then needs to be eliminated. In the normal mare, not susceptible to persistent post-coital endometritis, this is physically eliminated by uterine contractions induced by the release of PGF2α and oxytocin at mating (Madill *et al.*, 2000). In addition, an innate immune response involving PMN is mounted by the mare. This physical and immune response will ensure that within 36–48 h any inflammation has been resolved and the uterus is sterile in good time for the arrival of the embryo at 4–5 days post-coitum (Troedsson, 1999, 2006; Christoffersen and Troedsson, 2017). Mares susceptible to persistent post-coital endometritis are unable to clear the fluid and react to the immune challenge in time for the embryo to arrive, providing a non-ideal environment and so reducing sperm motility (Alghamdi *et al.*, 2001) and survival of the conceptus (Knutti *et al.*, 2000; Watson, 2000; Rigby *et al.*, 2001a; Campbell and England, 2006; Christoffersen and Troedsson, 2017).

Post-coital prophylactic measures are often employed in such mares to reduce the incidence of inflammation by assisting uterine exudate clearance. Those sperm required for fertilization reach the Fallopian tube within 2–4 h of ejaculation and the fertilized ovum does not arrive in the uterus until day 5. In theory, therefore, uterine treatment is safe within these time limits. In practice, however, owing to the rapid rise in progesterone post-ovulation and as a result of a natural decline in uterine myometrial contractility and cervical closure (Stecco *et al.*, 2003), it is best not to attempt treatment after 48 h post-ovulation. Treatment can be

via uterine lavage using a saline plus antibiotic solution, which successfully removes uterine fluid and debris, enhancing neutrophil function and antibiotic efficiency. Lavage also stimulates uterine contractility and encourages the release of fresh neutrophils through irritation of the endometrium (Knutti *et al.*, 2000; Pycock, 2000; Card, 2005; Canisso *et al.*, 2016). As such, it is often the treatment of choice for such mares. Oxytocin may also be used, both alone and in combination with lavage, to encourage myometrial activity and hence fluid clearance (Allen, 1991; LeBlanc, 1994; Pycock and Newcombe, 1996; Campbell and England, 2002; Vanderwall and Woods, 2003; LeBlanc and Causey, 2009). PGF2α, by virtue of its similar action on uterine myometrial contractility, has also been used successfully (Combs *et al.*, 1996). These systems may be supplemented by AI using semen extended with antibiotic extenders. The addition of antibiotics significantly reduces any bacterial challenge, and the use of AI reduces the total number of sperm introduced into the uterus, further reducing the inflammatory response (Davies Morel, 1999; Nikolakopoulos and Watson, 2000; Sinnemaa *et al.*, 2003). Similarly, a reduction in inflammatory response has been reported with the use of corticosteroids just before or at covering (Bucca and Carli, 2011). For the same reason such mares should, ideally, only be covered once. It is also increasingly evident that teasing plays a role in encouraging uterine myometrial contractility. Work by Madill *et al.* (2000) indicated that uterine contractility is greatest in mares that are teased. It is increasingly less in mares that are covered by AI than in mares with sight of a stallion and least of all in mares that just hear the sound of a stallion call. The increased incidence of persistent post-coital endometritis and the success in using post-coital oxytocin and antibiotics in such mares has led to their prophylactic use, even though there is no evidence to support a benefit in normal mares (Cooke, 2015).

Chronic Endometritis

Chronic endometritis may be more accurately divided into chronic infective endometritis and chronic non-infective degenerative endometritis (now termed endometriosis, considered in Section 14.3.4.4).

Chronic infective endometritis can arise from an untreated or inappropriately treated acute uterine infection, or be due to a mare's inability to satisfactorily combat the initial infection (LeBlanc, 2008; Newcombe, 2011b; Tibary *et al.*, 2014). As with acute endometritis this may be due to fungal and yeast infection as well as to bacterial infection (Beltaire *et al.*, 2012; Nervo *et al.*, 2019). The condition is more often found in older multiparous mares, especially those with poor perineal conformation (where the breakdown in uterine defence mechanisms and possibly poor uterine myometrial contractility results in an inability to respond to introduced infection) and may also have allowed normal genital bacterial flora to contaminate the uterus. Such infection is often long term, but not as evident as a dramatic inflammatory response (LeBlanc, 2010, 2011). It can be extremely damaging to the endometrium, causing degeneration and necrosis, resulting in permanent infertility. Treatment, although not very successful, is as indicated for acute endometritis but with particular use of infusion and lavage. Large-volume infusion with a broad-spectrum antibiotic is advised, as often wide ranges of bacteria are present (Pycock, 2000; LeBlanc, 2010). Similarly, antimycotic agents are infused for fungal infections. Lavage using isotonic saline, followed by antibiotic and/or plasma infusion, is reported to be successful (Asbury and Lyle, 1993; Reghini *et al.*, 2016). At breeding, such mares should be treated in a similar manner to those susceptible to acute post-coital endometritis (Asbury and Lyle, 1993).

Acute Metritis

Acute metritis is potentially the most serious uterine infection. It is associated with a massive contamination of the whole uterus as a result of trauma, often associated with parturition involving retained placental or fetal tissue, or bacterial infection introduced via air inspired post-partum or via hands used to aid parturition. If it occurs post-partum it is commonly known as post-partum metritis (Blanchard, 2011). Decomposition of retained tissue encourages rapid bacterial growth along with toxin production. Occasionally, it may be evident post-coitum. The inflammation of the entire uterus then favours the passage of toxins into the main circulation resulting in toxaemia and, potentially, death.

Prevention is infinitely better than cure; and absolute hygiene at parturition, plus the complete expulsion of all placental and fetal tissue postpartum, is essential (Aoki *et al.*, 2014). Treatment must be immediate and normally involves large-volume lavage and possibly oxytocin to encourage uterine contraction and thus the flushing out of the uterine contents. Lavage should then continue until recovered fluids are relatively clear. Recovery is not possible until the source of the toxaemia is removed (Blanchard and Varner, 1993a; Threlfall,

1993; Canisso *et al.*, 2016). The prognosis is often poor and, even if the toxaemia is successfully resolved, long-term lameness from laminitis may result (Eustace, 1992; Pycock, 2000; Blanchard, 2011).

Pyometra

Pyometra is characterized by fluid accumulation in a large, pendulous uterus. In time the uterine walls may become leathery, tough and fibrous owing to continual infection. Such mares may appear healthy in themselves, but often do not show oestrous cycles due to the inability of the uterus to produce PGF2a, and hence persistence of the CL (Threlfall and Carleton, 1996; Satué and Gardón, 2016). Pyometra may be associated with a blockage of the uterus, fibrosis, adhesions, etc., resulting in a build-up of exudate within the uterus, with no normal drainage. It is often due to infection, but not necessarily so. Treatment normally involves drainage, followed by antibiotic infusion or lavage, but the prognosis for a breeding career is often poor (LeBlanc and McKinnon, 2011). If infection is not evident and breeding is not required, such mares may not require treatment if they show no signs of discomfort. However, the presence of infection poses problems and, if left untreated, infective pyometra may develop into septicaemia (Ricketts, 1978; Hughes *et al.*, 1979).

14.3.5.4. Cervical infections

Cervicitis (inflammation of the cervix) is usually associated with, and often precedes, endometritis. Such infection causes inflammation and possible pus accumulation (Sertich, 1993; Satué and Gardón, 2016).

14.3.5.5. Vaginal infections

Vaginal infections are often a prelude to endometritis, especially in mares suffering from poor perineal conformation (Satué and Gardón, 2016). Alternatively, they may be caused by chemical irritation of the vagina, for example from antimicrobial agents used in examination. These can also result in vaginal necrosis, which may also result from damage in cases of dystocia (LeBlanc *et al.*, 2004; McKinnon and Jalim, 2011). Systemic and topical antibiotic treatment is often successful and the prognosis, providing the infection is not long term or has developed into necrosis, is good.

14.3.5.6. Vulval infections

Vulval infections include equine coital exanthema (genital horse pox), which is evident as vesiculation and ulceration of the vulval lips or penis, and is caused by EHV3 (Section 14.3.5.7). It causes blister-like lesions

5–7 days post-infection, both on the perineal area of the mare and on the penis and prepuce of the stallion. These resolve within 3–4 weeks, leaving scars. Although the direct effect on fertility is minimal, covering during the active phase may cause discomfort and bleeding, and is not advised in order to prevent transmission (Samper and Tibary, 2006; Barrandeguy and Thiry, 2012). It is sexually transmitted, and symptomless carriers are reported (Barrandeguy et al., 2008). Treatment with antibacterial creams or powders prevents secondary infections and helps the natural healing process (Seki et al., 2004; Metcalf, 2011).

14.3.5.7. Viral infections

The incidence of viral abortion is 1–5%, and mainly occurs in late pregnancy. Two main viruses have a major effect on reproductive performance in the mare: equine arteritis virus (EAV), the causal agent for EVA; and EHV, the causal agent for equine rhinopneumonitis (a cause of equine abortion).

EAV is an acute contagious disease of the horse which came to particular attention in 1984 when it affected a number of Thoroughbred studs in the USA. It is not life-threatening but is of reproductive significance as it causes abortion in mares (Castillo-Olivares et al., 2003; Balasuriya et al., 2018) and illness and death in young foals (Del Piero et al., 1997). The virus can be spread via the venereal (natural covering and AI) and the respiratory route, and also from the placenta of aborting mares and the urine of infected animals (Acland, 1993; Timoney, 2011b; Balasuriya et al., 2018). EVA is evident worldwide with the exception of Japan and Iceland and, until relatively recently, the UK (Wood et al., 1995; Samper and Tibary, 2006; Holyoak et al., 2008). Many countries have strict regulations to limit its importation and spread. Stallions are the major route of infection as they can become asymptomatic carriers; the asymptomatic carrier state does not exist in mares and geldings, which only shed the virus during the initial infective phase. Mares and geldings eliminate the virus within 60 days but remain seropositive owing to the previous infection. Similarly, all stallions become seropositive, but 30–60% do not eliminate the virus and become persistently infected and so persistent shedders, the virus lodging in the accessory glands and then being shed in semen (Glaser et al., 1997; Balasuriya et al., 2018). Seropositive stallions – which it is suggested can account for up to 80% in some countries – can, therefore, be classified as shedders and non-shedders and it is the seropositive shedder stallions that are a risk to mares. The carrier state and the shedding of the virus through semen are testosterone dependent; therefore, gelding of a stallion removes the risk. Similarly, it has been reported that shedding stallions treated with gonadotrophin-releasing hormone (GnRH) antagonist stopped shedding the virus, although a return to the shedding status was resumed after the end of treatment (Fortier et al., 2002). Shedding stallions can be classified as short-term shedders (only excreting the virus in the initial infective period, as seen in mares and geldings), long-term shedders (excreting the virus for 3–9 months) or chronic persistent shedders (which will permanently excrete the virus). It is these later stallions that are the biggest risk: 85–100% of seronegative mares mated by a seropositive shedder stallion will become infected (Samper and Tibary, 2006), whether mating be via natural service or AI. Infected mares may not show clinical signs but shed the virus for around the first 60 days via nasopharyngeal secretions, urine and the infected placenta if abortion occurs. Infection does not affect fertility per se but can cause abortion, usually in months 3–10 of pregnancy, due to severe oedema and necrosis of the endometrium (Balasuriya et al., 2018). Mares aborting owing to EAV do so as a result of contact with an acutely infected horse via the respiratory route. Mares do not abort as a result of venereal transfer at covering. Mares and geldings normally recover spontaneously and so treatment beyond supportive care is not required and is largely unsuccessful. There is no treatment for carrier stallions. Prevention and management of control measures is, therefore, very important. The status of all mares and stallions should be ascertained by blood sampling; strict hygiene precautions should be practised; and, ideally, shedding stallions should not be used for covering although it may be acceptable to use them to mate seropositive or vaccinated mares. Mares and stallions can be vaccinated. Both modified live vaccines and an inactivated vaccine are available (Timoney and McCollum, 1993; Parlevliet and Samper, 2000; Holyoak et al., 2008; Balasuriya et al., 2018), which will give protection for several years (Timoney, 2011b). It is important, however (and required by some breed societies), that all animals are blood tested prior to vaccination, to certify that their subsequent seropositive status is due to the vaccination and not to infection (Timoney and McCollum, 1993, 1997; Holyoak et al., 2008; Balasuriya et al., 2018). In the UK, EVA is a notifiable disease under certain circumstances and, as such, is now included in the Horse Race Betting and Levy Board Codes of Practice.

Five main strains of EHV infect the horse (EHV 1–5) of which EHV1 and 4 are the most important as regards reproductive performance, although EHV3 is the causal agent for equine coital exanthema, which is primarily transmitted venereally (Section 14.3.5.6; Thein, 2012). EHV1 and 4 are of more concern, especially EHV1; this is the causal agent of equine rhinopneumonitis which is associated with, among other things, abortion in mares and pneumonia in young foals (Timoney, 2011a). Virus transfer is via the respiratory route, from allantoic and amniotic fluids at birth, soiled bedding, placental tissue, etc. It may also be found in semen (Acland, 1993; Davies Morel, 1999). The virus causes placental separation, resulting in fetal suffocation and abortion, with 96% occurring in the last 4 months of pregnancy. It can have a devastating effect, causing abortion storms in mares, plus neonatal losses. As with EVA, EHV1 is now included in the Horse Race Betting and Levy Board Codes of Practice and is as yet of minor concern in the UK. Vaccination against EHV1 and 4 is available, although of limited effectiveness. Despite this, vaccination use is advocated as it reduces the severity of the disease and the duration of virus shredding (Wilson, 2005; Timoney, 2011a; Thein, 2012).

There are other viruses whose major effects are not on fertility but may be a minor cause of reduced reproductive function. One example is West Nile virus, a mosquito-borne virus that primarily causes encephalitis (inflammation of the brain) and/or meningitis (inflammation of the lining of the brain and spinal cord), but indirectly affects reproductive ability (Bunning et al., 2002; Long et al., 2002; Wilson, 2011).

14.3.5.8. Protozoa infection

Dourine was thought to be caused by *Trypanosoma equiperdum* but is now thought to be caused by a related *Trypanosoma* strain, *T. evansi* (Claes et al., 2003). It is a sexually transmitted protozoan, now eradicated from the UK, most of Europe and North America, but still prevalent in the temperate regions of many countries in Africa, South and Central America, the Middle East and Asia (Claes et al., 2003). It causes intermittent fever; depression; progressive loss of body condition; and vaginal and vulval infection and inflammation, along with discharge. Infected horses also develop characteristic subcutaneous lesions (areas of thickened skin). If left untreated it will develop systematically to form raised rings within the mare's coat, along with depigmentation of the genitals, plus fever and death

in 50–75% of cases (Brun et al., 1998; Brown, 1999; Yasine, 2019).

Piroplasmosis, caused by the tick-borne haemoparasites *Theileria equi* or *Babesia caballi*, may also be a potential risk to mares and stallions. Present worldwide, except for the UK, Ireland, Japan, the USA, Australia and Canada, it is most often transmitted by ticks as a blood-borne protozoan; however there is a chance of transfer of infection to mares if semen of an infected stallion becomes contaminated with blood (Samper and Tibary, 2006), and transplacental transmission has been reported (Georges et al., 2011).

14.3.5.9. Fungal and yeast infection

Mycotic or fungal infections can potentially be transferred venereally and may cause endometritis (Dascanio, 2000; Dascanio et al., 2001; Coutinho da Silva and Alvarenga, 2011; Beltaire et al., 2012; Satué and Gardón, 2016). The most commonly isolated fungi are *Chlamydia* spp., which have been associated with endometritis, salpingitis, reduced fertility and abortion, and also balanitis (inflammation of the penis) in the stallion (Herfen et al., 1999; Coutinho da Silva and Alvarenga, 2011; Nervo et al., 2019). Yeasts may also cause problems to both mares and stallions and be transferred venereally; these include *Candida* spp. and *Aspergillus* spp. (Satué and Gardón, 2016). Over-use of antibiotics, including their use in semen extenders, has been suggested to be the reason why the incidence of fungal infections has increased (Dascanio et al., 2001; Satué and Gardón, 2016). Although present occasionally in semen, the greatest risk is transfer at AI, if strict hygiene procedures are not adhered to.

All these infective agents, as with bacterial infections, disrupt the ability of the uterus to support a developing embryo. If present later in pregnancy they can cause abortion via placentitis and occasionally fetal infection. The majority of fungal abortions occur around 10 months of pregnancy (Acland, 1993). Treatment is via infusion of antimycotic agents such as povidone-iodine, nystatin or lufenuron but the success rate is low (Hess et al., 2002). Acidic agents, such as vinegar and acetic acid, have also been used with some success (Pycock, 2000). If the mycotic growth cannot be arrested the prognosis is hopeless.

14.3.6. Fetal congenital deformities

Many fetal developmental deformities have been reported (Leipold and Dennis, 1993). Many of these are *not* compatible with fetal life, and so cause abortion.

Chromosomal defects also occur normally, leading to EED rather than to abortion (Ricketts *et al.*, 2003).

14.4. Conclusion

The causes of infertility in the mare are numerous. The prime time of biggest risk is EED prior to day 15 of pregnancy and, second, EM between days 15 and 40, caused by degenerative or infective endometritis. Identification of the causal agent of any infertility is essential, not only to ensure optimum chance of conception, but also to eliminate the risk of transmitting any infective agents.

Study Questions

Having identified that your maiden mare is not showing any ovarian activity despite it being the middle of the breeding season, evaluate what the causes may be.

Having identified that your mare habitually suffers from persistent post-coital endometritis, discuss the ways in which this may be alleviated and her pregnancy rates improved.

Discuss the reproductive issues that may face a multiparous mare over 20 years of age, and how these may be addressed.

You suspect your mare has contracted a uterine infection. Discuss how you would confirm this, the bacteria that may be involved and the consequences of such an infection.

You are presented with a mare that has a large amount of uterine luminal fluid. Evaluate the possible reasons for this and the options to manage the problem.

You have just received confirmation from a uterine biopsy of your mare that she is a grade III for uterine histology (very poor). Discuss the reasons for this and evaluate the management options available.

Suggested reading

Hurtgen, J.P. (2011) Uterine abnormalities. In: McKinnon, A.O., Squires, E.L., Vaala, E. and Varner, D.D. (eds) *Equine Reproduction*, 2nd edn. Wiley-Blackwell, Philadelphia, London, pp. 2669–2673.

Hurtgen, J.P. (2011) Abnormalities of cervical and vaginal development. In: McKinnon, A.O., Squires, E.L., Vaala, E. and Varner, D.D. (eds) *Equine Reproduction*, 2nd edn. Wiley-Blackwell, Philadelphia, London, pp. 2719–2720.

LeBlanc, M.M. and McKinnon, A.O. (2011) Breeding the problem mare. In: McKinnon, A.O., Squires, E.L., Vaala, E. and Varner, D.D. (eds) *Equine Reproduction*, 2nd edn. Wiley-Blackwell, Philadelphia, London, pp. 2620–2642.

Troedsson, M.H.T. (2011) Endometritis. In: McKinnon, A.O., Squires, E.L., Vaala, E. and Varner, D.D. (eds) *Equine Reproduction*, 2nd edn. Wiley-Blackwell, Philadelphia, London, pp. 2608–2619.

Satué, K. and Gardón, J.C. (2016) (June 29th 2016). Infection and Infertility in Mares, Genital Infections and Infertility, Atef M. Darwish, IntechOpen, DOI: 10.5772/63741. Available from: https://www.intechopen.com/books/genital-infections-and-infertility/infection-and-infertility-in-mares

Pasolini, M.P., Del Prete, C., Fabbri, S. and Auletta, L. (2016) Endometritis and Infertility in the Mare – The Challenge in Equine Breeding Industry–A Review, Genital Infections and Infertility, Atef M. Darwish, IntechOpen, DOI: 10.5772/62461. Available from: https://www.intechopen.com/books/genital-infections-and-infertility/endometritis-and-infertility-in-the-mare-the-challenge-in-equine-reeding-industry-a-review.

Christoffersen, M. and Troedsson, M.H.T. (2017) Inflammation and fertility in the mare. *Reproduction in Domestic Animals* 52 (Suppl 3), 14–20.

McCue, P.M. and Ferris R.A. (2017) Review of ovarian abnormalities in the mare. *Proceedings of the American Association of Equine Practionners* 63, 61–68.

Allen, W.R. and Wilsher, S. (2018) Review Article: Celebrating 50 years of Equine Veterinary Journal Half a century of equine reproduction research and application: A veterinary tour de force. *Equine Veterinary Journal* 50, 10–12.

Rose, B.V., Firth, M., Morris, B., Roach, J.M., Verheyn, K.L.P. and de Mestre, A.M. (2018) Descriptive study of current therapeutic practices, clinical reproductive findings and incidence of pregnancy loss in intensively managed thoroughbred mares. *Animal Reproduction Science* 188, 74–84.

Section

D

Management of the Stallion

Section D applies the stallion anatomy and physiology considered in Section B to the management of the stallion throughout his breeding career. It also considers infertility and the reasons for reproductive failure. Various management options are discussed to enable you to make informed decisions with regard to managing a working stallion within a stud environment, ensuring optimum reproductive success, and also welfare.

Selection of the Stallion for Breeding

15

The Objectives of this Chapter are:

To begin to apply the reproductive physiology knowledge you have gained from Section B to stud management.

To consider the criteria that need to be assessed when selecting a stallion, based on his reproductive competence, to maximize the chance that he will successfully cover a mare.

To evaluate the methods by which these criteria can be assessed and their appropriateness for different breeding establishments.

To introduce some of the causes of infertility in the stallion and the methods by which they can be investigated; infertility will be developed further in Chapter 18.

15.1. Introduction

As with the mare, the choice of stallion for breeding can be a time-consuming process, and often not enough importance is placed upon this selection. This results in an oversupply of mediocre or poor stock with unnecessary breeding difficulties.

In common with the mare, one of the most obvious selection criteria is that of performance, which is fully justified as the horse should be bred for a specific market or use. However, regardless of the performance criteria used, stock should also be selected on reproductive competence. This is often neglected, leading to potentially serious consequences for the individual breeder and the equine population as a whole. Regardless of the type of horse you intend to breed, reproductive competence (i.e. the ability to cover a mare safely and efficiently and produce healthy offspring with minimal risk to mare, stallion and handlers) should also be of prime importance. Today's horse, unlike other farm livestock, has been selected primarily for performance ability, often at the expense of reproductive competence. As a result, there are many potential reproductive problems that the breeder should be aware of in selecting a working stallion.

As in Chapter 8, when selecting the mare for breeding was considered, this Chapter will assume that performance selection criteria have been met and so will concentrate solely upon the criteria and techniques that can be used in the selection for reproductive competence. A wide range of techniques will be included, many of which are costly in terms of time and money. Parts of this Chapter will overlap with infertility (Chapter 18). Many of the more intrusive techniques may not be justified for use when selecting a stallion, but more applicable to investigating infertility; however, they have been included for completeness. The extent to which these techniques are used when selecting a stallion (as with the brood mare) depends on personal choice and the value of the breeding stock concerned and of the potential offspring. It will also depend on whether you are selecting a stallion for purchase, when a much more detailed examination is warranted, or one just to cover a single mare, when all that is required is reassurance that he is capable of covering the mare and has a good general temperament.

Breeding soundness evaluations (BSE) are necessary prior to purchase, but may also be used routinely prior to each breeding season, or if a problem is suspected (Thompson, 1994). It must also be remembered that a BSE is not able to predict fertility levels with any accuracy, but can certainly be used to identify infertile stallions and provide an indication of the stallion's likely fertility, workload or number of insemination doses.

Even if this information does not preclude the stallion from a breeding career, much of it can be used to inform his future breeding management. Further information specific to infertility, and hence an expansion of some of the issues raised here, is included in Chapter 18.

The selection criteria for reproductive competence in the stallion are similar to those of the mare and are:

- history;
- temperament and libido;
- age;
- general conformation;
- reproductive tract examination;
- semen evaluation;
- chromosomal abnormalities;
- blood sampling;
- infections; and
- general stud management.

15.2. History

Records of a stallion's history are invaluable in aiding selection and, as with the mare, can be divided into his breeding and general history. Records for stallions do not tend to be as detailed or as readily available as those for mares, although all should have a passport with basic details recorded.

15.2.1. Reproductive history

Records of his past breeding performance, if available, should answer questions such as:

- When does his season normally start and end?
- How many mares is he used to covering in a season?
- What are his return rates like?
- What is his semen quality like?

The answers to these questions will indicate his reproductive ability (Van Buiten *et al.*, 1999; Love, 2003, 2011a). A stallion with a short season will be less able to cover as many mares and may suffer from low libido; he will be of particular concern if mares are to breed early in the season. The number of mares he has served per season in the past and the return rates, along with

semen analysis, will give an indication of what workload he will be capable of. If his return rates are high, especially if a significant decrease is seen with an increase in workload, this may indicate the natural limit of the number of mares he is able to cover. The routine of covering may affect performance and can be tailored to suit the stallion. Routines may involve one or two covers per day for 6 days with a day's rest, or two covers per day for 8 days followed by 2 days' rest, or numerous variations on these themes. Most stallions do need a rest day but should be able to cover mares at the rough frequency of the systems given above; some may be able to cover up to four mares/day. If there are indications that a stallion is not capable of such workloads and requires more rest days to maintain his fertility rates, then his selection should be queried, especially if you are looking for a stallion to purchase. Return rates are a good guide to a stallion's ability, but it must be remembered that the fertility of a stallion is only as good as the fertility of the mares he is presented with (Van Buiten *et al.*, 1999; Love, 2003; Varner, 2016).

Any previous semen analysis should also be detailed in his records. Many valuable stallions have a routine semen analysis carried out at the beginning of each season. This, along with a blood sample (which is normally taken at the same time), allows any potential problems to be identified in time for remedial action to be taken before the breeding season starts. Any past reproductive tract infections should also be detailed in a stallion's records, along with any treatment given and the outcome. Any long-term effects of infection should be evident in the stallion's workload and return rates for the rest of that season and for any subsequent seasons.

15.2.2. General history

The stallion's general history should indicate his vaccination and worming status, along with the incidence of injuries and accidents. Damage to his hindquarters or limbs may restrict his ability to mount a mare, as may laminitis and neurological disorders (Griffin, 2000). Artificial insemination (AI) may be an alternative (Davies Morel, 1999); even so, he is likely to need the occasional mount for the collection of semen samples, although the number of mounts per mare fertilized will be significantly reduced and the unpredictability of mounting a mare avoided. Such stallions are not advised for purchase. As with the mare, in the event of suggestions that any damage or weaknesses may be heritable, selection would not be advised. Injuries to a stallion's genitalia, usually as a result of a kick from a mare, will cause degenerative and scar tissue within the penis and/or testes, which will reduce his fertility rates and his ability to mate a mare. Severe damage resulting in the removal of a testicle should also be noted in a stallion's records to reassure potential purchasers that he is not a cryptorchid or rig. Such stallions are capable of fertilizing a mare, but the workload may have to be reduced. Severe injuries to a stallion during mating often have long-lasting psychological effects, reducing his libido, possibly to such an extent that he is unwilling to cover naturally.

Past illnesses should also be indicated in his records. Illnesses associated with the respiratory or circulatory systems may indicate that the stallion will not be capable of working a full season, limiting the numbers of nominations that can be sold. Again, if there is a possibility that such weaknesses could be heritable, the stallion should be avoided. Any illnesses resulting in a fever can disrupt spermatogenesis owing to the elevated testicular temperature (Johnson *et al.*, 1997). This may result in temporary infertility or subfertility, although

this may not be evident for several weeks as the spermatogenic cycle takes 57 days (Davies Morel, 1999). Systemic infections such as strangles or influenza can cause inflammation within the testes and, if this results in a significant amount of tissue degeneration, permanent sub-fertility or even infertility may result.

15.3. Temperament and Libido

The temperament of the stallion is very important for ease of management and as a heritable trait (Hellsten *et al.*, 2009). A stallion of a quiet and kind disposition is a great asset and will be much easier and safer to handle (Fig. 15.1). A stallion that is rough to his mares will not only run the risk of inflicting permanent damage to them but may also be hurt himself if they retaliate. A rough stallion, who savages his mares, will prove unpopular and it may be difficult to get him enough mares to make his use economic. Some protection, in the form of neck guards, can be given to mares that are mated to stallions that tend to bite during covering, but no protection can be given against stallions that are

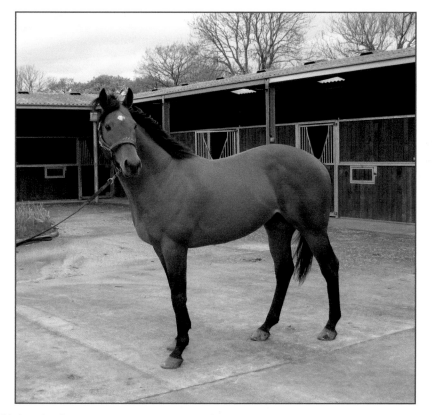

Fig. 15.1. A well-behaved stallion is an asset to any stud, easing his management and reducing the danger to his handlers.

downright vicious, and they should be avoided at all costs. There is some evidence to suggest that stallions brought up in an intensive/isolated environment with little social interaction are more likely to show such traits, as well as demonstrating poorer libido, than stallions brought up in a more natural herd environment (McDonnell and Murray, 1995; Christensen *et al.*, 2002a; Jackson, 2011).

Ideally, records should indicate the stallion's temperament and any specific characteristics he might have. It is to be hoped that his bad habits, especially those that might prove dangerous, will also be indicated. To be forewarned is to be forearmed and might lead you to reject an unsatisfactory stallion.

Bad behaviour in many stallions is a direct result of the conditions and management under which they are kept (Chapter 17). Therefore, especially in the case of a stallion that seems to have developed bad habits later in life, or after a change of owner or management, the conditions under which he is kept should be assessed before he is rejected for covering a mare. However, as a potential purchase he is not a good choice, as such habits are difficult to break. Bad behaviour tends to perpetuate itself as, owing to the potential danger, such stallions are often kept confined for longer periods of time and hence away from companions. Their boredom is therefore exacerbated and their bad habits develop further. Stereotypies (repetitive bad behaviour or habits) to be aware of include: weaving, crib-biting and wind-sucking, all signs of boredom and/or elevation of stress. Additionally, there is a commonly held belief, although not supported by scientific research, that other horses may copy stereotypies.

Stereotypies such as self-masturbation (Section 17.6.3) were once frowned upon but are now considered natural behaviour, of no consequence except the potential embarrassment to owners. Some stallions also indulge in self-mutilation (Section 17.6.2), especially after mating, biting themselves in areas where the smell of the mare lingers. Although thorough washing post-mating can reduce the incidence, the potential for self-harm – and the added management time and expense – may preclude their selection.

A stallion's libido partly determines his reproductive potential. Libido is governed, like all other sexual activity, by season (Section 7.3.1). Hence, those stallions with longer seasons tend to show a higher libido and, therefore, willingness to mate early on in the season and so extending the time in which they can be worked. This has particular advantages in the Thoroughbred industry and for those wishing to have foals born early.

Ideally, if selecting a stallion to purchase, he should be seen teasing and covering a mare (Varner, 2016). A stallion with a low libido will need to mount a mare several times before ejaculation, often taking 20 min or more to cover a mare, or he may fail completely; he may also show initial interest very reluctantly. Such 'time wasting' can be a considerable inconvenience on studs with a high throughput of mares. The number of mounts per ejaculation and the time between actual intromission and ejaculation are also good indications of libido. The number of mounts per ejaculation should be as near to one as possible and the time between intromission and ejaculation a matter of seconds (McDonnell, 2000a,b; Turner and McDonnell, 2007; McDonnell, 2011a,b).

15.4. Age

The age of the stallion is less important than that of the mare, as far as reproductive ability is concerned. The significance of age in the selection of the stallion depends on what that stallion is required for: that is, for a single mating to a selected mare or as a potential purchase for long-term future use. If you are selecting him for service of a single mare then, as far as you are concerned, he will be required to perform on just a couple of occasions; his age is of limited importance provided he is capable of covering. However, if you are looking to select a stallion for purchase and, therefore, long-term future use, you have to ensure that he is young and fit enough to give you plenty of seasons but old enough to have proved his worth and know his job.

As far as a lower limit is concerned, most colts reach puberty at 18–24 months of age (Section 7.2; Clay and Clay, 1992; Heninger, 2011). A colt can, in theory, be used as soon as he reaches puberty, but care must be taken to introduce him to the job gradually and not to overwork him too soon or give him awkward mares, which may affect his – as yet delicate – ego and reproductive confidence (Johnson *et al.*, 1991). Further details on early stallion management are given in Section 17.4. The purchase and use of such young stallions is risky, as they have no proven performance record; however, sperm production, as indicated by testis size, may continue to increase up to 8 years of age and particularly in late-maturing stallions such as draft horses (Parlevliet *et al.*, 1994).

As far as an upper age limit is concerned, this really depends on the stallion's general health and condition. If he has no problems such as lameness, limited stamina, respiratory system problems or injury he may well be capable of working well into his teens and even twenties, although in the later years his workload may have to be reduced. The use of AI may further prolong his breeding life, necessitating fewer mounts per mares covered. There is reported evidence that reproductive capability is inherently reduced with age (Naden *et al.*, 1990; Dowsett and Knott, 1996; Fukuda *et al.*, 2001; Madill, 2002; Darr *et al.*, 2017). However, other work disputes this, suggesting that any decline in reproductive performance with old age is indirect, due to reducing libido from problems such as injury and arthritic conditions, and is not a decline in spermatogenesis per se (Johnson, 1991a).

As discussed in the case of mare selection, if an older ex-performance horse is being considered, it must be borne in mind that he will require a prolonged period of time to adjust physically and psychologically to his new role in life. Details of the problems associated with using performance horses as stallions are given in Section 16.2.

15.5. General Conformation and Condition

A stallion's general conformation is of importance, not only as it will be passed on to his offspring, but also to ensure that he is capable of withstanding a full breeding season. A stallion with poor limb conformation (especially in the hindquarters) will also be weak in this area and may, therefore, be unable to withstand the heavy workload of a full breeding season, limiting his economic viability.

Particular note should be made of his physical ability to cover mares. He should be free of all signs of lameness, especially in the hind limbs. His legs should be checked before and after exercise and a comparison made, to ensure that there is no sign of swelling, a sign of possible weakness. He should be free of all conditions such as arthritis, spinal or limb injury, wobbler syndrome, laminitis or any neurological disorder, all of which could cause pain, especially at covering (Griffin, 2000). A stallion's feet should also be in excellent condition, regularly trimmed to ensure they stay that way. Adequate heart room in a broad chest is also desirable and, if doubt is placed on the stallion's cardiovascular system, electrocardiography may be conducted.

Good general condition and physical fitness are very important for the breeding stallion. The condition

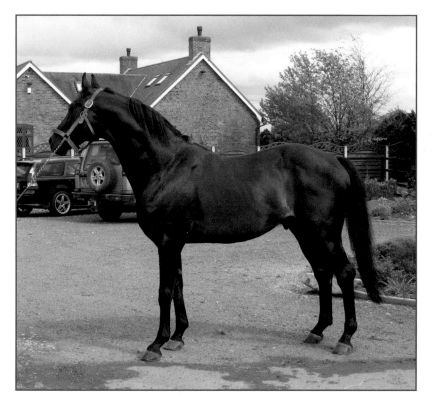

Fig. 15.2. A stallion in good, fit, well-muscled working condition (body condition score 3) ready for the breeding season.

of a stallion, like that of the mare, can be classified on a scale of 0–5 (0 emaciated, 5 obese; Figs 8.1–8.4). The optimum body condition for a stallion in work is 3; that is, he is well muscled-up and in fit working condition (Fig. 15.2). Stallions in condition score less than 3 tend to have lower libido and are physically less able to stand a heavy workload (Jainudeen and Hafez, 1993). If the stallion's condition is very poor, spermatogenesis may also suffer. At the other extreme an obese stallion also tends to have low libido and to be lazy, and may be incapable of mounting a mare. In addition, the extra weight puts additional strain on his hind legs and on the mare at mating, and may cause damage to both. It is to be remembered that the nutritional demands during the breeding season are similar to those of a performance horse, the workload of the two being approximately equivalent (Thompson, 1994; Griffin, 2000). Further details on stallion nutritional management are given in Section 17.5.3.

15.6. External Examination of the Reproductive Tract

An external examination of the stallion's reproductive genitalia is an essential selection procedure, as his ability to perform is naturally a function of the condition of his reproductive organs (Griffin, 2000; Varner, 2016). He should have two normally functioning testes, which may be felt through the scrotum and palpated to ensure they are of a similar size and consistency, move easily within their tunicae and are not warm to the touch. They should be oval in shape, lying in a horizontal plane, although when retracted may assume a more vertical position. They should be symmetrical, although occasionally the left testis is slightly larger than the right, but the difference should only be slight and should not be accompanied by an increase in heat (Sertich, 2011). It has been suggested that testicular temperature can be assessed using infrared (Neto *et al.*, 2013; Rode *et al.*, 2016). Differences in testicular size of greater than 50% can indicate late descent of a testis and, therefore, decreased sperm production (Stout and Colenbrander, 2011). The surface of the testis should feel smooth, with the occasional blood vessel being felt running under the skin. Any adhesions preventing the testes moving up and down easily within the tunicae are likely to indicate scar or fibrous tissue due to past injuries. This not only reduces the volume of functioning testicular tissue but may also interfere with spermatogenesis within the remaining tissue. Indeed, testicular

size is a good indicator of the spermatozoa-producing capacity of the stallion, and hence his potential workload. As such, testicular volume has been advocated as an assessment criterion when selecting for reproductive potential (Fig. 18.1; Love *et al.*, 1991; Pickett and Shiner, 1994; Parlevliet, 2000; Stout and Colenbrander, 2011). Excessive fat within the scrotum as a result of excessive body condition will increase the insulation of the testes and there is the danger of increasing testicular temperature and, therefore, of decreasing sperm production.

Malignant or benign growths within the testes are rare but may be evident (Caron *et al.*, 1985; Schumacher and Varner, 1993). The skin of the scrotum should be checked for dermatitis, which can cause an increase in testicular temperature. The position of the epididymis should also be felt. Their normal position in the non-retracted relaxed testes is on the dorsal (horizontal to the abdomen) side of the scrotum with the tail of the epididymis at the caudal end. The epididymis may assume a more vertical position when the testes are retracted. Positioning elsewhere may indicate testes torsion or twist (Threlfall *et al.*, 1990; Love, 2011a). Further details on testicular conditions is given in Section 18.3.4.The vas deferens leaving the testes, plus the testicular blood, nerve and lymphatic supply, passes up into the body of the stallion through the inguinal canal, which should be free from adhesions and hernias (Love, 2011a).

The penis and prepuce of the stallion should also be examined for any sign of injury or scarring, and also for haematomas, squamous cell carcinoma, summer sores, sarcoids and general infections or injury (Rochat, 2001; Carleton, 2011; Sertich, 2011). The glans penis should be examined in detail, including the urethral opening and fossa area. Examination can be carried out at washing prior to semen collection, or when testing the stallion's libido by presenting him with an oestrous mare, and should be a routine selection procedure. Details on venereal disease (VD) infections and penile conditions are given in Sections 18.3.4.9 and 18.3.5.3.

15.7. Internal Examination of the Reproductive Tract

As with the mare, examination of the internal reproductive tract of the stallion is a skilled veterinary surgeon's job. Information given by internal examination can be very useful in assessing the reproductive potential of a stallion, although internal examination is harder to perform and less informative than in the mare, and may be limited by financial implications and the need for experienced personnel.

Access to the internal parts of the stallion's reproductive tract is also very difficult. Some appreciation may be gained by rectal palpation and ultrasound (Little, 1998). Via rectal palpation, the vas deferens can be felt entering the body cavity at the inguinal canal and both, one on either side, should feel smooth and of uniform diameter. Alongside the vas deferens as they enter the body cavity lies the spermatic artery, the pulse of which should also be checked. An appreciation of testicular blood flow may also be gained by standard ultrasound and colour Doppler ultrasound (Pozor and McDonnell, 2002, 2004). Very low blood pressure, or a drop between successive examinations, may be indicative of a haemorrhage, blood clot or tumour, or the release of body fluids into a localized infection site. The accessory glands may also be palpated individually and their texture, size and shape assessed. Paired glands, such as the seminal vesicles, should be checked for symmetry. Ultrasound may be used to give an indication of physical abnormalities of the scrotum contents (testis and surrounding structures) such as cryptorchidism, testicular degeneration or enlargement, abscesses, neoplasia, hematoma, fluid accumulation, cysts, etc. (Blanchard *et al.*, 2000; Pozor and McDonnell, 2002; Brito *et al.*, 2009), and also abnormalities of the accessory glands such as occlusion, enlargement, neoplasia, cysts, etc. (Weber and Woods, 1992, 1993; Pozer and McDonnell, 2002). Additionally the iliac arteries and testicular blood supply can be assessed for blood flow and in particular for thrombosis (Varner *et al.*, 2000; Turner, 2007, 2011b). Ultrasound may also be used to indicate accessory gland function (Varner *et al.*, 2000). Finally endoscopy, although not as popular today with the advent of ultrasonography, still remains the best method of assessing the lumen and walls of the urethra, accessory glands and bladder. Although its use as a means of selecting stallions is not justified, it is certainly useful in investigating known infertility, and especially conditions such as haemospermia, urospermia and pain on ejaculation or urination (Carleton, 2011). An indication of the function of the accessory glands may also be gained by semen evaluation, and will be discussed in the following section.

15.8. Semen Evaluation

Semen evaluation is a routine selection procedure. If a stallion is to cover mares throughout the breeding season with consistent success, his semen has to meet various minimum parameters (Colenbrander *et al.*, 2003; Baumber-Skaife, 2011). In many studs, all stallions routinely have their semen evaluated at the beginning of each season, and if a problem is suspected. The quality of his semen has a direct effect on the stallion's ability to consistently and successfully cover a number of mares throughout the season (Jasko *et al.*, 1990a,b, 1991; Gastal *et al.*, 1991; Pickett, 1993a; Parlevliet and Colenbrander, 1999; Love, 2011c; Varner, 2016). Semen evaluation results are affected by a stallion's use in the last 7–10 days. For an accurate evaluation, therefore, samples should ideally be taken either as: (i) one after 3 days' sexual rest preceded by a collection 1 h prior to test collection; (ii) the last collection of a series of seven daily collections, preceded by a collection taken 1 h prior to test collection; or (iii) the second of two collections taken 1 h apart after 1 month's sexual rest (Ricketts, 1993; Davies Morel, 1999; Baumber-Skaife, 2011). In most commercial enterprises/AI programmes such regimes are not economically viable, and single sampling (interpreted with caution) can provide adequate information for most routine practices.

Collection of semen is normally by means of an artificial vagina (AV). Details of the collection and evaluation procedure are given in Sections 21.3, 21.4 and elsewhere (Davies Morel, 1999; Baumber-Skaife, 2011; Brinsko, 2011a). The normal parameters for semen are given in Table 21.3.

15.9. Infections

Like the mare, the stallion is susceptible to sexually transmitted diseases, and so all stallions should be tested for infections prior to purchase, either to eliminate them or to allow treatment to commence prior to their use.

As with the mare, swabs can identify infections of the genital tract; these are taken from the urethra, the urethral fossa and the prepuce of the stallion's penis. Swabs should be taken from the erect penis, erection being encouraged by an oestrous mare or tranquillizers. Three different swabs must be used and it is best to take the urethral fossa sample last, as this one can cause considerable discomfort and hence objection. Swabs of semen samples can be cultured to test for bacterial growth or used for cytology assessment. The stallion's semen and penis have a natural microflora of bacteria and fungi and these should be distinguished from VD pathogens. The most noteworthy bacteria, classified as VD causers of acute endometritis, are *Klebsiella pneumoniae*, *Pseudomonas aeruginosa* and *Taylorella equigenitalis*

(Section 14.3.5.3; Couto and Hughes, 1993; Parlevliet *et al.*, 1997; Metcalf, 2011; Petry *et al.*, 2018).

Swabbing is routinely carried out in many studs on all their stallions well before the season starts. This allows time, if infections are identified, for treatment to begin and take effect before the breeding season. Further details of infection of the stallion's reproductive tract and the effect upon reproduction are given in Section 18.3.5.

15.10. Blood Sampling

Blood sampling of stallions can be used to assess their general health and can indicate low-grade infection, blood loss, cancer, nutritional deficiencies or parasite burdens (Pickett, 1993c). Details of the information that can be gathered from blood sampling have been given in the previous section on the selection of the mare (Section 8.9 and Table 8.1) and are the same for the stallions. Any stallion showing these characteristics should not be considered for use until the problem has been identified and appropriate treatment commenced.

Blood samples are rarely used for hormone analysis because the considerable inter-stallion variation reduces the accuracy of such testing to assess potential reproductive performance (Roser, 1995). Additionally, the episodic nature of testosterone release also necessitates a period of sequential blood sampling, from which an average should be taken rather than a single sample. Low plasma testosterone concentrations have been associated with low libido and poor semen quality (Watson, 1997).

15.11. Chromosomal Analysis

Chromosomal abnormalities are well documented in the mare but less so in the stallion. However, they are potentially of greater importance, as a single stallion can have a greater effect on the genetic make-up of subsequent generations than a single mare. As with the mare most abnormalities appear to be associated with the sex chromosomes: conditions such as XX male syndrome (64XX), chimerism or mosaic (64XX: 64XY), Klinefelter's syndrome (65XXY) and 13 quarter/deletion (64XY), which are associated with an inability to impregnate mares or very low fertility rates, often despite apparently normal genitalia (Bowling, 1996; Makinen *et al.*, 2000; Paget *et al.*, 2001; Kakoi *et al.*, 2005; Brito *et al.*, 2008). Autosomal defects (those associated with non-sex chromosomes)

have been reported; these may not directly affect fertility but, through genetic abnormalities of the offspring, result in early embryonic death, abortion or the trait being passed on to subsequent generations (Durkin *et al.*, 2011).

Recently attempts have been made with mixed results to identify a candidate gene, possibly a polymorphism within the equine CRISP3 gene, that is linked to semen quality (Hamann *et al.*, 2007).

15.12. General Stud Management

If your selection of a stallion is not for purchase but rather for use on one of your mares, you will also be interested in the management at the stud at which he stands, especially if your mare is to board at the stud. There are several things that will concern most owners selecting a stud to send their mare to, and these will be discussed in turn.

The system of breeding used is of prime importance. Is the stud appropriately equipped to house visiting mares, or are you expected to 'walk in' your mare; that is, bring her in for the day, having detected at home whether or not she is in oestrus, and take her away the same day after covering? Some studs allow mares to stay a few nights but have only limited facilities and may well expect mares to live out. This obviously has a bearing on the distance it is possible to travel. You should also consider the method of covering, varying from pasture breeding to intensive in-hand breeding. The various methods used are discussed in detail in Chapters 10 and 16. Some studs will expect the mare to be taken home as soon as she has been covered; others will allow her to stay for re-covering if necessary and will only allow her home after a positive pregnancy diagnosis at scanning and/or rectal palpation, usually 12–18 or 40 days post-mating.

'Walking in' mares necessitates mares being brought to stud very soon after foaling. This can be traumatic and dangerous for the foal, and may preclude using a stud that is too far away; or the foal may need to be removed from the mare prior to transportation. Some larger studs may have facilities to allow mares to be brought in to foal, normally 4–6 weeks prior to foaling. This allows the mare to be covered on her foal heat without the danger of travelling with a young foal; however, there have been recent concerns over cross-infections in young foals whose dams have been brought in from a wide geographical area, and so such arrangements are nowhere near as popular as they used to be.

The daily management at the stud should also be investigated and matched as closely as possible to the mare's normal routine. If not, her routine at home should slowly be altered to match that at the stud, to minimize the stress of change. All animals on the stud should be wormed regularly and vaccinated, and documented proof of adequate protection is usually required of all visiting mares. At some studs, particularly those standing valuable stallions, mares will also require negative certificates to a variety of VD bacteria (Horse Race Betting Levy Board, 2019).

A good impression of the standard of management of a yard can be gained by a general visit. The yard, whatever system in use, should be clean and tidy, all the mares and stallions should be in good condition, the pasture well tended and the animals contented. If the mare is to foal there, the foaling facilities should be clean, safe and roomy with a good system for 24-h monitoring by skilled staff. However, the facilities of the yard and the equipment and expertize available will reflect the type of stallion and his nomination fee.

The system that you choose is ultimately a personal choice depending on your priorities and the finances available. Traditionally, intensive systems tend to be associated with the Thoroughbred industry, where expense is of less concern but hygiene and protection of valuable stock are of paramount importance. In some intensive systems mares are taken to the stud to foal, are subsequently covered and possibly re-covered and remain at stud until pregnancy is confirmed, often at days 12, 25 and possibly as late as day 40. In such systems, the service fees are high and the costs of keep and veterinary attention are great, but this is offset by the value of the offspring and the risks are lower. At the other end of the spectrum, native studs will serve a mare that arrives in their yard, and within 30 min she can be on her way home. In such systems stallion fees are low, as are costs, but the offspring is often of low value and the risks are higher.

When examining potential studs it is as well to bear in mind that the ideal is not normally achieved. It is unrealistic to expect a yard standing a cheaper stallion, with stud fees of £50–100, to have the facilities found in a Thoroughbred stud standing stallions with nomination fees of £50,000 and above.

15.13. Conclusion

As for the mare, selection of stallions on the basis of reproductive competence, as well as athletic performance, it is essential to ensure that significant amounts of time, energy and effort are not wasted in breeding reproductively incompetent stock. This will also minimize frustration to breeders, and ensure that reproductive issues are not perpetuated in future generations.

Study Questions

Critically evaluate the criteria that should be considered when selecting a stallion based on reproductive competence. Include in your answer an evaluation of how reliable these criteria are in predicting the ease with which a stallion may be bred.

Evaluate what can be done by a lay person/non-veterinary professional to assess the reproductive competence of a stallion.

Discuss the necessity for, and the methods that might be used to conduct, an internal examination of the stallion when selecting on the basis of reproductive competence.

Suggested Reading

Little, T.V. and Holyoak, R. (1992) Reproductive Anatomy and Physiology of the Stallion. *Veterinary Clinics of North America: Equine Practice* 8(1), 1–29.

Thompson, D.L. (1994) Breeding management of stallions: breeding soundness evaluations. *Journal of Equine Veterinary Science* 14(1), 19–20.

Griffin, P.G. (2000) The breeding soundness examination in the stallion. *Journal of Equine Veterinary Science* 20(3), 168–171.

Love, C.C. (2003) Evaluation of breeding records. In: Blanchard, T.L., Varner, D.D., Schumacher, J., Love, C.C., Brinsko, S.P., Rigby, S.L. (eds) *Manual of Equine Reproduction*, 2nd edn. Mosby, St Louis, Missouri, pp. 229–237.

Love, C.C. (2011) Historical information. In: McKinnon, A.O., Squires, E.L., Vaala, E. and Varner, D.D. (eds) *Equine Reproduction*, 2nd edn. Wiley-Blackwell, Philadelphia, London, pp. 1429–1434.

Love, C.C. (2011) Relationship between sperm motility, morphology and the fertility of stallions. *Theriogenology* 76, 547–557.

Baumber-Skaife, J. (2011) Evaluation of semen. In: McKinnon, A.O., Squires, E.L., Vaala, E. and Varner, D.D. (eds) *Equine Reproduction*, 2nd edn. Wiley-Blackwell, Philadelphia, London, pp. 1278–1291.

Carleton, C.L. (2011) Endoscopy of the internal reproductive tract. In: McKinnon, A.O., Squires, E.L., Vaala, E. and Varner, D.D. (eds) *Equine Reproduction*, 2nd edn. Wiley-Blackwell, Philadelphia, London, pp. 1448–1457.

Turner, R.M. (2011) Abnormalities of the Ejaculate. In: McKinnon, A.O., Squires, E.L., Vaala, E. and Varner, D.D. (eds) *Equine Reproduction*, 2nd edn. Wiley-Blackwell, Philadelphia, London, pp. 1119–1129.

Turner, R.M. (2011) Ultrasonography of the genital tract. In: McKinnon, A.O., Squires, E.L., Vaala, E. and Varner, D.D. (eds) *Equine Reproduction*, 2nd edn. Wiley-Blackwell, Philadelphia, London, pp. 1469–1490.

Varner, D.D. (2016) Approaches to breeding soundness examination and interpretation of results. *Journal of Equine Veterinary Science* 43, 37–44.

Preparation of the Stallion for Breeding and Mating Management

16

The Objectives of this Chapter are:

To detail the preparation of the stallion in the months leading up to breeding.

To appreciate the various challenges presented when breeding young stallions, ex-performance stallions and those established in their breeding career.

To understand how and why management of the stallion prior to breeding can affect reproductive success.

To apply the reproductive physiology and behaviour knowledge gained in Section B to understand how the stallion's reproductive activity can be manipulated.

To evaluate the various management options practised for mating stallions, and so enable you to make informed management choices.

To enable you to appreciate the challenges that various breeding management options pose, and how these affect reproductive success and animal welfare.

16.1. Introduction

It is essential that preparation of the stallion starts in plenty of time prior to breeding. Planning ahead will help ensure that a stallion is able to perform to the best of his ability, optimizing his health and well-being as well as that of his mares. This Chapter will concentrate mainly on the 6-month preparation period prior to the breeding season, along with stallion management at mating. Details of general management, particularly from the point of view of the mare, are given in Chapter 10 and so will not be repeated here.

16.2. Preparation of the Stallion

Stallions used for breeding will either be those that have been brought up with that intention (and bred on the basis of their genetics) or stallions that have had a previous performance career and have proven their ability prior to being retired to stud. Both types of stallion can present challenges. Further details on general stallion management appear in Chapter 17.

If a colt is destined to become a working stallion, and not have a performance career, he must be brought up during his early life with this aim in mind, especially with regard to discipline. Many stallions become hard to handle, and in some cases downright dangerous, because discipline and respect for authority have not been established in early life. A stallion cannot be expected to deal with a full book of mares until he has reached physical maturity (usually around 5 years of age, although this will depend on the breed) (Johnson *et al.*, 1991, 2008), and pushing him to cover too many mares too early will affect his physical and psychological ability to breed; his introduction to covering is, therefore, very important (Section 17.4).

In stallions that have had a previous athletic career (Fig. 16.1) one of the major problems can be behavioural abnormalities. These stallions will have had several years during which they will have been actively discouraged from displaying any sexual behaviour. As a result, they may be severely inhibited at their first sight of an oestrous mare, anticipating punishment. They will often find it hard to revert to natural stallion behaviour and need varying amounts of time to adjust to their new career (Van Dierendonck and Goodwin, 2005). Many stallions take a few seasons to completely adjust and

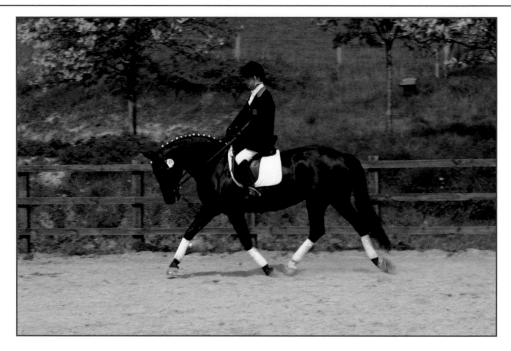

Fig. 16.1. Many successful stallions are currently, or have been, performance horses. As such, they need careful management in order to perform well at both jobs.

some never really do achieve complete adjustment. A stallion's libido may also be affected and such stallions may, as a result, always prove to be slow to react to an oestrous mare and show clumsy mounting behaviour. Attention should be paid to a stallion's nutrition and exercise, as well as to his psychological adjustment, during this preparation period. He must be fit, not fat. A heavy covering season places significant demands on the stallion, especially in terms of energy, and he will often lose condition over the season. This loss in condition is minimized if the stallion's energy intake is increased by enhancing the concentrate proportion of his diet, and if he is fit and in a body condition score (CS) 3 as the season commences (Fig. 16.2). Both excess and low body weight reduce a stallion's libido. Exercise helps a stallion maintain good condition, preventing obesity and maintaining muscle tone and stamina. Stallions have a tendency to become obese, as they are regularly kept individually in stables or paddocks away from each other, and from mares, whereas in natural conditions they would be free to exercise at will. If stallions are badly behaved, it is tempting to keep them confined, with only limited turnout. This only serves to perpetuate the problem and boredom accentuates any misbehaviour. Some stallions can be safely ridden or driven, which provides an excellent form of exercise as well as

good discipline (Fig. 16.3). In the less-intensive studs some quiet stallions can be turned out in July at the end of the season with either their mothers, an old mare or other quiet pregnant mares. They can then be brought back into riding work over the winter. This system allows a rest period after the season, followed by a fitness regime prior to the start of the next season. It also provides them with another purpose in life, which greatly helps discipline. However, this is not popular with many owners, who are understandably reluctant to put valuable stallions into any environment of perceived danger.

Increasingly, particularly with the widespread use of artificial insemination (AI) in performance horses, stallions are fulfilling the roles of being both breeding stallions and athletes at the same time. For these stallions discipline is particularly important, and a clear demarcation in their two roles is required: for example, different handlers, tack and facilities.

Regardless of their background, all stallions should be brought into the stud environment at least 4–6 weeks prior to their first mare of the season. They should then be introduced or reintroduced to the yard, handling systems, buildings, surroundings and especially the covering area, with plenty of time to allow familiarization prior to the first covering. Any changes in diet should be introduced slowly, before the season

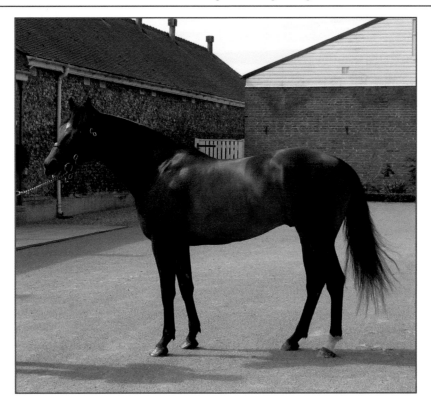

Fig. 16.2. A stallion should be in a fit, not fat condition; that is, in condition score 3 at the beginning of the breeding season.

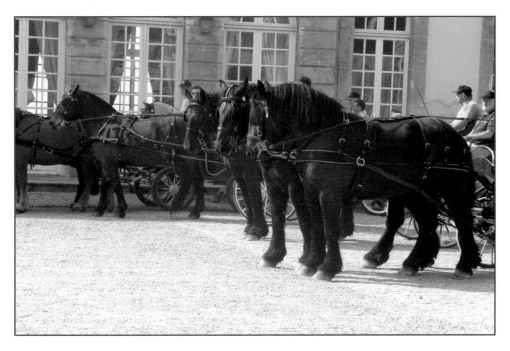

Fig. 16.3. Riding or driving provides an excellent form of exercise as well as good discipline.

starts, along with any new companions. Further details regarding stallion management are given in Chapter 17.

16.3. General Aspects of Preparation for Breeding

Several aspects of general management need to be considered when preparing the stallion for breeding.

16.3.1. Drugs

Many performance horses may have been on various drug regimes during their performance careers. Corticosteroids, used as anti-inflammatory drugs to treat various injuries, can have serious detrimental effects on the reproductive performance of stallions (McCue and Ferris, 2011). This also applies to anabolic steroids, used to boost muscle development, which detrimentally affect both libido and spermatogenesis (Nagata *et al.*, 1999). The effects of most of these drugs is usually temporary and, as long as sufficient time is allowed for them to be eliminated from the system, there should be no long-term adverse effects.

16.3.2. Testing for infections

To prevent transfer of infections that will be detrimental to reproductive performance, testing for infections needs to be carried out in stallions as well as in mares (Metcalf, 2011). Stallions, however, are normally only tested at the beginning of the season; providing they are only presented with certified clean mares, and no problem becomes evident during the breeding season, that should suffice. In a similar way to mares (Section 9.4.2) all stallions should be swabbed to test for bacterial infection. It is advised that they have two sets of swabs taken at an interval of no less than 7 days soon after 1 January in each covering season. Swabs should be taken from the urethra, urethral fossa and the sheath of the penis. For high-risk stallions, clitoral swabs may be taken from their first four mares of the season at 2 days after covering. Although not normally required, some studs also swab stallions in the middle of the season, and they should certainly be swabbed if/as soon as any problem is suspected (Kristula and Smith, 2004). As with the mare (Section 9.4.2) swabs are tested primarily for the venereal disease bacteria: *Taylorella equigenitalis*, the causal bacteria for contagious equine metritis (CEM; Timoney, 2011c), plus *Klebsiella pneumoniae* and *Pseudomonas aeruginosa*. Other bacteria such as *Escherichia coli*, *Streptococcus zooepidemicus* and *Staphylococcus aureus*, all present in the environment but which may still cause problems, may be also tested for. The exact requirements should be checked against breed requirements, for example the Horse Race Betting Levy Board (HBLB) Codes of Practice for Thoroughbreds, which forms the basis of requirements for other breeds. It is important not only to test the stallion, but also to ensure that testing is adequately carried out for all mares being covered, and that clear documentation is used. The owner/manager of the stallion determines the exact testing mares must undergo within any breed guidelines, and so it is essential that mare owners are correctly informed of all requirements when stallion nominations are agreed. As with the mare, CEM is a notifiable disease in the UK and so must be reported to the Department for Environment, Food and Rural Affairs (DEFRA). If other infective bacteria are isolated, then covering should be immediately stopped and advice/treatment sought. Some stallions are long-term carriers of CEM and so can need prolonged periods of treatment (Kristula and Smith, 2004). It should be remembered that the stallion's penis should never be sterile, as a natural microflora balance should be evident. Infective bacteria, however, are a concern. Equine viral arteritis (EVA), as with the mares, is a notifiable venereal disease (VD) in the stallion. It is advised that all stallions are blood-sampled at the beginning of the season, at least 28 days before their first mare, and the blood tested for antibodies. If no antibodies are present, then the stallion is free of infection and can be safely used for covering. However, if antibodies are identified, this may not necessarily mean that the stallion has an active infection. The antibodies may be the result of vaccination and veterinary advice should, therefore, be sought as to whether the stallion can be used (Section 14.3.5.7; MacLachlan and Balasuriya, 2006; Holyoak *et al.*, 2008).

Again in common with the mare, equine herpes virus (EHV) and strangles are potential infections (Lu and Morrese, 2007). Neither is notifiable but any animals suspected of having contact with EHV or strangles must not be allowed onto a stud. If either is confirmed in a stallion, the stud must be closed, and veterinary advice sought as to whether covering can recommence that season. There are effective current and newly developing vaccines against EHV (Section 14.3.5.7; MacLachlan *et al.*, 2007; Metcalf, 2011). The HBLB Codes of Practice also provide advice on these conditions (Ricketts *et al.*, 1993; Horse Race Betting Levy Board, 2019). Further details on VD are given in Section 18.3.5. Once swabs have been taken and the stallion is declared clean, the laboratory certificate confirming the stallion's disease-free status should be available to all mare owners.

16.3.3. Nomination forms

Mare owners book a covering (or nomination) with a specific stallion by completing a nomination form from the stud at which the stallion is standing. This is a legal agreement between the stallion owner and the mare owner for a nomination to a specific stallion. The exact information and agreement made varies with the stud, but it will lay out the basic conditions. These will include any health/testing requirements that the mare must satisfy before she arrives on the stud; what the nomination fee is; and how it will be paid. It may also include other selection criteria for mares (performance, general conformation, etc.) and ask for a rough date when it is planned the mare will be covered. The HBLB Codes of Practice often form the basis of the requirements regarding mare health, even if the breeding stock are not Thoroughbreds, and it is the mare owner's responsibility to satisfy all the requirements before presenting the mare to the stallion. As far as the stallion is concerned the returned nomination agreements allow the stallion owner to manage the stallion work load, spreading it as evenly as possible through the season, and provide a measure of financial security as to the income that stallion will generate.

The nomination fee is paid in a variety of different ways and depends on the stud. Some studs will require a fee or deposit to be paid at the time of submitting the nomination form with the balance due later. Some require a straight fee to be paid post-covering, regardless of whether the mare is in foal or not; this is often the case in native pony studs and those charging a lower fee. Alternatively, arrangements such as 'no foal, no fee October 1st' terms may apply, under which agreement fees are paid on covering but if the mare is proven not to be pregnant on 1st October the stud fee (excluding any keep fees) is returned. A similar arrangement is termed 'no foal, free return October 1st', in which instead of the fee being returned, the mare has a free cover to the same stallion or a replacement the following year. For the most expensive stallions, a part-payment arrangement may be made whereby 50% of the fee is due on covering and the balance paid if the mare is pregnant on 1st October. Alternatively, a 'live foal' arrangement may be made whereby the stud fee is returned or a 'free return' given if the mare does not have a live foal, or one that survives for 48 h. Occasionally concessions can be given to certain mares in the form of a reduced fee to encourage good mares whose offspring will be a good advertisement for the stallion. This is a useful way of getting good mares to a promising young stallion.

16.3.4. General preparation

The stallion should enter the breeding season in a fit condition (CS 3). Ideally, immediately prior to the season, he should have all shoes removed to minimize damage to mares at mounting. He should be up to date with his vaccinations, including influenza and tetanus and any other necessary vaccinations (EVA, EHV etc.), as well as recently wormed. The stallion should be well turned out and in good condition, especially in studs where the mares are walked in for covering by their owners: he should be a good advertisement for himself.

16.4. Manipulation of the Breeding Activity in the Stallion

Manipulation of stallion reproduction is not as essential as manipulation in the mare, as it is the mare's reproductive cycle that is normally the limiting factor to the time of breeding. Additionally, given enough encouragement, a stallion will naturally breed during the non-breeding season, but less efficiently. For this reason, research work in the area is limited. As in the mare, the breeding season of the stallion is governed by photoperiod, and the stallion reacts to increasing day length in a manner similar to that seen in the mare; light treatment can, therefore, be used to advance the breeding season (Deichsel et al., 2016). Introduction of a 16 h light/8 h dark regime in November/December will result in coat loss within 4 weeks followed shortly after by increased reproductive activity and libido (Argo et al., 1991). This is particularly useful in systems where mares are to be covered early in the year and especially in stallions of low libido. Simply putting stallions under the same light regime as the mares on the stud works well. Continual stimulation, however, produces refractoriness and a return to normal seasonal changes, despite the altered photoperiod (Argo et al., 1991). This can be an issue in stallions shuttled from northern to southern hemispheres. As with the mare, rugging up stallions and increasing nutritional intake (so moving them from CS 2.5 to CS 3 in the 6 weeks prior to the start of breeding), has additional benefit by ensuring stallions can breed early in the season.

Manipulation of reproduction in the stallion is also used to suppress reproductive activity as a possible temporary alternative to gelding (Stout, 2005). Although this is not of direct relevance to stud management, it is interesting to note that gonadotrophin-releasing hormone (GnRH) immunization/antagonists have been used successfully to temporarily suppress reproductive activity. This is also true of an GnRH overdose which, as a result of flooding the system with GnRH, down-regulates the pituitary response (Turkstra et al., 2005). GnRH has also been used to try to alter stallion behaviour, such as to improve libido, but with limited and varied success (Stout and Colenbrander, 2004; Stout, 2005). Finally, microencapsulated testosterone propionate (MTP) has been used in an attempt to suppress pituitary production of luteinizing hormone (LH) and follicle-stimulating hormone (FSH). An effect on spermatogenesis has been reported, but only limited effect on behaviour (Turner and Kirkpatrick, 1982).

16.5. Management at Mating

The management of mating, both general and specifically from the mare's point of view, is covered in depth in Section 10.2.2.4. However, it is worth noting a few things that particularly relate to the stallion (Umphenour *et al.*, 2011). Owing to the influence of testosterone, and the presence of mares, a stallion's behaviour during the covering season can be particularly unpredictable and, therefore, dangerous. Management techniques can reduce this danger, such as a regular routine including turnout as much as possible. Tying up (racking up) of stallions in their stables as a routine (Fig. 16.4) while they are being groomed/mucked out can be beneficial, as catching an enthusiastic stallion can be made much safer when a mare arrives on the yard if he has been/is used to being tied up and is familiar with the routine. The use of a specific bridle for different activities is very useful

(i.e. different tack for exercise, turnout and covering), so a stallion knows what is required of him by the tack presented. For covering in intensive in-hand systems, a stallion is normally presented with his shoes removed (in particular the front shoes), and tacked up with his covering bridle and long rein. Some suggest

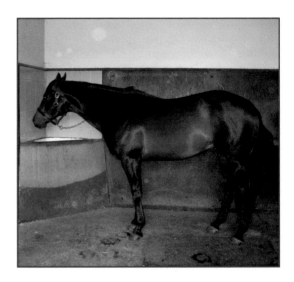

Fig. 16.4. A tie ring at the back of the stallion's stable to which the stallion can be tied (racked up) as part of his daily routine can be good idea.

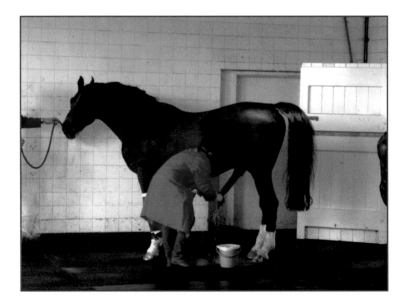

Fig. 16.5. Prior to covering, a stallion's penis and genital area should be washed; erection can be encouraged by the close proximity of an oestrous mare or environment associated with breeding.

using a pole to give a greater degree of control, allowing you to push a stallion away from you as well as moving him towards you, although this is perceived by some to be more dangerous. A stallion's penis, genital area, belly and inside hind legs should be washed with warm, clean water immediately before covering (Fig. 16.5). Many yards have a wash-down area particularly for the purpose. Ideally, the penis should be erect at washing. Erection may occur naturally, owing to the anticipation of covering; others may require initial teasing. Antiseptic and/or soap solutions, once very popular, should be used with care and rinsed off thoroughly. Their use may be questioned, not only because of their spermicidal effects, but also because of the detrimental effect they may have on the natural penile microflora (presenting an opportunity for colonization by opportunistic bacteria, which, while not VD bacteria, can still cause endometritis) (Betsch *et al.*, 1991; Clement *et al.*, 1995). The stallion is then led to join the mare waiting in the covering area ready for mating. Details of the mating management are given in Chapter 10 and in particular in Section 10.6.

16.6. Conclusion

It is evident that, in order to maximize reproductive success and so optimize a stallion's use, it is essential that a stallion is prepared in good time for his breeding career. Additionally, the management of the stallion at covering needs to also be considered carefully. A number of options are available, their use depending on value of stock, personal choice and facilities available.

Study Questions

Evaluate the factors that need to be considered when planning to breed an ex-performance stallion to maximize the chances that he will perform appropriately.

'When considering the manipulation of reproduction there is little that can be done with regard to the stallion, as the mare is the limiting factor'. Discuss.

Detail the preparations that need to be made, and management that needs to be considered, from autumn onwards when starting to breed a stallion in February.

Discuss the means by which the transfer of disease can be prevented, with particular reference to the stallion.

Detail the management of the stallion during the mating process.

Suggested Reading

Stout, T.A. (2005) Modulating reproductive activity in stallions: a review. *Animal Reproduction Science* 89(1–4), 93–103.

Varner, D.D. (2005) *Handling the breeding stallion.* Proceedings of the 51st Annual Convention of the American Association of Equine Practioners, pp. 498–505.

Metcalf, E.S. (2011) Venereal disease. In: McKinnon, A.O., Squires, E.L., Vaala, E. and Varner, D.D. (eds) *Equine Reproduction*, 2nd edn. Wiley-Blackwell, Philadelphia, London, pp. 1250–1260.

Umphenour, N.W., McCarthy, P. and Blanchard, T.L. (2011) Management of stallions in natural-service programs In: McKinnon, A.O., Squires, E.L., Vaala, E. and Varner, D.D. (eds) *Equine Reproduction*, 2nd edn. Wiley-Blackwell, Philadelphia, London, pp. 1208–1227.

General Stallion Management

The Objectives of this Chapter are:

To apply the anatomy, physiology and behaviour knowledge gained in Section B to stallion management.
To enable you to consider alternative ways of keeping stallions by understanding the challenges of managing them.
To understand how and why management of the stallion can affect his success as a breeding animal.

17.1. Introduction

Management of the stallion should not be neglected in the enthusiasm to obtain optimum mare and foal management. It has already been considered in some depth in Chapters 15 and 16. However, it is also worth considering the introduction of the stallion to his work as a breeding animal, and the general training and management principles that should be borne in mind when keeping stallions.

17.2. Early General Training

Early training, well in advance of the stallion's first introduction to a mare, is very important to reduce the chances of injury to both horses and handlers. It will also reduce the risk of him developing potentially dangerous bad habits.

It is very important that a stallion is taught discipline and respect from a young age. Once a good grounding has been established, this can be built upon. It is nearly impossible to start disciplining a 3–4-year-old stallion without the considerable risk of injury to both parties, and it will inevitably lead to conflict and not respect. In training a stallion the handler's attitude and competence are of real importance, as rough handling and incorrect and inconsistent training can cause many

problems, from poor breeding behaviour and performance to dangerous vices (McDonnell, 2000b).

Basic discipline includes acceptance of the handler, bridle and leading; and obeying voice commands to halt, stand, walk on and back up, etc. The stallion should also accept boxing, shoeing, veterinary inspection and general handling. Once this basic discipline has been achieved, he may be trained further in a specific area or discipline, or maintained at this level for breeding. Further training for riding or driving is advantageous, as it provides the stallion with another constructive outlet for his energies other than just covering. This advanced level of discipline normally leads to greater respect and subsequently an easier stallion to handle working in a less stressful environment, which enhances stallion semen quality and reproductive success, as well as human safety (Graham and Card, 2007).

17.3. Restraint

Several means of restraint can be used to control a stallion. The method used depends on the stallion's temperament, the facilities available and the handler's personal preference. The effect of the handler on the behaviour of the stallion cannot be overemphasized.

A nervous and insecure handler will transfer these feelings to the stallion which, in picking them up, is more likely to act uncharacteristically and unexpectedly, and be perceived as requiring greater restraint. It is especially important that the handler dealing with young stallions is calm and confident and has had plenty of experience. The overuse of restraint or punishment to compensate for nervousness is a trap that can, all too easily, be fallen into. If a stallion needs to be reprimanded, it should be immediate and effective. Continuous ineffective and half-hearted attempts – often due to a lack of experience or confidence on the part of the handler – leads to the stallion resenting the handler.

Stallions are by nature proud and courageous, attributes much to be admired and often selected for in breeding. It is important, therefore, that they are treated with respect in order to maintain these attributes; they should, however, be channelled into a safe expression and not into conflict (Varner, 2011). Ideally, the stallion should be restrained for day-to-day management by a good, strong leather or webbing head collar or halter, and a lead rope (Fig. 17.1). These must be checked regularly as, owing to his strength, a stallion may break away easily from inadequate restraint and has the potential to wreak havoc in a yard. He should have been taught acceptance of the halter and leading at a young age so that this is not a problem. However, it is inevitable that he will become more boisterous as he gets older and, especially if he has been inappropriately trained in early life, he may need a more substantial means of restraint. This may consist of a halter plus chain either under or over the nose, so that a pull on the chain applies pressure to the nose and provides extra restraint (Conboy, 2011b).

Many stallions are restrained, especially for covering, by means of a snaffle or stallion bit and, again, a chain may be attached in one of several positions (Fig. 17.2a–d). Passing the chain under the chin is popular but is thought by some to encourage rearing, and so an alternative is to pass the stallion chain over the nose and looped through the noseband. This is reported to discourage rearing by encouraging the head to come down when pressure is applied (Fig. 17.1b). The more severe forms of restraint should only be used as a last resort (Varner, 2011).

The effective use of the handler's voice also should not be underestimated. A clear, confident voice command is just as effective as a physical reprimand to a well-trained stallion. A halter for everyday use and a snaffle bridle for covering, along with the effective use of the voice, are all a well-trained stallion should require (Fig. 17.2). Whatever restraint is chosen, ideally a stallion should have different tack for varying occasions such as turnout, riding or covering, so that he knows what is expected of him by the restraint used.

17.4. Introducing the Stallion to Covering

A young stallion should not be expected to cover mares until he is at least 3 years old. A 3-year-old stallion should be capable of covering mares successfully in his first season, but only a few. A 4-year-old is capable of covering a full book of mares (50 per season) but his fertility rates and libido cannot be expected to be consistent. By 5 years of age he should have reached his full reproductive potential which, for most stallions, is 50–100 mares per season and up to three mares per day with rest periods (Johnson *et al.*, 1991; Dowsett and Knott, 1996; Turner and McDonnell, 2007; Johnson

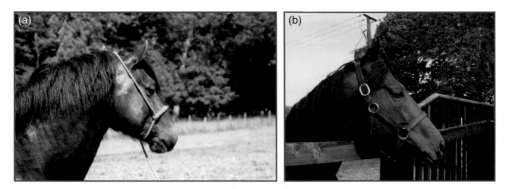

Fig. 17.1. All a well-behaved stallion should require for restraint on an everyday basis is a halter (a) or head collar (b).

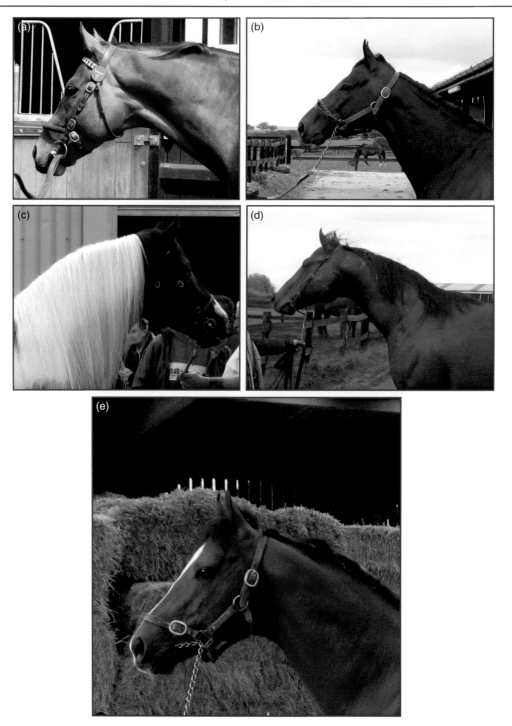

Fig. 17.2. There are numerous forms of restraint for a stallion including (a) stallion bit with chain or lead rope under the chin; (b) stallion bit with chain or lead rope over the nose; (c) stallion bit with chain under the chin but attached to both left and right ring; (d) a Chifney bit; and (e) chain passed through the mouth and acting as a bit.

et al., 2008). The workload that he is capable of at 5 years of age (full maturity) is likely to be that which can be expected of him at least until his 20s, barring unforeseen circumstances. It is advised, therefore, that during his first season a stallion should be limited to 15 mares or so spread out over the season, and he should not be expected to cover more than one per day. The owner of a young stallion should also be prepared to cancel further nominations in the first season if the stallion is showing signs of losing interest and lacks libido or gets injured. All mares for young stallions should be individually picked, as only mature mares of quiet disposition well in oestrus should be chosen. Such mares are often offered on a 'no foal, no fee' basis as, even if a semen evaluation has been conducted, the stallion has as yet no proven fertility record.

A stallion's first covering should be with an experienced handler who knows the stallion well. Even if the stallion is eventually to be used in pasture breeding, or other non-in-hand breeding situations, it is advisable that his first cover is in hand, or in more controlled conditions, to ensure that evasive action can be taken in the event of emergencies. This first cover is extremely important and its success can seriously affect a stallion's long-term ability and behaviour. It is essential that the mare to be covered is experienced, quiet and in full oestrus. Maiden mares are not advisable as they themselves may be unpredictable and it is enough of a job watching an inexperienced and, therefore, unpredictable stallion, without having the added complication of an unpredictable mare. Ideally, the mare should be slightly smaller than the stallion, making it easier for him to mount (Pickett, 1993d).

The stallion and mare should be prepared for covering as detailed in Section 16.5, although some omit washing the genitals for the first few covers (Samper, 2000). The stallion should be familiar with the covering area, having been introduced to it beforehand, and extra care should be taken to ensure that the floor is non-slip and that there are no protrusions that may injure him or cause him to fall (Conboy, 2011b).

The handler should be experienced in the normal sequence of events when mating mature stallions, as ultimately the novice will need to behave in a similar fashion. An inexperienced stallion cannot be expected to conform immediately. At the first covering it is best to more or less allow him his head. Excessive interference by humans discourages the stallion, and at this stage excessive guidance or discipline should be avoided; he should be allowed to gain confidence in his own ability before he is taught manners as well (discussed in Section 10.2.2.3 and 10.2.2.4). However, potentially dangerous habits such as kicking or biting should be corrected immediately as, if allowed to persist, they could render the stallion unusable.

At his first few coverings, the stallion may need prolonged teasing, and may mount the mare several times before ejaculation is achieved. He should not be hurried or forced in any way, as this will only serve to upset him, put him off his stride and result in long-term problems. If he seems unable to ejaculate properly, he should be taken away and returned to his box, and either tried again with the same mare later on in the day or – better still – with another mare. There is no reason why such setbacks in the first few covers should have any effect on his long-term performance. This first season is all about building up the stallion's confidence in his ability and gradually instilling manners for the sake of safety. It is a gentle balancing act between the two aims, and the rate of progress very much depends on the individual stallion. You must always be prepared to suspend all attempts at covering if he has a bad experience, and to start again at the beginning to restore his confidence. A bad experience may mean he develops an aversion to a particular type of mare (for example colour, size or age) or even a permanent reduction in his libido (Conboy, 2011b).

The aim of the stallion's first season is to ensure that he associates his new job with pleasure, in a calm and secure atmosphere, so that he will be able to deal with the occasional less cooperative mare in later life. It is essential that everything is carried out calmly and that any incident is dealt confidently. Panic and insecurity in the handler will affect the stallion's attitude and performance. Confidence in his handler and surroundings can only serve to enhance his own self-confidence and, therefore, his ability.

17.5. General Stallion Management

The general management of the stallion is extremely important in ensuring that he is fit, able and willing to do his job. It also helps to prevent the acquisition of bad habits and increases safety. The main areas of stallion management that need to be considered are housing, exercise, nutrition, feet care, dental care, vaccination and worming programmes.

279

17.5.1. Housing

Naturally, a stallion would roam wide areas of land, migrating over new pasture with his mares. He could, therefore, exercise himself at will and was always provided with fresh, clean grazing (Fig. 17.3; McDonnell, 2005, 2011a). Domestication has largely put paid to this, except in some pasture breeding systems. A stallion's management needs to compensate him for this loss and so optimize his welfare and performance. Ideally, a stallion should be turned out in a large paddock, but this is not always possible. Climate and limited grazing in many areas preclude the use of all-year turnout.

Most stallions are confined to a stable for at least some period of time. This stable must be large, at least 5 × 5 m for a 15-16 hh horse, and be light and airy. It should have a strong, secure door, with top and bottom sections, plus a top grid that can be shut to provide extra safety but still allow ventilation. Details such as the stallion's pedigree can be displayed, adding interest, especially on yards where visitors are catered for (Fig. 17.4). The stable should have a tie ring at the back to which the stallion should be tied (racked up) as part of his general daily routine, normally when his stable is mucked out, and the water and hay replenished (Fig. 16.4). It is a good idea to rack up stallions routinely, as it makes them easier to handle if visiting mares are around in the yard, and allows them to be easily caught if required. A consistent routine enhances their discipline.

As with all horses, a stallion's stable should be kept clean and free of flies. Regular cleaning of water troughs and feed mangers is essential.

To reduce boredom and the development of vices such as crib biting, weaving and stable walking, the stable door should overlook a busy part of the yard. Chains, plastic bottles, etc., hung from the ceiling; a

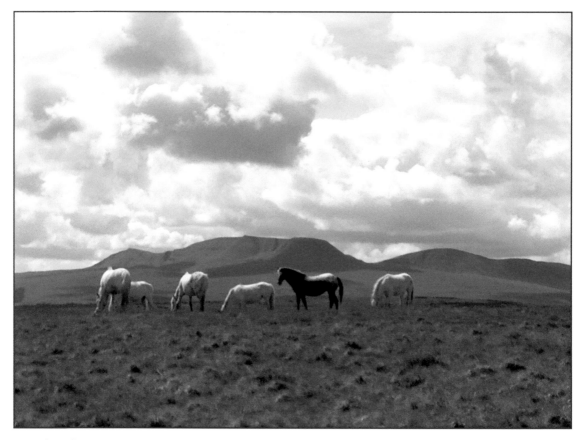

Fig. 17.3. Stallions would naturally roam over large areas of land, exercising at will. Ideally, intensive management needs to compensate the stallion for the loss of such freedom. (Photo courtesy of Dr Jill Bullen.)

football; or even a cat have been used successfully to provide the stallion with entertainment and, therefore, reduce boredom. The box should have easy access to a paddock, which is normally exclusively for his use. Two

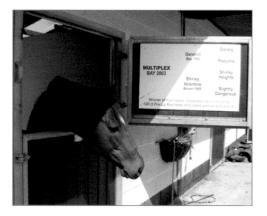

Fig. 17.4. A stallion box at the National Stud, Newmarket, UK, showing the stallion's pedigree displayed on the inside of the upper door.

acres per stallion is ideal and allows plenty of room for exercise. The cost of fencing can be minimized, as only this paddock needs to have strong, high, stallion-proof fencing. For larger stallions, fencing should be post and rail, and at least 2 m high. An electric fence, run along the top or projecting into the field about 15 cm from the top of the fence, may be added to provide extra security. Provision of a field shelter is also advocated to provide protection in inclement weather (Fig. 17.5).

Research indicates that the housing of stallions has a direct effect upon reproductive performance. Housing stallions in close proximity to other stallions mimics the natural bachelor herd scenario (McDonnell and Murray, 1995; Christensen *et al.*, 2002a,b). Stallions in such bachelor groups have lower testosterone levels and, therefore, a lower libido than harem stallions. Social interaction with mares in the absence of other stallions results in elevated testosterone concentrations. It is, therefore, advised that stallions are best housed individually with a group of mares, as an imitation of the natural harem situation, rather than on the traditional stallion yards. Pasture-bred stallions are reported to

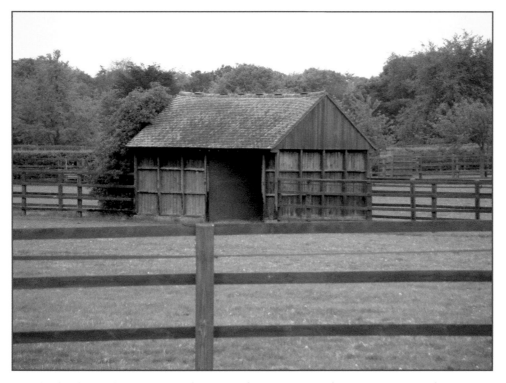

Fig. 17.5. A paddock with a 2-m-high post and rail fence, and a field shelter, is ideal for a stallion. An electric fence running along the top or inside the fencing provides extra security.

have higher libido and exhibit higher fertility rates than stabled, in-hand-bred stallions (McDonnell and Murray, 1995). In general it is advantageous for stallions to be turned out under natural daylight as much as possible, with plenty of exercise and – within the constraints of safety – any social interactions should be with mares rather than with other stallions, at least during the breeding season (McDonnell, 2000b).

17.5.2. Exercise

Exercise, as for all horses, is essential for the physical and psychological well-being of the stallion. It helps to reduce boredom and to maintain basic fitness and muscle tone (Jackson, 2011; Popescu et al., 2019). Fitness is especially important, as stallions undergo short, sharp periods of extreme exercise when covering. Exercise improves the cardiovascular system and reduces the chances of conditions such as azoturia (tying up) and also improves general well-being (Popescu and Diugan, 2017; Popescu et al., 2019). It also helps digestion and promotes a healthy appetite. The stallion can either be free or forced (i.e. turned out or ridden/lunged). Many stallions are unbroken, in which case the only option is free exercise. As such, they should be turned out for as long as possible each day (Fig. 17.6; Popescu et al., 2019).

Free exercise is fine for those stallions willing to exercise themselves. However, some refuse to move around the paddock, or at the other extreme charge around madly and pace the fence, spending no time grazing and so losing condition. The exercise of these stallions has to be controlled by means of forced exercise, which also improves discipline, especially in nervous and highly strung animals. Riding and lunging are popular forms of forced exercise. Other forms include swimming, which is particularly beneficial to the cardiovascular system and for lame horses. Treadmills or horse walkers provide an effective means of forced exercise but should be restricted to stallions accustomed to them (Fig. 17.7). On a slight note of caution, some evidence reported by Taylor et al. (1997) suggested that high workloads may be associated with poorer sperm morphology and by implication, therefore, poorer fertility rates. However, there was much variation between stallions in their study.

Some stallions, especially native types, can be turned out with mares and foals. This system has the added advantage that mares returning to oestrus after unsuccessful covering can be detected and re-covered by the stallion turned out with them (Fig. 17.8). This system should be confined for use with well-behaved, older stallions which are well into their working season.

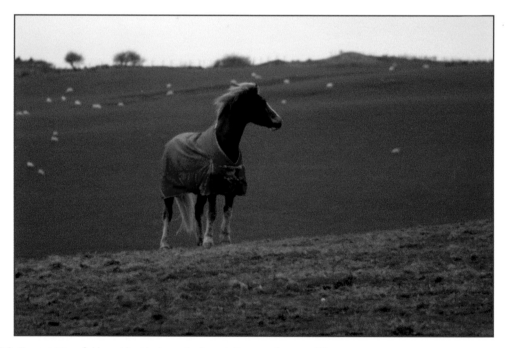

Fig. 17.6. Turnout into a field provides ideal exercise for a stallion, weather permitting.

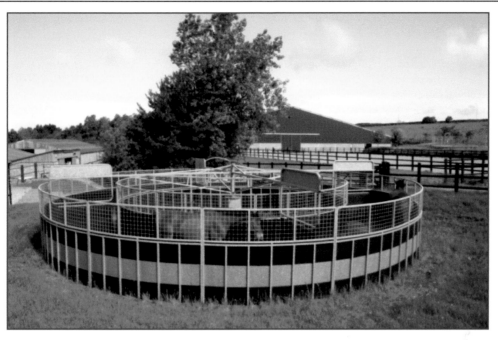

Fig. 17.7. Treadmills or horse walkers are a good means of forced exercise but should be restricted to stallions that are used to them.

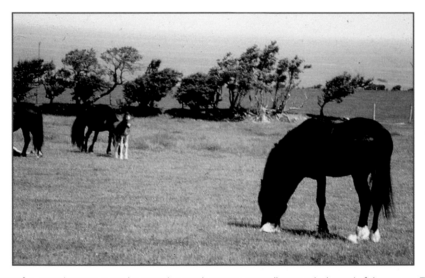

Fig. 17.8. Stallions of a quiet disposition can be turned out with mares, especially towards the end of the season. This relieves boredom in the stallion and allows mares returning to service to be re-covered. (Photo courtesy of Derwen International Stud.)

Recently, work by the Swiss National Stud demonstrated that working stallions can be safely turned out as a group during the non-breeding season, provided that a large area of land is available (Freymond *et al.*, 2013).

Exercise must be closely monitored, along with nutrition, to ensure that the stallion remains in body condition score (CS) 3. He must not be over-exerted or he will not have enough energy for the real job in hand.

17.5.3. Nutrition

A properly balanced diet is essential for a stallion's well-being. Each stallion should be fed individually according to factors such as his size, condition, work-load and temperament. He should be in CS 3 and his feed should be carefully monitored throughout the year to maintain this. One of the problems encountered with older stallions is obesity. Good nutrition and exercise management can prevent this. During the breeding season the workload of a stallion with a full book of mares is, in nutritional terms, as great as that of a performance horse. As a general rule, a stallion should have a daily dry matter intake (DMI) of 2–3% of body weight; at least 50% of this should be of good-quality roughage (Hintz, 1993b; Jackson, 2011). Young, growing stallions may require a slightly higher proportion of concentrates (i.e. a ratio of 6:4 concentrates:roughage).

17.5.3.1. Energy

For a 500-kg stallion daily digestible energy (DE) levels of 21.8 Mcal, similar to those for horses in heavy work, are recommended during the breeding season and 18.2 Mcal day^{-1} for the non-breeding season (Tables 11.2, 17.1, 17.2; Hintz, 1993b; Hurtgen, 2000; National Research Council, 2007). DE is particularly important in stallions in heavy work, with a difference of up to 15% in requirements being reported between a stallion with a breeding load of 70 mares per season and one serving 14 mares per season (Siciliano et al., 1993).

17.5.3.2. Protein

For a 500-kg mature, working stallion, a crude protein (CP) daily intake of 789 g is recommended, with higher levels for young stallions. In the non-breeding season requirements are 720 g day^{-1}. As with feeding mares and youngsters, the quality of protein is assumed to be as important as quantity; however, there has been no scientific work carried out in stallions. It is assumed that, in common with other horses, lysine may well be the most limiting amino acid and as such should be monitored in the diet (Tables 11.2, 17.1, 17.2; Hintz, 1993b; Hurtgen, 2000; National Research Council, 2007).

17.5.3.3. Vitamins and minerals

Many breeders feed a vitamin and mineral supplement on a free-access basis to stallions, regardless of feed analysis. This is not always necessary, but can be used as a precaution. The only vitamin that is likely to be short in a well-balanced diet is Vitamin A (Ralston et al., 1986). However, the inclusion of roughage in the diet in the form of leafy green forages, which are high in Vitamin A, helps to address this potential shortfall (Hintz, 1993b; Hurtgen, 2000). There is no research that indicates that any single nutrient can improve sperm quality or quantity (Steiner, 2000).

Inappropriate nutrition is one of the major causes of low libido and poor reproductive performance. Correct monitoring of a stallion's condition and adjustment of nutrition and exercise, accordingly, cannot be overemphasized. However, sudden changes to feeding immediately prior to the breeding season can have as detrimental an effect on performance as over- or under-nutrition per se (Hintz, 1993b).

17.5.3.4. Water

As with all horses, access to a clean, reliable water source is essential. A working stallion of 500 kg in an ambient temperature of 20°C may well require in excess of 50 l day^{-1} (10 l 100kg^{-1} body weight day^{-1}). In comparison, a similar stallion not in work (i.e. maintenance requirement only) would require only 25 l day^{-1} (5 l per 100 kg body weight per day; Frape, 2004; National Research Council, 2007). Water is particularly important in stallions as (unlike mares) they tend to be housed, and so fed more conserved forage and concentrate feeds.

Table 17.1. Daily nutrient requirements of stallions of varying weights. (From National Research Council, 2007.)

Animal	Weight (kg)	DE (Mcal)	CP (g)	Lysine (g)	Ca (g)	P (g)	Mg (g)	K (g)	Vitamin A (10³ IU)
Stallion (working)	200	8.7	316	13.6	12	7.2	3.8	11.4	8
	500	21.8	789	33.9	30	18.0	9.5	28.5	20
	900	39.2	1421	61.1	54	32.4	17.1	51.3	36
Stallion (non-breeding)	200	7.3	288	12.4	8	5.6	3.0	10.0	8
	500	18.2	720	31.0	20	14.0	7.5	25.0	20
	900	32.7	1296	55.7	36	25.2	13.5	45.0	36

DE, digestible energy; CP, crude protein; Ca, calcium; P, phosphorus; Mg, magnesium; K, potassium; IU, international unit.

Table 17.2. Expected feed consumption by stallions (percentage of body weight). (From National Research Council, 1989.)

Animal	Forage	Concentrate	Total
Mature stallion	1.0–2.5	1.0–1.5	2.0–3.0
Young stallion	0.75–2.25	1.25–1.75	2.0–3.0

17.5.4. Feet care

The feet of a stallion should never be neglected. Lameness can severely reduce and restrict the stallion's ability to cover. This is especially evident in hindlimb lameness and is often first evident as uncharacteristically low libido. Ideally, a stallion should not be shod during the breeding season, as shoes can inflict more damage than unshod feet. Regular trimming at 6–8-week intervals should be carried out to ensure that the feet remain clean and un-cracked. Any problems should be dealt with immediately to avoid long-term complications. Appropriate feeding and regular turnout is conducive to good-quality hooves, again reinforcing the ideal of keeping stallions in paddocks for at least part of the day (Hurtgen, 2000).

17.5.5. Dental care

Rough and uneven teeth, along with lesions or abscesses, can reduce a stallion's appetite because of pain. They can also cause food to pass into the stomach without full mastication, reducing the efficiency of digestion. If a stallion starts to lose condition for no obvious reason, one of the first things to check is his teeth and mouth. In any case, a stallion's mouth should be checked annually to see whether attention is required (Fig. 17.9).

17.5.6. Vaccination

Vaccination is an essential part of a preventative medicine routine that should be developed and implemented regularly for a stallion throughout his life. The vaccinations required depend upon the country in which the stallion resides and on the prevalence of various infections. In the UK, stallions should have up-to-date influenza and tetanus inoculations. Vaccination against equine herpes virus 1 (EHV1) is becoming more popular in UK, and is also available now for equine viral arteritis (EVA; Timoney and McCollum, 1997; Wilson, 2005; Holyoak *et al.*, 2008; Timoney, 2011a; Thein, 2012; Balasuriya *et al.*, 2018). In other parts of the world vaccination for rabies, botulism, eastern and western encephalomyelitis, African horse sickness and Potomac horse fever may be considered; vaccination against strangles is possible but not popular because of side

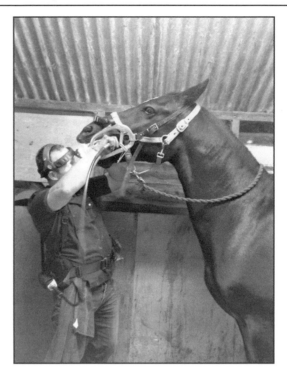

Fig. 17.9. Regular dental care for all breeding stock is essential to ensure optimum use of feed and general welfare.

effects (see Section 14.3.5.7). In general, it is advised that any vaccination is administered at least 60 days before breeding starts, to ensure that any resultant fever does not affect breeding performance (Hurtgen, 2000; Steiner, 2000; Wilson, 2011).

17.5.7. Swabbing

Swabbing of the stallion's genitalia to test for pathogenic bacteria, as detailed in Section 16.3.2, is practised more and more. An annual series of swabs is a compulsory requirement for Thoroughbreds and is increasingly demanded by other breed societies. Swabs are normally taken from the prepuce, urethral fossa and sheath at the beginning of each season, and if a problem is suspected.

17.5.8. Parasite control

Worming is another essential part of a preventative medicine routine. As with all wormers in all horses, the key to success is regular use in combination with good grazing management, dung removal and rotation of the product to ensure that resistance does not develop. *Strongylus vulgaris* (one of the three large strongyles) used to be the biggest problem for adult horses, including stallions (Kaplan and Nielsen, 2010) (Section 11.5.3). However, *S. vulgaris* is now rarely seen in managed horses, and the parasite of biggest concern is cyathostomins (small strongyles) (Shideler, 1993d; Love *et al.*, 1999; Nielsen, 2016). Parasite control must, therefore, be geared to addressing this challenge (Section 11.5.3). In common with any other parasitic infection, a high worm count causes listlessness and hence low libido and reduced reproductive performance. Targeted worming, in combination with faecal egg count monitoring, should be part of any worming regime (Lyons *et al.*, 2011). Some wormers are themselves reported to cause listlessness and reduced libido, but only for a few days after administration. Bearing this in mind, some studs try to organize their worming regime so that stallions are not wormed at the height of their covering season.

17.6. Stallion Vices

Many stallions are in danger of developing bad habits, stereotypies or vices owing to boredom and isolation (Visser *et al.*, 2008), largely because of current management practices. Prevention is infinitely better than cure and it is, therefore, essential that the stallion's management is geared appropriately (McBride and Hemmings, 2005). A regular routine of work, exercise, feeding, etc., and a stable in an area of the yard where activity can be observed, goes a long way to achieving this. A frustrated and bored stallion releases his energies and tensions in the only way possible to him, by developing vices. These vices can be harmful to the stallion himself, dangerous to the handler and may also affect his reproductive performance. If prevention has failed, and vices have developed, it is often beneficial for aesthetic and occasionally for health reasons to discourage them, and there are certain practices that can help control them and/or their effects.

17.6.1. Stereotypic behaviour

The cause of stereotypic behaviour is unknown (McGreevey *et al.*, 1995; McGreevey, 2011; Roberts *et al.*, 2017). Initially it was considered to be solely the result of poor management, isolation and boredom. Indeed, such behaviour is at least in part a means by which horses cope with such stress (Mason and Latham, 2004; McBride and Hemmings, 2005). However, stress and stereotypic behaviour themselves have been linked to reduced reproductive success (Graham and Card, 2007; Benhajali *et al.*, 2014). This, along with the involvement of gastric ulcers/acidity in stereotypic behaviour,

make such behaviour of increasing concern to stallion owners. Additionally, over time stereotypic behaviours become increasingly divorced from their initial cause, as they continue to be expressed even though management has changed.

17.6.1.1. Crib biting and wind sucking

Crib biting and wind sucking are related stereotypies, one often developing from the other. During crib biting the horse bites part of the stable structure or other convenient object (Fig. 17.10). It is thought to develop from the horse's natural urge to eat or graze regularly. The condition is exacerbated when feed is delivered in small concentrate meals with limited roughage. Increasing roughage and allowing *ad libitum* availability will certainly reduce the chance of this vice developing and will help alleviate the condition in sufferers. The habit can be discouraged by removing all objects that can be grasped by the teeth, or by painting structures with one of the several deterrent substances available. Wind sucking can develop on from crib biting and, in this more serious condition, the horse – while grasping the projecting structure – arches his neck and gulps in air. If the habit is allowed to continue unchecked it can lead to colic and reduced appetite, as well as to excessive wear and tear on the upper incisor teeth. A muzzle can be used to prevent both vices, or a cribbing strap can be placed around the horse's throat. This prevents the stallion from tensing the neck muscles used in wind sucking and may also help (Fig. 17.11).

A more extreme method of preventing wind sucking is to sever the neck muscles attaching the hyoid bone to the base of the tongue. Alternatively, the nerves serving these muscles can be severed. Such a procedure will effect a cure in the majority of cases and, in the remainder, considerable improvement is obtained; but these are drastic solutions to a problem that is largely avoidable with appropriate management (McGreevey *et al.*, 1995).

17.6.1.2. Weaving and stable walking

Weaving involves the lateral swaying of the horse's head and neck rhythmically from side to side, often over the stable door. This can cause damage to the forelegs as the horse's weight is repeatedly shifted from side to side. The condition is thought to develop from the horse's natural urge to move continuously, associated with grazing in groups over large tracts of land. Confinement and removal of companions are reported by some to be the trigger, hence housing in social groups or close to others (or even the provision of a mirror to simulate company) have all been reported to reduce the incidence of weaving (Cooper *et al.*, 2000; McAfee *et al.*, 2002; Mills and Riezebos, 2005). A chronic weaver may weave himself to the point of exhaustion. The condition can be alleviated by anti-weave bars over the lower stable door (Fig. 17.12).

Unfortunately, chronic weavers will often continue to weave within their boxes. Furthermore, stable walking may develop, in which the stallion continually paces around his box, seemingly chasing his tail. There is little that can be done to cure this behaviour except to turn the horse out into a paddock to relieve the boredom, but such horses often then fence walk and usually revert to stable walking as soon as they are stabled again (Mills and Nankervis, 1999).

17.6.2. Self-mutilation

Self-mutilation is not strictly a stereotypic or abnormal behaviour but nevertheless can be extremely distressing to the stallion and his owner. The stallion bites his own legs, shoulders and chest, causing himself some considerable damage. It is normally particularly evident after mating. If evident only then, thorough washing of the stallion after dismount reduces expression of the vice, which in this case is thought to be due to the smell of the mare. If, however, the stallion is a habitual self-mutilator, there is very little that can be done to cure him, although the use of a muzzle or cradle can prevent him from inflicting damage (McDonnell, 2011b).

17.6.3. Masturbation

Masturbation by a stallion is considered by some to be a further vice, thought to originate from boredom,

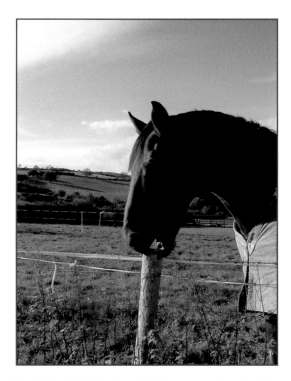

Fig. 17.10. Crib biting is a relatively common stereotypic behaviour, and involves the grasping of protruding surfaces such as stable doors, but may also be seen in horses turned out. (Photo courtesy of Dr Sebastian McBride.)

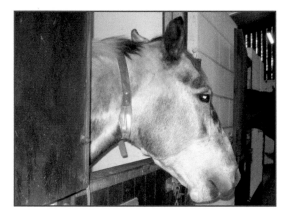

Fig. 17.11. A cribbing strap may be used to prevent the stallion from tensing the neck muscles required for wind sucking.

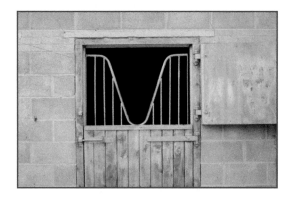

Fig. 17.12. When the top door of the stable is open, anti-weave bars may be used to discourage the stallion from weaving over the bottom door.

especially if sexually frustrated. However, it is evident that feral and wild ponies also demonstrate such behaviour. It has been suggested, therefore, that it is a natural behaviour rather than a problem, and any problem lies with human perception and potential embarrassment. The old-fashioned use of penile rings, etc., is now frowned upon as unnecessary. Masturbation is expressed by the stallion rubbing the extended penis along the underside of his abdomen. In extreme cases masturbation may result in ejaculation and concern over the loss of valuable sperm. Providing the stallion's workload is not too high, such behaviour should not affect his fertility rates; indeed, increasing his workload may go some way to reducing it (Pickett, 1993d; McDonnell, 2000b, 2011b).

17.6.4. Aggressive behaviour

Some stallions develop extremely aggressive behaviour and become a danger to both handlers and mares (McDonnell, 2000b, 2011b). Occasionally this behaviour is associated with certain conditions or restraint, or is directed towards certain people, and can be averted by avoiding such situations. However, more often than not, it is expressed generally and is due to mismanagement during his formative years. If the behaviour is beyond control, the stallion can be gelded. In the vast majority of cases, gelding significantly reduces aggressive tendencies. If the stallion must remain entire then certain measures can, and should, be used to protect handlers and mares. He should be muzzled and a neck guard used on the mares to prevent him savaging them during covering, and possibly should be controlled by a pole attached to his bit, giving his handler more control. The only option for some stallions may be artificial insemination (AI). In deciding whether to continue to use an aggressive stallion, it must be certain that his behaviour is management induced and not inherited, as it is very important that such behaviour is not perpetuated in subsequent generations.

Rearing and striking out with the front feet constitute a relatively common vice, although potentially very dangerous to handlers. This should be corrected, especially in young stallions, where the vice can be cured. To avoid being kicked, the handler should always stand to one side of the stallion, and never in front. A long lead rein should be used so that contact can still be maintained from a distance if the stallion rears. As soon as the stallion starts to rear, his lead rein should be jerked sharply, along with a verbal reprimand. Backing the stallion at the first signs of rearing can also help to avert the situation. The use of a chain under the chin is one of the more popular forms of stallion restraint, but has been reported to be associated with a higher incidence of rearing, and hence may be best avoided.

Finally, biting is another relatively common vice in stallions. This should be corrected at a young age by a short, sharp jerk on the lead rein, or a sharp tap on the muzzle, and verbal reprimand as punishment. If allowed to continue, a stallion can become almost impossible to handle. Some stallions only bite in certain situations, such as when they are eating, after mating, when they are being groomed or when fed by hand. Such situations should, therefore, be reduced to a minimum and any handlers warned of the problem.

17.7. Conclusion

Stallion management from a very early age has important implications for reproductive ability, behaviour and safety. Many problems encountered in stallions that either do not perform to their full potential or exhibit antisocial or dangerous behaviour stem from mismanagement at an early age. One of the major problems encountered with stallions is boredom and stress due to confinement and isolation. This can directly affect libido, performance and other behavioural characteristics. Unfortunately, this often becomes a self-perpetuating downward spiral that is very difficult to break. Many of the problems encountered in the management of stallions can be averted by consistent discipline and providing turnout, social interaction and activity.

Study Questions

Ideally the working stallion should have a body condition score of 3. Discuss the management of the stallion to achieve this.

Confinement of stallions is a major welfare concern. Discuss why stallions traditionally are confined and evaluate the management options available to address this concern.

Discipline is essential in the stallion. Discuss how this can be achieved, and the consequences of having an ill-disciplined stallion.

Critically evaluate the central role that housing and exercise play in a stallion's mental and physical well-being.

Suggested Reading

Conboy, H.S. (2011) The novice breeding stallion. In: McKinnon, A.O., Squires, E.L., Vaala, W.E. and Varner, D.D. (eds) *Equine Reproduction*, 2nd edn. Wiley-Blackwell, Philadelphia, London, pp. 1396–1401.

Jackson, S.G. (2011) Nutrition and exercise for breeding stallions. In: McKinnon, A.O., Squires, E.L., Vaala, E. and Varner, D.D. (eds) *Equine Reproduction*, 2nd edn. Wiley-Blackwell, Philadelphia, London, pp. 1228–1239.

Varner, D.D. (2011) Handling the breeding stallion. In: McKinnon, A.O., Squires, E.L., Vaala, W.E. and Varner, D.D. (eds) *Equine Reproduction*, 2nd edn. Wiley-Blackwell, Philadelphia, London, pp. 1391–1395.

Popescu, S., Lazar, E.A., Borda, C., Niculae, M., Sandru, C.D. and Spinu, M. (2019) Welfare quality of breeding horses under different housing conditions. *Animals* 9 (3), 81.

18 Infertility in the Stallion

The Objectives of this Chapter are:

To apply the anatomy and physiology knowledge gained from Section A to identify abnormalities and causes of infertility.

To gain an appreciation of why fertilization might fail.

To provide you with the knowledge that enables you to have an informed discussion with veterinarians when reproduction fails, and to make appropriate management choices.

18.1. Introduction

Infertility is a vast topic and so this Chapter will provide just an introduction to stallion infertility and provide a basis from which further information can be sought. Infertility may have its root cause in either the stallion or the mare. A similar approach has been taken with respect to mare infertility in Chapter 14. On average, a stallion might be expected to cover 1–2 mares per day during the breeding season, with a rest day every 7–10 days. This gives reasonable results, with fertilization rates of about 60–80% (Baker *et al.*, 1993; Morris and Allen, 2002b; Allen *et al.*, 2007b; Allen and Wilsher, 2018; Rose *et al.*, 2018). These figures are only an average and are affected by many things, as discussed for the mare (Chapter 14), including the type and condition of mares presented to a stallion and also by the characteristics of the individual stallion. Some stallions are capable of much heavier workloads: it is not uncommon for popular Thoroughbred stallions to cover 3–4 mares per day, but some struggle with fewer (Pickett and Shiner, 1994). One of the major responsibilities of the stallion manager is to be aware of the limitations of their individual stallion and to work within these constraints (Kenney, 1990).

Research into the causes of infertility in the stallion is relatively limited because of previous concentration on the mare. However, in any breeding programme, 50% of the outcome is determined by the stallion, and so deserves fair discussion. The difficulty in obtaining standard figures for fertility (Section 14.1) and the reluctance of the majority of stallion owners to select for reproductive performance and to assess for breeding soundness have led to relatively low average fertility rates. Before discussing the subject further, the following glossary should be noted to prevent confusion in terms:

- sterility – permanent inability to reproduce;
- infertility – temporary inability to reproduce;
- subfertility – inability, either temporary or permanent, to reproduce at full potential;
- impotency – temporary or permanent inability to ejaculate semen (sperm capable of fertilizing an ovum may, however, be produced).

As with the mare, reproductive failure may be due to extrinsic and/or intrinsic factors.

18.2. Extrinsic Factors Affecting Reproductive Efficiency in the Stallion

Extrinsic factors affecting the reproductive efficiency of a stallion include lack of use, the presentation of subfertile or infertile mares, poor mare management, poor stallion management, imposition of an artificial breeding season and dual hemisphere covering. Each of these factors will be discussed in turn in the context of reproductive efficiency/infertility. It will be noted that many aspects have already been discussed in previous chapters, especially those concerning management, and so such details will not be repeated here.

18.2.1. Lack of use

Reproductive efficiency in any animal reflects its use. A stallion may not be used in a particular year by design, or because of financial or management considerations. Disease may also preclude a stallion from use for part or all of a season (owing to the risk of direct disease transfer to mares in the case of venereal or contagious diseases) or may limit his ability to perform (in the case of non-contagious diseases). Alternatively, the stallion may have suffered from disease or infection during the previous year and is not to be used in the following season to allow full recovery, or because the long-term effects of disease on his reproductive performance make it inappropriate to use him until he has fully recovered. Diseases of the stallion's reproductive tract will be discussed later as intrinsic factors (Section 18.3.5).

Finally, semen evaluation is part of good practice, and should be carried out regularly at the beginning of each season. Poor semen quality may lead to the stallion being taken out of use until the cause has been isolated and the problem solved.

18.2.2. Subfertile or infertile mare

Both mare and stallion are equally responsible for fertilization. A stallion is only as good as the mare he is to cover, and vice versa. It is essential that any mare presented to a stallion is capable of reproducing and does not suffer from any of the factors affecting reproduction discussed in Chapter 14. If the mare herself is subfertile or infertile, lack of success cannot be blamed on the stallion.

18.2.3. Poor mare management

Mare management is discussed in detail in Chapters 8–14. Inappropriate management will adversely affect the mare's ability to conceive and, therefore, the apparent fertility rates of the stallion that covered her. The most important management area as far as stallion reproductive efficiency is concerned is during the time of covering. Service at an inappropriate time, due to a failure to detect oestrus and ovulation accurately, will obviously be reflected in poor fertility rates. Failure to detect oestrus is usually a result of either prolonged dioestrus preventing oestrus from being displayed, or of infrequent or inaccurate teasing, along with lack of records and mare observation. In such cases, veterinary examination by means of rectal palpation and/or scanning have been shown to significantly improve fertility rates by allowing more accurate detection of ovulation.

18.2.4. Poor stallion management

Stallion management is discussed in detail in Chapters 15–17. All aspects of a stallion's management will affect his ability to cover mares successfully. Stallion management, as far as it directly affects reproductive efficiency, can be subdivided into the following categories.

18.2.4.1. Excess workload

The amount of work or number of mares a stallion may be expected to successfully cover during a season is highly variable (Pickett and Shiner, 1994), as discussed previously. It is one of the responsibilities of stallion managers to know the capabilities of their stallions. The workload of a stallion depends upon the ability of his testis to produce sperm and on epididymal sperm storage reserves. Among other things, this is a function of testis size, which can be assessed by calipers or ultrasonically (Fig. 18.1; Love *et al.*, 1991). Twenty years ago the normal expected workload was 40–50 mares per season. Today, popular stallions may cover up to 200 mares per season by natural service, and artificial insemination (AI) increases this number significantly.

Stallions with large testes have larger daily sperm outputs and can cope with a heavier workload than stallions with smaller testes. Testis size is positively correlated with age (at least until mature body size is reached) and so, therefore, with workload (which has an important bearing on fertility) (Douglas and Umphenour, 1992; Pickett and Shiner, 1994; Dowsett and Knott, 1996). It is a good idea, especially with new stallions, to carry out a full semen analysis to give a guide to daily sperm production (Section 21.4).

Sperm concentrations are usually in the range of $100–300 \times 10^6$ sperm ml^{-1} and, for successful fertilization, $300–500 \times 10^6$ sperm are required (Squires, 2011a). On average, 50–60% of sperm produced can be classified as normal progressively motile sperm capable of fertilizing an ovum. The average daily sperm production for a stallion is $0.6–6 \times 10^9$ depending upon season, environment, age, etc. (Parlevliet *et al.*, 1994; Colenbrander *et al.*, 2003; Ball, 2014; Barrier-Battut *et al.*, 2016). From these figures it is apparent that, in theory, a stallion could be expected to perform an average of 1–3 successful services per day. There are, however, other considerations to take into account when looking at workloads.

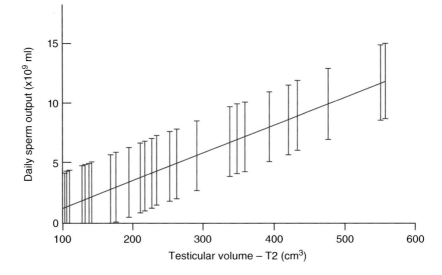

Fig. 18.1. The relationship between testicular volume and daily sperm output. (From Love *et al.*, 1991.)

It is interesting to note that total sperm production per week is the same, regardless of whether a stallion is used daily or on alternate days. However, daily use results in a lower concentration of sperm per millilitre (Pickett *et al.*, 1975). This may be of no consequence in stallions with high daily sperm production rates, as concentrations will still be acceptable, but daily use of stallions with lower daily sperm production figures may have a detrimental effect on fertility rates. More recent work by Sieme *et al.* (2004a) indicates that optimum fertility rates are achieved with heavier workloads, in excess of one mating or AI collection per day, and that infrequent use (less than one mating 48 h⁻¹) is detrimental to semen quality.

Excessive workloads may, however, result in a lack of libido. As a result, the stallion will be slow to breed or may even fail to ejaculate. In such cases, it is best to take the stallion out of work for a short period of time and reintroduce him a week or so later. If libido is still low, it may well be indicative of further problems.

In an ideal world, a stallion would be used just once or twice a day and given regular periods of rest of 1–2 days every 10 days or so; this is particularly important in young stallions. However, there are many pressures, not least financial, that entice stallion managers to increase workloads. Individual variation means that some stallions can cope with up to four mares per day, during periods of excessive use in a busy season, provided they are given adequate periods of rest.

18.2.4.2. *Training management and behaviour*

Early training is of utmost importance in the long-term ability of a stallion to perform to his full potential (Section 17.2). A stallion brought up in a relaxed, unstressed environment with consistent, fair discipline and respect is much more likely to perform to his full potential in later life.

One of the major problems encountered as a carry-over effect from early life, which is often unappreciated, is stallion isolation. Many managers isolate stallions to ensure the safety of personnel, other stock on the yard and the stallions themselves. This is a self-perpetuating problem, and such treatment often results in boredom, vices and excessive excitability and unpredictability, which in turn results in further isolation in the interests of safety. A happy medium between safety and stallion participation in the general yard activities has to be achieved.

Breeding behavioural abnormalities and, with these, an inability or lack of willingness to cover a mare and ejaculatory dysfunction may be seen (McDonnell, 2011b). They can have several causes including inappropriate early training, presenting a young stallion with challenging mares or too high a work load, and all can have a negative effect on breeding behaviour. Physical abnormality (often genetic in origin) as well as psychology may be the cause of ejaculatory dysfunction. Overuse in older stallions has also been associated with poor libido. Reducing workloads and/or presenting a stallion to a mare in a more natural scenario (such as natural mating) and then gradual retraining, particularly in the case of the young stallion, can work. Stallions can also be completely removed from breeding for that year and reintroduced the following year; or, sometimes, simply a change in routine can have a positive effect. Finally, letting the stallion watch a mature stallion covering a mare may also invigorate mating behaviour (Ball, 2014). Androgen therapy, such as testosterone or gonadotrophin-releasing hormone (GnRH) along with xylazine and/or imipramine for ejaculatory dysfunction have been reported to be successful but should be a last resort (McDonnell 2001, 2011c,d). Behavioural issues are not be restricted to low libido: slow breeders or overzealous stallions may also be a problem. These stallions require careful, experienced handling and their management emphasizes the importance of good discipline and respect for all working stallions.

18.2.4.3. Breeding discomfort

Full physical examination of the stallion is essential before purchase to ensure that no abnormalities are present (see Chapter 15 for details). It is also advisable that stallions undergo regular examinations at the beginning of each season to ensure that no problems have arisen since the last season. Pain associated with the act of covering can cause a permanent reduction in libido. Poor feet care or conditions such as laminitis or navicular disease cause pain on mounting, especially if the problem is in the hind feet. Muscular or skeletal problems, including arthritis, may also limit the stallion's ability to mount as a result of pain. Irritation and soreness of the penis or sheath area may also cause pain at covering, especially if smegma has accumulated, or soap or antiseptic wash has not been rinsed thoroughly. Breeding accidents involving inadequate erection at intromission, kicking by a mare and rough handling will discourage a stallion from future covering, as he will associate covering with pain. Finally, when using an artificial vagina (AV), care should be taken that the internal temperature is not too hot, as this will cause pain and will reduce his future willingness, not only to use an AV, but also in natural service.

18.2.4.4. Nutrition

Appropriate nutrition throughout the year is essential to ensure that the stallion is in optimum physical condition for the season (Section 17.5.3). Obese or excessively thin stallions suffer from low libido, and nutrition – along with exercise – is a major determinant of body condition. A body condition score (CS) of 3 on a scale of 1–5 is to be aimed for.

Only limited research has been carried out into specific deficiencies. It is known that, in general, severe nutritional deficiency is associated with a delay in puberty, testicular atrophy and a reduction in sperm production. Deficiencies in energy and, to a lesser extent, protein, have also been associated with low reproductive efficiency (Jainudeen and Hafez, 1993; National Research Council, 2007; Jackson, 2011). Severe deficiencies in Vitamins A and E and selenium are specifically associated with a reduction in spermatogenesis in other farm animals and have been suggested to have a similar, but as yet unproven, effect in stallions (Ralston et al., 1986). In addition, low dietary intake of copper (Cu), iron (Fe) and/or cobalt (Co) results in a reduction in appetite with accompanying weight loss and anaemia and, via these, a potential decline in semen production (Jainudeen and Hafez, 1993).

Obesity will result in a loss of libido and may also cause a reduction in spermatogenesis. Obesity is associated with excess fat deposition within the scrotum, increasing scrotal insulation and hence causing an increase in testicular temperature, with an associated decline in spermatogenic efficiency.

18.2.4.5. Chemicals and drugs

It is essential that, if a stallion has been on any drug regime, time must be allowed for the drug to be eliminated from his system prior to use (Section 16.3.1).

Although illegal in many countries, and/or in competitions, anabolic steroids (testosterone derivatives) are sometimes used in an attempt to improve male characteristics such as weight gain, muscle growth and performance in young horses. They have also been used in attempts to improve stallion libido. In humans and other animals, such use of anabolic steroids is known to be associated with infertility, and a similar association has been indicated in stallions (Snow, 1993; Amann, 2011c). Anabolic steroids have been reported to result in a decrease of up to 40% in testicular size and weight (Blanchard et al., 1983; Snow, 1993; Koskinen et al., 1997) and a change in testicular vascularization (Teubner et al., 2015). Spermatogenesis is also reduced, with fewer sperm per gram of testicular tissue being produced, and lower sperm motility rates (Squires et al., 1982; Blanchard et al., 1983; Snow, 1993). Anabolic steroids have been successful in improving libido; however, this is invariably accompanied by an increase in aggression, which is a significant drawback and limits their breeding use (Snow, 1993).

Anabolic steroids are, therefore, not recommended for stallions in breeding work. Not only do these drugs have an immediate effect, but they may also have a long-term effect, certainly until they are completely eliminated from the stallion's system.

Testosterone itself has been used to improve libido in stallions, and with some success, but it has serious potential side effects as far as fertility is concerned as well as increasing aggression. Chapter 7 outlines the fine control and delicate hormonal balance controlling male reproductive functions. If one component of the system is altered, the delicate balance of the whole system is affected. Hence, if a stallion is treated with testosterone (or similar compound), this increases circulating levels, which in turn act as a negative feedback on the hypothalamus and pituitary, reducing gonadotrophin-releasing hormone and in turn luteinizing hormone (LH) and follicle-stimulating hormone (FSH) release, so reducing stimulation of the testes including sperm production (Squires *et al.*, 1997; Nagata, 2000; Nagata *et al.*, 2000). Testosterone therapy is, therefore, associated with low fertility owing to reduced sperm counts, and hence is not advised for use in stallions in work, unless under veterinary supervision (Amann, 2011c).

Little work has been done to investigate the effect of other drugs such as corticosteroids, wormers, antiparasitics and antibiotics. It is known that, in mares, such drugs can have an adverse effect (Section 9.4.1). The limited evidence in stallions indicates that, at therapeutic doses, these drugs do not have an effect (Juhász *et al.*, 2001). However, the use of any drug or treatment that causes appetite depression, diarrhoea or lack of condition is ill-advised during the breeding season and should only be used under veterinary supervision. The fear and anecdotal reports that some wormers are associated with a temporary decline in fertility mean that many breeders arrange their parasite control regimes to ensure that stallions are not treated during the breeding season.

18.2.5. Imposed breeding season

Reproductive activity in the stallion, as in the mare, is naturally limited by a breeding season, although with enough encouragement most will cover mares out of season (Pickett and Shiner, 1994). Season affects the number of sperm per ejaculate, total sperm number, number of mounts per successful ejaculation and reaction times (Section 7.3.1). As a result, fertilization potential

out of season is significantly reduced. The natural breeding season, with its optimum fertilization rates and libido, is nature's way of ensuring that foals are born during the spring and early summer to maximize their chances of survival.

Unfortunately, this natural breeding season does not coincide with the arbitrary breeding season man has imposed in an attempt to achieve foaling as near as possible to 1 January. This is the official registered birth date of all foals in several breed societies, the Thoroughbred being the most well known. The arbitrary breeding season in the northern hemisphere starts on 15 February, as opposed to the natural breeding season that starts in April/May. In the southern hemisphere the imposed season starts 15 August, as opposed to the natural season in October/November. Stallions are, therefore, expected to cover mares at a time of the year when their libido and fertilization rates are naturally low and when they are unable to perform to their full potential. The adverse effect of season on reproductive efficiency is increasingly evident in older stallions (Johnson and Thompson, 1983).

Reduced use at either end of the non-breeding season can be quite successful, but a full workload can in no way be expected. Exact performance depends on the individual animal, but improved fertilization rates and libido can be obtained by the use of artificial lighting in the stallion's stable from November onwards, to give 16 h light and 8 h dark, so mimicking the early onset of spring and advancing the breeding season (Section 16.4; Clay and Clay, 1992; Deichsel *et al.*, 2016).

18.2.6. Dual hemisphere covering

Since the 1990s many popular stallions, in particular Thoroughbreds, are shuttled annually from the northern to the southern hemisphere, and vice versa. This allows them to have two breeding seasons, covering mares in the northern and southern breeding seasons (Digby, 1996). Not a lot of work has been done on the effect of shuttling on reproductive performance; however, it is evident that libido in particular may suffer, and that stallions should be carefully selected so they can withstand the physical and psychological stress of shuttling. It is unclear whether shuttling affects sperm quality; initial work by Pickett and Voss (1998a,b) indicated no adverse effect and more recent work by Walbornn *et al.* (2017) supported this. However, other reports, plus anecdotal evidence, have suggested that for some stallions at least an adverse effect may be seen (Umphenour *et al.*, 2011).

18.3. Intrinsic Factors Affecting Reproductive Performance in the Stallion

These include age, and chromosomal, hormonal, physical and semen abnormalities. These will be discussed in turn in the context of reproductive performance.

18.3.1. Age

Age is important in considering the potential fertility of a stallion. Young and old stallions may have problems with taking on a full workload with consistent success.

A young stallion is still learning the job and can easily be adversely affected by his handlers and/or management. He may, therefore, be slow to breed, mounting several times per successful ejaculation, failing to ejaculate, ejaculating prematurely or exhibiting enlargement of the glans penis before intromission. Careful treatment and handling during this period is essential to ensure that any such behavioural problems are not perpetuated (Naden *et al.*, 1990). As far as physical capabilities are concerned, puberty (18–36 months) heralds the beginning of sexual activity (Clay and Clay, 1992; Fukuda *et al.*, 2001). Three year-old stallions may, therefore, be used for covering and are perfectly capable of fertilizing a mare, but they have a limited sperm-producing capacity. By 4 years of age they are capable of producing adequate numbers of sperm to cover as many mares as an adult stallion, but fully consistent fertilizing capacity is not attained until full mature size, around 5 years of age on average (Berndston and Jones, 1989; Johnson *et al.*, 1991; Fukuda *et al.*, 2001). From this time sperm numbers have been reported by some to increase slightly, until 16 years of age, or to remain stable until old age (20 years) (Pickett *et al.*, 1989; Fukuda *et al.*, 2001).

At the other end of the spectrum, old age may be a problem. An age-related decrease in semen quality after 20 years of age has been reported by some (Johnson and Thompson, 1983; Amann, 1993a,b), but this is not supported by other work (Johnson *et al.*, 1991). More recent sperm genetic evaluation does suggest a decrease in sperm quality with age, with older stallions having a higher frequency of sex chromosome aberration and a significant positive correlation between age and disomy of XY, XX, YY and trisomy of XXY (Bugno-Poniewierska *et al.*, 2011). Additionally, age is reported to have a negative effect on sperm mitochondria and hence sperm motility (Darr *et al.*, 2017). Conditions such as epididymal fibrosis, which reduces epididymal sperm reserves and hence daily sperm production, have been linked to old age. However, a decline in fertility may well, at least in part, be is associated with general age-related problems such as arthritis, many of which cause pain on mounting, a major cause of low libido and, therefore, of low fertilization rates. If such problems are encountered they may be alleviated, to a certain extent, by the use of breeding platforms, or AI, as well as allowing the stallion extra time. The effect of age is very variable between different stallions, and older stallions should not automatically be precluded from use, as such animals have had many years in which to prove their worth as far as their own performance and that of their progeny are concerned. Older stallions often tend to be more gentlemanly to handle, know their job well and are good to use on maiden, shy or nervous mares, giving them confidence. When using an older stallion, it is particularly important that his semen should be evaluated regularly and monitored closely, to allow a reduction in his workload if a decline in semen quality is detected.

18.3.2. Chromosomal abnormalities

The normal chromosomal complement for the stallion is denoted as 64XY. Chromosomal abnormalities or genetic inadequacies may be the cause of infertility in stallions that otherwise appear fit (Millon and Penedo, 2009). These may be associated with semen abnormalities, or more obvious abnormalities of the genitalia. As with the mare (Section 14.3.2) the most common abnormalities involve the sex chromosomes. Intersex conditions occur where individuals are genetically male but show abnormal genitalia; these include hermaphrodites (both ovarian and testicular tissues are present internally with an intermediate male/female external genitalia) and pseudohermaphrodites (either ovarian or testicular tissue is present internally with an intermediate male/female external genitalia) (Keifer, 1976; Varner and Schumacher, 1999). Chromosomal abnormalities are very rare but the most common involve the X chromosome such as genetic chimeras or mosaics (63XO:64XY or 65XXY:64XY), sex reversal such as male syndrome (64XX but phenotypically male) and Klinefelter's syndrome (65XXY) have been reported in stallions (Halnan and Watson, 1982; Bowling *et al.*, 1987; Bowling, 1996; Makinen *et al.*, 2000; Durkin *et al.*, 2011). Other genetic abnormalities are associated with cryptorchidism (rig; Section 18.3.4.1) and testicular hypoplasia, both directly affecting reproductive efficiency (Varner and Schumacher, 1991).

Some genetic deformities, such as umbilical and inguinal hernias, may not affect reproduction directly but may preclude the stallion from use. These may correct themselves naturally but the trait may well be perpetuated in succeeding generations. More recently, detailed genetic analysis has allowed the identification of genes that result in impaired sperm acrosomes, sperm carrying various sex chromosome aneuploidies, sex chromosome aberrations, etc., all of which may cause subfertility as opposed to infertility (Bugno-Poniewierska *et al.*, 2011; Kjöllerström, 2016). Physical abnormalities of the reproductive system that are possibly linked to genetic factors will be discussed under the specific areas of the tract detailed below.

18.3.3. Hormonal abnormalities

The endocrine control of reproduction is governed by a finely balanced system (Roser, 2008) (Chapter 7). Circulating concentrations of testosterone have a direct effect on reproductive performance, on both libido and sperm production; low testosterone levels are often, therefore, blamed for poor fertility rates (Nett, 1993c; Shiner *et al.*, 1993). Testosterone, human chorionic gonadotrophin (hCG) and gonadotrophin-releasing hormone (GnRH) therapy have been used, with mixed success, to address this problem. The lack of success may well be because depressed pituitary function is the cause of infertility in only 1% of cases (Boyle *et al.*, 1991; Roser and Hughes, 1991). Abnormal hormone levels may be associated with hypothyroidism, resulting in delayed puberty, smaller testes, decreased spermatozoa production, decreased libido and cryptorchidism. Feminization of the genitalia may also be observed. It has been postulated that changes in thyroid function may be the cause of stallion summer infertility associated with elevated environmental temperatures (Brachen and Wagner, 1983). In theory plasma concentrations of LH, FSH and testosterone would be indicative of testicular function, degeneration, etc. (Douglas and Umphenour, 1992; Roser and Hughes, 1992a,b; Brinsko, 1996). It has also been suggested that testosterone release in response to hCG could be used to indicate testicular function (Roser, 2001b). Unfortunately, results have been inconsistent. Most recently interest has been expressed in using anti-mullerian hormone (AMH) levels in young animals as a biomarker to indicate gonadal function and hence future fertility. A correlation between AMH and post-pubertal follicular development has been demonstrated in mares. Work by Scarlet *et al.* (2018) indicated that a correlation exists

between AMH in 2-year-old colts and abnormal testicular development, suggesting it could be used as an indicator of a stallion's future breeding potential.

18.3.4. Physical abnormalities

Numerous abnormalities of the stallion's genitalia have been reported. As with most anatomical abnormalities, they are caused either by disease or are inherited. It is reported that one in five males has an anatomical abnormality, the significance of which varies from life-threatening to a minor flaw that may be of little consequence as far as reproductive performance is concerned, but may still reduce his market value. Only those most commonly encountered will be considered in the following sections.

18.3.4.1. Cryptorchidism

A cryptorchid stallion or a rig is an animal in which either one or both of the testes have failed to descend into the scrotum. The passage of the testes from a position next to the kidneys should occur, as a gradual process, *in utero* or during the first few months of life (Fig. 6.13; Arighi, 2011a,b). A cryptorchid stallion may be further classified as unilateral (failure of descent of one testis), bilateral (failure of descent of both testes), inguinal (undescended testis located in the inguinal region) or abdominal (undescended testis in the abdomen) (Figs 18.2 and 18.3; Cox, 1993a,b; Coomer *et al.*, 2016; Pollark, 2017).

The failure of testes to descend is reported to occur in 2–5% of colts (Hayes, 1986; Arighi, 2011a; Almeida *et al.*, 2013) and may be temporary (most will descend within 3 years of birth) or permanent. Cryptorchidism has a heritable component and has a higher incidence in ponies (particularly temporary retention) and in Quarter horses and Paint horses (particularly permanent retention) (Leipold, 1986; Cox, 1993a; Pollark, 2017). The retention of one or both testes results in a significant decline in testes weight in the retained testis, often accompanied by relative increase in epididymis size, even if it does subsequently descend (Cox, 1982; Almeida *et al.*, 2013). The size may be reduced by up to 20-fold in the abdominally retained testis; the reduction in size of the inguinally retained testis is not as great, but a difference of up to sevenfold has been reported (Fig. 18.4; Bishop *et al.*, 1964; Vilar *et al.*, 2018). A unilateral cryptorchid is perfectly capable of successfully covering mares, although his total sperm output per ejaculate will be reduced and he will, therefore, be unable to bear a full workload. In practice,

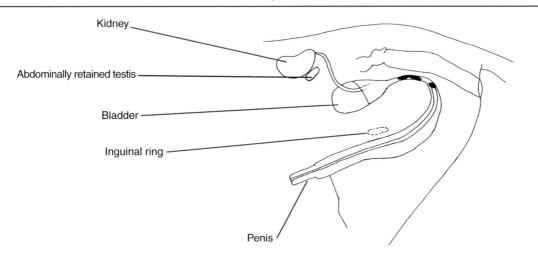

Fig. 18.2. An abdominal cryptorchid stallion is characterized by the testis lying up within the body cavity. In a unilateral abdominal cryptorchid, only one testis has failed to descend; in a bilateral, both remain in the body cavity.

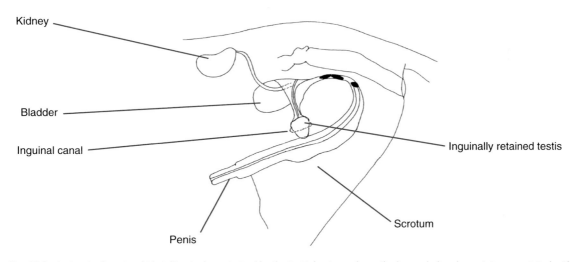

Fig. 18.3. An inguinal cryptorchid stallion is characterized by the testis having only partly descended and remaining associated with the inguinal ring. Failure of testis descent may be seen in both (bilateral) or only one (unilateral) testis.

however, it is not advised to breed cryptorchids owing to the possible heritability of the condition; indeed, several, but not all, breed societies do not allow such animals to be registered for use as a stallion. It is advised that cryptorchids are castrated; however, removal of the retained testis is not without complication, especially in abdominal cryptorchids, although the use of laparoscopic techniques now reduces the risks (Coomer *et al.*, 2016; Huppes *et al.*, 2017). Unfortunately it is, therefore, not uncommon for such animals to be unilaterally castrated, retaining the non-descended testis which, although it is not able to produce sperm, will continue to

produce testosterone (Cox *et al.*, 1973; Arighi, 2011a), and so an animal that outwardly appears to be a gelding will demonstrate stallion-like behaviour. Diagnosis of cryptorchidism is usually via blood test for oestrone sulfate. In animals aged 3 years or older, oestrone sulfate levels greater than 0.1 ng ml^{-1} indicate a retained testis (Cox *et al.*, 1986). In younger horses oestrone sulfate concentrations are less accurate. An alternative is to measure the release of testosterone in response to the challenge of a 6000 iu hCG injection. The presence of a retained testis is indicated by an increase in plasma concentrations of testosterone; in geldings no such reaction is seen (Silberzahn *et al.*, 1989; Lopate *et al.*, 2003). Others suggest that a simple test for plasma testosterone allows identification of cryptorchidism (Vilar *et al.*, 2018), as can serum AMH concentrations (Murase *et al.*, 2015), although these appear less accurate.

18.3.4.2. Hernias

Stallion hernias may be classified in a number of ways (Figs 18.5 and 18.6). All have the potential to affect spermatozoa production, due to an elevation in testicular temperature from the close proximity of the herniated part of the gastrointestinal tract (Cox, 1988; Frazer, 2008; Pollock and Russell, 2011; Ball, 2014).

Testicular hernias are usually due to accident or strain, but may also be congenital, owing to inherited

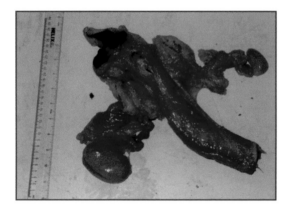

Fig. **18.4.** The testis dissected from a cryptorchid stallion post-slaughter. Note the significantly reduced size of the testis on the far right which was the inguinally retained testis.

abnormality (Varner and Schumacher, 1991; Cox, 1993a; Shoemaker *et al.*, 2004; Gracia-Calvo *et al.*, 2015). Testicular hernias may be further classified as inguinal or scrotal depending on the extent of herniation. Inguinal hernias result from intestinal tissue passing solely through the inguinal ring (Fig. 18.5; Stashak, 1993). Scrotal hernias result from further herniation where the intestine extends into the scrotum (Fig. 18.6; Varner and Schumacher, 1991). The most common form of hernia is the inguinal, especially in young foals, where large inguinal rings are the prime cause. Spontaneous recovery normally occurs within 3–6 months and no long-term detrimental effects have been reported (Varner and Schumacher, 1991). Surgical intervention is sometimes required; this is often unilateral or bilateral castration, at which time the inguinal canal can be closed. However, new procedures such as standing laparoscopic peritoneal flap hernioplasty (SLPFH) have been developed, to avoid reoccurrence of herniation and so preserve the stallion's breeding career (Van der Veldon, 1988; Gracia-Calvo *et al.*, 2015).

Apart from the mortal risk of intestinal strangulation if the intestine ruptures through the tunica vaginalis, the biggest problem associated with testicular hernias is the effect on testicular function, due to elevated temperature from the close proximity of the intestine (Varner and Schumacher, 1991; Cox, 1993a,b).

18.3.4.3. Testicular hypoplasia or degeneration

Both hypoplasia and degeneration are the terms given to an underdeveloped and, therefore, under-functioning

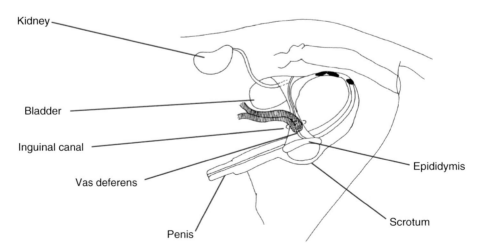

Fig. **18.5.** An inguinal hernia in the stallion, in which a loop of the intestine folds through the inguinal ring.

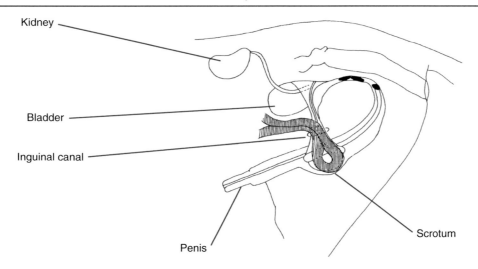

Kidney

Bladder

Inguinal canal

Penis

Scrotum

Fig. 18.6. A scrotal hernia in the stallion is a more extreme case of inguinal hernia, in which the loop of intestine has entered the scrotum and there is significant danger of complete ligation of the intestine, necrosis and death.

organ. Diagnosis is traditionally via physical examination of the testes plus stallion history. Ultrasound examination, testicular biopsy and serum AMH hormone concentrations have also been advocated as a means of diagnosis (Rode *et al.*, 2016; Pozor *et al.*, 2017, 2018).

Hypoplasia is generally the term given to a condition present from birth. Hence, in the case of testicular hypoplasia, the testes – for some reason – have never developed beyond an immature stage (Blanchard *et al.*, 1990; Varner and Schumacher, 1991; Varner *et al.*, 1991; Murchie, 2005; Turner, 2007). Its causes are many, including cryptorchidism and hernias, but also malnutrition, endocrine malfunction, infections, irradiation, toxins and chromosomal abnormalities, and it is often an inherited fault (Arighi, 2011a). The extent of the problem varies considerably from mild (where the testes appear normal, although possibly slightly small) to more severe cases (where the testes are significantly smaller than normal) and, if the condition is advanced, the testes may have become hard owing to the overdevelopment of connective tissue (Blanchard *et al.*, 1990; Ball, 2014). Spermatozoa production depends on the severity of the condition, varying from slight impairment to aspermic (no sperm at all). Any spermatozoa that are ejaculated have a higher incidence of abnormalities (Beard, 2011). In such cases the libido of the stallion is often not affected (Varner and Schumacher, 1991; Varner *et al.*, 1991).

Testicular degeneration refers to the condition where testicular development did originally occur to some extent but some subsequent problem has resulted in a degeneration of the tissue (Murchie, 2005; Turner, 2007). The testes are highly sensitive to extrinsic factors and so testicular degeneration is a major cause of infertility, especially in older stallions (Turner, 2018, 2019). Unlike hypoplasia, degeneration is an acquired condition. Degeneration may be temporary or permanent; it may be unilateral (affecting one testis, the cause being localized in origin) or bilateral (affecting both testis, so a systemic cause). The condition is evident as a shrinking of the testes, often showing small epididymides with a reduced number of spermatozoa within (Watson *et al.*, 1994a). Spermatozoa counts are depressed, and a decline in spermatozoa output is observed, with an increase in the percentage of morphologically abnormal spermatozoa (Friedman *et al.*, 1991; Blanchard and Varner, 1993b). The causes of testicular degeneration are many and varied. The prime causes are old age, elevated testicular temperature, scrotal/testicular injury (especially that associated with haemorrhage), increased scrotal insulation due to scrotal oedema, scrotal dermatitis (Varner and Schumacher, 1991; Blanchard and Varner, 1993b), cryptorchidism and autoimmune disease (Squires *et al.*, 1982a; Zhang *et al.*, 1990b). More minor causes include toxins, tumours, obstructions of the vas deferens and testicular torsion (Varner and Schumacher, 1991; Varner *et al.*, 1991). Testicular degeneration is, in most cases, reversible, providing that the duration of the problem is limited and the cause can be alleviated. However, age-related, infective and traumatic degeneration are more likely to be permanent (Burns and Douglas, 1985; Blanchard and Varner, 1993b; Turner, 2007, 2019).

18.3.4.4. Testicular torsion

Testicular torsion is the twist or rotation of the testis within the scrotum (Ball, 2014). The extent of the twist and the resultant effect is variable, although torsion occurs most commonly in younger stallions (those with larger scrotal sacks but small testes). The twist may be complete (i.e. occur through an angle of up to 360°), a condition difficult to detect immediately because the testes, on cursory examination, would appear to be positioned correctly. More commonly the twist is partial (i.e. through 90–180°), resulting in the epididymis being in a cranial position (towards the stallion's head) (Frazer, 2008). A minor torsion may be transient, presenting only a little pain and a slight decrease in ejaculated spermatozoa concentration (Pascoe *et al.*, 1981). Such torsions may have no long-term effects and may correct themselves (Threlfall *et al.*, 1990). Major torsion can result in symptoms similar to orchitis (Section 18.3.5.1) including acute colic pain, scrotal and testicular swelling, and obstruction of the blood supply. If present in a chronic case, this may lead to degeneration and permanent damage (Kenney, 1975; Threlfall *et al.*, 1990; Frazer, 2008). There is some dispute about the effect of the condition on semen quality. It is evident that if degeneration does result then semen quality will suffer.

18.3.4.5. Testicular tumours

Testicular tumours are rare in horses, although their exact incidence rate is difficult to ascertain, as the majority of stallions are gelded at a young age. Tumours or neoplasms can largely be divided into two (Frazer, 2008; Beard, 2011; Ball, 2014): (i) germinal neoplasms, including seminomas (most common; Hunt *et al.*, 1990; Weiermayer and Richter, 2009) and teratomas (seminiferous tubule in original and so may contain various tissues such as hair and teeth) (Fig. 18.7); and (ii) non-germinal neoplasms, interstitial cell or Sertoli cell tumours (Rahaley *et al.*, 1983; Schumacher and Varner, 1993). They are usually unilateral and are more likely to be observed in older stallions and cryptorchids (Farjanikish *et al.*, 2016). Often the condition is not associated with pain or elevated temperatures, but a firm swelling may be felt in the testicular tissue and is evident on ultrasound; the testis affected is also enlarged

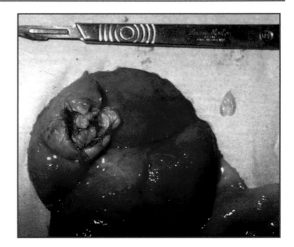

Fig. **18.7.** Testicular teratoma containing hair.

(Beck *et al.*, 2001). Neoplasms are causes of testicular degeneration and, therefore, associated with depressed spermatozoa counts and a high incidence of morphological abnormalities (Hurtgen, 1987; Weiermayer and Richter, 2009).

18.3.4.6. Testicular temperature

A rise in testicular temperature, whether from a fever, local infection (orchitis) or hernia, will have a detrimental effect on sperm production owing to the requirement for a lower temperature for maximum sperm production. Testicular temperature has much less of an effect on testosterone production (Section 6.6; Neto *et al.*, 2013). Once temperature has reduced to normal the effects may be seen for up to 56 days, the length of spermatogenesis in the stallion.

18.3.4.7. Hydrocele

Hydrocoele is a painless and often non-inflammatory accumulation of fluid between the visceral tunica vaginalis and parietal tunica vaginalis. The scrotum will appear enlarged because of the fluid accumulation. The reasons for the excess fluid accumulation is unclear but may be the result of trauma and may appear acutely or over time. The fluid accumulation causes a rise in scrotal temperature and this affects spermatogenesis, and so is of concern (De Vries, 1993; Frazer, 2008; Ball, 2014).

18.3.4.8. Vas deferens and accessory gland physical abnormalities

Physical abnormalities of the vas deferens and the accessory glands are rare but, if they occur, are invariably associated with a current or previous infection (Section 18.3.5.2) or inherited abnormalities (Varner *et al.*, 1991; Varner and Schumacher, 2011). The most common condition is blockage of the ampullae due to excessive accumulation of sperm. This can lead to aspermia as a result of complete blockage, or to poor sperm morphology due to sperm damage (Varner *et al.*, 2000). Varicocele (enlargement of the spermatic vein) may also be seen; this affects the functioning of the pampiniform plexus and hence testicular temperature control. Similarly, verminous granulomas, formed from parasitic migrations, affect testicular blood supply and pampiniform plexus function. Abnormalities associated with infection are manifest as fibrous growths or swellings at inflammation sites, which may cause obstruction and aspermia. Congenital abnormalities may be evident as immature, underdeveloped structures or complete absence. Most abnormalities can be identified by rectal palpation or ultrasonic scanning.

18.3.4.9. *Penis and prepuce physical abnormalities*

Abnormalities of the penis or prepuce are normally associated with trauma or injury (Frazer, 2008; Schumacher and Varner, 2011a). The penis, especially when erect, is very vulnerable to traumatic injury from a kick by an unreceptive mare (Vaughan, 1993). This causes vascular rupture and/or haemorrhage, making the return of the penis to within the prepuce difficult and painful. Haemorrhage of penile blood vessels (penile haematoma) may also occur if a stallion covers a mare with a Caslick's prior to episiotomy, or if the mare suddenly lunges to one side while being covered. The long-term effects of such trauma will depend not only on the physical recovery of the penis, but also on the stallion's psychological recovery. Such trauma can make a stallion, especially a young one, very reluctant to cover a mare again. Damage to the urethra within the penis is evident as blood contamination of semen, termed haemospermia (Schumacher *et al.*, 1995; Frazer, 2008). Congenital conditions such as small or short penis, stricture of the preputial orifice or hypospadias (displacement of the exit of the urethra) have been reported (Bleul *et al.*, 2007). Penile paralysis is a further condition, often caused by trauma, but also by neurological disease and general ill health. Other conditions may be observed such as priapism (persistent erection) caused by tranquilizer or anaesthesia;

paraphimosis or balanoposthitis (inability to retract the penis into the sheath) due to inflammation of the prepuce; and phimosis (inability to protrude the penis) due to penile lesions or tight preputial ring (Pearson and Weaver, 1978; Simmons *et al.*, 1985; Rochat, 2001; Lopate *et al.*, 2003; Murchie, 2005; Frazer, 2008; Resende *et al.*, 2014).

Tumours of the penis are not often malignant. The most common are squamous cell carcinomas (Howarth *et al.*, 1991), but lesions may also be due to melanomas, sarcoids and herpes virus (Section 14.3.5.6), which often burst and result in haemorrhage at covering and cause the stallion considerable pain. Blockage of the urethra or vas deferens has been reported, characterized by a normal libido but small-volume aspermatic semen, although testicular function is normal.

18.3.5. Infectious infertility

Infectious infertility in the stallion is not as evident as it is in the mare, as he is often an asymptomatic carrier of infection; but, as such, an understanding of stallion infectious infertility is essential.

18.3.5.1. *Testicular disease and infection; orchitis*

Infection and/or inflammation of the testes (orchitis) is relatively rare in the stallion and its cause may be infective or non-infective. In stallions orchitis is often associated with testis degeneration (Section 18.3.4.3). Infective orchitis may have a systemic or localized cause (Estepa *et al.*, 2006b; Frazer, 2008; Edwards, 2008). The usual point of entry for infection is the bloodstream, wounds, peritonitis or ascending infection, resulting in elevated testicular temperature and associated decline in spermatogenesis. The magnitude of the decline in fertility rates and the time period reflect the severity of the disease and the duration of the problem. When recovery occurs, it will be somewhat delayed, as the prime site of effect as far as spermatogenesis is concerned is the germinal cells. The spermatogenic cycle being 56 days, this period of time must be allowed after recovery for semen quality to return to anywhere near normal (Varner *et al.*, 1991; Tibary, 2004; Jahromi *et al.*, 2015).

Systemic disease causing orchitis normally results in bilateral inflammation of the testes and epididymis (Brinsko *et al.*, 1992). Bacterial agents causing such orchitis include *Streptococcus equi* (strangles), *S. zooepidemicus*, *Klebsiella pneumoniae*, *Actinobacillus equuli* and *Pseudomonas mallei* (glanders), *Escherichia coli* and possibly *Brucella abortus equi* (Timoney, 2011d). Viral agents may also be a systemic cause of orchitis: these include equine viral arteritis (EVA), equine infectious anaemia, equine influenza and equine herpes virus (EHV) (De Vries, 1993; Slusher, 1997). Systemic infections cause chronic, rather than acute, orchitis and have more of a chance of causing low-grade testicular degeneration and, with it, permanently depressed semen quality.

Localized infections may be caused via a wound, often to the scrotum, but also by descending infection via the inguinal canal (Varner and Schumacher, 1991). Such infections tend to cause acute orchitis (De Vries, 1993), which may be unilateral or bilateral, and present initially as soft, flabby, swollen testes. If the condition persists, chronic orchitis may result. Semen quality will be poor, with a decline in spermatozoa concentrations and an increased incidence of abnormalities. The major infective agents associated with localized orchitis are *Staphylococcus* spp., *E. coli*, *Streptococcus zooepidemicus* and *S. equi*. In cases of acute orchitis, rises in testicular temperature are also a potential hazard (Blanchard and Varner, 1993b).

Non-infective orchitis may be caused by testicular trauma (one of the commonest problems) or torsion, and by parasites (Jahromi *et al.*, 2015). The parasite most often associated is *Strongylus edentatus* larvae (Smith, 1973). These can migrate into the testicular tissue causing orchitis or obstruction of the testicular artery within the pampiniform plexus. This will have an additional detrimental effect upon the efficiency of the countercurrent heat-exchange mechanism (Roberts, 1986; Varner *et al.*, 1993; Wilson *et al.*, 2007).

Finally, orchitis may be caused as a result of damage to Sertoli cells and hence the blood–testes barrier, causing autoimmune orchitis. This will result in an autoimmune response to spermatozoa and testis inflammation (Papa *et al.*, 1990; Zhang *et al.*, 1990b). Orchitis not only has a negative effect on stallion fertility but in the case of infective orchitis (particularly bacterial), there is the opportunity of venereal transfer to the mare via both natural service and AI.

18.3.5.2. Vas deferens and accessory gland disease and infection

Inflammation/infection of the vas deferens and accessory glands is very uncommon but is frequently accompanied by inflammation of the epididymis and is often the cause of epididymitis. It is noteworthy, as such infections are often very persistent and so the stallion remains a carrier and of danger to mares he covers (for example he may transmit EVA) (Edwards, 2008; Carossino *et al.*, 2017). Infection or inflammation of the ampulla gland and seminal vesicles, although rare, is more likely than infection of the prostate and bulbourethral glands (Blanchard *et al.*, 1987) and can be due to ascending/descending infection, blood-borne infection or from surrounding infective tissue. The most common causes of accessory gland infection include *Corynebacterium pyogenes* and *Brucella abortus*, but *P. aeruginosa*, *K. pneumoniae*, *Streptococcus* spp. and *Staphylococcus* spp. have also been identified (Ball, 2014). Infection is often characterized by increased leucocyte concentrations within semen (especially in semen collected after rectal palpation) and bacterial contamination of semen, both of which affect motility as well as presenting a risk of infection transfer (Diemer *et al.*, 2003). Rectal palpation will also reveal that the seminal vesicles are swollen and painful (Varner *et al.*, 1991; Malmgren, 1992b). Treatment is problematic as it is very difficult for systemic antibiotics to reach significant concentrations in the accessory glands in order to have an effect. Flushing and local infusion with an appropriate antibiotic, although not easy (Reinfenrath *et al.*, 1997), gives the best success rates.

18.3.5.3. Penis, prepuce and urethral disease and infections

Infection or inflammation of both the penis (balanitis) and urethra (urethritis) may be due to non-infectious irritation (chemical) or infective agents, both often resulting in haemospermia. Contamination of semen with blood not only indicates the risk of possible infection transfer but is also associated with low fertility rates. Infective agents that may be evident on the sheath, prepuce or penis of the stallion include (i) parasites – *Habronema* larvae (habronemiasis or summer sores) (Schumacher and Varner, 2011a), myiasis (fly strike) (Hurtgen, 1987; Varner and Schumacher, 1991) and *Strongylus edentatus* larvae (Pickett *et al.*, 1981); (ii) protozoa – *Trypanosoma equiperdum* (dourine; Couto and Hughes, 1993; Ball, 2014); (iii) viruses – EHV3 (coital exanthema or genital horse pox; Ball, 2014) and EAV (EVA; Ball, 2014); and (iv) bacteria – *Streptococcus* spp., *K. pneumoniae*, *P. aeruginosa*, *Taylorella equigenitalis* and *E. coli* (Ball, 2014).

Not only may the penis itself be infected, but it is also the major means by which venereal infection can be passed from the stallion to the mare, and vice versa (Parlevliet and Samper, 2000; Samper and Tibary, 2006). The penis has a naturally balanced microflora that causes no problem to the stallion or to any mares that he covers. However, if this balance is disturbed because of systemic infection or disease, general ill health, impaired normal disease resistance or inappropriate use of soaps and detergents for penile washing, serious consequences can result (Bowen *et al.*, 1982). Similarly, if he comes into contact with a contaminated mare, his natural microflora balance may be breached and this may allow the invasion of foreign infective agents. The prepuce area protecting the penis then provides an ideal environment in which such organisms can multiply. Contamination of the stallion's penis may result from poor hygiene, especially at covering and during veterinary examination. Regular swabbing of the stallion and all mares to be covered, and washing of the stallion and mare during the preparation for covering, therefore, go a long way to preventing venereal disease transfer.

The stallion is often asymptomatic, failing to demonstrate any clinical signs of infection, but infection may be traced back through symptoms shown by mares he has covered (Samper and Tibary, 2006). Details of the organisms involved and their potential effect on reproductive performance have been given in Section 14.3.5.3, as their symptoms become manifest in the mare. Isolation and treatment of the stallion is the only course of action when such infections are suspected. Transfer from mare to mare via a stallion in a busy season is very easy and can have disastrous consequences.

Other conditions or infections may cause balanitis, as well as being transferred to the mare via the stallion at covering; for example, coital exanthema (caused by EHV3) which is often, but not always, characterized by lesions, particularly in the warmer climates of Asia, Africa, South America and south-eastern Europe (Couto and Hughes, 1993; Ball, 2014). EVA (Timoney, 2011b; Ball, 2014); EHV (EHV3, EHV4 and possibly EHV1) (Seki *et al.*, 2004; Timoney, 2011a; Ball, 2014); habronemiasis lesions (summer sores) (Philpott, 1993); and fungal infections (Zafracas, 1975) are other examples (see also Sections 14.3.5.7–14.3.5.9).

Complete prevention of venereal disease is difficult; it is aided by adhering to full hygiene precautions prior to covering, although complete disinfection of the stallion's penis is impossible and not advisable (Ball, 2014). Regular swabbing in accordance with the Horse Race Betting Levy Board (HBLB) guidelines (Horse Race Betting Levy Board, 2019) will greatly increase the chance that any pathogenic bacteria present are identified so that appropriate treatment can be given. Treatment itself can cause problems, as systemic antibiotics may affect the natural microfloral balance, which will take time to restore itself. Topical application of antibiotics and/or also dilute acidic preparations (*P. aeruginosa*) or sodium hypochlorite (*K. pneumoniae*) have been reported to be successful (Ball, 2014) but will also affect the natural microflora balance and, when applied to such a sensitive area, may also cause dryness and cracking, causing pain at covering. Semen for use with AI can be treated with an extender containing an appropriate antibiotic (Ball, 2014). Although not advised, natural service can be risked after thorough washing of the stallion's penis and with uterine lavage of the mare 4–6 h post-coitum followed by uterine infusion of an appropriate antibiotic (Samper and Tibary, 2006).

18.3.6. Immunological infertility

Semen contains many antigens, including those within seminal plasma and those that are spermatozoa bound. Under certain conditions, in particular as a result of traumatic damage to the blood–testis barrier, an autoimmune response to these antigens may occur, causing the destruction of spermatozoa within both the testis and the female tract (Wright, 1980; Teuscher *et al.*, 1994).

18.3.7. Semen abnormalities

Semen abnormalities are discussed in full in Chapter 21, along with an evaluation of semen. In summary, and as indicated throughout the previous text, most infections and trauma of the male reproductive tract have an adverse effect on sperm production and hence fertility. The normal parameters expected of a semen sample are given in Table 21.3.

Infection and/or abnormalities of the reproductive tract may affect any of these parameters, but usually cause a reduction in sperm concentrations, inadequate motility and poor longevity. Infection, rather than trauma, is often characterized by high leucocyte counts. If a semen sample does not meet the required parameters, the cause of the problem should be identified before the stallion is used, for his own protection and for that of any mare. In addition to poor sperm quality, urospermia (urine contamination), haemospermia (blood contamination) and bacterial contamination may be evident (Voss and McKinnon, 1993; Love, 2011c; Turner, 2011a; Al-Kass *et al.*, 2019).

Haemospermia, as mentioned previously, may be caused by a number of infective agents or by physical damage. A red blood cell count > 500 ml^{-1} or a white blood cell count > 1500 ml^{-1} will have an adverse effect on fertility. This effect appears to be modulated by the white or red blood cells themselves, rather than via the serum (Schumacher *et al.*, 1995).

Urospermia has a number of causes including neurological disorders (Leendertse *et al.*, 1990; Mayhew, 1990; Samper, 1995a; Griggers *et al.*, 2001; Lowe, 2001; Ball, 2014). Stallions suffering from urospermia may appear normal, with no neurological defects, and with adequate libido and mating ability. The condition may be continuous, intermittent and unpredictable. Contamination may occur at any time during ejaculation and may be as little as 1 ml or as great as 250 ml (Varner and Schumacher, 1991). Evidence suggests that contamination is not likely to be due to leakage alone but to an all-or-nothing effect. Urine contamination within a semen sample adversely affects spermatozoa motility and their capacity to fertilize an ovum (Varner and Schumacher, 1991; Ellerbrock *et al.*, 2016). Urine contamination may also affect semen pH (Samper, 1995a). The severity of the problem is dose dependent and stallion spermatozoa can tolerate minute amounts of urine without deterioration.

18.4. Conclusion

The causes of infertility or the failure to produce an offspring, whether on a temporary or permanent basis, are numerous. Some are treatable but, for many, the prognosis for the individual as a breeding animal is poor. It is essential, therefore, that all potential breeding stock are submitted to a thorough examination prior to purchase, to ensure that they are capable of fulfilling their reproductive potential.

Study Questions

You have identified that many of the mares covered by your stallion are returning as not pregnant, although it is the middle of the breeding season and has not happened in previous years. Critically evaluate what the causes may be.

You have had a semen evaluation done on your old stallion which reveals a much reduced sperm count from last year. Evaluate some of the reasons for this and whether there is anything that can be done.

Discuss the reproductive issues that may face an old stallion over 20 years of age and how these may be addressed.

You suspect your stallion has contracted an infection. Discuss how you would confirm this, the bacteria that may be involved and the treatments that could be given.

Suggested Reading

Murchie, T. (2005) Stallion infertility. Proceedings of the North American Veterinary Conference, Large animal. Orlando, Florida, USA, 19, 267–269.

Frazer, G.S. (2008) Stallion reproductive emergencies, Proceedings of the North American Veterinary Conference, Large animal. Orlando, Florida, USA, 22, 106–109.

Beard, W. (2011) Abnormalities of the testicles. In: McKinnon, A.O., Squires, E.L., Vaala, E. and Varner, D.D. (eds) *Equine Reproduction*, 2nd edn. Wiley-Blackwell, Philadelphia, London, pp. 1161–1165.

McDonnell, S.M. (2011) Abnormal sexual behavior. In: McKinnon, A.O., Squires, E.L., Vaala, E. and Varner, D.D. (eds) *Equine Reproduction*, 2nd edn. Wiley-Blackwell, Philadelphia, London, pp. 1407–1412.

Turner, R.M. (2011) Abnormalities of the Ejaculate. In: McKinnon, A.O., Squires, E.L., Vaala, E. and Varner, D.D. (eds) *Equine Reproduction*, 2nd edn. Wiley-Blackwell, Philadelphia, London, pp. 1119–1129.

Turner, R.M. (2011) Ultrasonography of the genital tract. In: McKinnon, A.O., Squires, E.L., Vaala, E. and Varner, D.D. (eds) Equine Reproduction, 2nd edn. Wiley-Blackwell, Philadelphia, London, pp. 1469–1490.

Ball, B.A. (2014) Applied andrology in horses. In: Chenoweth, P.J. and Lorton, S.P. (eds) *Animal Andrology: Theories and Applications*. CABI, Wallingford, Oxfordshire, UK, pp 254–296.

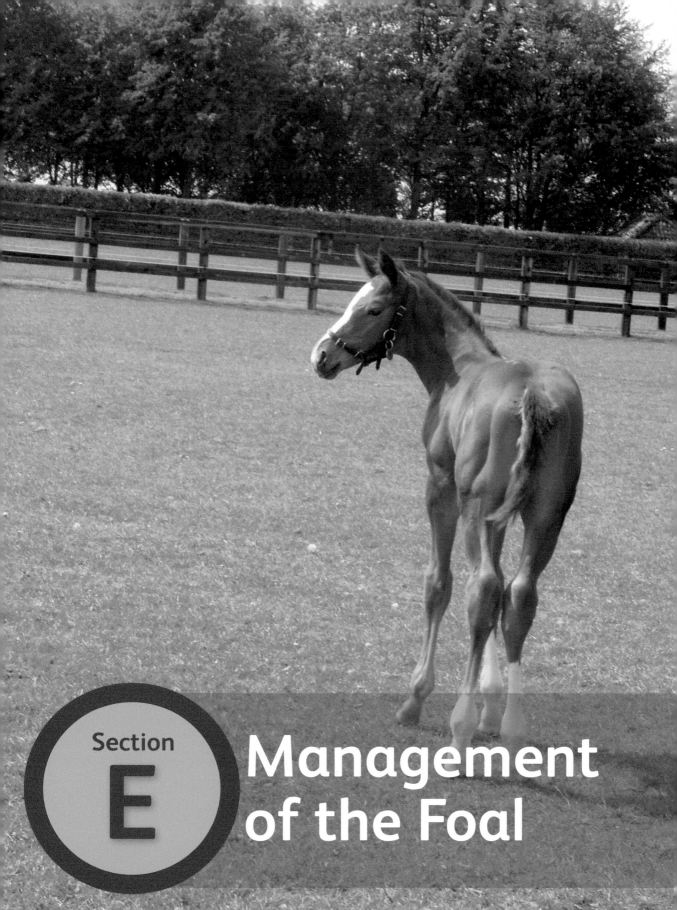

Management of the Foal

Section E considers the management of the foal, from the critical immediate adaptation to the extra uterine environment at birth, until after weaning. The physiology of adaptation is considered in some detail, along with a discussion of the various options available when managing the foal, in particular at weaning. Considerations of nutritional and general management are included, all geared towards ensuring optimum welfare.

19 Management of the Young Foal

The Objectives of this Chapter are:

To detail the adaptive process that the foal must undergo as it transitions from the inter-uterine to the extra-uterine environment.
To evaluate the management options for the young foal up to peak lactation at around 6 weeks of age.
To discuss the management of the older foal (after peak lactation at around 6 weeks) as the foal becomes increasingly independent.

19.1. Introduction

Correct management of the young and growing foal is crucial for its long-term survival and ability to meet its genetic potential. Adaptation from the intra- to the extra-uterine environment is crucial. The subject of neonatal complications and disease is vast and beyond the scope of this book. This Chapter will, therefore, concentrate on the normal foal in order that abnormal foals can be identified. More specific, detailed texts should be consulted on the problems that may be encountered in the neonate (Koterba, 1990; Madigan, 1990; Adams, 1993a,b; McClure, 1993; Reef, 1993; Roberts, 1993; Seltzer *et al.*, 1993; Traub-Dargatz, 1993a,b; Vaala, 1993; Welsch, 1993; Knottenbelt and Holdstock 2004a,b; Knottenbelt *et al.*, 2004; McKinnon *et al.*, 2011). Information on the management of the mare during this period is given in Chapter 13, which should be read in conjunction with this Chapter to give a complete picture of mare and foal management.

19.2. Foal Adaptive Period

Immediately post-partum the foal has to undergo substantial anatomical, functional and biochemical adaptive changes to survive in the extra-uterine environment; it is then classified as a neonate. In the normal foal, adaptive changes can be identified until puberty and even up until the achievement of mature size. However, in considering the true adaptive period for survival outside the uterus, the first 4 days of life are the most crucial. It is within this period of time that the majority of adaptive problems can be identified and, hopefully, rectified. If the foal satisfies all the normal criteria at this age, it has a very good chance of survival (Rossdale, 2004).

In a normal birth, the foal is born on its side, lying with its hocks still within its mother and the umbilical cord intact; it should rapidly sit up in sternal recumbency (Fig. 12.12). The newborn foal may be assessed within 3 min of birth on its appearance, pulse (rate), grimace (response to stimuli), activity (muscle tone) and respiratory rate (APGAR), and scored using the APGAR scoring system as normal, moderately depressed or markedly depressed (Table 19.1; Madigan, 1990; LeBlanc, 1997). The long-term prognosis for the foal is dependent upon this classification. As a rough guide the foal should weigh about 10% of the dam's weight and the placenta should weigh 10% of the foal's weight, so a 400-kg mare can expect to have a 40-kg foal with a 4-kg placenta. Within reason, the bigger the placenta the better, as foal weight is positively correlated to the surface area of the placenta (Wilsher *et al.*, 1999; Wilsher and Allen, 2003, 2012; Elliot *et al.*, 2009) which in turn is positively correlated with foal growth in the first 3 months of life (Allen *et al.*, 2002a,b) and final athletic performance (Rossdale and Ousey, 2002).

Table 19.1. The appearance, pulse rate, grimace, activity, respiration (APGAR) scoring system to aid in the classification of newborn foals. Score 7–8 normal, score 4–6 moderate depression and score 0–3 markedly depressed. (From Madigan, 1990.)

	Score		
Parameter	0	1	2
Appearance (A)	Recumbent and lifeless	Some attempts to move	Significant attempts to sit up (sternal recumbency)
Pulse rate (P)	Absent	< 60 min^{-1}	60 min^{-1}
Grimace (response to nasal stimuli) (G)	No response to stimulation	Grimace, slight rejection on stimulation	Cough or sneeze on stimulation
Activity (muscle tone) (A)	Limp	Some flexion of extremities	Sternal position
Respiration (R)	Absent	Slow, irregular	60 min^{-1} regular

19.2.1. Anatomical adaptation

Anatomical adaptations can be considered as the milestones that the foal should achieve within set periods of time in order to survive. These parameters can quite easily be observed by the foaling attendant and used to indicate foal viability and identify problems.

Passage through the birth canal compresses the foal's thorax and helps to expel excess fluid from airways, allowing and stimulating the normal foal to breathe within 30 s of final delivery (Acworth, 2003; Pierce, 2003; Stoneham, 2006). It may take a few sharp intakes of breath as its muzzle first reaches the air during passage through the birth canal, but a rhythm is normally established within 1 min of final delivery. If breathing does not occur within 3 min, there are serious consequences for the foal (Rose, 1988; Acworth, 2003; Wilkins, 2003). This initial breathing rhythm is normally a steady 60–70 breaths min^{-1} (Koterba, 1990; Acworth 2003; Pierce, 2003). The initiation of breathing results in a significant increase in blood oxygen levels. During this first minute of life, the foal's heart rate should be in the order of 40–80 beats min^{-1}, although others have reported lower rates. This can be measured by placing a hand on the left side of the chest near the heart. The foal's body temperature should be 37.5–38.5°C (Koterba, 1990; Traub-Dargatz, 1993a; Vaala, 1993, Medica *et al.*, 2018). The foal's mucous membranes should appear pink and moist and have a refill time of 1–2 s within the first 2 h (Curcio and Nogueria, 2012). Within a few hours the respiratory rate declines to 30–40 breaths min^{-1}. The heart rate rapidly increases to 120–140 beats min^{-1} when the foal moves in its attempts to stand, plateauing at 80–100 within the first week (Lombard, 1990; Pierce, 2003). The foal's temperature should stabilize at 37–39°C (99–102°F) (Medica *et al.*, 2018).

The significant increase in blood oxygen concentrations as a result of breathing activates the first reflexes and muscle movements. Within 5 min of birth the normal foal should be in a sternal recumbency position (Fig. 19.1). It will respond to pain and begin to show evidence of the reflexes associated with rising to its feet, in the form of raising its head, extending its forelimbs, blinking and possibly whinnying (Madigan, 1990; Traub-Dargatz, 1993a). It will also demonstrate the suckling reflex if offered a finger or bottle (Vaala, 2000; Pierce, 2003; Stoneham, 2006).

The next major event is the breaking of the umbilical cord, on average 5–9 min after birth (Pierce, 2003). It is important that the cord is left to break naturally; early work by Rossdale (1967) suggests that premature breakage results in the loss of up to 1 l of blood by preventing drainage from the placenta (Smith, 2006), although work done by Doarn *et al.* (1985, 1987) failed to support such a blood loss. Breakage naturally occurs at a constriction about 2–3 cm from the abdomen of the foal. The umbilical artery and vein have thinner walls in this area, and so collapse and constrict naturally at this point, as the pressure of blood circulating within these vessels declines. The decline follows a change in the foal's circulatory system, diverting blood away from the placenta and allowing a clean seal of the blood vessels to occur, so minimizing blood loss. This clean seal also reduces the chance of bacteria entering the umbilicus and causing an infection (Acworth, 2003). The mare may be recumbent postpartum for up to 20 min and, therefore, the cord is usually broken by the movements of the foal in its first attempts to rise to its feet, the increased tension resulting in the cord breaking at the constriction, the weakest point. Once the cord has severed, the navel must be dressed. Traditionally, iodine-based preparations have

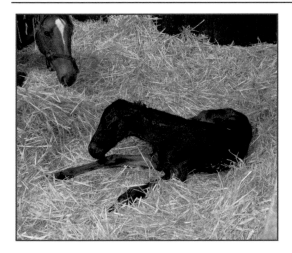

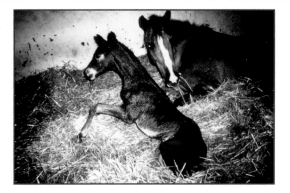

Fig. 19.2. Soon after the end of second-stage labour the foal makes concerted efforts to rise to its feet; at this time the umbilical cord breaks. (Photo courtesy of Mr Stephen Rufus.)

Fig. 19.1. Very soon after the foal's hips have been born the foal should sit up in sternal recumbency.

been used. However, there is a suggestion that treating with iodine causes a sloughing of skin cells and a risk of reopening the navel to infection (O'Grady, 1995). It is suggested by some that 0.5% chlorohexidine is a better alternative.

Around the time of umbilical cord breakage, the foal makes concerted efforts to raise itself to its feet (Fig. 19.2). The exertion of standing causes the heart rate to increase to up to 150 beats min^{-1}. Heart rate continues to fluctuate with activity around a normal resting heart rate of 80–100 beats min^{-1} in the first few days. When attempting to stand, the series of movements is the same as in the mature horse: stretching forwards of the head and neck, extending the forelegs; flexing the hind legs and raising the front end off the ground first, followed by the hindquarters. Many initial, unsuccessful attempts are made, which form part of the process of developing reflexes and muscle coordination and control. At this stage the foal is at risk of damage from projecting objects such as buckets, hay racks or automatic water feeders. Successful standing normally occurs in ponies within 35 min post-partum but may take an extra 30 min or more in Thoroughbred foals (Fig. 19.3; Wulf et al., 2017; Medica et al., 2018). Differences also exist with other breeds and between genders, colts taking longer than fillies (Vaala, 2000; Pierce, 2003; Stoneham, 2006; McCue and Ferris, 2012). Failure to stand within 2–3 h is indicative of a problem and veterinary assistance should be sought (Madigan, 1990). This remarkable ability to stand and walk so quickly is the result of the evolutionary development evident in plain-dwelling

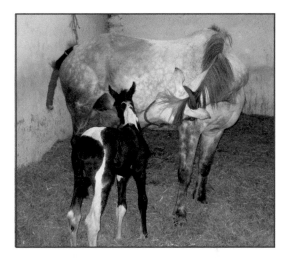

Fig. 19.3. Successful standing in the pony foal takes on average 35 min compared to up to 1 h in the Thoroughbred. The foal then searches for the udder; encouraged by the mare, the suckling reflex is already present and is elicited by contact with soft, warm, dark areas.

animals such as the horse, to enable them to flee from potential predators as soon as possible after birth.

Although the suckling reflex is evident within 5 min post-partum, successful suckling can obviously not occur until after standing and locating the udder. The actual reflexes involved in suckling are elicited by contact with soft warm surfaces; hence, foals are seen to suckle and nuzzle their dam's flanks while searching for the udder. It has also been suggested that an appeasing pheromone is produced by the mare which also acts as an attractant to the foal and may have a role to play in initial bonding (Mills, 2005). As soon as the foal stands it demonstrates directional movement, moving along the mare's flanks towards the udder, located by the dark and warmth. This process of locating the mare's udder can easily be disrupted by human interference. It is very tempting to try and help a foal, and frustrating to watch it suckling at the hock or chest and seemingly unable to locate the teat. However, it is much better to resist the temptation to interfere. The mare will normally assist the foal by gently nudging it and moving her hind leg away from her body to allow the foal easier access (Fig. 19.3). Occasionally, a primiparous (maiden) mare may need to be held to allow the foal to reach the udder, appearing ticklish and initially objecting to the foal's attentions. However, she will soon settle down and should be left alone. Foals normally take 30 min to successfully suckle after standing, although this varies with breed and fillies suckle significantly more quickly than colts (Fig. 19.4; Vaala, 2000; Pierce, 2003; Stoneham, 2006; McCue and Ferris, 2012; Wulf *et al.*, 2017; Medica *et al.*, 2018). At suckling, a real affinity develops between mother and foal, which develops into a very strong bond. Human interference at this stage may well disrupt this bonding process (Chavatte, 1991). Throughout its first few days of life the foal will suckle for about 2 min at 10–15-min intervals. In the first 24 h it will consume 5–10% of its body weight and by day 2 it will be consuming 20–25% of its body weight; later on, the intervals between suckling lengthen (Carson and Wood-Gush, 1983a; Ousey *et al.*, 1996). If during the first few days of life a foal is not seen to suckle for 3 h or so, problems should be suspected.

During the first 12 h the foal should be seen to pass meconium, its first bowel movement. It may well be passed earlier than this and is sometimes seen within a few minutes of the first feed (Fig. 19.5; Vaala, 2000; Pierce, 2003; Stoneham, 2006; McCue and Ferris, 2012). Meconium consists of bowel glandular secretions collected during the foal's inter-uterine life, along with digested amniotic fluid and cell debris, which are passed through the foal's digestive tract *in utero*. Meconium is stored in the colon, caecum and rectum ready for expulsion after birth. Premature expulsion may occur under stressful conditions during, or immediately prior to, delivery. Meconium staining of the amniotic fluid or the perineum area of the foal is, therefore, indicative of fetal or foal stress. Meconium should be brown to greenish brown in colour and is usually all expelled within the first 2 days. Meconium is followed by the characteristically yellow- or tan-coloured milk dung, which indicates correct gut function (Fig. 19.6). The routine use of enemas using medicinal paraffin or warm soapy water is advocated by some within 12–18 h post-partum (Madigan, 1990). However, their repeated use can irritate the mucosal lining of the gut and there is no evidence that they reduce the incidence of meconium compaction. Routine enemas are becoming less popular as the adverse effect of such stresses on the newborn foal is increasingly understood. Enemas may be considered appropriate if meconium is not passed within 48 h and/or the foal is showing signs of meconium retention. Colt foals should urinate for the first time within 5–6 h, whereas filly foals urinate later, on average at 10–11 h. Regular urination of large volumes, up to 150 ml kg^{-1} day^{-1} (6 l for a 40-kg foal) of near colourless hypotonic urine should be observed in the

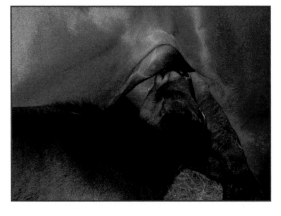

Fig. 19.4. Foals will normally have found the mare's udder and successfully suckled within 30 min of standing.

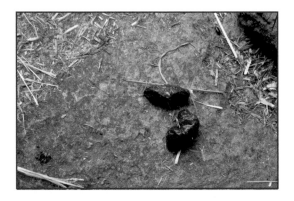

Fig. 19.5. Within 12 h the foal should have passed greenish brown meconium, the first bowel movement.

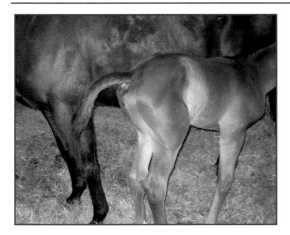

Fig. 19.6. The passage of the yellow milk dung by the foal follows the passage of meconium and is a good indicator of correct gut function.

normal foal in the first 48 h (Brewer *et al.*, 1991; Traub-Dargatz, 1993a; Stoneham, 2011).

19.2.2. Functional adaptation

This section will consider how the functions of the pulmonary, cardiovascular, temperature-control, immune and renal systems adapt to accommodate the change from the intra- to the extra-uterine environment. The change in their functions is reflected in the observed anatomical changes, or foal milestones, discussed previously.

19.2.2.1. Pulmonary ventilation

Successful gaseous transfer within the lungs across the air–blood interface depends upon their functional and structural maturity. One of the major events is the laying down of surfactant. Surfactant is a complex lipoprotein produced by type II alveolar pneumocyte cells, which provides the alveoli with a surface film, so reducing the surface tension and increasing the efficiency of gaseous exchange and reducing lung collapse (Lester, 2005; Curcio and Nogueira, 2012). Surfactant maturation occurs in the last third of pregnancy, particularly around day 300 onwards, and may not be complete until after delivery (Pattle *et al.*, 1975; Lester, 2005; Curcio and Nogueira, 2012). Maximum respiratory efficiency is not possible until superfactant development has been completed, and this creates a problem with premature foals.

The foal takes its first breath while *in utero* as mechanical practice for post-partum functioning of the muscles involved in respiration. Successful extra-uterine breathing then relies on removal of fluid collected within the lungs during pregnancy, which is expelled by compression of the thorax during delivery, and by evaporation and spluttering during early breaths. There are three triggers to respiration: chemical (the main one), tactile and thermal. The foal is born hypoxemic (low circulating plasma oxygen concentrations, PO_2) and hyercapnic (high circulating plasma carbon dioxide concentrations, PCO_2). These chemical stimuli, which occur during labour, activate the respiratory centre of the medulla and so stimulate the first proper extra-uterine breaths and the subsequent breathing rhythm. The decrease in PO_2 and blood pH, correlated with the increase in PCO_2, are the result of placental separation and the occlusion of umbilical cord blood supply as the foal is forced through the birth canal (Acworth, 2003; Curcio and Nogueira, 2012). It should be noted that the peripheral set point for PO_2 (oxygen pressure/blood concentration) is relatively low in foals compared to adults for the first 2–3 days. Because of this they can tolerate a greater reduction in O_2 than adult horses before increased respiration is initiated (Wilkins, 2003). Cold shock (thermal stimulus) from the invariably cooler atmosphere, and tactile stimuli such as rubbing and mare's licking, are secondary respiration stimuli and help to also initiate breathing. The first breath should occur within 30 s of the foal's hips appearing through the birth canal (Stewart *et al.*, 1984; Ousey *et al.*, 1991; Acworth, 2003; Pierce, 2003; Stoneham, 2006). After birth, as a breathing rhythm is established, the alveoli continue to expand and develop, induced by lung expansion and stretching of the bronchi (Vaala, 1993). Initial breathing has a tidal volume (volume of air inspired per breath) of 520 ml, resulting in minute volume (volume of air inspired min^{-1}) of 35 l (Koterba, 1990). After a few hours the tidal volume increases to 550 ml and the minute volume reduces to 20 l and may stay at this relatively high breathing rate compared to adults (8–12 min^{-1}) for a few days (Rossdale and Ricketts, 1980). At birth, the efficiency of gaseous exchange is low but this is compensated for by rapid breathing rate. Over time, as the bronchi are stretched and alveolar development continues (so increasing inspiration volume and surface area/air ratio), more efficient gaseous transfer is achieved and the breathing rate declines (Lester, 2005; Stoneham, 2011). Calcification of the initially compliant (soft) chest wall also makes breathing more effective with time (Koterba and Kosch, 1987). After 7 days there is a significant improvement in the foal's respiratory reserve and efficiency (Stewart *et al.*, 1984; Stoneham, 2011). At this stage alveoli and bronchial development is complete in most horses, but there is evidence that development may continue until 12 months in Thoroughbreds (Beech *et al.*, 2001). During initial breathing sternal recumbency is to be encouraged as this is the most efficient position for respiration, allowing the lungs to hang within the thoracic cavity, as opposed to one lung being squashed by the other in lateral recumbency.

19.2.2.2. Cardiac and circulatory systems

In utero the placenta acts as the 'lungs', in being the major site of oxygen and carbon dioxide exchange, as well as nutrient uptake. To supply the placenta, blood must pass from the pulmonary artery via the ductus arteriosus to the aorta, so bypassing the pulmonary system (the lungs) and passing directly to the placenta (Fig. 19.7). Only a small supply of blood to the

pulmonary system is required, just enough for pulmonary growth and development. Additionally, the foramen ovale allows blood to pass from the right atrium directly to the left atrium and ventricle, and hence immediately around the body via the aorta, rather than to the right ventricle. Blood enters the placenta via the two umbilical arteries and leaves via the single umbilical vein, to pass to the liver, and then back to the right side of the heart. The bypassing of the lungs is aided by the relatively high pulmonary vascular resistance compared to the systemic resistance. Both ventricles work in parallel, with the right ventricle dominating in size and output (MacDonald *et al.*, 1988; Vaala, 1993).

Immediately post-partum, the circulatory system of the foal must change dramatically to redirect blood through the pulmonary system to the lungs, and away from the umbilical system to the placenta (Fig. 19.8). The trigger for this change is unclear, but a decrease in

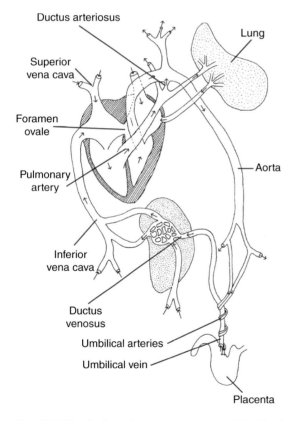

Fig. 19.7. The fetal circulatory system in utero. The blood passes through two openings, the foramen ovale between the left- and right-hand sides of the heart and the ductus arteriosus, hence bypassing the lungs.

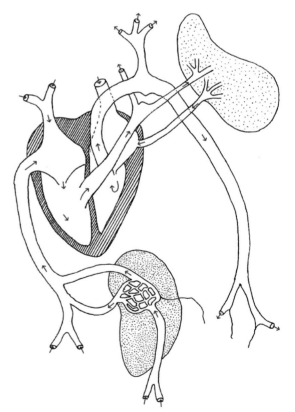

Fig. 19.8. The circulatory system of a normal foal post-partum. The foramen ovale and the ductus arteriosus will close within a few days of birth.

pulmonary resistance plays a significant role. As the foal takes its first few breaths the collapsed lungs inflate, stretching the alveoli and rapidly reducing pulmonary resistance by up to tenfold, resulting in increasing blood perfusion of the lungs (Kullander *et al.*, 1975; Curcio and Nogueira, 2012). As pulmonary resistance declines, blood is drawn up directly through the pulmonary artery to the lungs and not across the ductus arteriosus to the aorta. As more blood is drawn away from the right-hand side of the heart and more blood enters the left side of the heart from the pulmonary vein, blood pressure in the left-hand side of the heart becomes greater than that in the right. In addition, as blood flow to the placenta decreases, less blood enters the right atria, further decreasing blood pressure on the right-hand side of the heart. As a result of this differentiation in blood pressure the foramen ovale closes. Some blood leaving the right-hand side of the heart in the pulmonary artery may still continue to pass through the ductus arteriosus to the aorta and vice versa. This continues until the physiological closure of the ductus arteriosus at around 24 h; complete anatomical closure may take up to 4 days (Lombard, 1990; Stoneham, 2011; Curcio and Nogueira, 2012). The trigger for closure of the ductus arteriosus is unclear but is suggested to be associated with increasing plasma oxygen concentrations and decreasing tissue concentrations of prostaglandins (Lombard, 1990; Vaala, 1993; Curcio and Nogueira, 2012). Until its complete closure, it may reopen in response to stress or hypoxemia (Livsey *et al.*, 1998; Stoneham, 2011). Delayed closure is often associated with caesarean section births, or induced parturition, as final preparation for closure of the ductus arteriosus has not been allowed to occur (Machida *et al.*, 1998). In the newborn foal blood should now be pumped from the right side of the heart via the pulmonary artery to the lungs for oxygenation and back via the pulmonary vein to the heart for circulation around the body (Figs 19.7 and 19.8).

Many newborn foals initially suffer from arrhythmia (irregular heartbeat) but this soon settles down naturally (Yamamoto *et al.*, 1992; Stoneham, 2011). Many foals show signs of asphyxia during the second stage of labour, evident as a blue tongue and mucous membranes of the eyes caused by a reduction in blood flow and, therefore, oxygen to the head. Such constriction of the head, neck and chest during passage through the pelvis is of no long-term significance providing the foal continues to be delivered normally and parturition is not delayed. The foal can tolerate reduced PO_2 for short periods of time. After birth, the mucous membranes may remain blue/grey in colour for a short while, but should be the normal pink colour within 2 h. The fetal medulla is only able to produce norepinephrine (a vasodilator); however, the neonatal medulla is able to produce epinephrine (a vasoconstrictor) as well norepinephrine. This enables the neonate to balance perfusion of the core and the extremities and, in situations of low PO_2, enables preferential perfusion to the animal's core and hence support the functioning of vital organs (MacDonald *et al.*, 1988).

At birth the foal's blood pressure is elevated (Holdstock *et al.*, 1998), and the red blood cell count is also elevated ($9–13 \times 10^{12}$ l^{-1}) compared to that later on in life ($7.5–10.5 \times 10^{12}$ l^{-1}), although haemoglobin levels are similar to those seen in adults. This is unusual, as in most mammals haemoglobin levels are elevated in the newborn (Knottenbelt *et al.*, 2004; Axon and Palmer, 2008). Elevated red blood cell counts are thought to be due to fetal stress during birth, as levels are further elevated in foals born with difficulty. Within 2 h of birth, red blood cell counts decline and white blood cell counts rise to normal levels (Table 19.2; Chavatte *et al.*, 1991).

19.2.2.3. Thermoregulation

The foal is born with a relatively well-developed thermoregulation (temperature-control) mechanism, unlike many other mammals and especially primates, which cannot effectively control their body temperature for several weeks after birth. At birth, the foal can maintain a steady body temperature of 37–37.5°C (100°F; Vaala, 1993; Medica *et al.*, 2018), which increases to 38–38.5°C within 1 h despite a cold environment. This is due to the high metabolic rate of newborn foals (200 W m^{-2}), which is three times that of a 2-day-old foal (Ousey, 1997). The prime metabolic energy resource is glycogen and so premature foals and those born with low birth weight owing to limited fat and glycogen stores are at a disadvantage (Acworth, 2003; Morresey, 2005; Curcio and Nogueria, 2012). A body temperature below 37°C or above 40°C is a cause for concern. The exact mechanism by which it maintains this steady body temperature is unclear. Foals are invariably born into a relatively cold environment and so heat generation and conservation is critical. Foals are able to shiver within 3 h post-partum and this, plus muscular activity and the strain of the foal's first movements, contribute to heat generation whereas the foal's insulating layers of fat and its hair coat help to conserve the heat generated.

Table 19.2. The major haematological and biochemical parameters for foals from parturition to 7 days of age. (From Irvine, 1984; Stewart *et al.*, 1984; Vivrette *et al.*, 1990; Knottenbelt *et al.*, 2004.)

	Abbreviation	Units	Birth	24 h	7 days+	Adult
Haematology						
Haemoglobin	Hb	$g\ l^{-1}$	120–180	130–155	115–175	130–170
Haematocrit	PCV	ll^{-1}	0.40–0.52	0.34–0.46	31–40	34–44
Erythrocytes	RBC	$\times 10^{12}\ l^{-1}$	9.0–13.0	8.0–11.0	7.5–10.5	8.5–11.0
Leukocytes	WBC	$\times 10^{9}\ l^{-1}$	5.5–11.5	–	7.0–12.0	6–12
Lymphocytes	L	$\times 10^{9}\ l^{-1}$		1.8–3.0	2.0–4.0	1.5–4.0
Metabolites						
Glucose	Gluc	$mg\ 100\ ml^{-1}$	50–70	100–110	100–110	75–120
Lactate	Lact	$mmol\ l^{-1}$	3–4	2–3	–	0.5
Fibrinogen	Fibrin	$g\ l^{-1}$	< 2	2.0–3.0	1.6–2.8	1.5–3.7
Total protein	TP	$g\ l^{-1}$	45–47	52–70	60–65	46–69
Electrolytes						
Calcium	Ca	$mmol\ l^{-1}$	–	2.5–4.0	2.4–3.4	2.7–3.4
Phosphates	P	$mmol\ l^{-1}$	–	2.2–5.2	–	0.6–1.7
Iron	Fe	$mmol\ l^{-1}$	72–88	18–63	18–54	18–50
Blood gases						
Bicarbonate		$mmol\ l^{-1}$	23	27	24	
Carbon dioxide	pCO_2	$mmol\ l^{-1}$	21–34	37–50	22–32	24–31
Oxygen	pO_2	$mmol\ l^{-1}$	77	75–98	75–106	
pH			7.36–7.4	7.39	7.43	
Minerals						
Copper	Cu	$\mu mol\ l^{-1}$	–	9–12	–	
Selenium	Se	$\mu mol\ l^{-1}$	–	1.2–1.6	–	
Hormones						
Cortisol		$ng\ ml^{-1}$	120–140	60	30	30
Thyroxine	T_4	$nmol\ l^{-1}$	6–10	–	8–20	

RBC, red blood cells.

Unlike the human baby, the foal does not have brown heat-producing adipose (fat) tissue. Its ability to shiver earlier in life negates this requirement. The presence of brown fat is associated with neonates unable to shiver and those that have less fine control over their body temperature (Ousey *et al.*, 1991). Hypothermia can occur in newborn foals; its onset may be rapid and can result from infection or dystocia as well as a cold environment. Hypothermia may cause hypoxemia and acidosis, causing an attempted reversion to fetal cardiac and circulating patterns and altered gastrointestinal function (Savage, 2011).

19.2.2.4. Neurological control

Neurological control of the foal is highly sophisticated at birth, allowing escape from predators in the wild. Despite this there are some differences between the foal and the adult which may persist for several days. The forelimbs, and to a lesser extent the hind limbs, demonstrate marked cross extensor reflex (failure of the contralateral limb to compensate for loss of support when the ipsilateral limb withdraws from a stimulus), and a marked resting extensor tone (limbs over extended) when the foal is lying in lateral recumbency. The hind limbs in particular tend to hyperflex (over flex, with foals appearing down on their heels; Fig. 19.9). In general, the foal's gaits and its head movements are hypermetric (exaggerated) and jerky. Despite these challenges foals are able to coordinate their limbs effectively enough to run at high speed within a few hours of birth, a major evolutionary adaptation to survival as a predated animal. In addition, the menace response (blinking of the eyes in response to fast-moving object) is not complete until 14 days of age and the eye itself does not appear to be fully operational for the first few days. Foals have a slower biphasic pupillary light response (the two-part blink response to light: first a small but fast response, followed by a second slow and complete response) than adults and the pupil position is more ventromedial than dorsomedial for the first 4 weeks of life. These continued developments of the eye post-partum may be why foals are considered by many to have relatively poor eyesight for the first few days, and is a reason often given for not turning foals and dams out until 3 days post-partum, and then into small secure paddocks to prevent separation (Fig. 19.10; Enzerink, 1998; Knottenbelt *et al.*, 2004; Morresey, 2005; Stoneham, 2011).

19.2.2.5. Immune status

The equine placenta is epitheliochorial and, as such, presents a considerable barrier to the passage of blood components from mother to fetus *in utero*, especially those of large molecular size such as immunoglobulins (antibodies) (Section 3.2.3). In the foal, therefore, the attainment of immunoglobulins *in utero* is limited and so colostrum is vitally important for achieving adequate

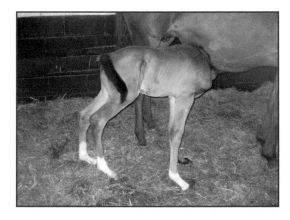

Fig. 19.9. Hyperflexion of the hind limbs, in particular, is often seen in young foals for the first few days until the extensors tighten.

immunity for survival in the extra-uterine environment. At birth the foal is plunged from sterile conditions into an environment of varying immunological challenge. The foal's system is perfectly capable of meeting this challenge by producing its own antibodies over time, but is born immunologically naive (without antibodies) apart from a small concentration of immunoglobulin M (IgM) and so has no 'safety net' to protect it until it has produced enough antibodies to protect itself. This safety net is provided by the immunoglobulins in colostrum. Equine immunoglobulins can be subdivided into IgG, IgM and IgA. The most predominant in colostrum is IgG and these are most evident in the circulation of the young foal (Stoneham, 2011). Adult levels of immunoglobulins are not immediately evident in the foal; these are reached only after the foal starts to actively produce its own immunoglobulins. For the first 24 h post-partum, enterocyte cells lining the foal's small intestine are able to absorb by pinocytosis large protein molecules such as immunoglobulins (Curcio and Nogueira, 2012) which appear in the foal's blood 6–8 h after colostrum ingestion (Stoneham, 2011). The ability to absorb whole proteins is seemingly enhanced by other components of colostrum, and controlled in part by cortisol, though the exact mechanisms are unclear. Over time, the enterocytes are replaced by cells incapable of absorbing proteins. It is, therefore, essential that newborn foals receive at least 500 ml of colostrum within the first 24 h of life, and preferably within the first 12 h, when absorption is most efficient (Sellon, 2006) and ensures that the foal obtains maximum protection from infection via maternal antibodies. Efficiency of immunoglobulin absorption declines from 51% at 2 h to 1% at 22 h post-partum (Stoneham, 2011). Several tests to ascertain the immunological status of the foal in terms of IgG are available (Bertone and Jones, 1988; LeBlanc, 1990; Madigan, 1990; Cash, 1999; Curcio and Nogueira, 2012). The amount of colostrum required depends on the size of the foal and concentration of immunoglobulins in the colostrum. It is generally agreed that foal IgG serum concentrations of 4–8 g l^{-1} are appropriate. Colostrum may also be tested, and it has been suggested that a specific gravity of >1060 is indicative of an IgG concentration of > 30 g l^{-1}. In a 50-kg foal with approximately 5 l blood volume this will, if the foal ingests 800 ml, result in a foal serum concentration of > 5 g l^{-1}. This is the minimum requirement and so ideally the foal should ingest more to bring its IgG levels up to 8–10 g l^{-1} by 24 h (LeBlanc *et al.*, 1986;

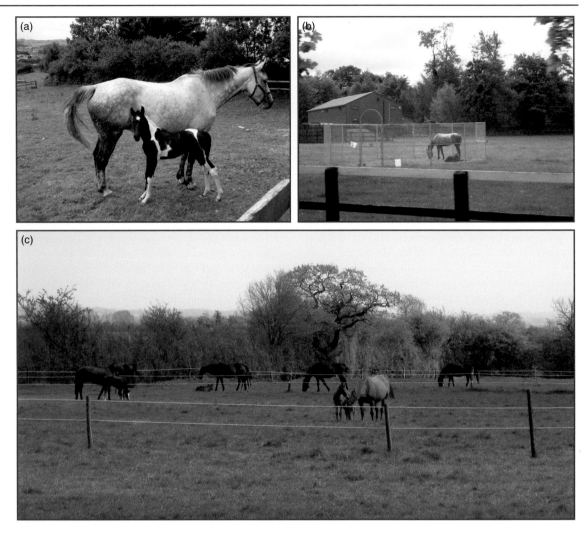

Fig. 19.10. After 3 days a foal's eyesight should have developed enough to allow it to be turned out with its mother. This can be in (a) a small safe paddock; (b) an enclosure, several within a paddock (although these must only be used for the first few days or with mares and foals with problems); or (c) paddocks with electric fences.

Stoneham, 1991; Curcio and Nogueira, 2012). If the colostrum is of poor quality then the foal will need to ingest more, and vice versa if the colostrum has a higher IgG concentration.

The foal's own immune system does start to function to a very limited extent during pregnancy; hence, a small concentration of IgM is evident at birth, but it does not reach maximum capacity until 3–4 months of age (Cullinane *et al.*, 2001). Colostrum, therefore, provides protection in the interim until the foal's own immune system is fully functioning. Colostrum also contains maternal lymphocytes, hormones, cytokines,

growth factors, etc., which may also act to pump prime the foal's immune system and help to ensure rapid activation of the foal's immune system (Stoneham, 2011). However, immunoglobulins derived from colostrum have a varying half-life (IgG 176 days, IgA 3.44 days) so the foal experiences a trough in antibody levels around 2 months of age when it is particularly susceptible to disease, and it may not be apparent until then that the foal's initial immunoglobulin intake via colostrum was inadequate (McTaggart *et al.*, 2005; Wagner *et al.*, 2006; Stoneham, 2011). If the mare is immunized during late pregnancy then the antibodies raised pass to her colostrum and are available to the foal, providing it with essential temporary protection. For this reason immunization and introduction to the foaling environment is advised 4–6 weeks prior to expected delivery.

19.2.2.6. Renal function

Newborn foals will initially urinate frequently (around 150 ml^{-1} kg^{-1} day^{-1}), producing more hypotonic (more dilute) urine than adult horses (Brewer *et al.*, 1991; Curcio and Nogueira 2012). The dilute nature of the foal's urine is indicative of the fact that the fetal kidney is not mature at birth. This reduced ability to concentrate urine can be of concern in dehydrated foals, and has implications on the use of renally excreted drugs,

including antibiotics (Holdstock *et al.*, 1998). This is another reason to be cautious about the prophylactic use of antibiotics in newborn foals.

Table 19.3 illustrates the main physiological parameters, or milestones, that a foal should reach at set times post-partum as an indication of well-being. Alternatively, a behaviour inventory proposed by Grogan and McDonnell (2005) (Table 19.4) can be used in conjunction with the APGAR score (Table 19.2) to assess neonatal well-being and future prognosis.

19.2.3. Biochemical adaptation

At birth, the foal's metabolic system undergoes dramatic alterations from a dependent to an independent

Table 19.3. The major parameters or milestones that should be achieved by the foal in the first few hours of life.

Parameter or milestone	Average values for the healthy foal (minimum and maximum duration)
Foaling	
Duration of stage 1 labour	30 min (10 min to 48 h)
Duration of stage 2 labour	30 min (5–60 min)
Duration of stage 3 labour	2 h (20 min to 8 h)
Placenta	
Weight	1% of mare's post-foaling body weight, 500 kg mare = 5.0 kg (4.5–5.5 kg)
Foal	
Weight	7%–10% of mare's post-foaling body weight 500 kg mare = 35–50 kg foal
Heart rate - at birth	40–80 beats min^{-1}
Heart rate - resting (> 24 h)	80–100 beats min^{-1}
Heart rate - active (> 24 h)	Up to 150 beats min^{-1}
Birth to first breath	30–60 s
Respiration rate - birth	60–70 breaths min^{-1}
Respiration rate - resting (> 4 h)	30–40 breaths min^{-1}
Time to ability to shiver	Within 3 h
Birth to umbilical cord breakage	5–10 min
Birth to sternal recumbency	5–15 min
Birth to standing	30–90 min
Birth to suckling reflex	5–20 min
Birth to successful suckle	60–120 min
Suckle frequency in 24–96 h	1–2 h^{-1}
Birth to first meconium	0–12 h
Birth to first milk dung	48–72 h
Birth to first urination	1–12 h
Body temperature - at birth	37–37.5°C
Body temperature - at 4 h	38–38.5°C

status (Ousey *et al.*, 1991). While *in utero* it is dependent entirely upon the maternal system via the placenta; post-partum, this dependency is removed and replaced by reliance upon the pulmonary and gastrointestinal systems controlled by the foal's endocrine system.

At birth, the foal goes through a transitional period after the severing of the maternal connection (umbilical cord) and before suckling. This period of time is one of considerable stress and exertion for which energy is required, provided by hepatic (liver) glycogen stores laid down during the later stages of gestation; the equine fetus only stores limited glycogen within the brain. Mobilization of glycogen (its conversion to glucose) is via the process of glucogenesis. One of the major enzymes in this pathway is glucose-6-phosphate, which the liver only produces after birth. Hence, glycogen reserves can only be mobilized post-partum. Full glycogenic ability is not reached until 1 month post-partum (Ousey *et al.*, 1991). Glucose levels can be measured in the plasma of newborn foals and used to indicate the availability of these glycogen stores. However, these stores are finite and are quickly depleted in cases of stress/hypoxemia, etc. The foal's body fat can then be used as energy and should be enough for the first 24 h of life (Buchanan *et al.*, 2005). Immediately post-partum, glucose concentrations should be in the order of 50–70 mg 100ml^{-1} blood. Levels lower than 50 mg 100 ml^{-1} are critical and indicate hypoglycaemia. Once the foal has suckled, glucose levels increase and in a normal foal that is 36 h old they reach values of 100–110 mg 100ml^{-1} blood. Glucose levels then increase over the next 48 h to 120–210 mg 100ml^{-1} and remain relatively high compared to the adult horse (75–120 mg 100ml^{-1}) for the first 6 months of life (Bauer, 1990).

Bicarbonate levels rise steadily over the first 36 h of life from 23 mmol l^{-1} evident at birth to 27 mmol l^{-1} (Fowden *et al.*, 1991). Lactate concentrations also rise immediately post-partum to 3–4 mmol l^{-1} and decline to normal adult levels (0.5 mmol l^{-1}) within 72 h; greater than 5 mmol l^{-1} indicates a problem (Franklin 2007; Castagnetti *et al.*, 2010). The initial increase in lactate coincides with a fall in venous pH (7.4 post-partum to 7.35 at 30 min) and may be a result of the energy demands during the transition period. This fall in pH rectifies itself within 12 h when pH increases to 7.39 (Stewart *et al.*, 1984). Table 19.2 illustrates the major haematological and biochemical parameters for foals from parturition to 7 days of age.

Hepatic function is thought to be good at birth but does not fully function until 4–6 weeks of age, unlike pancreatic function which appears to be fully functional at birth (Knottenbelt *et al.*, 2004; Ousey, 2011). Renal function can also be indicated by urea and/or creatinine plasma concentrations which are high in the first 24 h, with values of 15–30 mg dl^{-1} and 2–4 mg dl^{-1} for urea and creatinine, respectively (Harold, 2011). Creatinine may remain high in the first 36 h of life before it drops to levels typical of adult horses; urea levels are generally reduced at levels on the low side for adult horses for the first 24 h of life (Edwards *et al.*, 1990; Harold, 2011).

Endocrine function can also be indicated via blood sampling. Two hormones of particular interest are cortisol and thyroxine. In the normal fetus adrenal cortex activity increases significantly in the last 4 days of gestation, cortisol concentrations rising to 70–80 ng ml^{-1}. In the first few hours of life this again increases significantly to 120–140 ng ml^{-1} before declining to 60 ng ml^{-1} within 6 h of birth, finally declining to normal basal levels, 30 ng ml^{-1}, within 3 days (Silver and Fowden, 1994). Such a pattern of cortisol release is not evident in premature foals, in which cortisol concentrations may not reach above 30 ng ml^{-1} and reaction to adrenocorticotropic hormone (ACTH) is very poor (Silver *et al.*, 1984; Gold *et al.*, 2007). The proposed link between cortisol and final organ maturation pre-partum would explain the compromised nature of premature foals.

The newborn foal has higher circulating concentrations of thyroid hormones, T3 and T4, than most other domestic animals. At birth, these may be up to 10–20 times those seen in adults (T3 3.36 ± 0.65, T4 8.05 ± 2.09 nmol l^{-1}). Concentration then drops in the first few days but rises again (T3 0.86 ± 0.4, T4 14.34 ± 6.7 nmol l^{-1}) 4–6 days post-partum; levels then drop again over the next 3 months (Irvine, 1984; Vivrette *et al.*, 1990; Knottenbelt *et al.*, 2004). Thyroid hormones are known to be involved in many physiological functions and also integrally linked to metabolic rate. This is noteworthy, as the metabolic rate of the newborn foal is particularly high.

The significant changes in both cortisol and thyroxine in the later stages of gestation and during early life make them very likely candidates as the main drivers of final fetal development and neonatal adaptation.

The biochemical changes apparent in the newborn and very young foal can only be assessed via blood sampling and vary considerably. They must, therefore, be viewed with a certain amount of caution when used as a diagnostic aid (Jones and Rolph, 1985; Fowden *et al.*, 1991).

19.2.4. Post-partum foal examination

Within 1 h of birth it should be evident whether or not the foal is adapting to the extra-uterine environment appropriately, though there is variation between foals about when various milestones are met. If problems are suspected a veterinary surgeon should be called. The prognosis for foals that fail to adapt to the extra-uterine environment appropriately has improved over the last 10 years due to advances in intensive care, but they are still not good (Fig. 19.11). Assessment of parameters in Tables 19.1, 19.3 and 19.4, which include the following, will give a very good indication of foal well-being:

Foal:

- heart rate;
- respiration;
- ability to stand;
- vigour;
- ability to suckle;
- straight legs;
- body weight; and
- general demeanour.

Placenta:

- weight;
- integrity; and
- abnormalities.

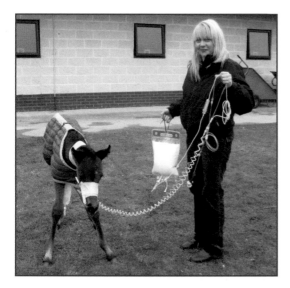

Fig. 19.11. Foal receiving total parenteral nutrition (TNP) as part of intensive care treatment. The prognosis for such foals has greatly improved over the last 10 years but is still relatively poor. (Photo courtesy of Dr Mel Lean.)

Mammary gland function:

- colostrum quantity and quality.

19.3. Early Foal Management: the First 6 Weeks

Early management has a significant effect on the foal's long-term prospects (Simpson 2002; Lansade *et al.*, 2004), and so needs to be discussed with the stud owner if the mare is to foal away from home; if she is to foal at home the subject needs serious consideration. Immediately after foaling and foal examination the following management procedures may be carried out:

- Navel dressing (Fig. 12.19).
- Administration of broad-spectrum antibiotics (penicillin/streptomycin), a precautionary method taken by some. However, indiscriminate use is not encouraged owing to the potential for bacterial resistance; disruption in the microbial colonization of the small intestine and caecum; diarrhoea; and selection for *Salmonella* antibiotic-resistant organisms (Madigan, 1990).
- Administration of vitamin supplements.
- Blood testing for haematology and blood biochemistry (see Table 19.2).
- Isoerythrolysis (mare–foal compatibility) test.
- Immune status test/immunoglobulin uptake.
- Enema – still practised routinely by some but generally not advised unless meconium impaction is identified. If an enema is routinely used, it is best administered during the first passage of meconium or at 12 h. Administration too early may be ineffective if no meconium has yet passed beyond the pelvic inlet (Madigan, 1990).
- Vaccination, particularly for tetanus, is practised by some. It is not advised if the mare is adequately protected, as colostral antibodies many reduce the efficiency of some vaccines (such as tetanus) if foal's vaccination occurs within 4–5 months of birth.

Apart from this, the foal should be left in peace with its mother for the all-important maternal–foal bond to form. Regular, unobtrusive observation is then advised so any issues can be identified and acted upon as soon as possible. A radiant-heat lamp may be used to provide warmth for the foal if the environment is particularly cold, but care should be taken to ensure that the lamp is high enough to provide all-round heat, not 'spot' heat.

Table 19.4. An alternative scoring inventory to assess neonatal well-being by assessing behaviour rather than physiology. Total score of greater than 10 is high normal, 4–6 is average to low normal and less than 4 is slower than usual, indicating a compromised foal. (From Grogan and McDonnell, 2005.)

Behaviour	Slower than usual = 0	Average to low normal = 0.5	High normal = 1
Sternal recumbency	> 5 min	3–5 min	< 2 min
Shake response (head or body)	> 10 min	3–10 min	< 3 min
Attempts to stand begins	> 30 min	10–30 min	< 10 min
Stands successfully (with steps)	> 60 min	30–60 min	< 20 min
Standing – udder seeking	> 10 min	3–10 min	< 3 min
Suckle	> 90 min	45–90 min	< 45 min
Locomotor burst of speed	> 2 h	1–2 h	< 1 h
Circle dam at speed	> 2 h	1.5–2 h	< 1.5 h
Organized recumbency	> 3 h	2–3 h	< 2 h
Autogrooming	> 3 h	2–3 h	< 2 h
Organised gaits (walk, trot, plus)	> 4 h	2–4 h	< 2 h
Retreat from approaching human	> 4 h	2–4 h	< 2 h

19.3.1. Exercise

For the first 3 days of life the eyesight of the foal is considered by many not to be good enough to safely allow it out of the stable or small foaling paddock. The foal is born with poor eye reflexes, low corneal response and slow pupillary light responses, which gradually improve over the first few days of life (Section 19.2.2.4.; Enzerink, 1998; Knottenbelt et al., 2004). After 3 days it should have developed adequate appreciation of distance and depth to be turned out with its dam for 1–2 h during the day, providing the weather is good (Fig. 19.10a,b,c).

It is best to avoid turning out young foals if it is wet or very cold and windy. Such weather will easily soak the foal through and, as both mare and foal will be reluctant to move around in such weather, it defeats one of the main objectives of turning them out, that of exercise (Back et al., 1999). In inclement weather turnout into an indoor school or exercise area, if available, is a good alternative. The paddock provided for foals should be small: 0.5 acre is ideal. It should have strong, well-constructed fences, ideally post and three rails with no wire. There should be no protruding objects, old machinery, wire, holes, low branches, etc., as these can prove death-traps to young foals still unsure on their feet. Ideally, mares and foals should be turned out in mixed gender groups and kept in these groups until weaning. An alternative system is electric fence paddocks. Providing mares are accustomed to electric fences, large fields can be subdivided into small paddocks with electric tape (Fig. 19.10c) or even moveable enclosures (Fig. 19.10b), allowing some association with other mares and foals but security in the first week.

Water should be provided in a bucket. Streams or large water troughs can also prove lethal for a very young foal. The paddock should have plenty of good grass as this, along with exercise, will encourage the mare to eat. It will also improve gut motility, which is especially important in mares whose appetite has declined after parturition.

Persuading the foal to leave its stable for the first time can be a challenge, but should be made as free from trauma as possible, otherwise nervousness will be perpetuated. During the first 3 days of life the foal should have been handled gently, stroked all over and got used to having arms put around it. When the big day comes, therefore, it should be used to human contact. The best day to turn a foal out for the first time is a day that is sunny but not too bright, for bright sunlight may discourage the foal from leaving the much darker stable environment. It should not be too hot, or flies will be a problem. There should be at least two handlers. The mare should be led ahead slowly by one handler and another should cradle the foal in his/her arms, one arm behind its hindquarters and the other around its chest, and encourage it to follow its dam (Fig. 19.12).

Some foals will follow easily; others prove more difficult. A foal should never be pulled from the head by means of a halter, as this may seriously damage its neck and head. A soft twisted cloth, bandage or thick rope can be put around its neck initially and can be replaced later with a soft leather or webbing halter. Leather is preferred, as it will stretch and eventually break under strain. Some people like to leave head collars on foals while they are out; this can be very convenient for catching them and gives the foals time to get used to them. However, the collar must be very well fitting to ensure that it will not get caught on anything or allow the foal to catch its feet in it (Fig. 19.13).

19.3.2. Handling

Initial handling in the first few days before turnout should consist of gentle stroking over the whole body and general familiarization to humans (Fig. 19.14). Once a foal can be led, it must start to learn how to be tied. This is best done by using a round pole with no projections, so the foal cannot get itself twisted up or caught on fences. A rope can then be attached to its head collar and on to the pole. As mentioned earlier, there is a risk of damage if the foal is pulled by a rope attached to its head. Hence, an alternative is to loop the rope around the foal's girth and up through its head collar and on to the pole. This method of restraint means that all the pull is taken on the girth and not on the foal's head. However, foals will soon learn that they cannot escape and that it is easier to stand still.

Once the foal has learnt to accept tying up, the general stroking and handling can progress to grooming and attention to feet and, eventually, travelling. These are particularly important if you intend to show the foal. Grooming can develop slowly and the foal will soon come to enjoy it, providing all progression is done slowly and patiently.

Providing the weather is good, a foal can be bathed, again of great use if it is to be shown. The weather must

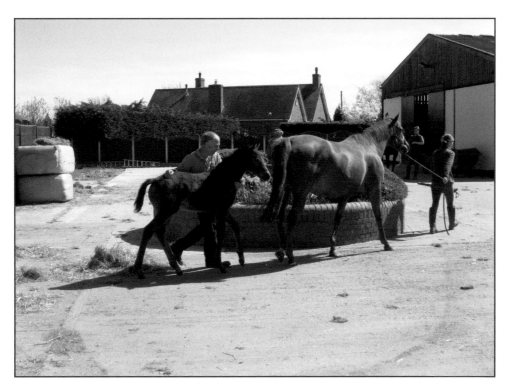

Fig. 19.12. The foal may be encouraged to lead for the first few times if you cradle it in your arms, one arm behind its hindquarters and the other around its chest.

be warm and it should not be bathed very early or late in the day, to avoid it catching a chill.

Introduction to a trailer or lorry can also be done in the first 6 weeks of life. The mare can be used to encourage the foal and many take to it easily, providing the mother is a good loader. If she is not, there is danger of the foal picking up her bad habits or her fear. In such cases, leaving the trailer in the foal's paddock with the door open and feed in the top end can encourage it to investigate and get used to going in and out at will. If this is done, the foal must be watched at all times to ensure it does not hurt itself. Once the mare and foal have been successfully loaded and unloaded a couple of times they can be taken for a short ride. A foal will sometimes travel better if there is no central partition dividing the trailer (Fig. 19.15). If there is a top door, it should be closed or a bar or cover used, to prevent the foal from trying to escape over the tailboard if it panics. Early handling may have a beneficial effect, not only on how easy the foal is to handle, but also in its interaction with humans at a later date, potentially making it more trainable (Sondergaard and Jago, 2010).

19.3.3. Feet care

The foal's feet should need little attention in early life unless they have a significant deformity. Nevertheless, picking up the feet, picking out the hooves and grooming the legs should be done regularly, and – along with ensuring a general acquaintance with the blacksmith when the mare's feet are attended to – will ease work on the foal's feet later on. Regular inspection of the feet will allow examination for injury and damage, and light trimming every 6–8 weeks from 3 months onwards can be done.

19.3.4. Behaviour

During the first 6 weeks of life the foal shows quite significant development in behaviour and social interaction, and is very inquisitive (Fig. 19.16). Initially the

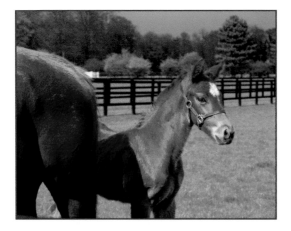

Fig. 19.13. A leather halter is preferred as a first-time halter as it will stretch and eventually break under strain.

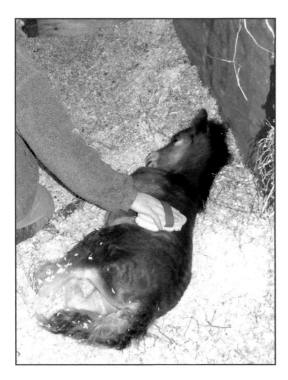

Fig. 19.14. A foal should learn to be handled, for example groomed, from an early age. (Photo courtesy of Ms Helen Tench.)

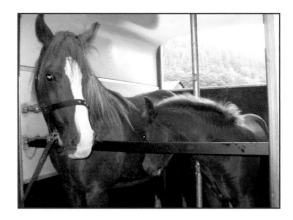

Fig. 19.15. Foals should learn to load and be transported in a trailer or lorry; they will often travel better with the central partition removed.

foal's whole world and social experience just revolves around its mother. This includes play, which may consist of rubbing her mane and tail, and kicking. Through this, it begins to learn how far it can push it before being reprimanded, and so what is acceptable and what is not. Once the foal has developed more steadiness on its feet, normally after about 1 week, it will start to explore further away from its mother, but never straying far. Over the next few weeks the circle gets bigger and it spends more time away from its mother, investigating and playing alone (Fig. 19.17).

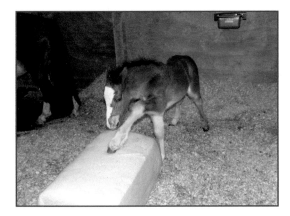

Fig. 19.16. Foals are very inquisitive and so care must be taken regarding what is left in their stables or field. (Photo courtesy of Ms Helen Tench.)

If at this stage the foal has access to other foals it will begin to interact with them and play will gradually include them rather than with its mother. By 8 weeks it spends up to 50% of its time playing with other foals and only 10% playing around its mother. If, however, the foal has no contact with others, it will play with its mother much longer and may try to play with other older horses present, or even with dogs or other animals regularly in its company (Fig. 19.18). If its mother is particularly possessive, or shy, these characteristics can be passed on to the foal and it will not integrate as well with other foals. In general the foal tends to hold a position in the foal hierarchy similar to that of its mother in the mare hierarchy, particularly if the mare is the alpha mare or right at the bottom of the hierarchy (Carson and Wood-Gush, 1983b; Mills and McDonnell, 2005).

Apart from play, the foal spends a significant amount of time lying down and resting (Fig. 19.19). These are normally short periods of rest, particularly in warm sunlight, between periods of play.

The remainder of its time is spent suckling. These periods of suckling in the first week are short and may occur as often as every 15 min. With time, the intervals between sucklings become longer, 35 times day^{-1} by week 10, but the periods of time spent suckling and hence the intake increases (Fig. 19.20; Carson and Wood-Gush, 1983a; Mills and McDonnell, 2005).

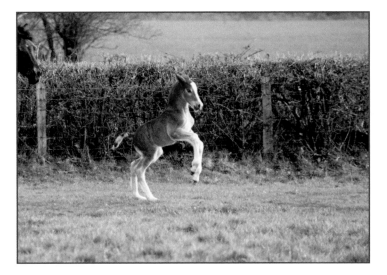

Fig. 19.17. Play is a very important aspect of a foal's early behaviour, and through play it will explore its environment and capabilities. (Photo courtesy of Penpontbren Welsh Cob Stud.)

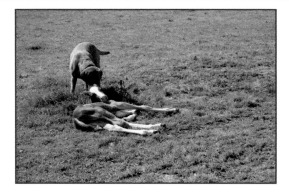

Fig. 19.18. Turning out a foal with other mares and foals is ideal but, in the absence of other foals, it may well play with other animals (such as a dog) that are regularly in its company.

19.3.5. Nutritional requirements and the introduction to solids

It is hard to ascertain the exact nutritional requirements of the newborn foal, but extrapolation from milk composition would suggest that the newborn foal requires 120–150 kcal kg^{-1} day^{-1} energy and 5.5–6.0 g kg^{-1} day^{-1} protein (Knottenbelt *et al.*, 2004; Vaala, 2011) in the first few weeks. This then declines and by 5–6 weeks foal requirements have declined to 98 kcal kg^{-1} day^{-1}, and 3.7 g protein kg^{-1} day^{-1} and 4–5 g kg^{-1} day^{-1} of fat (Oftedal *et al.*, 1983). In early life milk will satisfy these requirements; however, the foal will soon need to supplement this and so may be first seen investigating concentrate feeds, and even ingesting some, as early as 3 days of age. Investigation of the mare's feed at an early age (Fig. 19.21) is to be encouraged, as the mare's milk is naturally short of iron (Fe), copper (Cu) and zinc (Zn), which invariably results in anaemia in very young foals (Brommer and Van Oldruitenborgh-Oosterbaan, 2001). Cu and Fe are vitally associated with red blood cell function and haemoglobin levels. Adequate levels of Cu, Fe and Zn can be achieved by the foal picking at the mare's feed (Fig. 19.21), although oral supplementation is sometimes given. Anaemia may persist in foals too weak to nibble hay or concentrates until they are treated or are able to eat. Foals may also be observed nibbling the mare's dung (coprophagy) in the first 5 weeks or so (Fig. 19.22). The reason for this is unclear but may be a means of addressing mineral deficiency or of populating the gut with the microflora (bacteria and protozoa) for digestion. This coprophagic behaviour does, however, run the risk of parasite ingestion by the foal and so monitoring of faecal egg counts and appropriate worming of mares with young foals at foot are particularly important. Vitamin requirements are unclear but milk appears to provide what is required. Despite this, vitamin supplementation is often practised, but there is no evidence that this is to the advantage of any other than compromised foals.

In theory, the mare's milk up until peak lactation (on average week 8) provides the vast majority of the nutrients required by the developing foal. During this time, however, gradual investigation and ingestion of its dam's feed provides an increasing amount of nutrients, but this is not significant until after weeks 6–8. This interest in the mare's feed can be capitalized upon by introducing creep feed (concentrate feed formulated for feeding to young foals). The amount of extra creep feed that a foal will require in the first few weeks depends largely on the mare's milk yield. Creep feed can be introduced as an optional extra as early as week 1, but the foal should never be forced to eat it. The progression from milk to solid food must be gradual and can start slowly at an early age. Providing the mare is producing enough milk and is correctly rationed herself then the foal should not need to have creep feed until 10–12 weeks of age (Pagan, 2005). Many proprietary creep feeds are available, specially formulated to ensure the foal gets the adequate nutrients for a healthy start in life. If you mix your own, there are a few considerations to bear in mind. Protein should be relatively high in foal diets (to provide up to 6 g^{-1} kg^{-1} day^{-1}, often up to levels of 20%) when compared to adult diets. In particular, these proteins should be digestible and contain the ten essential amino acids for horses: lysine, methionine, leucine, isoleucine, histidine, arginine, tryptophan, valine, phenylalanine and threonine. Many legumes, grains and pulses lack lysine, and so soybean meal and linseed meal can be added within reason, as they are good suppliers of lysine. Other dietary components of special importance in growing animals are calcium (Ca) and phosphorus (P). A ratio of these two minerals of 2:1 should be aimed for. These minerals are essential for healthy growth of bones, cartilage, tendons and joints (Pagan, 2005). Excess Ca or P can cause problems. Excess P causes Ca to be mobilized from the foal's bones in order to maintain the ideal 2:1 ratio, causing bone weaknesses and epiphysitis, so delaying growth. Many people supplement Ca in the form of limestone flour or equivalent as numerous legumes, grains and pulses have a relatively high concentration of P. Low Cu concentrations are reported to be associated with angular limb deformities and high Zn concentrations

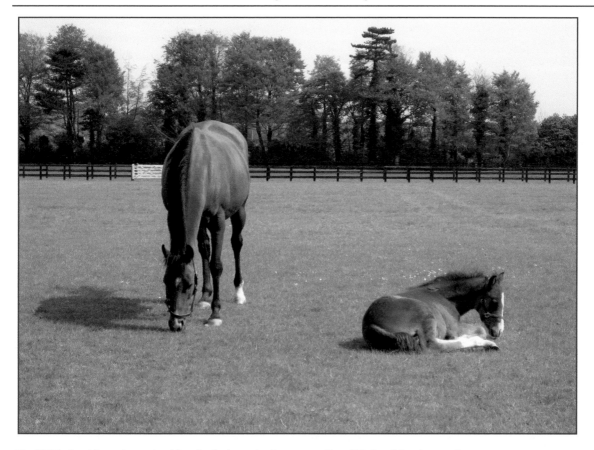

Fig. 19.19. Apart from play and suckling, the foal spends a large proportion of his time lying down resting.

with developmental orthopaedic disease (DOD) (Section 19.5; Savage *et al.*, 1993).

In addition to concentrates, the foal must be introduced to roughage in the form of grass or hay, as a diet of concentrates and milk alone can cause diarrhoea. Lucerne (alfalfa) is good, as it is relatively high in digestible protein and Ca. Hay may be fed, but it must be of a good quality, with no evidence of dust, mould, dampness, etc. Best of all is free access to fresh grass, which provides an *ad libitum* supply of continually fresh material.

Once the foal starts to pick at its mother's food, care must be taken that, when its intake becomes significant, she receives enough to meet her own requirements. Foal and mare should now be fed separately, ideally using a creep feeder (Fig. 19.23) to ensure that the mare does not gain access to the high-protein feed that the foal requires. By 3–4 months the foal should be eating 1 kg day^{-1}, about

0.3–0.5% of body weight. Careful monitoring of the foal's feed is required to prevent obesity and resultant conditions such as DOD (Ralston, 1997; Coleman *et al.*, 1999).

Water intake should not be ignored during this period of early life. In the first 3 weeks the foal's fluid intake will be satisfied by milk. However, as it takes in more solid food, it will increasingly require access to clean water. At 4–6 weeks the foal will require approximately 2–4 l water day^{-1} (approximately 2 l per 100 kg body weight per day) (Martin *et al.*, 1992).

19.3.6. Dentition

Providing the teeth of the foal erupt as expected and at the correct angle, there is no need to do anything with the teeth in the first 6 weeks. Most foals are either born with the central incisors or they erupt within 8–9 days. The middle incisors should then erupt at 4–6 weeks (Table 19.5; Dixon, 2017).

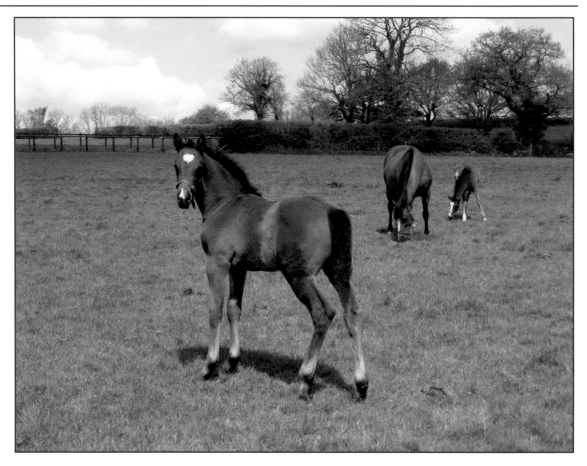

Fig. 19.20. As the foal grows up it spends less time suckling and with its mother, the intervals between suckling getting longer as it explores its wider environment.

19.3.7. Immunization and parasite control

Foals historically have been routinely immunized against tetanus in the first few days of life. However, colostrum from a suitably immunized mare is a much more effective method of providing protection against tetanus and numerous other diseases. Vaccinations have now been developed for a whole range of infections and the appropriate ones to consider depend on prevalence of the infection and geographical location of the foal (Wilson, 2011). Vaccination of young foals is now not thought to be appropriate, as work suggests that immunization of young foals (less than 2–3 months of age), born to mares that are adequately protected by vaccination, may suffer a detrimental effect on their long-term protective response to subsequent immunization, known as maternal antibody interference (Van Maanen *et al.*, 1992; Cullinane *et al.*, 2001; Wilson *et al.*, 2001). Vaccination of foals is not recommended, therefore, but the best protection is conferred by vaccination of the mare in the 8th, 9th and 10th month of pregnancy (Wilson, 2011). Vaccination as an older foal, or if the mare has not been adequately immunized, may be considered. Tetanus may in particular be considered, as foals throughout the world are particularly susceptible to it; additionally, vaccination against botulism and rotavirus, to which foals are more susceptible than adult horses, may also be advised.

Worming can be done first at 7 days of age, although ideally it would be delayed until 6–10 weeks of age. Good managerial control of parasites including monitoring faecal egg counts (FEC) should be practised to minimize the need for anthelmintics; the foal should

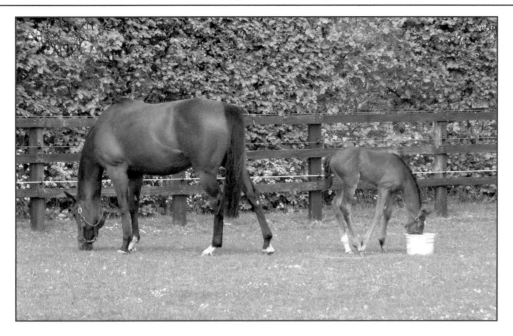

Fig. 19.21. A foal will soon be seen investigating its mother's feed. This is to be encouraged, as it provides the foal with essential copper and iron.

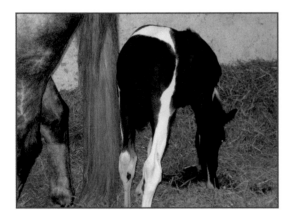

Fig. 19.22. Coprophagy is common in young foals and may be a means by which the foal addresses mineral deficiencies or populates the gut with microflora.

then follow a regular monitoring and worming regime. Monitoring for – and, if needed, worming against – *Strongyloides westeri* in both the mare and young foal is particularly important to prevent transmammary passage. Appropriate pre-partum worming may be justified as a routine to reduce FEC immediately post-partum (Craig *et al.*, 1993; Shideler, 1993d). *Parascaris equorum* (ascarids) are also considered to be a particular problem for young foals. By 6 weeks of age ascarids are reported to be prevalent in 30–60% of foals, and so appropriate wormers should be selected (Knottenbelt and Pascoe, 2003; Lyons and Tolliver 2004; Lyons *et al.*, 2011). There is, however, an increasing school of thought that foals should be allowed to develop a limited worm burden (FEC up to 200) as this encourages them to develop immunity to worms (Brown *et al.*, 1997). Hence FEC should be monitored and anthelmintics only given if they exceed 200.

19.4. Management of the Foal at Covering

The management of the foal at foal heat covering or at covering at any time while the mare has a foal at foot presents challenges with respect to managing the foal, and various options are practised. These, along with further discussion of the challenges in covering the mare on foal heat, are discussed in Sections 10.2.2.1. and 10.3.

19.5. Developmental Orthopaedic Disease

DOD is the generalized term given to disturbances in skeletal growth and development of foals and young stock such as angular limb deformities; contracted

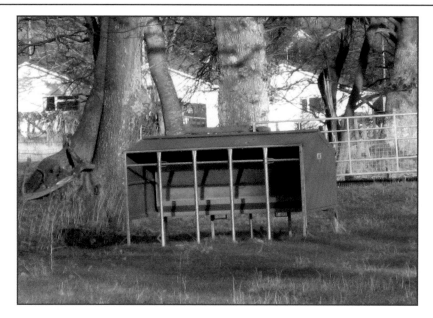

Fig. 19.23. Mares and foals should be fed separately, ideally using a creep feeder.

Table 19.5. The ages of eruption of equine teeth. (From H. Tremaine, Wales, 2002, personal communication.)

Tooth	Deciduous	Permanent
1st incisor	< 1 week	2.5 years
2nd incisor	4–6 weeks	3.5 years
3rd incisor	6–9 months	4.5 years
Canine	–	4–5 years
Wolf tooth	5–6 months	
1st cheek tooth	Birth–2 weeks	2.5 years
2nd cheek tooth	Birth–2 weeks	3 years
3rd cheek tooth	Birth–2 weeks	4 years
4th cheek tooth	–	9–12 years
5th cheek tooth	–	2 years
6th cheek tooth	–	3.5–4 years

tendons; incorrect calcification of bone; bone and joint inflammation (osteochondritis dissecans, OCD); epiphysitis; vertebral abnormalities (wobblers syndrome); and general abnormalities in bone and joint structure and development (Coleman *et al.*, 1999; Mackie *et al.*, 2008; McIlwraith, 2011). It is beyond the scope of this book to discuss these in detail but some general information is pertinent as it has been reported that up to 66% of Thoroughbreds are affected and it it is becoming increasingly evident in Warmbloods and Standardbreds (Jeffcote, 2005). There are several reasons for DOD including inherited conditions, limb trauma from excessive work on growing limbs, endocrine dysfunction, toxicity, fast growth rates and malnutrition (Thompson, 1995; Van Weeren *et al.*, 2003). The last two are due to incorrect feeding, which can have several effects. First, general overfeeding of both energy and protein results in overweight, and this leads to excessive strain on young, still-growing limbs and joints, causing deformities. Second, incorrect feeding (both too much and too little) of specific nutrients can have specific effects. For example, excessive energy appears to have a direct effect on the hormone regulation of bone growth and development (Thompson *et al.*, 1988a; Brown-Douglas *et al.*, 2011). This effect is made worse if animals are fed large carbohydrate (glucose) meals infrequently; that is, feeding once a day is more likely to cause DOD than feeding three times per day (Raub *et al.*, 1989; Lepeule *et al.*, 2009; Siciliano, 2011). Similarly, feeding low-quality protein (especially when it is low in the essential amino acid lysine) predisposes to DOD (Staniar *et al.*, 2001). Minerals such as Ca and P are also important, as deficiencies of either will cause DOD; additionally, the ratio of Ca to P needs to be correct. If P levels are relatively high this imbalance will tie up Ca reducing the amount available for bone growth and, therefore, cause DOD, even if Ca levels in the diet appear correct (Savage *et al.*, 1993; Van Weeren *et al.*, 2003). Finally, Cu and Zn are important for bone growth and development, inadequate levels leading to DOD (Pearce *et al.*, 1998; Savage and Lewis 2002; Siciliano, 2011). Along with nutritional management DOD can be limited by ensuring correct exercise; consistent, low-grade exercise is best and can be achieved by turning youngsters out. Acute, sudden exercise from intermittent exercise can contribute to DOD and should be avoided (Rogers *et al.*, 2008; Lepeule *et al.*, 2009) It is, therefore, very important that youngsters are fed a correctly rationed quality diet in several meals per day and that exercise (ideally turnout) is provided, but not excessively so, to prevent limb trauma.

19.6. Foal Management: 6 Weeks of Age Onwards

From 6 weeks onwards, the foal becomes increasingly independent of its mother and its management should reflect this.

19.6.1. Exercise

Continued turnout is essential to help muscle coordination and development, fitness, gastrointestinal and cardiovascular system function, and independence (Fig. 19.24). Ideally, mares and foals should be turned out together in mixed gender groups, to help the foal's development of social awareness and appreciation of

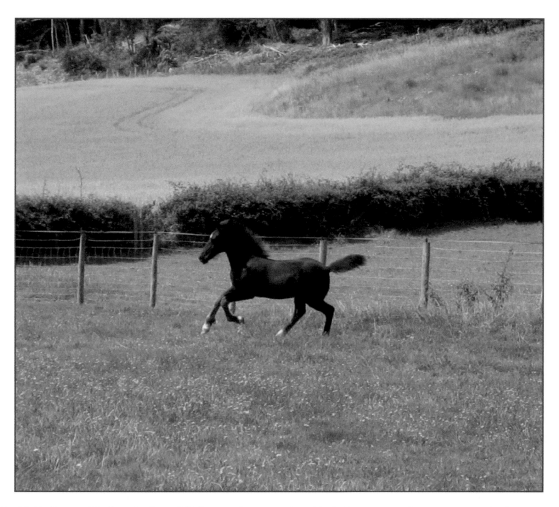

Fig. 19.24. Exercise (ideally in the form of 24-h turnout) is essential in older foals to maintain fitness, cardiovascular function, etc., and – not least – to help prevent developmental orthopaedic disease. (Photo courtesy of Penpontbren Welsh Cob Stud.)

hierarchy. Group turnout is an ideal starting point for gradual weaning systems.

19.6.2. Handling

The foal's handling at this stage should develop from that started in the first 6 weeks of life, remembering patience and reward. Halter breaking should have been established by now (Fig. 19.25). Late halter breaking can lead to confrontation. Leading lessons should develop and the foal should learn to lead without resistance. The process can be aided by a rope around the foal's hindquarters that can be pulled to encourage it to walk forwards. Well before weaning, the foal should be happy to be led without resistance or fuss, both behind its mother and away from her. This can only be achieved by continual and patient training, using short and frequent lessons (Fig. 19.26). The foal should also become further accustomed to travelling, leading on to travelling alone.

19.6.3. Feet care

Foot problems can be identified and possible correction considered within the foal's first year of life. In addition to regular trimming and handling, this can ensure that minor faults and problems can be identified before training begins. Overzealous attack on a foal's feet in attempts to correct leg problems should be avoided, as it exacerbates existing problems. Indeed, if left alone, many such deformities often prove to be self-correcting.

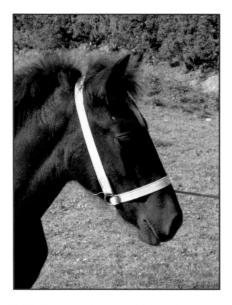

Fig. 19.25. Halter breaking should have been started by 6 weeks of age. (From Penpontbren Welsh Cob Stud.)

Corrective trimming should be done only by a trained and experienced farrier or veterinary surgeon. Deformities, such as an incorrect hoof/pastern angle, can within reason be corrected by specific trimming to change the length of the horse's heel. Toes out or toes in result in uneven wear of the hoof wall, and corrective and compensatory trimming can alleviate the problem. Excessively long toes (or the opposite, club foot) can be corrected by ensuring that any trimming done is adequate, not overzealous.

19.6.4. Behaviour

From 6 weeks of age the foal continues to develop its independent traits, spending more and more time away from its mother, playing and interacting with other foals. This is invaluable in developing social awareness and learning about hierarchies within a group, in preparation for survival alone with its peers and without its mother for protection.

19.6.5. Nutrition

From about 8 weeks of age creep feed becomes increasingly important to the foal as a source of nutrients. From this stage onwards milk quality declines and this encourages the foal to seek nutrients elsewhere. The quality of creep feed that is fed must be assessed carefully to ensure it provides all the nutrients required for optimum growth and development. However, it should be borne in mind that optimum growth is required, not maximum growth. As a rough guide, a foal destined to make 150–160 cm may gain up to 2 kg day^{-1} but by 1 year of age it should not weigh in excess of 80% of its expected mature weight (Frape, 1998; Brown-Douglas et al., 2011). Excess weight gain causes strain on muscles, tendons, joints, the circulatory system, etc. It is especially important when these structures are still developing that undue stress does not cause permanent deformity.

The protein requirement of the foal for growth is high and it becomes the first limiting factor as far as nutrient supplied by milk is concerned. Creep feeds have been discussed previously (Section 19.3.5) but, for the older foal, the feed should contain 20% protein. At 4 months, a foal destined to make a mature weight of 500 kg requires 669 g crude protein (CP) day^{-1} in a highly digestible form. In addition it requires 39.1 g day^{-1} Ca and 21.7 g day^{-1} P, although a Ca:P ratio within the range of 1:1 and 3:1, respectively, is acceptable. The importance of Zn and Cu is increasingly evident (Frape, 2004; Brown-Douglas et al., 2011).

As far as quantity of feed is concerned, 0.5 kg day^{-1} at 2 months is adequate, gradually increasing as weaning

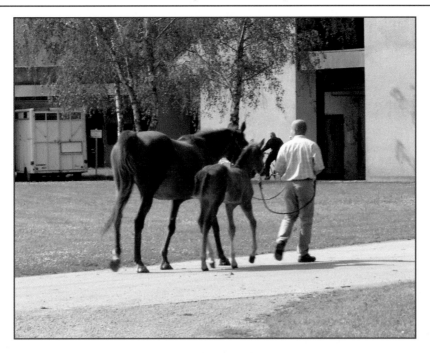

Fig. **19.26**. The foal should learn to be led without resistance from an early age.

approaches. As a guide foals of 3 months of age should be consuming 0.25–1.0 kg 100 kg⁻¹ body weight day⁻¹, which is normally about 1 kg day⁻¹ (Frape, 2004; Brown-Douglas *et al.*, 2011).

It is important that the mare does not have access to the foal's creep feed, as this may discourage the foal from feeding. Specially designed creep feeders permit the foal to feed alone without danger that the mare can have access to the feed (Fig. 19.23). The amount of feed per foal should also be controlled and, if several are run together, it is best if they are fed individually. This may prove difficult but will ensure that each foal is fed according to need and monitored against weight gain. Free access allows greedy foals to gorge themselves at the expense of smaller, less-dominant individuals.

If foals are fed outside in a creep feeder, then food should be checked regularly to avoid mould developing. Free access to fresh grass or lucerne is essential, and access to a mineral supplement is good practice.

Water must not be forgotten and foals of 8–10 weeks in age require at least 5 l water day⁻¹ (Fig. 19.27). This will increase in warm environments and with exercise, and the dry matter content of feed (Martin *et al.*, 1992).

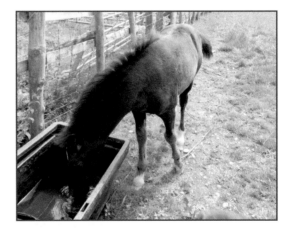

Fig. **19.27**. At 8–10 weeks the foal will require ad lib access to clean water to supplement the fluid obtained from milk. Water intake at this age is 5 l water day⁻¹.

19.6.6. Dentition

By 6 weeks the foal's first and second incisors should have erupted. These are then followed by the wolf-teeth at 5–6 months and then the third deciduous incisors at 6–9 months (Table 19.5). Attention to teeth beyond familiarization with opening the mouth to allow the teeth to be viewed should not be required at this stage.

19.6.7. Immunization and parasite control

Immunization against tetanus and influenza can be instigated at 5–6 months of age. Vaccination against strangles, rabies, equine viral encephalitis and African horse sickness may be considered at this time, depending on the prevalence of the diseases, although the side effects of immunization (such as abscessed vaccination site with strangles inoculation) make some unpopular as part of a general routine (Wilson, 2011).

A regular worming regime can be established from 2 months of age but is better informed by using FEC. FEC > 200 suggests that worming is required. Wormers against strongyles and ascarids are particularly important, as these specifically affect young horses (Rossdale and Ricketts, 1980; Lyons *et al.*, 2011).

19.7. Conclusion

In summary, the management of the foal is particularly important during the first few hours post-partum. Once this initial adaptation of the foal to the extra-uterine environment has been successfully achieved, the likelihood of the foal surviving is high. From this stage onwards, focus should be on the management of the foal so that it grows into a healthy, well-disciplined individual.

Study Questions

Detail the functional adaptations made by the foal in the first 12 h of neonatal life.

Discuss the implications that equine placenta anatomy has on the neonatal foal.

Milk provides the main source of nutritional support for the neonate. Discuss the foal's reliance on milk and how this can be reduced as the foal approaches weaning.

Discuss how the foal becomes increasingly independent of the dam and how management can help prepare the foal for this eventuality.

Suggested Reading

Knottenbelt, D.C. and Holdstock, N. (2004) The role of colostrum in immunity. In: Knottenbelt, D.C. (ed.) *Equine Neonatology and Surgery*. Saunders, Edinburgh, pp. 15–18.

Knottenbelt, D.C. and Holdstock, N. (2004) Methods of assessing colotrum quality. In: Knottenbelt, D.C. (ed.) *Equine Neonatology and Surgery*. Saunders, Edinburgh pp. 393–394.

Knottenbelt, D.C., Holdstock, N. and Madigan, J.E. (2004) *Equine Neonatology and Surgery*. W.B. Saunders, Philadelphia, Pennsylvania, pp. 508.

Grogan, E.H. and McDonnell, S.M. (2005) Mare and Foal Bonding and Problems, *Clinical and Technical Equine Practice* 4, 228–237.

Stoneham, S.J. (2006) Assessing the newborn foal. In: Paradis, M.R. (ed.) *Equine neonatal medicine*. Elsevier Saunders, Philadelphia, Pennsylvania, pp. 1–10.

Stoneham, S.D.L. (2011) The normal post partum foal. In: McKinnon, A.O., Squires, E.L., Vaala, E. and Varner, D.D. (eds) *Equine Reproduction*, 2nd edn. Wiley-Blackwell, Philadelphia, London, pp. 63–68.

Wilson, W.D. (2011) Vaccination of mares, foals and weanlings. In: McKinnon, A.O., Squires, E.L., Vaala, E. and Varner, D.D. (eds) *Equine Reproduction*, 2nd edn. Wiley-Blackwell, Philadelphia, London, pp. 302–330.

Brown-Douglas, C.G., Huntington, P. and Pagan, J. (2011) Growth of horses. In: McKinnon, A.O., Squires, E.L., Vaala, E. and Varner, D.D. (eds) *Equine Reproduction*, 2nd edn. Wiley-Blackwell, Philadelphia, London, pp. 280–291.

Lyons, E.T., Ionita, M. and Tolliver, S.C. (2011) Important gastrointestinal parasites. In: McKinnon, A.O., Squires, E.L., Vaala, E. and Varner, D.D. (eds) *Equine Reproduction*, 2nd edn. Wiley-Blackwell, Philadelphia, London, pp. 292–301.

Curcio, B.R. and Nogueira, C.E.W. (2012) Newborn adaptations and healthcare throughout the first age of the foal. *Animal Reproduction* 9(3), 182–187.

Stoneham, S.J., Morresey, P. and Ousey, J. (2017) Nutritional management and practical feeding of the orphan foal. *Equine Veterinary Education* 29(3), 165–173.

20 Management of Weaning

The Objectives of this Chapter are:

To enable you to understand the challenges faced by the foal at weaning.
To critically evaluate the different ways in which the weaning of foals can be managed.

20.1. Introduction

Correct weaning management is critical in ensuring the foal's long-term good health, physical growth and development, psychological development, social interaction with fellow equids and humans, and long-term productivity.

20.2. Weaning

Weaning is essential to allow the mare's mammary gland to recover in order to ensure an adequate milk supply for the forthcoming foal. Naturally, the foal would be weaned at 9–10 months of age, giving the mare at least 1 month to recover before the birth of the new foal. By 9 months of age the foal will normally be consuming a large quantity of solid food, with minimal reliance on milk. The resultant dry period, after weaning and before the new lactation, allows the mare's system to recover, concentrate on supporting the foal *in utero* and replenish body reserves (Waran *et al.*, 2008).

20.2.1. The timing of weaning

Naturally, during the last 3 months of lactation, the foal (now over 6 months of age) derives most of its nutrients from grass and herbage. It is, therefore, quite possible with appropriate management and the provision of supplementary feed (concentrates and/or creep feed) to wean foals at 6 months of age (Coleman *et al.*, 1999; Xiao *et al.*, 2015). Weaning at 6 months is the practice in most studs and coincides, for most, with the autumn when mares may be beginning to be housed. Housing foals and mares separately is easier and so weaning at 6 months is primarily driven by management. However, weaning should ideally not be considered unless it is certain that the foal is in good physical condition as well

as taking in adequate amounts of feed. The effective time of weaning will also depend upon the mare's behaviour, month of parturition and the dependence of the foal upon the mare (Apter and Householder, 1996; Waran *et al.*, 2008). Early weaning, as soon as 4 months of age, may be practised if the mare is ill or suffering. This requires planning and good management but, providing the foal is well prepared, introduced to solids in good time and is in good physical condition, it should not suffer significantly as a result. Early weaning can cause complications; for example, foals cannot be run out with other foals, which will either not yet be weaned or will be older and so dominate the foal and not allow it adequate access to concentrate feeds. An alternative companion needs to be provided to give psychological security and development; a small, quiet donkey or pony can be ideal. Whether weaning occurs at 4 months or 6 months an immediate depression in average daily liveweight gain (DLG) is seen. This suppression of growth normally lasts for 2–3 weeks and is particularly evident as a reduction in bone mineral density, heart girth and wither height (Reichmann *et al.*, 2004). In younger weaned foals a reduction in cannon bone growth specifically has also been reported (Warren *et al.*, 1997, 1998a,b; Rogers *et al.*, 2004; Brown-Douglas *et al.*, 2005; Dubcová *et al.*, 2015). In extremes (death of mare, vicious mare, etc.) foals can be weaned at a very young age, but these foals are in essence brought up as orphan foals.

20.2.2. Weaning stress

Weaning is a very stressful process, both physically and psychologically (Apter and Householder, 1996; Waran *et al.*, 2008). The foal will be separated from its dam, milk will be eliminated from its diet, it will be introduced to strange horses and there will be more handling and contact with humans. Careful management, however, can ease these stresses and thus reduce the stress of weaning.

The physical stress of weaning can be reduced by ensuring that the solid food intake of the foal prior to weaning is adequate, to minimize any setback due to the sudden removal of milk from the diet (Waran *et al.*, 2008; Fig. 20.1). Sudden changes in diet at all ages can cause digestive upsets, and in foals they can also lead to growth and developmental retardation (Warren *et al.*, 1998a,b; Waran *et al.*, 2008). To ensure a gradual change, some studs advocate milking the mare for a few days after weaning and feeding the milk to the foal along with its concentrate diet. This is also reported to reduce the risk of mastitis, but is time-consuming, and some mares will object violently to being milked by hand. Alternatively, foals can be fed milk pellets for a while after weaning. Such artificial inclusion of milk into a weanling's diet, however, defeats one of the main objects of weaning: that of removing milk from the diet. In addition, if the foal has naturally significantly reduced its intake of milk prior to weaning, the addition of milk

post-weaning will be a retrograde step and may adversely affect newly established gut microflora and so cause digestive upsets.

A foal being considered for weaning must be in good health. Any animals showing signs of illness such as runny nose, coughing, listlessness, starry coat, diarrhoea, etc., must not be weaned until their condition improves. Young animals can suffer quite dramatically from seemingly small problems, resulting in considerable setbacks to their development and possible permanent damage. If in doubt, it is advisable to call a veterinary surgeon. In exceptional cases, and only under veterinary supervision, foals suffering from ill health may be weaned, as some medicines are easier to administer and are more effective in a foal not on a milk diet. Psychological stress can be reduced by introducing the foal to his post-weaning companions and regular handling prior to removal from its mother (Chapter 19). At around the time of weaning it is common to also castrate, vaccinate and worm foals. Such an onslaught on the foal at the same time can have a significant detrimental effect on health, growth and development, and so it is advocated that foals are vaccinated, wormed and castrated either 1 month before or after weaning.

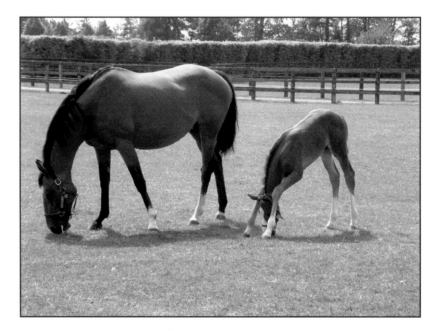

Fig. 20.1. Intake of solid food must be adequate prior to weaning, to minimize the upset to the digestive system as a result of the change from a liquid, milk-based to solid, concentrate- and forage-based diet. This intake of solid food can be slowly introduced from a few weeks of age when foals are turned out on to grazing.

20.2.3. Methods of weaning

Plans for weaning foals should be considered well in advance of the actual event. There are four main types of weaning: sudden or abrupt; gradual; interval or paddock; and weaning in pairs. The method employed is often dictated by the facilities available, the numbers of foals and young stock, and also by personal preference. Traditionally, foals were weaned suddenly and individually by removing the mare abruptly and leaving the foal in a stable or loose box out of earshot of its mother. More recently, other methods have been advocated, which are based on a more gradual removal of the mare or the introduction of substitute companions, and so are considered to be less stressful (Apter and Householder, 1996; Waran *et al.*, 2008).

20.2.3.1. Sudden or abrupt weaning

Sudden or abrupt weaning involves the abrupt separation of the mare and foal (Fig. 20.2; Apter and Householder 1996; Erber *et al.*, 2012). If this system of weaning is to be employed, then a safe and secure stable is required for the foal. It must be free from any projections likely to cause damage; water buckets should either be fixed to the wall or not left unattended. Hay should be fed in a hay rack off the ground. A hay net is not advised as the foal may strangle itself; hay on the floor is better but can be wasted. The bed should be deep, ideally made of straw, providing good protection as the foal launches around the box. The stable door should be secure, with an upper grill or metal-mesh door as well as a solid upper door (Fig. 20.3).

At weaning, the mare is abruptly removed from the loose box, leaving the foal behind. The foal should by now be accustomed to handling and can be held in the stable while the mare is removed. She must be kept moving even though she is likely to be very reluctant; the quicker she is removed and with the least fuss, the better. As soon as she is out of the stable, both solid doors top and bottom should be shut and a light left on in the stable. The foal should be relatively safe under these conditions for a short while until the mare has been attended to (Heleski *et al.*, 2002).

The mare should be taken to a field out of earshot of the foal, with limited grass cover (Fig. 13.5). The field should be secure, with safe boundaries. Some mares are very disturbed for the first few hours and can easily damage themselves by careering around; others appear to consider weaning a relief. The mare should be watched until she has settled down and started to graze. The foal should then be checked. It should be given water, as it will have invariably worked itself into a good lather. Hay should also be made available *ad libitum,* along with a small feed which is fed as soon as it has calmed down. The foal should remain in the box for the first few days to allow it to get used to life alone. A large stable is, therefore, advantageous. For these first few days the upper mesh door should be closed at all times to prevent the foal attempting to jump out and yet still provide ventilation and allow the foal to see activity in the yard. Foals are notoriously unaware of danger and will launch themselves at obstacles that an adult horse would not dream of attempting. They are, therefore, very prone to damage and extra care should be taken to avoid potential hazards: prevention is infinitely better than cure. The foal should be handled and mucked out regularly.

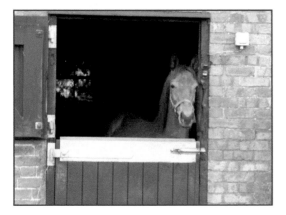

Fig. 20.2. Traditionally foals are weaned by sudden removal of the mare, leaving the foal in a secure stable.

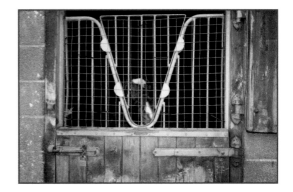

Fig. 20.3. The stable where the foal is left after removal of the mare should be very secure and have an upper grill or mesh as well as a solid upper door.

These first few days are very stressful and the foal is susceptible to physical damage and disease; this is one of the main disadvantages of this system. After a few days, providing the foal is calm, it may be turned out for short periods of the day with a companion in a small, secure paddock (Henry *et al.*, 2012). The length of turnout can be increased gradually to all day and night if appropriate. In many systems, foals are still brought in at night until the following spring, as weaning does not occur until late summer or autumn.

20.2.3.2. Gradual weaning

Gradual weaning is a newer and increasingly popular method, as it attempts to reduce the stresses of sudden weaning. It can be practised in yards with single mares or groups. As with abrupt weaning, if two stables are to be used for the mare and foal, they must be safe and secure and ideally have an interconnecting, barred window. More commonly, adjacent paddocks are used and, providing these are well fenced and secure, there should be no problems. It is advised that the fencing should be post-and-rail, rather than wire, to reduce the chance of injury. If two paddocks are to be used, it is normal to select the lusher pasture for the foal, as its requirements will be greatest and eating will provide a distraction. Initially, the mare and foal are turned into the separate paddocks or stables for a short period of time, 30 min or so. Over the next couple of weeks this time of separation increases, until they are turned out separately all the time. The close proximity of the foal to the mare allows physical contact and interaction, and so psychological support, but does not allow suckling. Independence and a reduction in the reliance on milk are developed over a period of time so the stress of abrupt and complete separation is much reduced. An additional advantage is that, as the time of separation is gradually increased post-weaning, mastitis is not a problem (Fig. 20.4).

20.2.3.3. Paddock or interval weaning

Paddock weaning requires careful planning and is not possible with single foals or with foals of vastly differing ages. Ideally, the foals should be born in batches within 2 weeks of one another and brought up together in the same paddock after the first couple of weeks (Fig. 20.5). This allows them to develop a hierarchy while their mothers are still around to dilute any aggression. In such systems some mares may be seen allowing a foal other than their own to suckle, providing her own foal is not also demanding milk. Near the projected time of weaning, all foals should be checked for physical condition and adequate solid food intake. In an ideal system on large studs there will also be other batches of younger foals born later and following behind, so any foals not ready for weaning in one batch can be transferred to the next one, giving them 2 weeks more or so to become prepared.

Once all the foals are ready for weaning, the most dominant mare or the dam with the most independent foal can be removed on one day, followed by the next dominant the next day, and so on until all have been

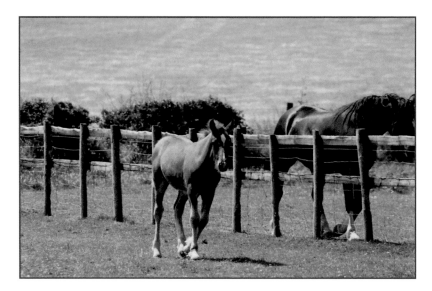

Fig. 20.4. Gradual separation of mare and foal over time can help minimize the stress of weaning. (Photo courtesy of Penpontbren Stud.)

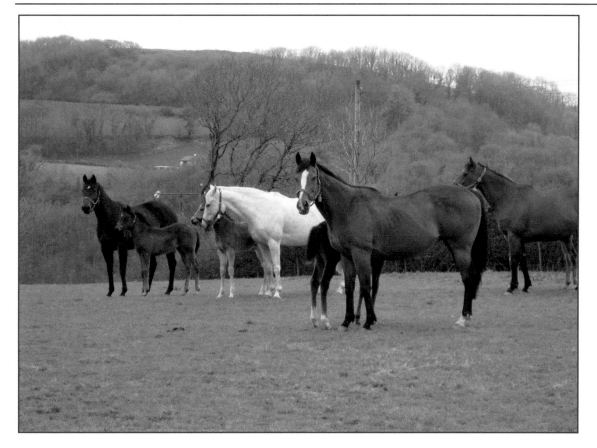

Fig. 20.5. In a paddock or interval weaning system, the groups of mares and foals of similar ages are run together, in preparation for the gradual removal of the mares at weaning.

removed. Occasionally, a gentle dry (barren, so not lactating) mare or gelding may be introduced as a companion. The mares must be taken well away from the foals and out of earshot. In this system, the foal that has lost its mother is solaced by the security of its fellow foals and the other mares. Mares should be turned out on to poorer grazing and be watched for mastitis (Fig. 13.5).

20.2.3.4. Weaning in pairs

A final alternative not used widely in practice, but an area of some research, is paired weaning. Based upon the sudden weaning system, foals are weaned abruptly in pairs rather than as singles, two foals being left in a stable together (Hoffman *et al.*, 1995) (Fig. 20.6). However, this system does potentially put two foals that are unaccustomed to each other in close proximity, and requires the two foals to be 'weaned' from each other at a later stage, which may be as stressful as initial sudden weaning alone would have been.

20.2.4. Variable stresses of weaning systems

More recent discussion has addressed the issue of weaning stress and the possible long-term consequences (Waran *et al.*, 2008). As indicated, gradual and paddock weaning are considered the least stressful, as the foals are solaced by familiar surroundings and companions and any change is gradual (De Ribeaux, 1994). This is supported in work by McCall *et al.* (1985, 1987) who, using vocalization as an indicator of stress, suggested the following ranking of weaning methods, listing the most stressful first and then decreasing stress involved: sudden weaning with no creep feed; sudden weaning with creep feed; gradual weaning with no creep feed; and gradual weaning with creep feed. Work by Holland *et al.* (1996 and 1997) agreed with this conclusion, although Waren *et al.* (2008) cast some doubt on this, stating that the behavioural and physiological consequences

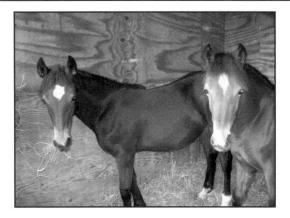

Fig. 20.6. Paired weaning is based on the principles of sudden weaning but leaves two foals together in a stable.

of weaning were still not fully understood. Work by Wulf *et al.* (2018) demonstrated that salivary cortisol quadrupled in abruptly weaning foals within 30 min of weaning, indicating considerable stress. A two-stage approach to abrupt weaning has been suggested – use of udder covers for 4 days followed by abrupt removal of foals – and is reported to be less stressful than single-stage, abrupt weaning (Merkies *et al.*, 2016). Paired and paddock weaning are advocated by some as less stressful; however, they require the foal to be 'weaned' from its other foal companions at a later stage, prolonging the stress. This is of particular concern in paired weaning systems. Indeed, work by Hoffman *et al.* (1995) and Malinowski *et al.* (1990) indicated that paired sudden weaning was in fact more stressful than single sudden weaning, as measured by plasma cortisol levels and foal behaviour. Malinowski *et al.* (1990) also indicated that lymphocyte proliferation to a challenge of concanavalin A was suppressed in foals weaned in pairs compared to singles. This would indicate a lower disease resistance. This suppression, however, could be reduced by human contact (McGee and Smith, 2004), and it has been suggested that paired weaned horses (or at least those weaned in small groups with regular human contact) are easier to train in later life than singly housed weanlings (Søndergaard and Ladewig, 2004). The introduction of an adult horse post-weaning is also reported to reduce weaning stress, and so future aggression and stress behaviours (Henry *et al.*, 2012). Paddock-weaning systems appear less stressful but are not possible with a single, or a few foals, as age-group batches are required. The use of equine appeasement pheromone has been suggested as a way to reduce stress as reflected

in the foal's reaction to an immunological challenge (Berger *et al.*, 2013). In addition to the immediate physical and psychological stress, work by Nicol *et al.* (2002) among others has suggested that weaning stress has a long-term effect, predisposing horses to gastric ulcers and depressed growth rates as a result. This is not supported by all workers; some (Rogers *et al.*, 2004) reported no difference in daily live-weight gain (DLG) between foals abruptly or gradually weaned, although all foals did experience some reduction in DLG post-weaning. Any depression in DLG may be due in part to an effect on the gut microbiome; the effect is reported to be greater in abruptly weaned foals as opposed to gradually weaned foals (Mach *et al.*, 2017). However, gastric ulcers are of increasing concern in intensively managed youngsters and have been linked to stress, in particular weaning stress, as well as to non-steroidal anti-inflammatory drugs (NSAID) and infection (Barr, 2011). A link between stable weaning and confinement post-weaning, and the development of stereotypic behaviour has also been suggested (Heleski *et al.*, 2002; Waters *et al.*, 2002). Diet at weaning may also be linked to stress levels, with creep feed and fibre diets being less stressful than high sugar and starch diets (Nicol *et al.*, 2005), and foals on complete pelleted diets having greater DLG than foals on grain and hay diets (Flores *et al.*, 2011). More recent work indicates that not only does foal management at weaning have an effect on the weaning stress, but so does management immediately after weaning. Dubcová *et al.* (2015) demonstrated that removing foals from their pre-weaning social and physical environments immediately after abrupt weaning resulted in a greater effect on short-term acute stress, but less of an adverse effect on growth rate, than delaying moving foals to 1 week after weaning.

It is increasingly evident that careful management of weaning is required to minimize any effects on the foal's psychological development as well as on growth and development, including bone growth predisposing to injury (Coleman *et al.*, 1999; Fletcher *et al.*, 2000). However, weaning need not always lead to problems; with good management, maintenance of familiar surroundings and routines, gradual preparation in diet and handling for the event, stress can be minimized as can any setback in growth, even in foals weaned as early as 4 months (Warren *et al.*, 1998a,b; Waran, 2008). Physical damage to the foal can also be minimized by ensuring that it is in safe and secure surroundings, and health promoted by exercise and access to sunlight and fresh air (Holland *et al.*, 1997).

20.3. Conclusion

Considerable thought should be invested in the method of weaning. Management at this young age can have long-term repercussions on the foal's physical and psychological development and so affect its ability to fulfil its potential in later life.

Study Questions

'Weaning is the most stressful time in a horse's life'. Discuss this statement with reference to weaning methods, stresses and consequences. How may the physical stress of changing diet at weaning be alleviated? What may the consequences be if you do not get it right?

Suggested Reading

Apter, R.C. and Householder, D.D. (1996) Weaning and weaning management of foals: a review and some recommendations. *Journal of Equine Veterinary Science* 16(10), 42.

Nicol, C.J., Badnell-Waters, A.J., Bice, R., Kelland, A., Wilson, A.D. and Harris, P.A. (2005) The effects of diet and weaning method on the behaviour of young horses. *Applied Animal Behaviour Science* 95(3–4), 205–221.

National Research Council (2007) *Nutrient Requirements of Horses*, 6th edn. Revised. The National Academies Press, Washington, DC, pp. 315.

Waran, N.K., Clarke, N. and Farnsworth, M. (2008) The effects of weaning on the domestic horses (*Equus caballus*). *Applied Animal Behaviour Science* 110, 42–57.

Advanced Reproductive Techniques

Section F considers the various techniques that can be used to breed horses as an alternative to natural mating. These include artificial insemination (AI), embryo transfer (ET) and advanced reproductive techniques (ART). Many of these methods are now commercially available and hold exciting prospects for breeding horses in the future. However, many raise ethical concerns and their use is subject to considerable debate, on the basis of both welfare and fair competition.

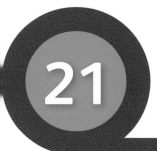

21 Artificial Insemination

The Objectives of this Chapter are:

To detail the process of artificial insemination (AI), from collection through to insemination, evaluation and storage.
To enable you to make informed decision about whether AI is appropriate for any breeding scenario or requirement.
To provide you with the knowledge to enable you to have an informed discussion with an AI practitioner on the procedure and its uses.
To enable you to appreciate both the limitations and future use of AI within the equine industry.

21.1. Introduction

Artificial insemination (AI) was first developed in horses and dogs in the later part of the 19th century but, as the horse was increasingly replaced by the combustion engine, AI in horses dwindled while its use in other farm livestock, especially cattle, increased significantly (Heape, 1897; Perry, 1968). Research specifically into AI in equids is still some way behind that of cattle, the other major commercial user of AI, as historically many breed societies were reluctant to accept for registration progeny conceived in this way. Although all equine breed societies do all now accept AI, the Thoroughbred Breeders' Association remains the notable exception, still refusing to accept for registration any progeny conceived through AI. The Thoroughbred Breeders' Association has a significant influence on the equine industry and is a major cause for the slowness of the technique being adopted by other breed societies, and for the relative lack of research. All other breed societies within Britain and worldwide do now accept the progeny of AI, but many set strict regulations, such as a limit on the number of foals that can be registered per stallion per year, the use of semen after the stallion's death, etc. In Europe, Australia, China, South Africa and the USA, equine AI is now widespread (Kowalczyk *et al.*, 2019). In 2019 Mizera reported that 43% of European mares were covered by AI compared to figures of up to 90% for other parts of the world (Nath *et al.*,

2010). Despite its increasing popularity it still has some way to go before it reaches the sophistication of cattle AI. More detailed accounts of equine AI may also be found in Brinsko and Varner (1993), Davies Morel (1999), Pickett *et al.* (2000), Samper (2000) and Kowalczyk *et al.* (2019).

21.2. The Uses of AI

There is a variety of reasons why equine AI is practised. Some of these are dependent upon and limited by the regulations set out by the countries and breed societies involved. The reasons for using AI include:

1. Removal of geographical restrictions.
2. Minimization of disease transfer, both venereal and systemic, by the removal of direct contact between the mare and stallion. Semen can still provide a means of transferring venereal disease (VD) (e.g. equine viral arteritis (EVA), equine herpes virus (EHV), VD bacteria, etc.) but it may also be treated with extenders containing antibiotics to minimize the bacterial content and so reduce the number of potentially pathogenic organisms. Such semen is, therefore, useful for mares that have an increased susceptibility to uterine infection (Clement *et al.*, 1993; Metcalf, 2001; Timoney, 2011d).
3. Reduction in injury risk to both handlers and horses by the removal of direct contact between mare and stallion. The risk is further reduced if the stallion can be persuaded to mount a dummy mare.

4. Increasing the number of mares that can be inseminated per ejaculate.

5. Improvement of native stock through semen importation (Ghei *et al.*, 1994).

6. Development of gene banks for future reintroduction of genetic material (Zafracas, 1994).

7. Breeding of difficult mares: those with physical abnormalities, especially caused by accidents, infection, poor perineal conformation, psychological problems, etc. However, care must be taken to ensure that such problems are not heritable.

8. Breeding from difficult stallions: those with physical problems, injury, infection, inadequate semen characteristics, psychological problems, etc. (McDonnell *et al.*, 1991; Love, 1992). As with the mare, care must be taken to ensure that such problems are not heritable.

9. Reduction in labour costs (Boyle, 1992).

10. Semen sexing (Lindsey *et al.*, 2001; Seidel, 2003; Allen, 2005).

11. Research and assisted reproduction techniques (ART) (Chapter 23).

Several concerns have also been expressed over the use of AI, including the reduction in the genetic pool, with overemphasis on 'fashionable' strains, the technical skill required and the infection risks if adequate screening is not practised (Morrell, 2011); however, many of these can be overcome with expertize and legislation.

21.3. Semen Collection

Semen collection can be carried out using one of several methods. The easiest method is the collection of dismount samples. The drips of semen are collected into a sterile jar from the stallion after withdrawal from the mare. This method is unreliable, as the quality of sample is very variable and the majority of the sample is left within the mare. Samples often contain low sperm concentrations and are relatively high in pathogenic organisms. Semen can also be collected from the anterior vagina immediately after mating. However, the semen at collection has already come into contact with the acidic, and hence spermicidal, secretions found within the vagina. The sperm may also become contaminated by pathogenic organisms. Neither of these methods of collection allows the assessment of the total volume of semen produced nor true appreciation of semen quality.

Condoms have been developed for use with horses. They can work very well, but do have a tendency to burst or become dislodged (Perry, 1968; Boyle, 1992).

Finally, the best, and now most commonly used method of semen collection, is the artificial vagina

(AV). Usually the stallion is encouraged to ejaculate into the AV by mounting an oestrous jump mare or a dummy. Stallions with musculoskeletal problems can be taught to ejaculate while standing using manual stimulation (McDonnell and Love, 1990; McDonnell and Turner, 1994; Davies Morel, 1999). Alternatively, pharmacological ejaculation (chemical stimulation) using xylazine, imipramine or clomipramine plus manual stimulation (McDonnell and Love, 1991; McDonnell and Turner, 1994; Davies Morel, 1999; Brinsko, 2011a; McDonnell 2001, 2011c) can be used with some success. Electroejaculation is used in some animals but is reported to be unsuccessful and/or too dangerous in stallions. However, Collins *et al.* (2006) report some success. The first AV was developed for use with horses in Russia at the beginning of the 20th century. Various models, including the Cambridge, Colorado, Missouri, Nishikawa and Hannover, are now available for use and they are all based on the same principles (Davies Morel, 1999; Brinsko, 2011a). They provide a warm sterile lumen surrounded by a water jacket, under some pressure, with a collecting vessel at the end, in an attempt to mimic the natural vagina (Figs 21.1 and 21.2).

Most AVs consist of a solid outer casing with two rubber linings, an outer and an inner. The outer lining and the casing form a jacket, into which warm water and/or air is passed by means of a tap or valve. The temperature inside the AV should be slightly above body temperature at 44–48°C. The amount of water used must be adequate to ensure that the pressure within the lumen of the AV mimics, as closely as possible, the pressure against the insertion of the penis within the natural vagina. Some models (the Missouri) allow the lumen pressure to be increased by inflating the water jacket; as air is lighter than water, this minimizes the final weight of the AV. The inner lining of the AV is often protected by an additional disposable inner liner, so ensuring sterility. The disposable liner, or in some cases the inner liner itself, is connected to the collecting vessel. Before use, this liner is lubricated with sterile obstetric lubricant to aid the stallion. It is most important that the collecting vessel and the lumen of the AV are also kept warm during collection, at the slightly lower temperature of 38°C, to prevent cold shock (see Section 21.6.5.1; Kayser *et al.*, 1992; Amann and Graham, 2011; Conboy, 2011a). If the temperature of the AV is too hot, there is a similar detrimental effect on sperm; in addition, there is the risk of discouraging the stallion from using an AV, and also possibly from carrying out natural service. The stallion seems less sensitive to

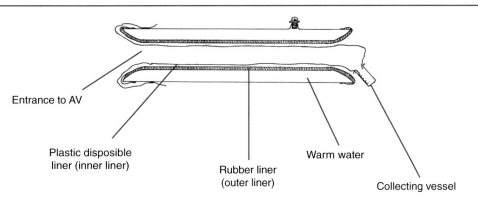

Fig. 21.1. A diagrammatic representation of an equine artificial vagina (AV).

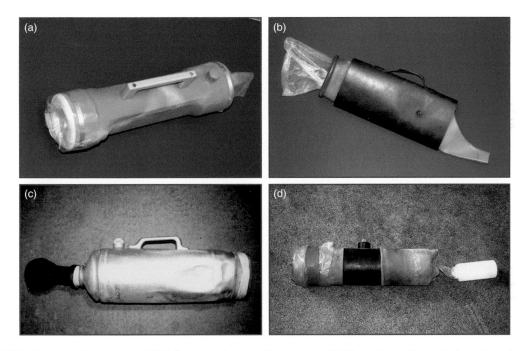

Fig. 21.2. Various artificial vaginas (AVs) for use in horses: all, except the Nishikawa, have disposable inner liners in place. (a) Cambridge; (b) Missouri; (c) Nishikawa; and (d) Hannover.

temperature than other farm livestock, but temperatures above 48°C must be avoided (Hillman *et al.*, 1980), although sperm themselves seem more sensitive to cold shock (Amann and Graham, 2011). A particular problem arises as the optimum temperature for semen is lower than the AV temperature preferred by the stallion. Hence it is important to encourage the stallion to thrust at collection to ensure semen is deposited rapidly into the collecting vessel and so has minimal contact with the higher temperature. Sperm are also susceptible

to ultraviolet light and so protection, as well as insulation, may be provided by enclosing the whole AV and collecting vessel within a protective jacket.

Stallions can be trained relatively easily to use an AV. Initial training uses a jump mare, a mare in oestrus either naturally or induced by treatment with oestradiol, to encourage ejaculation into the AV. The mare is prepared as for normal covering, including swabs in case of accidental covering; she must also be of a quiet and calm disposition.

Over time most stallions become quite happy to use a dummy (Fig. 21.3), especially if an oestrous mare is in the vicinity. Some stallions are not as keen, usually as a result of low libido; a possible consequence of coming into stallion work late in life after time as a performance horse; or as a result of incorrect AI management in the past. These stallions may never accept a dummy and will always require the extra stimulus of a jump mare.

A stallion is prepared for semen collection in the same manner as he would for natural covering (Section 16.5).

In readiness for collection all equipment must be at the right temperature for both collection and subsequent handling before the stallion is brought in for collection. Everyone involved must know what is expected of them. Collection of semen always carries a risk, owing to the unpredictable nature of stallions, especially when covering. As with in-hand covering, all handlers (especially the semen collector) are advised to wear hard hats. Up to three handlers will be needed if a jump mare is to be used: one to hold the stallion, one to collect the semen and one to hold the jump mare. All handlers should stand on the same side of the stallion. This ensures that, in the event of an accident, the stallion can be pulled away by his handler, and minimizes the chance of the semen collector or horses being kicked. The side used does not affect the sample collected, but once a stallion has got used to semen being collected from one side, it is best to try and stick to that side in future.

The stallion is allowed to mount the dummy or jump mare and the collector diverts the penis towards the AV (Fig. 21.4a–g). The stallion should be allowed to gain intromission and enter the AV of his own free will and not have the AV forced upon him. The AV can be stabilized by being held against the hindquarters of the

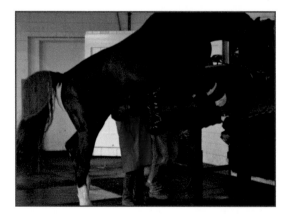

Fig. 21.3. Many stallions are trained to use a dummy mare. This eliminates the chance of accidental mating of a jump mare.

mare, if present, or the side of the dummy. The occurrence of ejaculation is noted, as in natural covering, by the flagging of the tail or by feeling for the contractions of the urethra and the passage of the semen along the ventral side of the penis.

After collection, the collecting vessel must be carefully removed from the AV, and speedily placed in an incubator at 38°C with minimal exposure to sunlight and agitation and then evaluated as soon as possible (Ball, 2014). If it is not possible to carry out semen assessment immediately, it can be extended and stored at 4–5°C for up to 24 h without appreciable reduction in its viability, and a reasonably accurate evaluation can still be obtained (Malmgren *et al.*, 1994; Batellier *et al.*, 2001).

21.4. Semen Evaluation

The gel fraction of semen has to be removed prior to evaluation. This gel fraction is the later secretion at ejaculation and has a very low concentration of sperm, which are invariably dead. The gel fraction is, therefore, of no consequence in AI and is removed by an in-line filtration system incorporated into the AV; by careful aspiration with a sterile syringe; by filtration through a gauze; or by careful decanting. Filtration is the most popular method used today and also ensures removal of debris (Davies Morel, 1999).

It is imperative that semen is kept warm at 37–38°C at all times, including during handling and evaluation. Sperm are very susceptible to cold shock (Section 21.6.5.1), and if any instruments, slides, microscope stages, etc., are not prewarmed then results obtained will be misleading. Semen can be evaluated under several categories (Baumber-Skaife, 2011) and not all evaluations involve all the assessments detailed below. They will vary according to what it is hoped to achieve by the assessments and the reasons for them being carried out. It is advisable for all the gross and microscopic assessments (Sections 21.4.1 and 21.4.2) to be carried out before a stallion enters an AI programme for the first time, and it is as well to repeat this at the beginning of every season.

When assessing the reproductive potential of a stallion, it is best to collect more than one sample for assessment. Several regimes are recommended to ensure the sample collected gives a true representation of the stallion's daily sperm output. The sperm produced by a stallion depends on his recent use. Suggested protocols include one for a stallion in breeding work within the breeding season: two ejaculates taken 1 h apart with the second ejaculate used, providing that the motility for

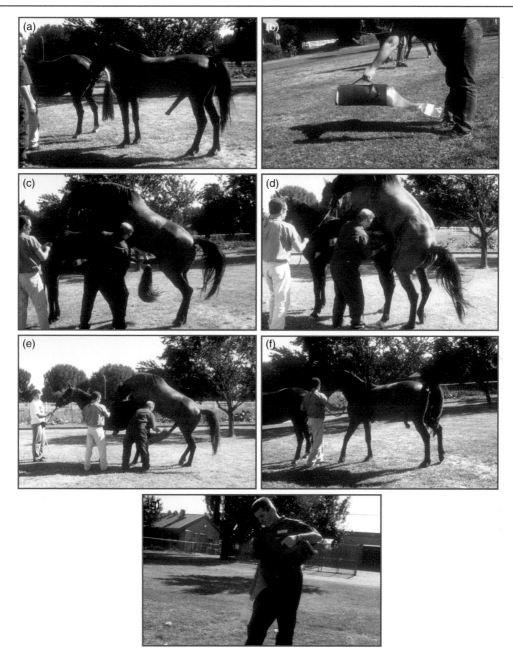

Fig. 21.4. Events involved in semen collection using a jump mare: (A) introduction or teasing of the stallion and jump mare; (B) artificial vagina (AV) ready for use; (C) guiding the stallion's penis into the AV and the correct positioning of handlers on the same side of the mare and stallion; (D) horizontal positioning of the AV to mimic the natural position of the mare's vagina; (E) dismount of the stallion and slow removal of the AV, ensuring all semen is collected; (F) after dismount the stallion should be turned away from the mare to reduce the chance of injury; and (G) the collected sample. (Photos courtesy of Dr Julie Baumber-Skaife and Mr Victor Medina.)

both samples is comparable and the second ejaculate has about half the number of sperm (Ball, 2014). At other times, or after a period of sexual rest, two ejaculates can be taken, followed 3 days later by a single ejaculate for evaluation; or two ejaculates collected 1 h apart, followed by daily collection of samples for 6–7 days with evaluation of the last sample (Rousset *et al.*, 1987; Thompson *et al.*, 2004). It is reported that it takes on average 4.7 days of daily collections to stabilize extragonadal sperm reserves after periods of prolonged sexual rest and so allow a truly representative sample to be obtained (Thompson *et al.*, 2004). However, these regimes take time and are rarely practical in many systems. In addition, any delays in testing are unpopular, as they delay the start of the breeding season. Therefore, in practice, most evaluation is carried out on a single ejaculation sample.

In addition to a full evaluation once a year, it is a good practice to perform a basic evaluation for semen quality assurance on each sample subsequently collected for AI. In this case, once the sample has been collected and filtered, a small volume (2–3 ml) is removed for evaluation of appearance, motility, concentration and possibly morphology, and the rest prepared for immediate insemination or storage.

21.4.1. Gross evaluation

The sample for gross evaluation is assessed untreated, immediately after collection. It is often advised that as soon as a sample has been collected a quick visual assessment is made to ascertain colour, smell, clarity, foreign debris, etc., after which it can be prepared for more detailed evaluation.

21.4.1.1. Appearance

Stallion semen is normally milky white/creamy white in colour with a thickness equivalent to single cream (Baumber-Skaife, 2011; Ball, 2014). It should not be pink (which indicates evidence of bloodstaining – haemospermia) or yellowish (an indication of urine contamination – urospermia) or contain clots (Varner and Schumacher, 1991; Samper, 1995a; Baumber-Skaife, 2011). The normal volume of semen produced by a stallion at each ejaculate varies considerably (30–250 ml) but, on average, most stallions produce 100 ml and, of this, the gel fraction is normally 20–40 ml. However, considerable variation is evident both between different stallions and the breeding season (Section 7.3.1; Ricketts, 1993; Davies Morel, 1999).

21.4.1.2. pH and osmolarity

Acidity/alkalinity is assessed using a standard pH meter. Acid conditions (low pH) are known to be spermicidal; elevated pH may also be indicative of extraneous material or infection. A pH of 6.9–7.8 is acceptable, with levels of 7.3–7.7 being best (Jasko, 1992; Oba *et al.*, 1993; Pickett, 1993a; Griggers *et al.*, 2001; McCue, 2014). There is a negative correlation between pH and

sperm numbers, so semen samples of high pH indicate low sperm concentration (Baumber-Skaife, 2011). The osmolarity of the stallion normally ranges from 300 to 350 mOsm l^{-1} but there is considerable variation between stallions (McCue, 2014).

21.4.1.3. Motility

A rough estimate of motility can be obtained by placing a drop of raw semen on a warmed microscope slide and viewed under ×10 magnification. It is not possible to track individual sperm with this method but a rough estimate of the percentage of motility can be gained with experience from the characteristics of the wave-like motion of the sample as the sperm within it move.

21.4.1.4. Concentration

A rough idea of concentration of sperm can be obtained by assessing the colour. Creamy white in colour, viscous with a thickness equivalent to single cream, indicates a good concentration of sperm. Milky in colour and watery in consistency indicates a low sperm concentration (Baumber-Skaife, 2011).

21.4.2. Microscopic evaluation

More detailed, and hence potentially more reliable, information on the quality of a semen sample may be gained by microscopic evaluation.

21.4.2.1. Semen extenders for evaluation

Prior to microscopic evaluation the sample is often extended (roughly 1:10 semen/extender), primarily to allow individual sperm to be observed, as sperm within raw semen tend to clump together. The exact dilution rate required depends upon the concentration of sperm and also the test being performed, but in general a sperm concentration of 20 ×10^6 ml^{-1} is aimed for. Extension of the sample also prolongs the life of the sperm, providing them with an additional source of energy and substrates for survival, while evaluation takes place (Morrell, 2011). Addition of the extender must be done immediately post-collection, ideally within 2 min, to reduce the chance of obtaining erroneous results from a loss of sperm viability caused by delay. There are numerous extenders available and used successfully during the evaluation process. In general, these are the same as those used in the preparation of semen for immediate AI and/or chilled semen storage (see Section 21.6.3). The most popular are those based upon either non-fat dried skimmed milk (NFDSM) or skimmed milk (Table 21.1).

Once diluted the sample is viewed under a light microscope with a magnification of ×40 or greater. Computer assisted sperm analysis (CASA) systems are now widely available and automate many of these evaluations. However, although the speed and repeatability of such systems are extremely good, they are only as good as the initial calibration, which often relies on traditional microscope methods (Zinaman *et al.*, 1996; Baumber-Skaife, 2011; Barrier-Battut *et al.*, 2017).

21.4.2.2. Concentration

Sperm concentration is a major determinant of the value of a semen sample and was traditionally assessed using a haemocytometer. A haemocytometer consists of a counting slide with etched grid and cover slip under which a set volume of diluted semen (usual dilution 1:100) can be trapped and viewed (Fig. 21.5). The number of sperm within the sample on the haemocytometer is counted by means of the counting grid. From this figure, and the dilution rate, the concentration of sperm can be calculated. This method gives a very accurate assessment, but is time-consuming and so cannot be easily done in the field (Ball, 2014). Hence the use of manual or automated spectrophotometers has become popular and now form part of complete CASA systems (Davies Morel, 1999; Baumber-Skaife, 2011; Barrier-Battut *et al.*, 2017). Spectrophotometers can be used anywhere; however, the results obtained can be variable and are only as

good as the initial calibration using a haemocytometer. The semen may be used raw or diluted in the order of 1:30; if diluted the diluent used must be optically clear, for example, 10% formalin plus 0.9% saline. The amount of light passing through the sample is then read by the spectrophotometer, from which the sperm concentration is calculated (Hurtgen, 1987; Davies Morel, 1999). Flow cytometers, electronic particle counters and photometers can also be used but are expensive in terms of both cost of equipment and of maintenance, and so are of limited commercial use (Hansen *et al.*, 2006). More recently, counters based on staining of sperm nuclear DNA by fluorescent propidium iodine have been developed and are reported to provide accurate, repeatable results (Hansen *et al.*, 2006; Johansson *et al.*, 2008). Finally, new on the market are portable analysers, such as the Ongo portable analyser, which analyse concentration and motility in the field and are reported to correlate well with CASA systems (Buss *et al.*, 2019).

The normal range for sperm concentration is 30×10^6 to 600×10^6 sperm ml^{-1} of undiluted semen (Stout and Colenbrander, 2011). A total number of at least 100×10^6 progressively motile sperm per inseminate is required for acceptable fertilization rates, although normally 300×10^6 to 500×10^6 is used (Brinsko, 2006; Sieme *et al.*, 2019). In practice, samples with a concentration greater than 50×10^6 to 200×10^6 ml^{-1} are considered to be normal and so acceptable for AI (Ricketts, 1993; Davies Morel, 1999).

Table 21.1. Examples of extenders used for semen evaluation.

Component	Quantity
(a) Non-fat dried skimmed milk glucose (NFDSM-G) extender, for use in semen evaluation. (From Kenney *et al.*, 1975.)	
NFDSM	2.4 g
Glucose	4.0 g
Penicillin (crystalline)	150,000 units
Streptomycin (crystalline)	150,000 µg
Deionized water	made up to 100 ml
(b) Non-fortified skimmed milk extender for use in semen evaluation. (From Varner and Schumacher, 1991.)	
Non-fortified skimmed milk	100 ml
Polymixin B sulfate	100,000 units
Heat milk to 92–95°C for 10 min in a double boiler, cool and add the polymixin B sulfate	

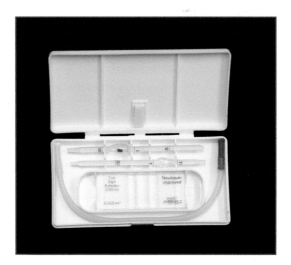

Fig. 21.5. A haemocytometer is traditionally used to measure sperm concentration.

21.4.2.3. Motility

Sperm motility is graded on a scale of 0–5 (Table 21.2). Motility must be assessed immediately, certainly within 5 min of collection, under a phase contrast microscope with a heated stage and on a heated slide, to get an accurate measurement. Ideally, a semen sample should be extended enough to give a concentration of 25×10^6 ml^{-1}, which allows the motility characteristics of individual sperm to be graded and particular note to be taken of progressive motility. However, dilution and handling may themselves affect motility, and so assessment tends to be subjective and dependent on the examiner's previous experience (Baumber-Skaife, 2011; Ball, 2014).

Owing to the subjectivity of microscopic assessment, other methods of assessing motility have been investigated, including the time-lapse dark-field photographic method (Van Huffel *et al.*, 1985), cinematographic techniques (Plewinska-Wierzobska and Bielanski, 1970) and computer analysis (Jasko, 1992; Burns and Reasner, 1995). The correlation between the results obtained by visual and computer analysis can be very good at 0.92, although this very much depends on the initial calibration (Bataille *et al.*, 1990; Malmgren, 1997). Despite this, CASA systems provide very repeatable results, and their convenience has driven their increasing popularity. Computer analyses have now become very sophisticated, not only providing data on progressive motility but also on

Table 21.2. Criteria for grading sperm motility.

Grade	Description
0	Immotile
1	Stationary or weak rotatory movements
2	Backward and forward movement or rotatory movement, but fewer than 50% of cells are progressively motile and there are no waves or currents
3	Progressively rapid movement of sperm with slow currents, indicating that about 50%–60% of the sperm are progressively motile
4	Vigorous, progressive movement with rapid waves, indicating that about 60%–70% of the sperm are progressively motile
5	Very vigorous forward motion with strong, rapid currents, indicating that more than 70% of the sperm are progressively motile

sperm velocity parameters (such as average path velocity, straight line velocity and curvilinear velocity), and they have been extended to give a full evaluation and not just of motility (Baumber-Skaife, 2011; Giaretta *et al.*, 2017). Although expensive, the ever-decreasing cost of these systems has led them to become increasingly popular. Most recently, portable analysers such as the Ongo portable analyser have been developed, and are reported to provide reliable results (Buss *et al.*, 2019).

Regardless of assessment method used, classification of type of movement, as indicated in Table 21.2, is important. Total motility (TM; % of sperm that are motile) and progressive motility (PM; % sperm moving across the microscope slide) are normally recorded. Progressive movement is important as oscillatory movement (movement on the spot) or movement in very tight circles is classified as abnormal and would not facilitate sperm progressing up through the mare's uterus. Some evaluators classify sperm motility as a ratio of those showing progressive movement/oscillatory movement, and CASA gives more detailed information on the velocity and paths of movement of individual sperm.

Semen containing at least 60% progressively motile sperm, which is grade 3 or better, can be considered as normal and adequate for AI (Colenbrander *et al.*, 1992; Ricketts, 1993; Davies Morel, 1999; Digrassie and Slusher, 2002). The correlation between motility and fertility is, however, variable and low (0.6–0.7; Samper *et al.*, 1991; Jasko *et al.*, 1992b; Heitland *et al.*, 1996; Love, 2011c). Although when compared with the other parameters evaluated it gives the best correlation, it cannot be relied upon to give an absolute indication.

21.4.2.4. Longevity

Assessment of motility over time has been used as an indication of viability. However, it must be remembered that longevity in a test tube does not necessarily equate to longevity within the mare's uterus, and so the test is less popular now. Longevity assessment involves the evaluation of initial motility and then at various intervals after storage at 5°C, 22°C or 37–38°C. For example, if motility is not less than 45% after 3 h or 10% after 8 h at 22°C, or > 30% at 24 h (or preferably 48 h) when stored at 5°C, then the semen may be classified as good enough for AI (Samper, 1995b; Baumber-Skaife, 2011). Testing longevity at 4–5°C is in many ways the most meaningful as this is the temperature of chilled semen.

21.4.2.5. Morphology

Morphological examination of sperm is a common method of trying to assess a stallion's fertility (Brito, 2007; Veeramachaneni, 2011). Individual sperm are examined and the overall percentage of abnormal sperm, along with the percentage of different abnormalities in the sample, is noted. Viewing of individual sperm can be enhanced by diluting a raw sample with formol-buffered saline (FBS) or by using a variety of stains, for example nigrosin:eosin stain, which stains dead sperm violet/purple (Dott and Foster, 1972), or cellular stains (such as Wright's (Diff-Quik), Giemsa and new methylene blue (Sperm Blue), all of which give reasonably similar results (Jouanisson et al., 2017; Murcia-Robayo et al., 2018). Finally, viewing under electron microscopy, although much less readily available, does allow various sperm components or abnormalities to be specifically identified (Reifenrath, 1994; Samper, 1995a; Veeramachaneni et al., 2006; Pesch et al., 2006; Baumber-Skaife, 2011). Staining of sperm to assess the integrity of specific areas may also be carried out, for example acrosome stains (Oetjen, 1988) immunofluorescence

tests (Zhang et al., 1990a) and labelled monoclonal antibodies (Blach et al., 1988). More recently, biochemical tests have been used to assess functional morphology (Section 21.4.3.1; Veeramachaneni, 2011). Figure 21.6 illustrates some examples of the abnormalities that may be seen.

Abnormalities can be classified as primary (failure of spermatogenesis, failure of sperm maturation), secondary (sperm damage occurring at ejaculation) and tertiary (inappropriate handling post-ejaculation). Failure of spermatogenesis is usually characterized by sperm with two heads, two tails, no mid-piece, no tail, rudimentary tails or excessively coiled tails and indicative of a long-term or even a permanent problem. Maturation failure is characterized by the presence of cytoplasmic droplets on the mid-piece of the sperm. As maturation proceeds, these cytoplasmic droplets should progressively move down the tail and disappear. This may well be only a temporary problem, a period of rest rectifying the problem. Damage occurring at ejaculation is normally characterized by tail abnormalities, bends, coils, kinks or swellings, detached heads and tails and protoplasmic

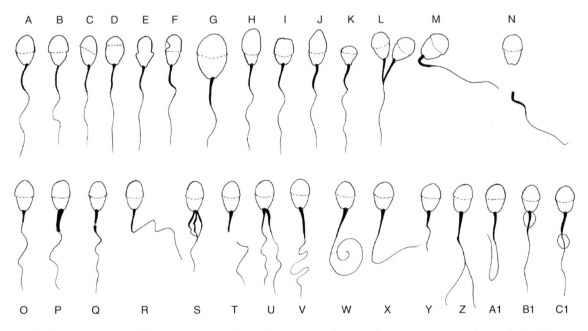

Fig. 21.6. Some examples of the more common abnormalities that may be seen when examining sperm for morphology. Top row from left to right: (A) a normal spermatozoon is followed by the following abnormalities in order. Acrosome defects: (B), swollen; (C), partially lifted; (D), small; (E), lifted; (F), part missing. Head defects: (G), big head; (H), elongated; (I), flattened; (J), lanceolated; (K), microhead; (L), double head. Neck defects: (M), bent; (N), broken. Second row: tail defects: (O), short; (P), fat; (Q), split/constricted; (R), bent annulus; (S), fibrous; (T), broken; (U), double; (V), convoluted; (W), corkscrew; (X), bent; (Y), small; (Z), double; (A1), shoehorn. Droplets: (B1), proximal; (C1), distal.

droplets. Finally, tertiary or post-ejaculatory damage is manifest as a loss of acrosome, fraying/thickness of the mid-piece and the bursting of sperm heads (Digrassie and Slusher, 2002; Veeramachaneni, *et al.*, 2006; Veeramachaneni, 2011).

The correlation between morphology and fertility is low (0.25–0.5; Malmgren, 1992a; Love, 2011c). Work has been carried out in an attempt to correlate specific abnormalities to fertility (see Section 21.4.3) but, again, correlations are poor. Moderate correlation (0.42) is reported between the percentage of normal sperm and per cycle pregnancy rate, whereas the correlation for specific morphological defects is weaker; for example abnormal heads (0.22), presence of proximal droplets (0.34), abnormal midpieces (0.30) and coiled tails (0.35) (Love, 2011c). Morphology is, therefore, not a very reliable indicator of the fertilizing potential, although (as with motility) it is used in the absence of anything else. Assessment for morphology does, however, allow problems to be identified such as testicular degeneration, abnormal spermatogenesis, orchitis, heat stress, etc., which in themselves may preclude a stallion or his semen sample from use in AI.

A normal semen sample would be expected to contain 50–60% morphologically normal sperm and as such would be appropriate for AI. This is much lower than the normal expectation in other animals (Jasko *et al.*, 1990a; Pickett, 1993a; Kenney *et al.*, 1995; Davies Morel, 1999).

21.4.2.6. Live/dead ratio

Motility gives an indication of the percentage of live sperm within a sample; however, differential staining of sperm gives a more accurate result. As used to assess morphology, staining with eosin–nigrosin stain in equal parts allows the differential staining of dead and live sperm. Dead sperm, as they are permeable to the stain, appear as violet/purple; live sperm remain clear (Johansson *et al.*, 2008; Foster *et al.*, 2011; Lacka *et al.*, 2016). Other stains such as Trypan blue and Chicago sky blue can be used in place of eosin–nigrosin. Alternatively, fluorescent stains (or probes) such as combined carboxyfluorescein diacetate (CFDA) and propidium iodide or calcein-AM and ethidium homodimer or commercially available stains such as LIVE/DEAD® Fixable Red Dead Cell Stain (Thermo-Fisher Scientific, Waltham, MA, USA) or Zombie Green® (Biolegend, London), differentially stain live and dead sperm and so can be used with flow cytometry to give a quantitative assessment of the live:dead

ratio (Sections 21.4.3.2 and 21.4.3.11; Hermenet *et al.*, 1993; Kutvolgi *et al.*, 2006; Baumber-Skaife, 2011; Ligon *et al.*, 2017; Fena *et al.*, 2018). The ratio, or percentage, of dead to live sperm is assessed in a number of samples from the collection. A live:dead ratio of 6:4 (60% live sperm) is acceptable for AI. However, a sample with a lower ratio may be considered to be usable, if it has a high total sperm count, as it can be diluted appropriately and it can still be ensured that the minimum number of live sperm for fertilization is inseminated (Ricketts, 1993; Davies Morel, 1999; Baumber-Skaife, 2011).

21.4.2.7. Cytology

Blood cells, leucocytes and erythrocytes can be identified in a semen sample using haematoxylin and eosin or Wright's stain, and viewed under a haemocytometer (Fig. 21.5; Ball, 2014). A count of leucocytes greater than 1500 ml^{-1} is indicative of a problem, possibly due to an infection, especially if the pH of the semen is also high. Such a sample would not be appropriate for use in AI (Ricketts, 1993; Davies Morel, 1999). Erythrocyte concentrations above 500 ml^{-1} are indicative of a problem such as haemorrhage or injury, and would also make a sample inappropriate for use in AI (Ricketts, 1993; Davies Morel, 1999).

21.4.2.8. Bacteriology and virology

Semen samples will potentially contain bacteria, both pathogenic and non-pathogenic (Clement *et al.*, 1995; Madsen and Christensen, 1995). Isolation and identification of pathogenic bacteria, in particular, is required to prevent passage of infection at insemination. Bacteria can be identified by direct plating of semen samples onto agar plates or by plating of swabs taken from semen or the genitalia. Incubation under various conditions then allows differentiation of bacteria (Madsen and Christensen, 1995). Genotyping of bacteria is now an affordable practice and so an alternative means by which bacteria can be identified. Long-term or acute infection may also be evident as high leucocyte counts in a semen sample or the evidence of pus. High bacterial counts in general reduce sperm motility (Diemer *et al.*, 2003); this, plus the identification of specific bacteria such as *Pseudomonas aeruginosa*, *Taylorella equigenitalis* and *Klebsiella pneumoniae* will preclude a semen sample from use, as they are potential VD bacteria, and also have an adverse effect on sperm quality (Scherbarth *et al.*, 1994; Davies Morel, 1999). High bacterial counts can be treated with antibiotics and, as such, antibiotics are very often added to semen extenders as a precaution (Clement *et al.*, 1995). Viruses such as EVA can also be passed from infective or carrier stallions to mares via semen and can now be identified by testing semen for the viral genome (Lazic *et al.*, 2015; Nam BoRa *et al.*, 2019). Stallions used for AI that are suspected to be viral carriers should be blood tested before use.

A summary of the acceptable semen parameters is given in Table 21.3. All the tests discussed so far are based upon gross or microscopic evaluation of sperm physical characteristics and all have their limitations. The future, therefore, may lie in functional tests (Varner, 2008).

21.4.3. Functional tests

Owing to the failure to find a physical characteristic of sperm that is consistently and highly correlated with fertility (motility being the best with a correlation of 0.6–0.7; Samper *et al.*, 1991; Jasko *et al.*, 1992b; Heitland *et al.*, 1996; Love, 2011c), attention has been drawn to the possibility of assessing the functional integrity of sperm (Neild *et al.*, 2005b). Many such tests have been investigated in isolation or as part of an accumulative model (Wilhelm *et al.*, 1996; Varner, 2008). However, many are still at the experimental stage and are also costly and labour intensive and so are not in widespread commercial use. They may, however, hold the key to the future of semen evaluation.

Table 21.3. The acceptable range for a normal stallion's semen parameters.

Parameter	Acceptable range
Volume of sperm produced	30–250 ml
Sperm concentration	$30–600 \times 10^6$ ml^{-1}
Morphology	> 50 % physiologically normal
Live/dead ratio	6.0:4.0
Motility	> 60 % progressively motile sperm
Longevity at room temperature	45 % alive after 3 h at 22°C 10 % alive after 8 h at 22°C
pH	6.9–7.8
White blood cells	< 1500 ml^{-1}
Red blood cells	< 500 ml^{-1}

21.4.3.1. Biochemical analysis

Biochemical analysis of semen may give indirect information on the quality of the sample. The total number of sperm present within a sample is reflected in the concentration of enzymes and substrates, such as aspartate amino transferase, lactate dehydrogenase (LDH), hyaluronidase, acrosin, adenosine triphosphate (ATP) and acetylcarnitine (Bruns and Casillas, 1990; Castro *et al.*, 1991; Stradaioli *et al.*, 1995; Varner, 2005). Many enzymes, such as LDH, acrosin and hyaluronidase, are located in the sperm head and specifically in the acrosome region, or in the mid-piece. As such, they can also be used to indicate sperm viability, as elevated free levels are indicative of sperm damage. For example, the total concentration of acrosin is reported to correlate with fertilization rates (Reichart *et al.*, 1993; Sharma *et al.*, 1993; Francavilla *et al.*, 1994; Varner, 2008). Although biochemical analysis can give an indirect indication of sperm numbers and damage, it is as yet very non-specific and it will remain so until more detailed work has been carried out to ascertain the normal concentration of these enzymes within the sperm and semen. Most recently it has been suggested that there is a positive correlation between sperm motility (and hence fertility) and oxidative stress parameters (such as lipid peroxidation and reactive oxygen species), and so identifying these within a sample could be used to indicate sperm viability (Hossain *et al.*, 2011; Luo *et al.*, 2013; Gibb *et al.*, 2014; Griffin *et al.*, 2019).

21.4.3.2. Membrane integrity tests

The integrity of the sperm membrane and internal organelles is a prerequisite for successful fertilization. Several tests have been investigated to evaluate sperm and mitochondria membrane integrity; these include the use of antibodies to various components of the sperm membrane, fluorescent probes or various stains, combined with light microscopy or flow cytometry (Section 21.4.3.3; Magistrini *et al.*, 1997; Silva and Gadella, 2006; Serafini *et al.*, 2013). Antibodies can be labelled with fluorescent dyes to allow the integrity of the membranes to be assessed visually (Blach *et al.*, 1988; Van Buiten *et al.*, 1989; Amann and Graham, 1993; Casey *et al.*, 1993; Neild *et al.*, 2005a).

Fluorescent probes such as calcein-AM:ethidium homodimer or CFDA:propidium iodide have been used (Garner *et al.*, 1986; Harrison and Vickers, 1990; Althouse and Hopkins, 1995). Both calcein-AM and CFDA are membrane permeable and so pass into live sperm where they fluoresce green. The counterstains, ethidium homodimer and propidium iodide, are membrane impermeable and can only enter membrane-damaged sperm, causing them to fluoresce red. The ratio of green to red fluorescing sperm, therefore, indicates the percentage of sperm with viable membranes. Additionally, the acrosome fluoresces more brightly than the rest of the head, allowing its integrity to be specifically assessed. Arguably the most important part of the sperm is the acrosome region of the head, which is critical for fertilization. In order for sperm to fertilize an ovum they need to go through the process of capacitation as they pass through the mare's reproductive tract and, on reaching the zona pellucida, they must undergo the acrosome reaction to penetrate the zona pellucida. Assessing the ability of sperm to undergo capacitation and the acrosome reaction is suggested to be a good way of assessing sperm fertilizing capacity. Additionally, they can be used to differentiate sperm that appear morphologically normal and pass membrane integrity tests but are still incapable of fertilization. The percentage of sperm that have undergone capacitation naturally or induced in the presence of capacitation inducers such as cyclic adenosine monophosphate (cAMP), bicarbonate, Ca ionophore or progesterone can be assessed by staining with chlortetracycline or Mercocyanine 540 (Meyers et al., 1995a,b; Rathi et al., 2001; Varner, 2008). Similarly, stains have been developed – for example Commassie blue or fluoresceinated lectins, or peanut agglutinin (PNA) to specifically stain the acrosome region and so assess the percentage of sperm that have undergone the acrosome reaction naturally or artificially induced. PNA can also be combined with a viability probe such as propidium iodide, which allows sperm that have undergone the acrosome reaction to be differentiated from those that have died and as a result lost their acrosome (Brum et al., 2006; Ball, 2014). This fluorescent technique is now becoming used in commercial AI laboratories as part of the evaluation procedure, particularly for post-thaw samples (Baumber-Skaife, 2011).

21.4.3.3. Flow cytometry

Light microscopy can be used to differentiate stained or fluorescing sperm but it is a time-consuming job. Flow cytometry, however, can be used to speed up the process and identify sperm that have undergone a variety of staining techniques, such as stains to test for membrane integrity or live:dead fluorescent probes, and so give a quantified result (such as a percentage of live or dead; or normal or abnormal sperm). Flow cytometry can be

used with both single and double staining of sperm and mitochondria (Wilhelm et al., 1996; Magistrini et al., 1997; Papaioannou et al., 1997; Love et al., 2003; Baumber-Skaife, 2011; Ball, 2014). The flow cytometer separates sperm passed through it on the basis of their colour (stains) fluorescence (fluorescent probes), giving a quantified value that indicates their functional capabilities. So, if the single stain or probe is used that specifically attaches to functional mitochondria, then the flow cytometer can give a reading for the percentage of sperm with optimum fluorescence, indicating the percentage of sperm with viable mitochondria (Papaioannou et al., 1997; Colenbrander et al., 2003). If a double stain is used, such as combined CFDA and propidium iodide – which differentiate live and dead sperm (Section 21.4.2.6) – then the percentage of live and dead sperm can be obtained. The results from flow cytometry work are encouraging and suggest a significant positive correlation between the number of stained sperm with optimally functioning mitochondria and viability, and with acrosome and fertilizing capacity. The use of flow cytometry is becoming a popular tool as it allows rapid, objective analysis of sperm which can be used to assess a number of analyses simultaneously, depending on the number and type of stains used. The variety of stains used continues to increase, but the technique remains expensive.

21.4.3.4. Filtration and density gradient centrifugation

Various filters including sephadex beads over glass wool; cotton, with or without sephadex; bovine serum albumin (BSA); and cellulose acetate have been used quite successfully to give an assessment of sperm viability. The passing of semen through such a filter delays the transit of the less-viable sperm which are held within the filter, resulting in a filtrate of highly viable sperm. A positive correlation exists, therefore, between the number of sperm in the filtrate and the fertilizing potential of the original sample (Strzemienski et al., 1987; Samper and Crabo, 1988; Samper et al., 1988). Such a filter can also be used to remove less-viable sperm and allow the concentration of sperm with high fertilizing potential (Samper et al., 1988; Casey et al., 1991; Sieme et al., 2003a).

Centrifugation through different concentrations of colloidal silica particles which form a range of density gradients has been used to successfully separate cells according to their specific gravity, which may relate to morphology, etc., allowing abnormal, non-viable sperm to be identified and ultimately discarded (Mortimer, 2000; Varner *et al.*, 2010).

21.4.3.5. Hypo-osmotic stress test

The hypo-osmotic test relies upon the fact that the sperm membrane is semipermeable, allowing the selective passage of water through it along an osmotic pressure (OP) gradient. A hypertonic solution has a lower water content, hence draining water across the membrane into it; a hypotonic solution is a weaker solution, allowing water to be drawn out of it. If stallion sperm are placed into a hypotonic solution (75–129 mOsm of either sodium chloride (NaCl) or sucrose for 15 or 60 min, respectively), water passes into the sperm resulting in a ballooning of the sperm head and deformation of the tail (Neild *et al.*, 1999; Nie and Wenzel, 2001; Baumber-Skaife, 2011). As a result the sperm tails show characteristic bending and coiling (Samper *et al.*, 1991). This effect is only observed in sperm with intact membranes. The test is widely used in other mammals, where significant correlation is reported between the swelling of sperm heads and the characteristic tail coiling with sperm motility and the percentage of sperm successfully penetrating an ovum (Jeyendran *et al.*, 1984; Correa and Zavos, 1994; Kumi-Diaka and Badtram, 1994; Revell and Mrode, 1994; Correa *et al.*, 1997). The test is used in stallions with some success (Zavos and Gregory, 1987; Samper *et al.*, 1991; Lagares *et al.*, 2000). Although its correlation to fertility is still unclear (Neild *et al.*, 2000; Nie and Wenzel, 2001), there is a suggestion of a good correlation between hypo-osmotic test results and post-thaw motility in frozen semen, making it a possible indicator of sperm freezing success (Magistrini *et al.*, 1997; Baumber-Skaife, 2011). Hyper-osmotic tests have also been investigated but with less success (De la Cueva *et al.*, 1997).

21.4.3.6. Cervical mucus penetration test

The ability of sperm to penetrate cervical mucus, the first major biological fluid that the sperm naturally come in contact with, has been used to indicate the viability of sperm from several species. A highly significant, positive correlation between penetration and acrosome integrity and also between penetration and total sperm integrity has been reported (Galli *et al.*, 1991). However, no correlation between penetration and fertility has yet been proved, and it is likely to be less successful in stallions, as sperm are naturally deposited into the top of the cervix/uterus and so bypass much of the cervical mucus.

21.4.3.7. Oviductal epithelial cell explant test

The effect of sperm on oviductal epithelial cell activity, including protein secretion, is reported to have a high correlation with sperm morphology, and to be a possible prognostic test for *in vitro* fertilization (Thomas *et al.*, 1995; Thomas and Ball, 1996). The number of sperm that bind to epithelial cell explants may also be a possible indicator of sperm viability (Dobrinski *et al.*, 1995; Thomas *et al.*, 1995).

21.4.3.8. Zona-free hamster ova penetration assay

The ability of a sperm to penetrate a zona-free hamster oocyte has been used successfully to indicate the viability of human (Yanagimachi *et al.*, 1976; Binor *et al.*, 1980; Overstreet *et al.*, 1980; Hall, 1981) and bovine (Amann, 1984) sperm. Successful penetration is dependent upon successful completion of capacitation and the acrosome reaction, and so gives an assessment of the sperm viability. Alternatively, sperm capacitation and the acrosome reaction can be induced artificially, and full penetration and fertilization of the oocyte assessed instead of just attachment. Some success has been achieved with the zona-free hamster oocyte test in stallions (Samper *et al.*, 1989; Zhang *et al.*, 1990a; Padilla *et al.*, 1991), including a reported correlation with conception rates (Pitra *et al.*, 1985). Incubation of non-capacitated stallion sperm with hamster oocytes results in activation of oocyte chromosomes, which has also been suggested as being an indicator of sperm viability (Ko and Lee, 1993; Avdatek *et al.*, 2010).

Similarly, fertilization of an ovum depends upon an increase in oocyte calcium (Ca) ion concentrations, which then oscillate at a specific frequency. Recently a sperm-specific oscillation factor phospholipase (PLC zeta) has been isolated in stallion sperm and is reported to correlate well with fertility in other species (Gradil *et al.*, 2006), but unreliable results have been reported in stallions (Wilhelm *et al.*, 1996).

21.4.3.9. Heterospermic insemination and competitive fertilization

Pooling of sperm from two males prior to insemination, or incubation with oocytes *in vitro*, allows direct assessment of the relative fertilizing ability of the two populations of sperm, usually sperm from a stallion of known fertility against a test stallion. This competitive assessment is termed heterospermic insemination. Identification of the source of each set of sperm is essential for the procedure to be successful. This may be achieved by the use of genetic markers or labelling of sperm (Fazeli *et al.*, 1993), However, batches of oocytes vary considerably in their ability to bind sperm, limiting the reliability of the test (Fazeli *et al.*, 1993).

21.4.3.10. Hemizona assay

A further development of the zona-free hamster penetration assay and heterospermic insemination is the hemizona assay, in which stallion sperm from different stallions are incubated with hemizona from a single oocyte. This eliminates the significant variation reported between the zona pellucida in different oocytes. This allows a stallion of known fertility to be compared to a stallion of unknown fertility. A significant relationship has been reported between the number of bound sperm for a particular stallion and the probability of pregnancy resulting from insemination with that stallion's semen (Fazeli *et al.*, 1995). Further development of this to assess the zona pellucida-binding ability of sperm has also been suggested as a means of assessing sperm viability (Pantke *et al.*, 1992, 1995; Meyers *et al.*, 1995b, 1996; Wilhelm *et al.*, 1996; Baumber-Skaife, 2011; Coutinho da Silva *et al.*, 2012).

21.4.3.11. DNA analysis, chromatin structure analysis

Finally, the total amount and structure of sperm DNA may also be assessed to give an indication of viability (Evenson *et al.*, 1995, 2002; Kenney *et al.*, 1995; Neild *et al.*, 2005b; Johnson, 2011). For example acridine orange can be used with flow cytometry to differentiate between single-stranded DNA (abnormal sperm) that fluoresces red and double-stranded DNA (normal sperm) that fluoresces green (Johnson, 2011).

21.5. Sexing Sperm

Many attempts have been made to preselect the sex of offspring in both man and animals. The first sex-selected offspring were rabbits in 1989 (Johnson *et al.*, 1989) and the first reported sex-selected foal was born in 2000 (Buchanan *et al.*, 2000). Preselection of sex in horses is driven by the popularity of different sexes for different disciplines: for example, geldings are most popular as event/leisure horses, and colts are most popular for racing, whereas fillies are more popular as polo ponies.

Sexing of sperm has been attempted by various methods with differing success in different animals (Morris, 2005, 2011), including the differential staining of the X and Y chromosome (Bhattacharya *et al.*, 1977; Ericsson and Glass, 1982; Windsor *et al.*, 1993), sperm karyotype analysis (Rudak *et al.*, 1978; Amann, 1989) and flow cytometry. Flow cytometry is now used successfully with stallion sperm (Johnson *et al.*, 1997, 1998; Cran *et al.*, 1995; Seidel *et al.*, 1998). In particular, fluorescence-activated cell separation (FACS), which is based on flow cytometry, is currently the method of choice for sex selection. FACS works on the basis that X- and Y-bearing chromosomes differ in their DNA content (3.7% difference in horses; Welch and Johnson, 1999). Sperm are diluted and incubated with the fluorescent dye bis-benzimidazole H33342; the amount of dye taken up depends upon the sperm DNA content (i.e. X-or Y-bearing chromosomes) (Morrell, 2011). They are then passed through an argon laser beam which induces fluorescence of the sperm without causing damage; and then through the flow cytometer's high voltage deflection plates, which separate them according to their fluorescence (i.e. whether they are X- or Y-bearing sperm) (Johnson, 2000; Morris, 2005; Sharpe and Evans, 2009). The accuracy of sex selection is reported to be 94–96% (Allen, 2005) and good conception rates (up to 60%) have been achieved using fresh or chilled sex-sorted semen (Lindsey *et al.*, 2002, 2005). However, there are two major drawbacks to this technology: first, work with frozen semen provides less encouraging results, with conception rates of around 20% (Lindsey *et al.*, 2001, 2002; Lee and Morris, 2005; Gibb *et al.*, 2017); second, the sorting rate of existing FACS machines. Current FACS machines can sort sperm at 20×10^6 h^{-1} for a limited period (2–3 h). Current technology will only provide doses of $40–60 \times 10^6$, which is well below the conventional insemination dose of $300–500 \times 10^6$; hence, low-dose insemination techniques are required if sex-sorted semen is to be successful (see Section 21.10.2). Alternatively, sperm can be preselected for viability by filtration or centrifugation, and only viable sperm sex-selected, making the process more viable.

Recent developments have suggested alternative means of sexing sperm, including the microfluidic dielectrophoretic (MF-DEP) system combining a microfluidic system (MF) and an dielectrophoretic system. Dielectrophoresis (DEP) is a non-invasive technique to separate cells, which uses non-uniform electric fields to control the movement of biological particles (such as sperm) to a particular position and so separate them from each another. Hence cells that possess different electrical surface properties, such as X- and Y-bearing sperm, can be separated under the electric field (Gonzalez-Castro and Carnevale, 2019). Additionally, sex-specific proteins on the sperm surface have been identified, to which antibodies have been raised; the idea is to use the antibodies to aggregate sperm-bearing specific sex chromosomes, and so to remove them from the sample (Morrell, 2011; Sang *et al.*, 2011; Yadav *et al.*, 2017).

21.6. Semen Storage and Use

Once the semen has been evaluated, it can be considered for insemination. Semen can be used in one of five ways: raw and undiluted to immediately inseminate a single or possibly two mares; diluted and used immediately for insemination into several mares; diluted and kept at room temperature for insemination within 24 h; diluted and refrigerated for use over the next 48–72 h; or diluted and frozen for indefinite storage. The method used depends on the stud system, the location of the mare(s) to be inseminated and personal preference.

21.6.1. Raw or undiluted fresh semen

Insemination of mares with raw, untreated semen is not usually carried out unless the indication for insemination is because of physical complications in either the mare or the stallion that preclude natural covering. Insemination with raw semen should be carried out up to 1 h after collection in order to obtain acceptable results. Insemination with raw semen provides none of the advantages of AI. Even the division of raw semen to allow the insemination of a number of mares with a single ejaculate is less successful than if the division of the sample occurs after the addition of an extender. The use of an extender is, therefore, recommended (Varner, 1986; Samper, 2011).

21.6.2. Diluted fresh semen

As with undiluted raw or fresh semen, the use of extender or diluted fresh semen defeats many of the objects of AI, but does allow several mares to be inseminated per ejaculate from a single stallion with a high workload. Many of the extenders appropriate for use with fresh semen are reviewed below (Section 21.6.3) and also in Aurich (2005).

The semen:extender dilution rate is an important consideration in all insemination. Inadequate dilution will not provide adequate support for sperm. On the other hand, excessive dilution has been associated with depressed fertilization rates (Katila, 1997). A minimum semen:extender ratio of 1:1 has been recommended (Brinsko and Varner, 1992). In general, fresh semen for immediate use is diluted in a ratio of between 1:1 and 1:4 depending upon the concentration of the raw semen sample (Section 21.7). A concentration of 2×10^6 to 50×10^6 sperm ml^{-1} is aimed for in the diluted sample (Samper, 2011).

Work by several authors indicates that conception rates for mares inseminated with extended fresh semen, immediately post-extension, are similar to or slightly better than those obtained with undiluted raw semen and vary from 60% to 75% depending upon the extender used (Jasko *et al.*, 1993b; Deng *et al.*, 2014). In general E-Z Mixin® (Animal Reproduction Systems Inc., Chino, California, USA) appears to be the most successful although many of the other extenders discussed in Section 21.6.3 are also successful.

Owing to the limited viability of fresh semen stored at body temperature or non-refrigerated, its use is limited. Stallion semen is, therefore, very often diluted then chilled or frozen, to allow storage for at least 2–3 days (see Sections 21.6.5 and 21.6.6).

21.6.3. Extenders for fresh ambient temperature or cooled semen storage and use

The use of extenders allows the number of mares inseminated per ejaculate to be increased significantly. It also prolongs the life of the sperm by providing additional energy for sperm metabolism; protein for membrane integrity; antioxidants to neutralize toxic by-products of metabolism; and antibiotics to counter infection. It also buffers changes in pH (6.8–7); maintains osmolarity (300–350 mOsm l^{-1}); and maintains chromatin integrity (Kotilainen *et al.*, 1994; Ball *et al.*, 2001; Love *et al.*, 2002; Aurich *et al.*, 2007; Aurich, 2011b). Extenders are also used to dilute semen prior to evaluation.

There is a plethora of extenders available; however, most used today are based upon milk products and/or egg yolk, as a source of protein and energy, with the addition of an antibiotic. Several other common components are added to maximize sperm survival (Section 21.6.3.5; Pickett, 1993b,c; Ball *et al.*, 2001; Aurich, 2011; Brinsko, 2011b).

In broad terms extenders in use today can, therefore, be divided into milk or milk product-based; cream and gelatin-based; or egg yolk-based.

21.6.3.1. Milk and milk product-based extenders

These extenders include non-fat dried skimmed milk glucose extender (NFDSM-G II) or Kenney extender (Table 21.4b), one of the most popular diluents used (Kenney *et al.*, 1975; Neuhauser *et al.*, 2018a), along with E-Z Mixin® (Table 21.4a), which is very similar in composition, plus variations on these (usually just changes to the sugar content and/or antibiotic added). These extenders are commonly used for extending semen prior to storage, but can also be used for evaluation as they are optically clear, and maintain sperm motility and fertility well. They are also relatively straightforward and cheap to prepare and can be frozen. Although slightly more expensive than the straightforward skimmed milk preparations (Table 21.4c) these extenders are normally the preferred option. The straightforward skimmed milk extender requires the milk to be heated to 92–93°C for 10 min to inactivate lactenin, an anti-streptococcal agent naturally found in milk which is toxic to equine sperm (Householder *et al.*, 1981).

Pregnancy rates with all milk-based extenders are reported to be quite acceptable at 52–62%, with little difference between the different extenders although E-Z Mixin® is considered by some to be more successful (Aurich *et al.*, 2007). Additionally, the milk-based extender INRA 82 (IMV Technologies, L'Aigle, France) (Table 21.4f), developed and widely used in France (Magistrini *et al.*, 1992), can be successfully used alone or with added egg yolk (INRA 83-Y® (IMV Technologies, L'Aigle, France); Rota *et al.*, 2004). This extender is reported to maintain sperm motility better than Kenney or E-Z Mixin® at 5°C (Ijaz and Ducharme, 1995).

Milk-based extenders are largely based on cow's milk; however, mare's milk has also been used successfully, both alone and with glucose (Table 21.4g,h; Lawson, 1996; Lawson and Davies Morel, 1996).

21.6.3.2. Cream-gel-based extenders

The addition of gelatin to an extender is thought to act as a membrane stabilizer and so increase pregnancy rates (Brinsko *et al.*, 2011; Table 21.5). The major disadvantage in using cream–gel-based extenders and the reason why they are not widely used as commercial semen extenders (despite their apparent success) is the difficulty in preparation and the presence of fat globules, which makes them inappropriate for use in microscopic examination.

21.6.3.3. Egg yolk-based extenders

Owing to their optical opacity egg yolk-based extenders are used primarily for storage rather than semen evaluation. However, it is evident that egg yolk has some cryopreservation properties, particularly at temperatures above freezing, when it appears to stabilize sperm membranes (Bergeron and Manjunath, 2006; Linden *et al.*, 2014); egg yolk is, therefore, particularly successful as part of an extender for semen destined for chilling or freezing (Moreno *et al.*, 2013). The specific use of egg yolk as a cryoprotectant will be discussed later under Section 21.6.6. There are many egg yolk-based extenders and many have found popularity for commercial use (Table 21.6; Jasko *et al.*, 1992a; Klug, 1992; Samper, 1995b; Pillet *et al.*, 2011; Neuhauser *et al.*, 2018a).

21.6.3.4. Defined component extenders

As discussed, most extenders for storage of equine semen are based on either milk or egg yolk and are then routinely stored at 4–6°C (Moran *et al.*, 1992; Aurich, 2005). Most recently work has been carried out into replacing some of the biological products, such as skim milk, with defined proteins (e.g. phosphocaseinates) in an attempt to include only substances beneficial to sperm, improve standardization and reduce the risk of microbiological contamination. These extenders are known as defined component extenders and are reported to be superior to traditional skim milk extenders (Batellier *et al.*, 1998, 2001; Pagl *et al.*, 2006a). As these extenders are not based on milk they have the advantage of allowing storage at room temperature (15°C) (Section 21.6.4; Batellier *et al.*, 2000). The most successfully defined component extender to date is INRA 96® (IMV Technologies, L'Aigle, France), which is reported to be appropriate for cooled (4–5°C) and ambient temperature (18–20°C) storage (Table 21.7; Batellier *et al.*, 1998, 2001). Commercial extenders such as EquiPro® (Minitube, Tiefenbach, Germany), based on defined casein and whey proteins, have also been produced and are proving successful both at ambient and cooled temperatures (Pagl *et al.*, 2006a; Aurich *et al.*, 2007; Price *et al.*, 2007, Price, 2008). Soybean-based extenders are also available but, after 24 h storage at 5°C, the quality of sperm is reported to be poorer

Table 21.4. Milk and milk-based extenders in use today.

Component	Quantity
(A) E-Z Mixin®. (From Province *et al.*, 1984, 1985.)	
Non-fat dried milk	2.4 g
Glucose monohydrate	4.9 g
Sodium bicarbonate (7.5% solution)	2.0 ml
Polymixin B sulfate (50 mg ml^{-1})	2.0 ml
Distilled water	92.0 ml
Osmolarity (mOsm kg^{-1})	375.00 ± 2
pH	6.99 ± 0.02
Mix the liquids first and then add the powders	
(B) Non-fat dried skimmed milk glucose extender II (NFDSM-G II) or Kenney extender. (From Kenney *et al.*, 1975.)	
Non-fat dried skimmed milk	2.4 g
Glucose	4.9 g
Gentamicin sulfate (reagent grade)	100.0 mg
8.4% NaHCO$_3$	2.0 ml
Deionized water	92.0 ml
Mix the liquids first before adding the NFDSM to avoid the antibiotic curdling the milk	
(C) Heated skim milk extender. (From Voss and Pickett, 1976.)	
Skimmed milk	100.0 ml
Heat to 92–93°C for 10 min in a double boiler. Cool to 37°C before use	
(D) Non-fat dried skimmed milk extender glucose I (NFDSM-G I). (From Kenney *et al.*, 1975.)	
NFDSM	2.4 g
Glucose	4.0 g
Penicillin (crystalline)	150,000 IU
Streptomycin (crystalline)	150,000 µg
Deionized water	made up to 100 ml
(E) Skimmed milk gel extender. (From Voss and Pickett, 1976; Pickett, 1993b; Householder *et al.*, 1981.)	
Skimmed milk	100.0 ml
Gelatin	1.3 g
Add the gelatin to the skimmed milk and agitate for 1 min	
Heat mixture in boiler for 10 min at 92°C, swirling mixture periodically	
(F) INRA 82. (From Magistrini *et al.*, 1992; Ijaz and Ducharme, 1995.)	
Glucose	5.0 g
Lactose	300.0 mg
Raffinose	300.0 mg
Trisodium citrate dehydrate	60.0 mg
Potassium citrate	82.0 mg
HEPES	952.0 mg
Penicillin	10.0 IU ml^{-1}

Table 21.4. Continued.

Component	Quantity
Gentamicin	10.0 µg ml⁻¹
Water	100.0 ml
UHT skimmed milk	100.0 ml
OP mOsmol kg⁻¹	326.0
pH	7.1
(G) Mare's milk extender. (From Lawson and Davies Morel, 1996.)	
Mare's milk	100 ml
Osmolarity (mOmol kg⁻¹)	303.00
pH	7.07
Heat the mare's milk at 62.8°C for 30 min	
(H) NFS mare's milk. (From Lawson, 1996.)	
Mare's milk	100.0 ml
Glucose	4.9 g
Streptomycin sulfate (crystalline)	0.1 g
Penicillin (crystalline)	0.1 g
Sterile deionized water	88.0 ml
Osmolarity (mOmol kg⁻¹)	307.00
pH	7.14
Heat the mare's milk at 62.8°C for 30 min	

NFS, non-fat skimmed.

than with other extenders (Aurich and Spergser, 2007; Nouri *et al.*, 2013).

21.6.3.5. Other major components within extenders

The four main types of extender for use with stallion semen have been considered. However, much work has been carried out on the addition of other components to improve what can be relatively poor and very variable conception rates. One of the major problems encountered in storing semen is the accumulation of metabolic by-products, or waste, including reactive oxygen species (ROS) which subsequently have a direct toxic effect on sperm and an indirect effect by altering pH (Sanocka and Kurpisz, 2004; Aurich, 2011, Aitken *et al.*, 2014). In an attempt to counteract this, antioxidants and buffers have been used. The most popular antioxidants in equine semen extenders are ascorbic acid or pyruvate (Bruemmer *et al.*, 2002). The most popular buffers include trisaminomethane (TRIS), HEPES (N-2-hydroxyethylpiperazine-N-2-ethanesulfonic acid), sodium bicarbonate, sodium phosphate, sodium citrate, citric acid and BSA. All of these have been used quite successfully over a range of temperatures and pH (Magistrini and Vidamnet, 1992). Citric acid and BSA, as well as superoxide dismutase (SOD) and glutathione peroxidase (GSH-Px), act as both buffers and antioxidants, reducing the peroxidation of lipids in the sperm plasma membranes and thereby reducing the detrimental effect of storage on membrane integrity (Kreider *et al.*, 1985; Padilla and Foote, 1991; Kankofer *et al.*, 2005; Pagl *et al.*, 2006b). Most recently the addition of antioxidants such as resveratrol (Res), a natural grape-derived phytoalexin, or epigallocatechin-3-gallate (EGCG), the

Table 21.5. Cream and gel-based extenders in use today.

Component	Quantity
(A) Cream–gel extender. (From Voss and Pickett, 1976; Lawson, 1996.)	
Gelatin	1.3 g
Distilled water	10.0 ml
Half and half cream	90.0 ml
Penicillin	100,000 IU
Streptomycin	100,000 IU
Polymixin B sulfate	20,000 IU
Osmolarity (mOmol kg^{-1})	280.00
pH	6.52
Add gelatin to distilled water and autoclave for 20 min. Heat cream in boiler at 92–95°C for 10 min and add cream to gelatin solution after removing scum from heated cream, to make a total of 100 ml	
(B) Skimmed milk gel extender. (From Voss and Pickett, 1976.)	
Skimmed milk	100 ml
Gelatin	1.3 g
Add gelatin to skimmed milk and agitate for 1 min. Heat mixture in boiler for 10 min at 92°C, swirling mixture periodically	

Table 21.6. Egg yolk-based extenders.

Component	Quantity
(A) Dimitropoulous extender. (From De Vries, 1987; Braun et al., 1993; Ijaz and Ducharme, 1995.)	
Solution A	
Anhydrous glucose	2.0 g
Fructose	2.0 g
Distilled water	100.0 ml
Solution B	
Sodium citrate dehydrate	2.0 g
Glycine	0.94 g
Sulfonilamide	0.35 g
Distilled water	100.0 ml
Egg yolk	20.0 ml
Osmolarity (mOsmol kg^{-1})	280.0
pH	6.9
Make up solutions A and B separately; mix 30 ml solution A and 50 ml solution B; to the combined solution add the egg yolk; centrifuge for 20 min at 1200 g. Use the resulting supernatant as the extender	
(B) Glucose–lactose egg yolk extender. (From Martin et al., 1979.)	
Glucose	30.0 g
Sodium citrate	1.85 g
Sodium EDTA	1.85 g
Sodium bicarbonate	0.6 g
Distilled water	100 ml
Add 50 ml of this solution to 50 ml of 11% lactose solution; supplement with 20% egg yolk and 4% glycerol	

EDTA, ethylene diamine tetracetic acid.

major polyphenol in green tea (*Camellia sinensis*), has proved promising. Their antioxidant properties help to maintain membrane integrity and mitochondria viability (Nouri *et al.*, 2018). Colostrum has also been used as part of an extender, again with good success (Alvarez *et al.*, 2019). Milk extenders also appear to have a better inherent antioxidant and pH buffering capacity.

Most extenders use glucose as the major source of energy (Katila, 1997). However, other sugars such as sucrose, fructose, pyruvate, lactose and raffinose have been used with some success. In addition to providing a source of energy, a cryoprotectant role for sugars has also been indicated (Arns *et al.*, 1987; Katila, 1997; Brinsko *et al.*, 2011).

21.6.3.6. Antibiotics

Many of the aforementioned extenders include antibiotics. The semen from mammals invariably contains a natural microflora which, under normal conditions, would pose no threat of infection to females mated. The inclusion of antimicrobial agents such as antibiotics

is necessitated not only by the risk of infection, especially in mares with a compromised uterine defence system, but also by the ideal nature of most extenders not only for sperm survival, but also for microbial growth. This microbial growth presents a risk of infection, and bacteria also compete for substrates within the extender and have a direct, detrimental effect on sperm motility (Aurich and Spergser, 2006). Despite all the precautions taken at collection, semen extension and handling, semen samples are invariably contaminated (Clement *et al.*, 1995). Thorough hygiene procedures

Table 21.7. Defined component extender INRA 96®. (From Batellier *et al.*, 1998, 2001.)

Component	Quantity
Glucose	67 mM
Hanks salt solution:	
CaCl	0.14 g
KCl	0.40 g
KH_2PO_4	0.06 g
$MgSO_4 \, 7H_2O$	0.20 g
NaCl	1.25 g
$Na_2HPO_4 \, 12H_2O$	0.118 g
$NaHCO_3$	0.35 g
Glucose	13.21 g
Lactose	45.39 g
HEPES	4.76 g
Distilled water	to make up to 1000 ml
Native phosphocaseinate (NPPC)	27 g l^{-1}
Penicillin	50 IU ml^{-1}
Gentamicin	50 µg ml-1

during preparation, at collection and during handling do reduce microbial counts but they cannot eliminate them. The use of antibiotics is, therefore, a safety precaution against such contamination and they are used whatever the storage method. The success of antibiotics is enhanced by cooling the sample to 5°C rather than to just 20°C (Vaillencourt *et al.*, 1993; Price *et al.*, 2007).

The most popular antibiotics, used either in isolation or as a combination, were traditionally penicillin, streptomycin and polymixin B. These still find favour. More recently ticarcillin, amikacin (both popular in the USA) and gentamicin (popular in Europe) have been used (Samper, 1995b; Hurtgen, 1997; Aurich, 2011b; Brinsko, 2011b; Brinsko *et al.*, 2011). The presence of both Gram-positive and Gram-negative organisms in stallion semen, and the recent suggestion that resistance to antibiotics is developing, has led to the use of new combinations of antibiotics such as amikacin sulfate, gentamicin sulfate, streptomycin sulfate, sodium or potassium penicillin, ticarcillin disodium and polymixin B sulfate (Varner, 1991; Clement *et al.*, 1995).

Although the use of antibiotics is undoubtedly beneficial, their use has been associated with an increase in extender pH and decreased sperm motility (Varner, 1991; Varner *et al.*, 1992; Jasko *et al.*, 1993a). The extent of adverse effects is dependent upon the antibiotics used and possibly on individual stallions (Varner *et al.*, 1992; Aurich and Spergser, 2006, 2007). Antibiotics such as gentamicin and amikacin are known to affect the pH of the extender, necessitating the addition of a buffer such as sodium bicarbonate to counteract this acidic effect (Jasko *et al.*, 1993a). This effect on the pH may also curdle the milk in milk-based extenders, so special precautions have to be taken during preparation (as indicated with some of the extenders given in Table 21.4). Antibiotics such as penicillin and streptomycin do not appear to have the same detrimental effect on pH.

Gentamicin sulfate and polymixin B sulfate, in particular, are reported to depress sperm motility, whereas amikacin sulfate and ticarcillin disodium have no such adverse effect (Jasko *et al.*, 1993a; Aurich and Spergser, 2007; Morrell and Wallgren, 2014; Samper, 2011). The exact mechanism by which the toxicity of antibiotics affects cellular mechanisms is unclear. However, it is evident that the significance of the effect increases with inclusion rates and length of storage (Varner, 1991; Clement *et al.*, 1993; Jasko *et al.*, 1993a). The adverse effects limit the applicability of some antibiotics in stallion semen extenders but they may still be used at low concentrations. When considering the use of precautionary or prophylactic antibiotics in any scenario, bacterial resistance needs to be considered; hence minimizing inclusion rates is important for this reason, as well as for possible adverse effects on sperm. Finally, the semen from different stallions may be affected differently by different antibiotics, and so tailoring for individual stallions may be required.

Concern about antibiotic resistance has also promoted the use of different antibiotics such as potassium penicillin G-amikacin disulfate (PEN-AMIK), ticarcillin disodium-potassium clavulanate (TICAR-CLAV), piperacillin sodium/tazobactam sodium (PIP-TAZ), or meropenem (MERO). All are reported to have a minimal effect on sperm viability (Hernández-Avilés *et al.*, 2019). In addition, alternatives to antibiotics have been investigated; these include single layer centrifugation (SLC), cationic antimicrobial peptides and cyclic hexapeptides. Of these SLC is the most promising, allowing the removal of bacteria post-centrifugation and so ensuring a much lower initial bacterial count within the sample than would naturally be evident (Morrell and

Walgren, 2014; Al-Kass *et al.*, 2018). Viruses such as EVA can also be removed via centrifugation on a density gradient followed by the 'swim up' method (Morrell and Geraghty, 2006).

21.6.3.7. Removal of seminal plasma

The components and function of seminal plasma have been discussed at some length in Section 6.3.1. Although it is reported that seminal plasma plays a role in sperm transport and survival in the female tract (Troedsson *et al.*, 2005), as far as semen storage is concerned it appears that some components have a detrimental effect on sperm, possibly causing premature capacitation and reducing their lifespan (Rigby *et al.*, 2001b; Pommer *et al.*, 2002; Akcay *et al.*, 2006). This effect is evident as a reduction in motility and subsequent fertility (Webb *et al.*, 1990; Jasko *et al.*, 1992a; Pruitt *et al.*, 1993), but not necessarily as a detrimental effect on sperm morphology (Sanchez *et al.*, 1995). Any effect of seminal plasma may vary between stallions. The fraction of seminal plasma responsible appears to originate from the seminal vesicles (Webb *et al.*, 1990), and has been suggested to be due to elevated concentrations of NaCl (which effect OP changes, especially during cooling and freezing) or a reaction of lipase in seminal plasma, specifically with milk-based extenders (Carver and Ball, 2002). Differing levels of NaCl and/or lipases may, therefore, account for some of the apparent differences in the ability of the semen of different stallions to survive chilling and frozen storage.

The removal of seminal plasma and its replacement with an appropriate extender may potentially allow the requirements of sperm to be met, but avoid the disadvantages of seminal plasma. Indeed, sperm survival rates increase as inclusion rates of seminal plasma decrease (Palmer *et al.*, 1984) and better longevity at 25°C, 5°C or –196°C is demonstrated in semen from which seminal plasma has been removed (Webb *et al.*, 1990; Sanchez *et al.*, 1995; Love *et al.*, 2005). However, these results are not supported by all (Pool *et al.*, 1993; Alghamdi *et al.*, 2004). This may in part be due to a particularly adverse reaction between egg yolk and seminal plasma (Bedford *et al.*, 1995a,b). Additionally, the composition of seminal plasma varies considerably between stallions (Jasko *et al.*, 1992b; Charneco *et al.*, 1993; Bedford *et al.*, 1995a,b), and therefore the adverse effects are also likely to vary (Katila, 1997). The ideal may, therefore, be that different extender regimes should be developed for different stallions. Despite the

adverse effects of seminal plasma, it may not be beneficial to completely remove it, as the inclusion of some has been reported to be advantageous (usually up to 20%; Pruitt *et al.*, 1993; Braun *et al.*, 1994).

There are several methods to remove seminal plasma: the most popular is centrifugation. Centrifugation at 400 g for 9–15 min successfully fractionates a semen sample, allowing the supernatant (mainly seminal plasma) to be aspirated off, leaving a soft plug of largely undamaged sperm-rich semen in the bottom (Jasko *et al.*, 1992a; Bedford *et al.*, 1995a,b; Heitland *et al.*, 1996; Sieme, 2011a). Centrifugation also allows accurate and standard dilution for cool storage and/or freezing, and gives a small volume of concentrated samples for efficient storage, which are then readily available at standard-dose rates for direct insemination. This is particularly important when considering the freezing of semen where small volumes of 0.5–4 ml are regularly used.

Although centrifugation may be successful, it runs the risk of damage to sperm, manifest as reduction in motility and adverse changes to sperm morphology; these are of particular concern in stallions with low sperm counts (Baemgartl *et al.*, 1980). There are a number of ways in which the detrimental effects of centrifugation can be reduced. These include the addition of a primary extender; minimizing the centrifugal force and/or minimizing the time of centrifugation; underlayering the semen with a dense, isotonic liquid (Equi Prep, Genus Plc, UK) that provides a protective cushion, reducing physical damage (Revell, 1997; Waite *et al.*, 2008); or density gradient centrifugation, where a series of colloids of increasing density act as a cushion under the sperm in a similar manner to Equi Prep; or, finally, the simpler single layer (of colloid) centrifugation (Morrell, 2012; Morrell and Wallgren, 2014). However, the extent to which sperm from different stallions are affected by centrifugation is variable (Cochran *et al.*, 1984; Pickett and Amann, 1993).

Once centrifugation has been completed, the pelleted sample is resuspended in an extender. Standardization of sample concentrations appropriate for insemination is made at this stage. Appropriate dilution rates can then be calculated to obtain the desired number of sperm per insemination dose: $100–800 \times 10^6$ (Hurtgen, 1997).

Alternatively, seminal plasma may be removed at semen collection using an open-ended AV. Such an AV allows isolation and collection of only the sperm-rich fraction (Heiskanen *et al.*, 1994b; Kareskoski *et al.*,

2006). This is reported to result in a significantly better sample (sperm motility) after cooled storage, compared to centrifuged unfractionated samples, but the successful use of an open-ended AV is a skilled job. A further alternative to centrifugation is filtration through a filter such as glass wool sephadex filter. Filtration appears particularly beneficial when freezing semen (Samper *et al.*, 1991), filtered semen showing better motility and conception rates (69.2% and 80.6%, respectively) than centrifuged semen (47.6% and 66.6%, respectively; Rauterberg, 1994). Filtration is also used to improve the overall quality of a semen sample subsequently prepared for cooling or freezing. Finally, the use of a 'swim up' method of separating highly viable sperm from seminal plasma and poor-quality sperm has also been reported to be successful (Casey *et al.*, 1991).

21.6.4. Ambient temperature storage

Cooling semen below 18–20°C exposes them to potential cold shock (see Section 21.6.5.1); hence, storage above this temperature would seem advantageous. Some success has been reported with storing diluted semen at 15–20°C, ideally in the dark, for 12–24 h (Varner and Schumacher, 1991). After 24 h, sperm motility declines rapidly compared to that stored at 5°C. It appears, therefore, that for short-term storage (24 h), cooling to 20°C provides a viable method, though for longer-term storage further cooling to 4–6°C is required (Zidane *et al.*, 1991; Love *et al.*, 2002). There are obvious advantages to storage at room temperature, especially in places where refrigeration is difficult. However, fluctuations in ambient temperatures are a risk, and ambient temperature is not cool enough to significantly reduce the sperm metabolic rate; this, therefore, limits the storage time. If storage at ambient temperature is to become widespread an alternative method of reducing metabolic rate is required. To this end various protocols have been investigated. Sperm storage in anaerobic conditions and oxygen-free extender successfully reduces sperm metabolism and prolongs life; however, these are difficult to prepare and require glass (gas-impervious) containers (Shannon, 1972). In cattle, carbon dioxide bubbled though egg yolk extender (illini variable temperature (IVT) extender) reduces oxygen availability and so successfully reduces the metabolic rate and increases sperm survival over a period of time (Salisbury *et al.*, 1978). Similarly, Caprogen® (LIC, Hamilton, New Zealand) diluents, which are saturated with nitrogen gas, successfully allow the storage of bull's

semen for up to 3 days at ambient temperature (Shannon, 1972; Graham, 2011a). There are few reports, however, of the use of such metabolic inhibitors with stallion semen, although Caprogen® has been used (Province *et al.*, 1985; Verberckmoes *et al.*, 2005) as have proteinase inhibitors (Katila, 1997), but with only limited success. As discussed in Section 21.6.3.4, defined component extenders have recently been developed and are particularly successful with ambient temperature storage, maintaining sperm viability longer than milk-based extenders (for up to 48 h; Batellier *et al.*, 1998, 2000, 2001).

Similarly, LeBoeuf *et al.* (2003) and Price *et al.* (2007) reported that storage of semen in the defined protein-based extender EquiPro® (Pagl *et al.*, 2006a,b) at 15°C gave comparable results to milk-based extenders also stored up to 48 h; beyond this the milk-based extender proved superior, especially when stored at 5°C. Storage at ambient temperature would have many advantages but, as yet, results are not consistent enough for it to be anything more than a potential for the future after more research work. In the last few years Gibb *et al.* (2018) have reported an extender (UoN) that is able to keep sperm alive for up to 7 days at ambient temperature (17°C).

21.6.5. Chilled semen storage

An alternative, and the most popular, method of reducing sperm metabolic rate and hence increasing viability is via cooling. No particularly sophisticated equipment is required and storage by this method allows adequate time (up to 72 h) for the transportation of semen over reasonably long distances.

As discussed previously the sample should be filtered, and seminal plasma normally removed, followed by addition of a semen extender (Section 21.6.3.7). Numerous extenders have been used, most of which are based on milk or egg yolk or are cream–gelatin-based (Section 21.6.3). Chilled semen is normally extended within a range of 1:1 to 1:10 concentrated semen:extender, although a tighter range of 1:2 and 1:4 is normally advised, but very much depends on initial sperm concentration. The aim is to have a sample ready for insemination with a concentration of 20×10^6 sperm ml^{-1}.

Chilled (5°C) semen will survive for 48 h without a significant decline in motility (Malmgren *et al.*, 1994) although some samples have been reported to survive for as long as 96 h (Hughes and Loy, 1970). In general, conception rates for cooled semen stored for any period of time in excess of 24 h are lower than those attained for insemination with fresh semen. Conception rates ranging from 50% to 76% are regularly reported for cooled semen in comparison to rates of 60–76% for insemination with fresh semen; this very much depends on the initial quality of the semen sample and inherent mare fertility (Jasko *et al.*, 1993b; Heiskanen *et al.*, 1994a; Samper, 2009, 2011; Deng *et al.*, 2014). Although chilling semen provides an efficient and successful means of reducing sperm metabolic rate, and hence allowing short-term storage, chilling itself has some adverse effects on sperm. These are manifested as a depression in survival rate, motility and conception rates (Braun *et al.*, 1994; Malmgren *et al.*, 1994; Graham, 2011a). These adverse effects of cooling are termed cold shock.

21.6.5.1. Cold shock

Cold shock is the term used to describe the stress response shown by sperm as a reaction to a drop in environmental temperature (in stallion sperm this is 20°C to 5°C) resulting in damage to the structure and function of the cell (Rota *et al.*, 2004). Damage is evident shortly after the drop in temperature has occurred and is affected by the rate of cooling and final temperature. Cold shock causes membrane alteration which is accompanied by a loss of intracellular components and a reduction in cellular metabolism. This damage to the cellular membranes, specifically changes in fluidity and distribution of the phospholipids, is of most significance and has a carry-over effect on other cellular structures and functions (Hammerstedt *et al.*, 1990; Parks and Lynch, 1992; Aurich, 2005), disrupting membrane function and permeability (Hammerstedt *et al.*, 1990; Graham, 2011a).

Unfortunately many of these changes to membrane configuration are irreversible and subsequent warming of the cooled sperm does not restore the original membrane configuration. Cold-shock damage manifests itself as a decline in cell metabolism, altered membrane permeability, irreversible loss of sperm motility and an increase in the number of dead sperm (Devireddy *et al.*, 2002a). As well as motility rates being adversely affected by cooling, the correlation between motility and fertility is also reduced, making motility – especially in frozen samples – an even poorer indicator of fertility (Watson, 1990). Sperm motion characteristics also change, with an increase in backward motion due to an over-bending of the tail area, arising from irreversible changes to the mid-piece and coiling of the tail (Watson, 1990).

The effects of cold shock are more evident when freezing semen, with sperm also undergoing changes similar to those of capacitation and senescence (Ball *et al.*, 1997; Neild *et al.*, 2003). Hence, when cryopreservation is considered in Section 21.6.6.1, cryoprotectants are discussed. For chilled storage the inclusion of components such as egg yolk, milk, glycerol, BSA, polyvinyl alcohol and liposomes in extenders affords some protection to sperm (Katila, 1997; Pillet *et al.*, 2012). It is increasingly apparent that the lipoproteins and phospholipids in milk have a significantly beneficial effect in protecting sperm in fresh and cooled storage, hence the continued popularity and success of milk-based extenders.

21.6.5.2. Cooling rates

The extent of sperm damage due to cold shock is not only dependent upon the temperature drop but also the speed and range of the drop. In general the faster the rate of cooling, the more severe the damage, and sperm are particularly vulnerable to irreversible cell membrane damage when temperature rapidly drops from 20°C to 5°C (Watson 1981; Graham 2011a); however, this also depends on the extender being used and temperature range.

Several regimes for the rate of cooling have been investigated, which try to accommodate the most critical temperature range of 20°C down to 5°C (Kayser *et al.*, 1992; Katila, 1997; Rota *et al.*, 2004). Therefore, a cooling regime consisting of rapid cooling from 37°C down to 20°C, followed by a slower cooling rate of 0.1–0.5°C min⁻¹ from 20°C down to 5°C for storage has been suggested. Further work in this area suggests that the critical range can be defined more specifically as 18°C down to 8°C, but this depends on extenders, egg yolk extenders affording more protection than milk-based extenders (Graham, 2011a). Outside this range of 18°C down to 8°C, rapid cooling rates could be resumed (Moran *et al.*, 1992; Katila, 1997). Unfortunately there also appears to be significant inter- and intra-stallion differences in ideal cooling rates, and so no hard and fast rule can be applied. Specific cooling regimes for individual stallions would, therefore, be ideal, but would pose serious difficulties for commercial work; hence, most practices use the simple protocol of a steady cooling rate of 0.3°C min⁻¹ across the whole range of 37°C down to 5°C (Douglas-Hamilton *et al.*, 1984). Semen can be cooled by a specialized cooling unit and kept in a refrigerator. However, more accurate control over cooling rates can be achieved by computerized cooling systems.

21.6.5.3. Storage temperature

Semen is commonly cooled to between 4°C and 5°C, but for short-term storage it may be cooled to room temperature (20°C; Section 21.6.4). Cooling sperm beyond 20°C risks cold shock; however, despite this, the best conception rates are generally obtained with storage at the lower temperature of 4–5°C (Kayser *et al.*, 1992). The benefit of reducing the temperature still further (0°C to –2°C) has been considered, but was associated with a greater adverse effect on motility (Moran *et al.*, 1992). Other storage temperatures have been investigated including 10–15°C, which have been suggested to be better than 0°C, 4°C and 5°C (Magistrini *et al.*, 1992).

21.6.5.4. Length of storage

Prolonged exposure to a cooled environment increases the effect of cold shock and although the metabolism of the sperm is depressed by cooling, it does not cease altogether, so eventually the build-up of toxins and the exhaustion of the nutrient supply results in death. Most studies indicate that insemination of mares with sperm that have been stored at 5°C for up to 24 h will result in good fertilization rates (60–70%; Metcalf, 1998; Love *et al.*, 2015; El-Badry *et al.*, 2017). Conception rates with storage beyond 24 h at 5°C result in depressed, but still acceptable, fertility rates (Love *et al.*, 2015) and there are several reports of successful insemination (73–87%) of mares with semen stored up to 96 h (Van der Holst, 1984; Heiskanen *et al.*, 1994a). This ability of semen to survive at 5°C for prolonged periods of time is used in the development of specialized insulated semen transport containers, the first of which was the Equitainer® (Fig. 21.7; Hamilton Research Inc., Ipswich, Massachusetts, USA), developed by Douglas-Hamilton *et al.* (1984).

21.6.5.5. Packaging and methods of transporting chilled semen

Sperm may be packaged for cool storage in a number of ways, including sterilized polyethylene bags (Whirl-Pak®, Cole-Parmer Instrument Co. Ltd, London), plastic bottles or baby-bottle liners. However, care should be taken as some types of plastic and rubber can be spermotoxic (Broussard *et al.*, 1990; Katila, 1997).

The presence or absence of air (oxygen) during storage is also reported to have an effect, storage in the absence of oxygen resulting in the best motility (Katila, 1997). It seems, therefore, that, for storage

at 4°C, air should be excluded and containers well filled prior to storage (Magistrini *et al.*, 1992). Additionally, storage of semen in tubes on a roller bench (five turns per min) may prolong survival (Katila, 1997).

If the advantages of chilling semen are to be fully realized then an effective means of storage and transportation needs to be devised. To this end several insulated transport containers of varying efficacy have been designed (Brinsko *et al.*, 2000). The one in most widespread use is the Equitainer® (Fig. 21.7).

The Equitainer® is designed to permit controlled cooling of the stored semen sample at 0.3°C min⁻¹ and subsequent maintenance of the sample at 4°C for up to 36 h. The semen should be diluted in a minimum ratio of 1:2 semen/extender and put in the plastic semen container which is put into the isothermalizing unit. The pre-frozen coolant cans are placed into the bottom of the container followed by the isothermalizer containing the semen container and then the foam rubber protective padding, and

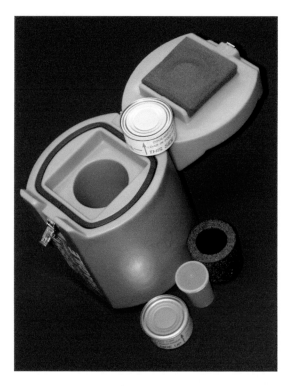

Fig. 21.7. The Equitainer® prior to assembly illustrating one of the coolant cans in the foreground, To the right is the plastic semen container and the black foam isothermalizing unit (which acts as a thermal impedance pad and protective padding). (From Hamilton-Thorn Research, Danvers, Massachusetts, USA.)

the lid is closed. Once closed, the contents of the iso-thermalizer gradually cool at an initial rate of −0.3°C min^{-1} to 4°C and then the content is kept at 4C for 36° h. This container is now a standard form of transporting semen. Other similar disposable containers include the Expecta Foal (Expecta, Parker, Colorado, USA) and Equine Express (MP and J Associates, De Moines, Iowa, USA), the Celle, popular in Germany and the Sarstedt (Leicester, UK), popular in The Netherlands, are also available and work on a similar basis. They allow transportation between countries via courier companies, postal services, etc., and in some countries by dedicated semen transport vehicles (Katila *et al.*, 1997). Work by Brinsko *et al.* (2000) and Guice *et al.* (2017) indicates that, of all the containers, the Equitainer® is superior in ensuring the correct temperature drop and maintenance despite varying environmental temperatures and so justifies its extra cost.

21.6.6. Frozen semen

The use of cooled semen is very successful for short-term storage, but long-term storage by this method is not possible. In order to realize many of the potential benefits of AI, long-term storage is necessary. This is only really possible by freezing, which halts the metabolic processes of the sperm and, in theory, allows indefinite storage. The discovery by Polge *et al.* (1949) of the cryoprotectant properties of glycerol made cryopreservation possible. As a result, the sperm of many species can today be stored at −196°C in liquid nitrogen for indefinite periods of time, while still retaining acceptable fertilization rates post-thaw. Significant variation in the success rates for frozen semen have been reported. In general pregnancy rates for frozen semen at best reach values approaching those of natural service, but are often much lower, and may result in complete failure despite the protocol for freezing apparently being unchanged (Thomassen, 1991; Pickett and Amann, 1993). Pregnancy rates from frozen semen vary enormously particularly with breed, season and between and within stallions (Vidament *et al.*, 1997) and so the prediction of success is inaccurate. However, it is apparent that, in general, pregnancy rates from frozen semen are not as high as those expected from using fresh semen, conception rates of 35–60% being acceptable in commercial AI practice (Thomassen, 1991; Pickett and Amann, 1993; Wockener and Collenbrander, 1993; Deng *et al.*, 2014). The biggest problem for commercial AI is this unpredictability of success and, in particular, the variation between stallions and even

between different ejaculates within the same stallion (Loomis, 1993; Torres-Bogino *et al.*, 1995; Vidament *et al.*, 1997); the reason for this is unclear (Aurich *et al.*, 1996).

21.6.6.1. The principles of cryopreservation

Even under ideal conditions, it is inevitable that some damage will occur to sperm during the freezing process. The main reasons for damage are extracellular and intracellular ice formation and accompanying dehydration causing membrane distortion (Hammerstedt *et al.*, 1990; Graham, 2011b; Sieme, 2011b). Changes in plasma membrane permeability to Ca has also been demonstrated, and is largely manifested as a depression in motility, and possibly acrosome morphology (Wockener and Collenbrander, 1993); hence, motility of sperm is an even poorer indicator of fertility in freeze–thaw samples than it is in fresh or chilled samples (Samper *et al.*, 1991).

Regardless of all these considerations, for cryopreservation to be considered a success the process should enable a sperm to retain its fertilizing capacity post-thaw. To achieve this the sperm must retain its ability to produce energy via metabolism; to show progressive motility; to maintain plasma membrane configuration and integrity (so it will survive in the female tract and attach to the oocyte plasma membrane); and to retain enzymes, such as acrosin, within the acrosome (to allow penetration of the ova). Disruption of any of these functions will significantly affect the sperm's ability to achieve fertilization. The formation of ice crystals and the resultant movement of water up osmotic gradients presents the greatest risk to the maintenance of these attributes.

During the process of freezing several biophysical changes are evident as the temperature drops from −15°C to −60°C. As water freezes, ice crystals form, between which small unfrozen channels exist. If the temperature continues to drop these unfrozen channels vitrify. Sperm can survive within these channels (any caught within the ice crystals die) and, once vitrified, remain undamaged. As an extended semen sample is frozen extracellular ice crystals begin to form from water within the surrounding medium. This ice formation increases the concentration of solutes (such as sugars, salts and proteins) in the fluid surrounding the sperm in the unfrozen, now hypertonic, channels. In response to this newly developed OP gradient, and the fact that water within the sperm is slower to form ice crystals than the water in the surrounding medium, water passes out of the sperm across the semipermeable plasma membrane. As a result the sperm becomes increasingly dehydrated and damaged. The rate of efflux of water from the sperm is also dependent upon the speed of temperature drop. The slower the drop, the greater the time allowed for the efflux of water out of the sperm, and hence the greater the dehydration. However, this does reduce the chance of internal ice crystal formation within the sperm, which can itself cause considerable damage (Amann and Pickett, 1987; Hammerstedt *et al.*, 1990; Graham, 1996, 2011b). This advantage (of reducing the likelihood of physical damage) has to be weighed against the greater damage due to increased intracellular dehydration and solute concentration. On the other hand, if the cooling rate is rapid, water has little time to move out of the sperm, across the plasma membrane, and hence large intracellular ice crystals form within the sperm, causing damage to cell membranes and components. However, the problems of dehydration and solute concentration are less evident with rapid cooling (Graham, 2011b). The aim, therefore, is to arrive at a compromise between all these factors. However, this optimum cooling rate, reported to be between $-10°C$ min^{-1} and $-60°C$ min^{-1}, changes with the composition of the medium surrounding the sperm, and hence the stallion and extender used (Graham, 1996, 2011b).

There are two main temperature ranges of concern regarding sperm damage during freezing. These are the period of supercooling (0°C to –5°C) and the formation of ice crystals (–6°C to –60°C). Excessive supercooling (0°C to –5°C) results in rapid ice formation, with the possibility of physical damage. This problem can be overcome by a technique termed 'seeding', which is designed to induce ice formation more gradually over a greater temperature range. However, there is variable evidence as to whether seeding a semen sample during the freezing process has any real advantages; the process remains complicated (Fiser *et al.*, 1991; Zirkler *et al.*, 2005; Saragusty *et al.*, 2007) and it is, therefore, not practised. The second area of concern is the formation of ice crystals (–6°C to –60°C) and accompanying change in OP and solute concentrations, as previously discussed. In an attempt to overcome this, cryoprotectants (or antifreeze agents) are used.

Cryoprotectants may be divided into two types, depending upon their action. They may be either penetrating (penetrating the plasma membrane of the sperm and acting intracellularly as well as extracellularly); or non-penetrating (and only acting extracellularly). Cryoprotectants act to lower the freezing point of the medium to a temperature much lower than that of water. Penetrating cryoprotectants act internally by replacing water, so reducing the chance of intracellular ice, and act externally to increase the size of the unfrozen channels in which sperm can survive. Non-penetrating cryoprotectants act only externally and induce cellular dehydration, so reducing intracellular ice. Some also interact with, and so stabilize, the membrane (Graham, 2011b). The first cryoprotectant identified was glycerol (Polge *et al.*, 1949), which remains one of the most favoured. Glycerol is a penetrating cryoprotectant, acting as a solvent and readily taken up by sperm, entering the cell within 1 min of addition to the surrounding medium (Pickett and Amann, 1993). Other penetrating cryoprotectants include dimethyl sulfoxide (DMSO) and propylene glycol. Examples of non-penetrating cryoprotectants include sugars, phenolic antioxidants, liposomes (in egg yolk, milk proteins and serum), detergents such as ethylene diamine tetracetic acid (EDTA), surfactants such as orvus ES paste (OEP) and lipids such as phosphatidylcholine (Denniston *et al.*, 1997; Ricker *et al.*, 2006; Wu *et al.*, 2015).

It has been evident for some time that cryoprotectants, both penetrating and non-penetrating, do themselves damage sperm (Demick *et al.*, 1976; Fahy, 1986; Fiser *et al.*, 1991). This may be due to both physical damage, as a result of the changes in OP gradients, and biochemical disruption of cellular components. The adverse effect of cryoprotectants is evident more as a reduction in motility rather than a reduction in fertility, hence the particularly poor correlation between motility and fertility rates in post-thaw samples. The use of motility as an indication of viability is not, therefore, a very accurate assessment in freeze–thaw samples. This effect may be due to a greater deleterious effect on mitochondria than on the acrosome membrane and region of the head (Schober *et al.*, 2007). The detrimental effects of glycerol on sperm function are more evident in stallion sperm than in other species such as cattle. A reduction in this effect may be achieved by altering the freezing protocol and timing of the addition of glycerol (Section 21.6.6.2).

The protocol for the use of cryoprotectants is ultimately a compromise between the advantageous and detrimental effects of their inclusion. Ideally, the exact protocol may well vary with individual stallions in order to obtain optimal results. However, such individual tailoring is not practical in a commercial situation, and hence further compromise is normally required.

21.6.6.2. Extenders for use with frozen semen

There are many commercial extenders for use in cryopreservation and they are based upon those used for cool storage (Section 21.6.3). Often a two-extender protocol is used: a primary extender for initial dilution after seminal plasma removal, which is then aspirated off after centrifugation, prior to the addition of a secondary extender which contains an added cryoprotectant for freezing. Numerous extenders have been used as both primary and/or secondary extenders.

The main function of a primary extender is to maintain sperm motility, but it also acts to protect sperm during the process of centrifugation (Knopp *et al.*, 2005; Moore *et al.*, 2005a). There is, therefore, no real requirement for a cryoprotectant in such extenders. Examples of primary extenders are given in Section 21.6.3.

The primary extender is added, usually in a ratio of 1:1; the sample is then centrifuged after which the primary extender is aspirated off; and then the secondary extender for freezing is added. Many of the secondary extenders are also based upon those given for fresh and cooled semen storage, and may be similar to the primary extenders used, but with a cryoprotectant added. These secondary extenders can also be used alone if semen is not centrifuged.

Glycerol and egg yolk-based extenders were among the first to be used for freezing semen (Nishikawa, 1975). Further, more recent work has demonstrated the cryoprotectant nature of many other components including sugars, liposomes and detergents (Heitland *et al.*, 1995; Squires *et al.*, 2004; Alvarenga *et al.*, 2005; Moore *et al.*, 2005b; Wu *et al.*, 2015). Many extenders used for freezing, therefore, contain a mixture of many components in varying ratios. Examples of extenders for freezing include those with added egg yolk, detergents, sugars, colostrum, glycerols and salts (Table 21.8) and are all commonly used as secondary extenders (Brinsko *et al.*, 2011; Neuhauser *et al.*, 2018a, 2019a; Alvarez *et al.*, 2019).

Glycerol remains the most popular cryoprotectant. However, as mentioned previously, the use of glycerol may itself be detrimental to sperm. Hence, a

Table 21.8. Examples of secondary extenders used for freezing stallion semen.

Component	Quantity
(A) Skimmed milk cryopreservation extender. (From Samper, 1995b.)	
Skimmed milk	2.4 g
Egg yolk	8.0 ml
Sucrose	9.3 g
Glycerol	3.5%
Distilled water	100.0 ml
(B) Detergent (Equex STM®, Nova Chemicals Sales, Scituate, Massachusetts, USA) based cryopreservation extenders. (From Cochran *et al.*, 1984.)	
Lactose solution	
(11% weight/volume)	50.0 ml
Glucose EDTA solution	
(EDTA glucose extender II primary extender)	25.0 ml
Egg yolk	20.0 ml
Glycerol	5.0 ml
Equex® STM	0.5 ml
(C) Lactose-, mannitol- and glucose-based cryopreservation extender. (From Naumenkov and Romankova, 1981, 1983.)	
Lactose	6.6 g
Mannitol	2.1 g
Glucose	0.7 g
Disodium EDTA	0.15 g
Sodium citrate dehydrate	0.16 g
Sodium bicarbonate	0.015 g
Deionized water	100.0 ml
Egg yolk	2.5 g
Glycerol	3.5 ml
(D) HF-20 extender which may be used as a primary extender (without the 10% glycerol) or as a secondary extender (with the 10% glycerol). (From Nishikawa, 1975.)	
Glucose	5.0 g
Lactose	0.3 g
Raffinose	0.3 g

(Continued)

Table 21.8. Continued.

Component	Quantity
Sodium citrate	0.15 g
Sodium phosphate	0.05 g
Potassium sodium tartrate	0.05 g
Egg yolk	0.5–2.0 g
Penicillin	25,000 IU
Streptomycin	25,000 μg
Deionized water (made up to)	100.0 ml
Glycerol	10%
(E) A simple sugar-based secondary extender. (From Piao and Wang, 1988.)	
11% sucrose solution	100.0 ml
Skimmed milk	45.0 ml
Egg yolk	16.0 ml
Glycerol	6.0 ml

EDTA, ethylene diamine tetracetic acid

compromise has to be reached in the concentration of glycerol and the length of time of exposure of sperm to glycerol prior to freezing, in order to maximize its beneficial effects but minimize its toxic effects. The efficiency of glycerol may be affected by the diluent to which it is added, as well as by the stallion. It is now known that 5–10% glycerol with an equilibration time of just a few seconds prior to freezing is adequate for cryoprotection to be achieved (Christanelli *et al.*, 1985; Pickett and Amann, 1993; Burns and Reasner, 1995).

21.6.6.3. Vitrification

It is increasingly evident that the physical damage caused by intracellular ice crystals that form at freezing has a significant detrimental effect; to address this, vitrification prior to freezing has recently been investigated. Vitrification (glass formation) requires sperm to be exposed to extender with high concentration of cryoprotectants (many of those discussed for freezing in Section 21.6.6.2 have been used) for a very short period of time. This causes dehydration of sperm prior to freezing (and so avoids the formation of ice crystals), followed by very rapid freezing by plunging into liquid nitrogen; thawing should also be very rapid. Dehydration or desiccation is achieved using a non-penetrating cryoprotectant. Often sugars such as sucrose are used: these are added to the extender in high concentrations, significantly increasing OP in the surrounding fluid,

causing water to be rapidly drawn out of the sperm which then become desiccated. The desiccated sperm are then plunged into liquid nitrogen (–196°C) cooling at 2,500°C min⁻¹ and so frozen immediately. The use of cryoloops allows even smaller droplets to be frozen, resulting in even more rapid temperature drop (up to 20,000°C min⁻¹). This results in an instantaneous transition to glass of both intracellular and extra cellular fluid. The faster the glass transition occurs, the less damage there is to sperm; however, the glass transition temperature depends to a certain extent on the concentration of cryoprotectant used, as well as the type of cryoprotectant. Different cryoprotectants have different toxicity, glass transition temperature and penetration rates, and so a balance has to be struck between the advantages and disadvantages of having higher cryoprotectant concentrations. In addition, very small volumes of extracellular fluid are also reported to be beneficial. Although some success has been achieved using vitrification it is not yet commercially available but it may prove to be a technique for the future (Arav *et al.*, 2002; Kelly *et al.*, 2003; Hossain and Osuamkpe, 2007; Saragusty and Arav, 2011; Hendriks *et al.*, 2014; Hidalgo *et al.*, 2018; Hinrichs, 2018; Consuegra *et al.*, 2018a,b, 2019).

21.6.6.4. Packaging for frozen semen

Several methods are available for the packaging of sperm for freezing. These methods include glass ampoules or vials; polypropylene, polyvinyl or plastic round or flat straws (usually 0.2–4.0 ml in volume) (Fig. 21.8); flat aluminium packets (10–15 ml); pellets (0.1–0.2 ml); and macrotubes (10 ml; Haard and Haard, 1991; Sieme, 2011b).

Initially semen was frozen in glass ampoules or vials with a volume of 1–10 ml. Subsequently the use of straws has become more widespread, having the advantage of being smaller in volume (0.25–5 ml) and, therefore, taking up less storage space. Semen may also be stored in pellets which, owing to their size, enable a more rapid decline in temperature to be achieved. Pellets are frozen by placing small drops (approximately 0.1 ml) of concentrated semen into small indentations in a block of solid carbon dioxide or a metal plate. Today straws are favoured by most and, although some work has suggested an effect of straw volume on subsequent fertility, straws of 0.5–5 ml are most commonly used, each containing adequate sperm so that either one or two straws can be used per insemination (Wockener and Schuberth, 1993; Heitland *et al.*, 1996). Once frozen, regardless of packaging, semen is held indefinitely at −196°C in flasks of liquid nitrogen (Fig. 21.9).

21.6.6.5. Cooling rates

Traditionally both ampoules and straws were frozen by suspension over, followed by plunging into, liquid nitrogen at −196°C. Most recently it has become evident that the rate of cooling is important (Section 21.6.6.1) and that the type of storage, extender and possibly stallion (Sieme, 2011a) has a bearing on this. Pelleted semen, for example, ensures a rapid, but rather uncontrolled, drop in temperature. The cooling of straws and aluminium packets can be controlled more easily by initial suspension in racks over liquid nitrogen (varying the heights and time of suspension allows some control of cooling rate), followed by plunging into the liquid nitrogen. Floating freezing racks, into which straws are placed and then floated on liquid nitrogen, have also been advocated along with programmable freezing units (Hurtgen, 1997).

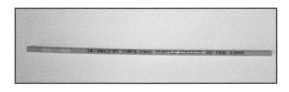

Fig. 21.8. A round plastic straw is one of the most common methods of storing frozen semen.

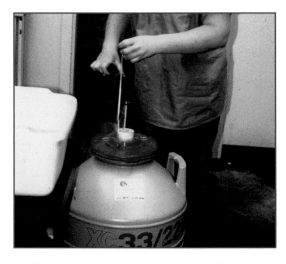

Fig. 21.9. Semen may be conveniently stored indefinitely in liquid nitrogen flasks. (Photo courtesy of Dr Julie Baumber-Skaife.)

The effect of various cooling rates has been investigated (Devireddy *et al.*, 2002b; Pugliesi *et al.*, 2014; Maziero *et al.*, 2019) and as a result a typical recommended equine cooling curve for a programmable freezer starting at 4°C is 10°C min⁻¹ to −10°C, 20°C min⁻¹ to −100°C and 60°C min⁻¹ to −192°C. This is normally achieved using a computer-controlled, programmable freezer. However, other cooling regimes have been suggested, and it is likely that different regimes suit different extenders and different stallions, and at different times of the year (Wrench *et al.*, 2010).

21.6.6.6. Thawing rates and extenders

Thawing rate is known to have an effect on post-thaw quality. The easiest and most commonly used method is to place the packaged semen in a warm water bath. Water bath temperatures of between 4°C and 75°C have been used successfully; however, this depends on the method of storage, volume of semen and conductivity of the packaging, etc. (British Equine Veterinary Association, 1991; Borg *et al.*, 1997; Sieme, 2011b).

Some protocols for thawing semen involve the addition of warmed thawing extender or seminal plasma to aid the thawing process and minimize the effects of OP changes. The extender may also increase the volume of inseminate and help maintain sperm viability until insemination. Thawing extenders may be used for semen stored in pellets, vials or straws, and often contain sugars such as sucrose, but have varying rates of success (Table 21.9; Al-Essawe *et al.*, 2018; Neuhauser *et al.*, 2019b).

Despite careful adherence to freezing and thawing protocols it is evident that there is considerable variation in success between stallions, and even between ejaculates from the same stallion. The reason for this is unclear. Ideally it would be possible to identify some marker that indicates the ability of sperm to survive the freezing process, but as yet no such reliable marker has been identified.

Table 21.9. A sucrose and milk diluent that may be used as a thawing extender. (From Piao and Wang, 1988.)

Component	Quantity
Sucrose	6.0 g
Powdered skimmed milk	3.4 g
Distilled water	100.0 ml

21.7. Semen Dilution

The extent of semen dilution depends on the initial concentration of the sample, the motility of the sperm and method of storage (Samper, 2011) and, therefore, means very little as a simple extension ratio. The aim of extension is to store the sample at an appropriate concentration and volume for survival and subsequent insemination, without the need for further treatment prior to insemination. Insemination of diluted semen containing 100×10^6 progressively motile sperm per insemination gives acceptable results, but normally 250×10^6 sperm per insemination is recommended to allow a margin for error. There appears to be no benefit of inseminating more than 500×10^6 sperm (Vidament et al., 1997; Samper 2009a, 2011). The optimal sperm concentration for fresh and cooled storage/insemination is considered to be $25–50 \times 10^6$ sperm ml^{-1} of extender (or extender plus seminal plasma; Webb et al., 1993; Samper, 2011). The insemination volume is calculated using the following formula:

$$\text{Insemination volume (ml)} = \frac{\substack{\text{Number of progressively motile} \\ \text{sperm (PMS) required}}}{\text{Number of PMS ml}^{-1}}$$

A greater number of sperm per insemination (800×10^6) is normally advocated for frozen semen, to compensate for loss during the freezing process (Samper, 1995b). Frozen semen can be inseminated in a very concentrated form direct from straws, or a thawing extender can be used and normally results in a sperm concentration of $50–100 \times 10^6$ ml^{-1}.

21.8. Insemination Volume

In addition to the total number of sperm, volume of inseminate also affects success. Volumes in excess of 100 ml or less than 0.5 ml appear to be detrimental to conception rates (Rowley et al., 1990; Jasko et al., 1992b; Katila, 2005). Usually the volume of inseminate varies from 10–30 ml for fresh semen, 5–40 ml for chilled and 0.5–5 ml for frozen (British Equine Veterinary Association, 1997). When deciding on dilution rates a happy medium needs to be struck between sperm concentration and inseminate volume (Newcombe et al., 2005; Samper, 2009a, 2011).

21.9. Insemination Timing and Frequency

When using fresh or chilled semen, insemination should occur (as with natural service) every 48 h, until the mare is no longer in oestrus or has ovulated. This is to ensure that she is inseminated around day 4 of oestrus and so is timed as close as possible to ovulation (Katila et al., 1996; Watson and Nikolakopoulos, 1996). With frozen semen timing is much more critical, as the longevity of sperm viability is much reduced, and so insemination needs to occur in the 6-h window prior to ovulation. This necessitates the use of hormones to advance ovulation (human chorionic gonadotrophin (hCG), gonadotrophin-releasing hormone (GnRH); Section 9.5.2) and/or frequent ultrasonic scanning monitoring (Woods et al., 1990; Heiskanen et al., 1994a,b; Sieme et al., 2003b, 2004b; Miller, 2008; Barbacini, 2011).

21.10. Insemination Technique

Owing to the cost and organization involved, the oestrous cycle of mares to be covered by AI is invariably manipulated to time ovulation so that the arrival of semen can be planned ahead. There are numerous ways in which this can be achieved (Section 9.5.2).

21.10.1. Conventional insemination

Mares are conventionally inseminated non-surgically. Semen, both diluted and undiluted, is usually deposited into the uterus by means of a plastic (rubber is spermicidal) sterile pipette with syringe attached (Figs 21.10 and 21.11), or by an insemination gun, guided in through the cervix to the uterus, using the index finger (Figs 21.12 and 21.13). Alternatively, the pipette can be guided in through the cervix as per rectal palpation, the cervix being felt through the rectum wall. Both methods have their merits and disadvantages. Per rectum-guided insemination reduces the risk of contamination of the reproductive tract, as no arm is introduced into the vagina and only a relatively small breach of the natural reproductive tract seals occurs, owing to the small size of the insemination pipette. However, it is more difficult to locate and manipulate the cervix per rectum. It is largely for this reason that the preferred method of insemination in the mare is guiding the pipette per vagina. Some pipettes have a flexible tip (Fig. 21.11) which allows direction into either of the uterine horns in the belief that deposition of the semen into the horn ipsilateral to (on the same side as) the ovulating ovary

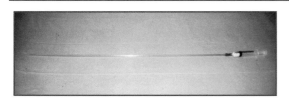

Fig. 21.10. In readiness for insemination, the filled syringe is attached to the end of the insemination pipette. (Photo courtesy of Dr Julie Baumber-Skaife and Mr Victor Medina.)

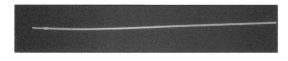

Fig. 21.11. Some insemination pipettes have a flexible end (far left) to enable it to be directed towards one uterine horn or the other.

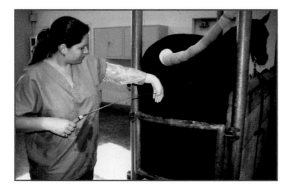

Fig. 21.12. The mare is restrained in stocks, with her tail bandaged and perineal area washed (Photo courtesy of Dr Julie Baumber-Skaife and Mr Victor Medina.)

may improve success rates, though there is no evidence to support this.

Once through the cervix the insemination pipette is pushed about 2 cm into the uterus. When it is in place the semen is slowly expelled by depressing the plunger, or the syringe or insemination gun (Fig. 21.14; Davies Morel, 1999; Conboy, 2011a). Conventionally, doses of 300–500 × 10⁶ progressively motile sperm are inseminated per mare (Brinsko, 2006), although more recent work suggests that a dose of 50–300 × 10⁶ is just as successful (Sieme *et al.*, 2003b).

21.10.2. Low-dose insemination

Recently, low-dose insemination methods have been developed to allow the use of smaller semen samples/ sperm numbers per insemination. This is potentially important in stallions with poor semen samples; that is, those that are low in concentration or in volume (Brinsko, 2006). It is also relevant in sex-selected semen where, owing to the limitations of current technology, only small samples of selected semen are available (Lindsey *et al.*, 2001) and with epididymal spermatozoa (Morris *et al.*, 2002). It may also have a role in frozen semen where success rates with conventional insemination techniques are lower and more variable (Samper, 1991; Barbacini *et al.*, 2000); reducing the distance the sperm need to travel through the tract to reach the Fallopian tube for fertilization may be beneficial. A progressive reduction in sperm numbers is reported to occur within the uterus (from immediately behind the cervix to the utero-tubular junction area) of many species, including the equine. This may reflect some form of selective gradient and so many non-viable sperm are lost during passage

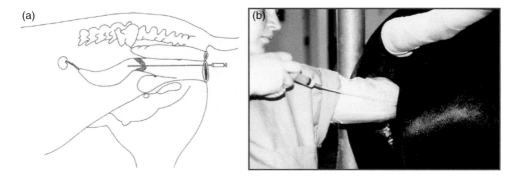

Fig. 21.13. (a) Diagram of artificial insemination (AI) in the mare guided per vagina. (b) A well-lubricated hand is introduced slowly into the vagina along with the insemination pipette. Once in place the plunger of the syringe or insemination gun should be slowly depressed to expel all the semen into the uterus. (Photo courtesy of Dr Julie Baumber-Skaife and Mr Victor Medina.)

through the reproductive tract (Parker *et al.*, 1975; Katila *et al.*, 2000; Scott *et al.*, 2000). It is reported that 0.0007% of sperm deposited into the tract actually make it through to the Fallopian tube (Rigby *et al.*, 2000) and that, despite the quality of sperm inseminated or deposited naturally at mating, 90% of sperm flushed from the oviduct are morphologically normal (Morris and Lyle, 2011). It would, therefore, seem possible that the insemination of a low dose of semen directly into the utero-tubular junction area would bypass this selection mechanism and give equivalent results. This ability to bypass the normal transit through the uterus may also be beneficial in mares with habitual persistent post-coitum endometritis. Three main methods are employed in low-dose insemination: ultrasound-guided deep uterine insemination; hysteroscopic or endoscopic insemination; and gamete intra-Fallopian tube transfer (GIFT).

21.10.2.1. Ultrasound-guided deep intrauterine insemination

Ultrasound-guided intrauterine insemination involves the deposition of as few as 10×10^6 sperm in a small volume of extender (200–1000 µl) directly into the uterine horn as near to the utero-tubular junction as possible. This is done by introducing the insemination pipette through the cervix as per conventional insemination; however, once the pipette end has passed through the cervix it is passed into the uterine horn ipsilateral to the ovulating ovary by palpation of the uterus per rectum. Alternatively, it can be visualized and its position monitored by the ultrasonic scanner; the pipette is then pushed further up into the uterine horn to the utero-tubular junction, where the semen is deposited (Buchanan *et al.*, 2000; Morris and Lyle, 2011). Success rates have been variable but conception rates of up to 50% have been reported (Morris *et al.*, 2000; Morris and Allen, 2002a; Petersen *et al.*, 2002; Morris and Lyle, 2011; Camargo *et al.*, 2018).

21.10.2.2. Hysteroscopic or endoscopic low-dose insemination

Hysteroscopic or endoscopic low-dose insemination is similar to ultrasound-guided deep intrauterine insemination, but uses even lower doses ($1–5 \times 10^6$ sperm) and volumes (10–500 µl; Morris *et al.*, 2000; Alvarenga and Leao, 2002; Allen, 2005). The position of the insemination pipette is monitored via an endoscope which is passed through the mare's cervix and up to the

tip of the uterine horn so that the utero-tubular junction can be visualized. A long catheter containing the small semen sample is then passed up the working channel of the endoscope until it is at the utero-tubular junction of the horn ipsilateral to the ovulating ovary, where the semen is then deposited (Morris *et al.*, 2000, 2003; Morris and Allen, 2002a). Conception rates are again variable but have been reported to be greater than 60% even at the lowest-dose levels (1×10^6 sperm; Morris *et al.*, 2000; Brinsko *et al.*, 2003; Sieme *et al.*, 2003b; Clulow *et al.*, 2007).

21.10.2.3. Gamete intra-Fallopian tube transfer

GIFT or oviductal insemination (Section 23.10) involves the surgical placing (via laparoscopy) of sperm directly into the Fallopian tube and has been used in attempts to reduce still further the number of sperm required for insemination, and to bypass any possible selection, storage and/or channelling function of the utero-tubular junction (Scott *et al.*, 2000). Doses as low as 2×10^5 sperm have been used successfully (Manning *et al.*, 1998; Morris, 2004).

21.11. Conclusion

The use of equine AI is widespread in many parts of the world, although the failure of the Thoroughbred industry to recognize and hence register progeny conceived by AI remains a limitation to its use, and to the development of associated techniques. Another major limitation is the relative lack of success and variability with frozen semen. Despite this, it is evident that equine AI is here to stay, and will continue to expand, opening up with it exciting opportunities in the selection and breeding of the equine species and reproductive technology.

Study Questions

Detail the processes involved in collecting semen from a stallion.

Evaluate the relative merits of assessing semen using microscopic evaluation versus functional tests.

Detail the challenges that cooling and freezing semen present and how these challenges can be managed.

You have collected a semen sample from your stallion: it measures 50 ml of gel-free fraction with a concentration of 200×10^6 sperm ml^{-1} with 50% progressive motility. How many mares would you expect to be able to inseminate with this sample when used for chilled AI? Describe the insemination process you would use.

What is cold shock and how does it affect sperm?

You have been provided with some very rare semen. Discuss how you could manage and inseminate it in order to maximize the number of foals that can be produced.

You have just collected a fresh semen sample, which is required for insemination in 7 days into a mare kept at a stud 500 miles away. How would you manage the sample in order to successfully inseminate the mare?

Suggested Reading

Davies Morel, M.C.G. (1999) *Equine Artificial Insemination.* CAB International, Wallingford, UK, pp. 406.

Pickett, B.W., Voss, J.L., Squires, E.L., Vanderwall, D.K., McCue, P.M. and Bruemmer, J.E. (2000) Collection, preparation and insemination of stallion semen. Bulletin No 10 Animal Reproduction and Biotechnology Laboratory. Colorado State University, Fort Collins, Colorado, pp. 1–15.

Samper, J.C. (2000) *Equine Breeding Management and Artificial Insemination.* W.B. Saunders, Philadelphia, Pennsylvania, pp. 306.

Baumber-Skaife, J. (2011) Evaluation of semen. In: McKinnon, A.O., Squires, E.L., Vaala, E. and Varner, D.D. (eds) *Equine Reproduction*, 2nd edn. Wiley-Blackwell, Philadelphia, London, pp. 1278–1291.

Conboy, H.S. (2011) Management of stallions in artificial insemination. In: McKinnon, A.O., Squires, E.L, Vaala, W.E. and Varner, D.D. (eds) *Equine Reproduction*, 2nd edn. Wiley-Blackwell, Philadelphia, London, pp. 1197–1207.

Samper, J.C. (2011) Breeding with cooled transported semen. In: McKinnon, A.O., Squires, E.L., Vaala, E. and Varner, D.D. (eds) *Equine Reproduction*, 2nd edn. Wiley-Blackwell, Philadelphia, London, pp. 1316–1322.

Sieme, H. (2011) Semen extenders for frozen semen. In: McKinnon, A.O., Squires, E.L., Vaala, E. and Varner, D.D. (eds) *Equine Reproduction*, 2nd edn. Wiley-Blackwell, Philadelphia, London, pp. 2964–2971.

Sieme, H. (2011) Freezing Semen. In: McKinnon, A.O., Squires, E.L., Vaala, E. and Varner, D.D. (eds) *Equine Reproduction*, 2nd edn. Wiley-Blackwell, Philadelphia, London, pp. 2972–2982.

Ball, B.A. (2014) Applied andrology in horses. In: Chenoweth, P.J. and Lorton, S.P. (eds) *Animal Andrology: Theories and Applications.* CABI, Wallingford, Oxfordshire, UK, pp 254–296.

Kowalczyk, A., Czerniawska-Piatkowska, E. and Kuczaj, M. (2019) Factors Influencing the Popularity of Artificial Insemination of Mares in Europe. *Animals* 9, 460.

22 Embryo Transfer

The Objectives of this Chapter are:

To detail the process of embryo transfer (ET), from embryo collection through to transfer into the recipient, along with evaluation and storage.

To enable you to make informed decisions about whether ET is appropriate for any breeding scenario or requirement.

To provide you with the knowledge to enable you to have an informed discussion with an ET practitioner on the procedure and its uses.

To enable you to appreciate both the limitations and future use of ET within the equine industry.

22.1. Introduction

Embryo transfer (ET) is an increasingly popular method by which horses can be bred and is now a commercially available technique in many parts of the world. The first reported successful equine ET was carried out surgically in UK between donkeys and horses (Allen and Rowson, 1972). Two years later workers in Japan (Oguri and Tsutsumi, 1974) reported the first successful non-surgical transfer and birth of a foal. Research since then has considerably improved the early low success rates, making ET a commercially successful practice (Squires *et al.*, 2003; Stout, 2006; Hartman, 2011; McCue and Squires, 2015). Nevertheless, the commercial application of ET in horses has yet to reach the sophistication and success of its application in cattle and sheep. One of the major constraints to the development of ET in horses is the continued reluctance of some breed societies, most notably the Thoroughbred, to register foals conceived in this manner. Of those that do, many will only allow one foal to be registered per mare per year, restricting many of the potential advantages of ET. ET in horses was first taken on board as a commercial procedure in Argentina, where it gained real popularity with breeding high-goal polo ponies, and more recently has grown in popularity in Europe (largely for breeding Warmblood sports horses) and in North America, helped by the lifting of the restriction on the number of foals per mare per year by the Quarter Horse Breed society, among others.

22.2. Embryo Transfer

ET may be used for a number of reasons (Samper, 2009b; Campbell, 2014) including:

1. To obtain foals from mares that are unable to carry a foal to term or to go through the process of parturition.
2. To obtain foals from older mares without risk.
3. To provide a genetically promising foal with the best maternal environment, both intra- and extra-uterine (maximum milk production).
4. To allow performance mares to breed without interrupting their performance career.
5. To provide embryos for freezing and so provide genetic diversity in the future.
6. To aid in the breeding of exotic equids.
7. To increase the number of foals/mare/lifetime.
8. To allow genetic testing prior to possible transfer.
9. For biotechnology and other related advanced reproductive techniques (ART).
10. To allow cloning, embryo sexing, etc.

Several concerns have been expressed with regard to the technique, including fear of the economic effect on certain sections of the industry; the possibility of inbreeding and reduction in the genetic pool perpetuating inherited traits that limit reproductive activity; the cost of the procedure (East *et al.*, 1999b,c); and how far should associated ART be allowed to progress.

22.2.1. Donor and recipient mares

The main principle behind ET is the transfer of elite embryos from a genetically superior donor mare, mated to a genetically superior stallion, into a normally, but not necessarily, genetically inferior recipient mare that is reproductively competent. This technique makes use of the fact that the genotype of the mare carrying the foal has no effect whatsoever on the characteristics of that foal. The foal's genotype and, therefore, its characteristics are determined by the mare that produced the ovum and the stallion whose sperm was used to fertilize it. The uterine environment of the recipient mare, her temperament and mammary gland function do, however, have an effect. For these reasons, as discussed later (Section 22.2.2.2), the choice of an appropriate recipient mare is important. The technique also makes use of the fact that, for the first 16–18 days of its life, the equine embryo is free-living within the uterus and has not yet formed an attachment. Therefore, moving it in early life to another mare's uterus can be carried out with reasonable ease.

In order for ET to be successful, the stage of the uterus into which the embryo is transferred must be similar to that of the uterus from which it was collected. This will ensure that the uterine secretions and development match the requirements of the embryo. To achieve this, the oestrous cycles of the donor and recipient mares must be synchronized. This can be achieved by having a large group of mares from which to select a mare at the correct stage of the cycle or, more conveniently, by using exogenous hormone therapy. Further details on the means of synchronizing and timing oestrus and ovulation in the mare are given in Section 9.5.2. Initial evidence suggested that the donor and recipient mares should ovulate within 24 h of each other, but more recent research has reported success over a much wider range of synchrony. The best results are reported if the recipient mare ovulates between 1 day before (+1 day) to 2 days after (–2 day) the donor mare. It is thought that, if an embryo is placed into a uterus that is a little behind the stage of the one from which it was removed, this compensates for any developmental retardation that may have occurred owing to the stress of transfer (Carnevale *et al.*, 2000b; McCue and Troedsson, 2003; Stout, 2003, 2006; Wilsher *et al.*, 2012; Cuervo-Arango *et al.*, 2018a). More recent work has

suggested good success with asynchrony as wide as +2 to –6 (Wilsher *et al.*, 2010).

22.2.2. Hormonal treatment of donor and recipient

For ET, both the donor and recipient mares may be similarly synchronized, using prostaglandin F2α (PGF2α), progesterone, often with human chorionic gonadotrophin (hCG) or gonadotrophin-releasing hormone (GnRH) (Section 9.5.2; Voss, 1993; Carnevale *et al.*, 2005b; Raz *et al.*, 2011; Greco *et al.*, 2012, 2016; Oliveira Neto *et al.*, 2018; Pietrani *et al.*, 2019). Alternatively, if a group of recipient mares is available, no hormone treatment may be necessary as if their cycles are closely monitored the best 'match' can be selected. Whatever protocol is used, close ultrasonic monitoring of follicular activity is essential to determine the exact time of ovulation (Hartman, 2011).

22.2.2.1. The donor mare

In an ideal transfer system, a large number of embryos are collected on one occasion from a single donor; that is, she is induced to produce many more embryos than she would during her natural oestrous cycle (i.e. she is super-ovulated) (Squires and McCue, 2007, 2011). However, only 50% of embryos are recovered on average, providing further impetus for super-ovulation (Roser and Meyers-Brown, 2012). In cattle and sheep super-ovulation is quite successful, although results vary. Equine chorionic gonadotrophin (eCG; also known as pregnant mare serum gonadotrophin (PMSG)) is often used as the super-ovulation agent; however, it has no effect on mares, even at very high doses. Originally the best success was achieved using equine pituitary extract (EPE), formerly known commercially as Pitropin (Douglas, 1979; Alvarenga *et al.*, 2000; Köllmann *et al.*, 2008). Injected daily over 7 days, Pitropin increases ovulation rates to an average of 3–4, yielding 1–2 embryos; however, the reaction is not consistent, either between different oestrous cycles in the same mare or between mares. This is likely to be due to the varying concentration of luteinizing hormone (LH) and follicle-stimulating hormone (FSH) in the crude preparation; a further disadvantage is the cost of collecting equine pituitaries and of extracting and purifying the preparation, plus the limited supply. Numerous protocols have been used to try and improve the response to EPE but variability remains a significant problem (Hofferer *et al.*, 1991; Dippert *et al.*, 1992; Alvarenga *et al.*, 2001), including in 2003 a commercially prepared standardized EPE which was, however, only available in the USA. Equine FSH (eFSH) has also been used, again with limited success; and, like EPE, as it is originates from equine pituitaries and so relies on slaughtered animals, it is of practical and ethical concern. Some success has been obtained using GnRH, although this also involves a series of injections (Harrison *et al.*, 1991). Further along these lines, some success has been reported using human menopausal gonadotrophins (hMG; Koene *et al.*, 1990), porcine FSH (pFSH; Fortune and Kimmich, 1993; Krekeler *et al.*, 2006) and inhibin vaccines. Most recently, commercially produced recombinant equine FSH (reFSH) has become available and appears promising (Niswender *et al.*, 2003; Squires and McCue, 2007; Köllmann *et al.*, 2008; Jennings *et al.*, 2009; Meyers-Brown *et al.*, 2010; Roser and Meyers-Brown, 2012). Although multiple injections are still required and a greater incidence of anovulatory follicles is reported, the use of reFSH can regularly result in 3–4 ovulations per oestrus, resulting on average in two embryos (Logan *et al.*, 2007; McCue *et al.*, 2007a, 2008b; Köllmann *et al.*, 2008; Roser and Meyers-Brown, 2012). This is still a long way off the 6–8 embryos/oestrus obtained in cattle, for example, but demonstrates that the equine ovary can respond to eFSH, and provides a positive start for future research. Even if equine ovaries are able to produce multiple pre-ovulatory follicles, the unique structure of the equine ovary (which dictates that ovulation can only occur through the ovulation fossa) may present a limitation. Competition is likely to exist between oocytes as they pass through the ovarian stroma towards the ovulation fossa and during actual passage through the ovulation fossa. As such, ovulation of multiple oocytes within a short period of time is unlikely to be possible. Using the protocols currently available, the best that can be expected is an average of 1.8 embryos/mare/flush (Allen, 2005).

A successful super-ovulatory agent would not only allow more embryos to be recovered per oestrus but also increase the likelihood of at least one viable embryo per collection. It may also have uses in providing more ova/oestrus in subfertile mares and in those to be mated by a subfertile stallion, so again increasing the chances of at least one ovum being successfully fertilized. Similarly, it may improve conception rates when using frozen semen, where fertility is naturally lower.

Many factors affect the yield and quality of embryos collected. For example, it has been reported that recovery rates of grade 1 embryos are much reduced in mares in training (Mortensen *et al.*, 2009). This is of particular concern, as one of the main commercial uses of ET is that it enables competition mares to breed without interrupting their athletic career (Campbell, 2014). This effect of training appears to be related to the vascular perfusion of the wall of the pre-ovulatory follicle on the day before ovulation, which is known to be linked to subsequent pregnancy rates (Kelley *et al.*, 2011; Smith *et al.*, 2012). A rise in cortisol, the hormone of stress, was also reported in exercising mares and this in turn is linked to a drop in LH (Kelley *et al.*, 2011). However, this link between training and ET success is not supported by all (Pessoa *et al.*, 2011). Providing breed societies will allow it, or if embryo freezing is successful, repeat collections from a mare within the season would allow multiple embryos to be produced. It is possible to perform up to four flushes per season; some have reported that more than this result in reduced recovery rates and embryo quality (Hoffman *et al.*, 2009; Carnevale *et al.*, 2005b) although, once again, this is not reported by all (Vasquez *et al.*, 2010; Aurich *et al.*, 2011).

Despite all the work being carried out, the lack of a reliable, effective, super-ovulation agent, and the restriction by some breed societies on registering more than one foal per year, remain the major challenges in the development and commercial use of equine ET.

A general routine that may be used to synchronize and attempt to super-ovulate a donor mare is given in Table 22.1.

22.2.2.2. The recipient mare

The ideal recipient mares are multiparous and have reached mature size; they are 5–10 years of age, and have a proven breeding record of reproductive soundness with no history of uterine infection or compromise. The tone of the recipient's uterus (an indication of dioestrous progesterone levels) and position and length of the cervix (ability to protect the uterus from infection) are also reported to be very important selection criteria (Carnevale *et al.* 2000b; Vita and Necchi, 2019). Recipient mares need be of no particular genetic merit, as they will in no way affect the genotype of the embryos transferred to them, but they should be musculoskeletally sound with a good mammary gland and known to be good mothers. Ideally they should be larger than the donor, to provide a larger uterus and so maximize fetal development *in utero*; this will have a positive carry-over effect on birth weight and future post-natal

Table 22.1. A general hormone routine that can be used to time and attempt to super-ovulate a donor mare for embryo transfer (ET).

Time	Drug to be administered/event
Day 0	PGF2α
Day 6	hCG
Day 10	Oestrus and ovulation in mares that had a CL at PGF2α administration
Day 14 (or identification of multiple follicles ≥ 25 mm)	eFSH
Day 15	eFSH and PGF2α
Day 16	eFSH
Day 17	eFSH
Day 18	eFSH, oestrus may start
Day 19	eFSH, oestrus
Day 20	eFSH, oestrus
Day 21 (or identification of follicles ≥ 30–35 mm)	hCG, oestrus
Days 22–24	Ovulation may occur – covering/AI
Days 30–32	Embryo collection (8-day-old embryo)

PGF2α, prostaglandin F2α; hCG, human chorionic gonadotrophin; CL, corpus luteum; eFSH, equine follicle-stimulating hormone; AI, artificial insemination

growth and development (Fig. 22.1; East *et al.*, 1999a,c; Allen *et al.*, 2004).

Recipients may be treated hormonally in a very similar manner to donors, except that no attempt is made to super-ovulate them and they are, of course, not mated. Some people advocate treating the recipient slightly behind the donor in order to be able to put the embryo into a recipient 24 h behind the donor uterus from which it was taken (Allen, 2001b, 2005; Greco *et al.*, 2016). An example of an exogenous hormone treatment regime used in recipients is given in Table 22.2.

Mares should be scanned to ensure that they have reacted to the synchronization programme and to determine time of ovulation. Work by Cuervo-Arango *et al.* (2018b) suggested that a better pregnancy rate to transfer is obtained in recipient mares with double ovulations. Ovariectomized mares have historically been used experimentally as recipients. These mares alleviate the need for synchronization and veterinary inspection but, because of the lack of ovarian progesterone, they require artificial progesterone supplementation for the first 120 days of pregnancy (Hinrichs and Kenney, 1988; McKinnon *et al.*, 1988a; Squires *et al.*, 1989).

22.2.3. Embryo recovery

Once ovulation in the donor is confirmed she is either covered naturally or by artificial insemination (AI) (Chapters 10 and 21). The age of embryos recovered varies with the chosen method of recovery. Equine embryos in general are collected at between 4 (morula) and 8 days (blastocyst) of age (Figs 3.3. and 3.4), although some success has been reported with embryos as old as 10 days (Wilsher *et al.*, 2010). They can be recovered at a relatively late stage compared to other farm livestock, as equine conceptuses do not expand into elongated trophoblasts but remain spherical and free-living within the uterus for a prolonged period of time (16–18 days; Section 3.2.3.1).

22.2.3.1. Surgical recovery

The initial method of recovery during early work was surgical. This technique is now rarely used. However, surgical collection allows the Fallopian tube to be flushed and so younger (prior to day 5) and so more robust embryos can be collected. It also avoids contact between the embryo and an infected or compromised uterine environment. Surgery was initially carried out under general anaesthetic with a ventral (abdomen) midline incision. This was replaced with the mare sedated

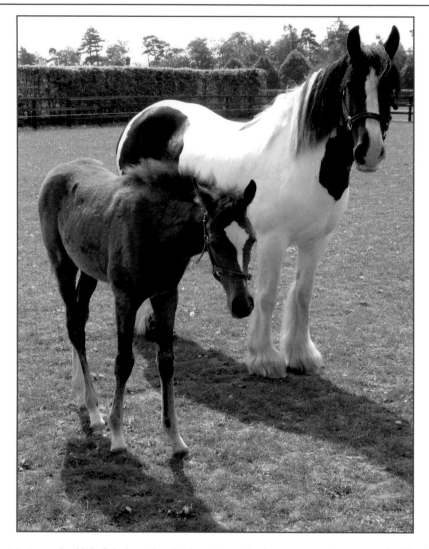

Fig. 22.1. The recipient mare should ideally be larger than the donor, to provide a larger uterus and so maximize fetal development *in utero*.

and held in stocks. The uterus is exteriorized through a ventral midline or flank incision. The uterine horn is then cannulated with a glass tube and the uterine horn is ligated (tied off) near to the uterine body, preventing fluid (and with it any embryos) passing into the body of the uterus. Approximately 50 ml of fluid is flushed, by means of a blunt-ended needle and attached syringe, from the Fallopian tube towards the uterine horn. As the fluid passes, it takes with it any embryos present and exits via the glass cannula to be collected in a warm collecting vessel (Allen and Rowson, 1975; Allen *et al.*, 1977; Castleberry *et al.*, 1980; Imel *et al.*, 1981). The fluid used is pre-warmed to 35–38°C and is often Dulbecco's phosphate-buffered saline, possibly with additional calf serum or oestrous mare serum and penicillin, to help prevent infection. Recovery rates in the order of 70–77% have been reported; these are similar to, or possibly lower than, the current commercial non-surgical techniques (Allen and Rowson, 1975).

22.2.3.2. Non-surgical recovery
Non-surgical embryo recovery was first used in horses with any consistent success in Texas, USA, in 1979 (Vogelsang *et al.*, 1979), although several other researchers had attempted it previously (Oguri and Tsutsumi, 1972; Allen and Rowson, 1975). It is now the

method of choice for commercial ET as there is no need for a general anaesthetic or opening of the abdominal cavity; hence the procedure carries much lower risks and is repeatable. Non-surgical collection allows only the uterus to be flushed and so is restricted to the collection of older embryos (older than 5 days). Younger

Table 22.2. An example of hormone regime used to time ovulation in a recipient mare.

Time	Drug to be administered/event
Day 0	PGF2α
Day 6	hCG
Day 10	Oestrus and ovulation in mares with a CL at PGF2α administration
Day 15	PGF2α
Day 18	Oestrus may start
Day 19	Oestrus
Day 20	Oestrus
Day 21	hCG, oestrus
Day 22	Ovulation may occur
Day 24	Ovulation may occur
Day 30	Embryo transfer
Day 31	Embryo transfer

PGF2α, prostaglandin F2α; hCG, human chorionic gonadotrophin; CL, corpus luteum

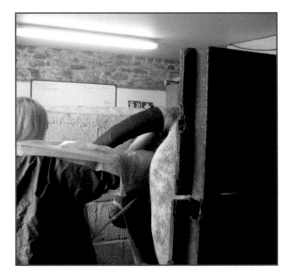

Fig. 22.2. A mare prepared for embryo transfer, with a foley catheter being inserted.

embryos are still within the Fallopian tube and cannot be recovered non-surgically.

The techniques for non-surgical recovery remain largely unchanged (Hartman, 2011). The mare is restrained in stocks, having been prepared and washed as for minimal contamination, natural covering (Fig. 22.2; Section 10.2.2.3). A three-way foley catheter (Fig. 22.3) is introduced through the cervix of the mare, guided per rectum or by inserting a hand into the vagina and guiding the catheter through the cervix using the index finger (Figs 22.2 and 22.3).

The catheter is passed as high up into the uterine horn as possible without undue pressure. Once in position, the cuff of the catheter (Fig. 22.3) is inflated with 15–50 ml of air via the inlet tube, so occluding the base of the uterine horn, and thereby preventing the escape of flushing medium through the uterus. The foley catheter has 'Y' shaped tubing attached, with taps (Figs 22.4a,b, 22.5 and 22.6). The taps enable the rate of flow, both into and out of the foley catheter, to be controlled. The end of the tubing is attached to a collecting vessel with in-line filter (Fig 22.4b). Fluid, usually Dulbecco's phosphate-buffered saline (PBS) as described for surgical transfer, is then flushed in through the entry catheter up into the top of the uterine horn. The fluid returns, along with any embryos present, via an opening into the outlet tube for collection in the warm collecting vessel (Fig. 22.4b). The collecting vessel has an in-line filter preventing the passage through of the embryo. The tap at the bottom of the collecting vessel can then be used to allow the fluid to slowly pass through the filter by gravity, always ensuring that a small amount stays within the collecting vessel above the filter bathing any embryos. Both horns may be flushed out simultaneously if the inflated cuff is drawn back against the internal os of the cervix, or independently if the cuff is placed in turn in each horn. The donor is usually flushed two or three times; the volume of fluid used depends upon the position of the inflated cuff and the size of the uterus, often

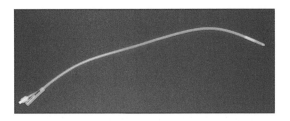

Fig. 22.3. A foley catheter used for non-surgical embryo flushing. Note the cuff area on the far right.

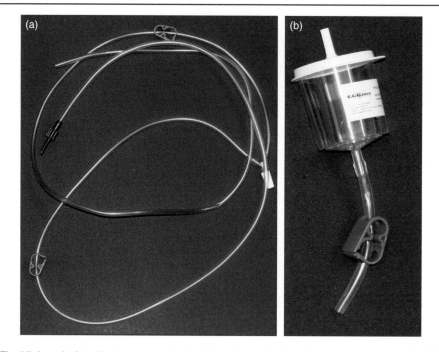

Fig. 22.4. (a) The 'Y' shaped tubing that is connected to the foley catheter (by the white plastic connector at the bifurcation of the tubing) allowing the flushing medium (attached to the black connector) to be flushed up and through the foley catheter and then to exit via the remaining tubing, which attaches to the top of the collecting vessel (Fig. 22.4b). The red tap controls the rate of flow of flushing medium in, and the blue tap controls the exit flow; and (b) the collecting vessel has an in-line filter, and the rate of flow through the collecting vessel and filter is controlled via the blue tap underneath.

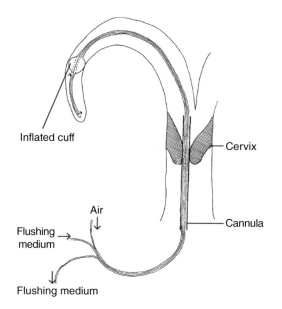

Fig. 22.5. A diagrammatic representation of the foley catheter illustrating the inlet and outlet tubes plus the air inlet for inflating the cuff.

larger in multiparous older mares. If the whole uterus is flushed then approximately 1 l of fluid per flush for ponies and up to 2 l per flush for older multiparous mares may be required. The aim is to introduce adequate fluid to stretch the uterus enough to ensure that fluid washes between the endometrial folds, optimizing the chance of dislodging any embryos (McCue *et al.*, 2010). Recovery of embryos can be improved by allowing the fluid to remain within the uterus for 3–4 min before opening the tap to allow it to pass out through the collecting vessel, and also by per rectum palpation of the uterus during flushing (Squires and Seidel, 1995; McCue *et al.*, 2003, 2010). Oxytocin may also be administered to encourage uterine myometrial activity and hence help in the evacuation of the fluid plus embryo (Jasko, 2002; Hudson and McCue, 2004). Complete evacuation of the uterus is important to not only optimize recovery but also reduce endometritis from retained fluid. After each flush a quick examination for embryos should be made. If no embryo is evident then a repeat flush up to four times is advised, and even leaving the mare for 24 h has resulted in embryos (McCue *et al.*, 2010). Recovery

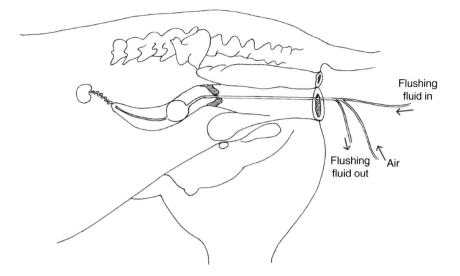

Fig. 22.6. The foley catheter in place ready for flushing and the collection of embryos.

rates are reported to be as good, if not better, than those for surgical recovery. They do, however, vary with the age of the mare; her reproductive health; the exact method of collection; age of the embryo; number of ovulations; semen quality; pre-collection hormone regime; and proficiency of the practitioner (McCue *et al.*, 2010; Pinto *et al.*, 2017). Recovery rates of 45–70%, roughly 10–15% below expected pregnancy rates (Squires *et al.*, 2003; Mortensen *et al.*, 2009; McCue *et al.*, 2010; Aurich *et al.*, 2011 are considered to be acceptable (Squires *et al.*, 1987; Ball *et al.*, 1989). Recovery rates of up to 80% have been reported for the collection of 6–7-day-old embryos (Oguri and Tsutsumi, 1980) and, as the technique has become more widely used and expertize improves, recovery rates of 100% and pregnancy rates of 80–90% have been reported (Hartman, 2011).

Both methods of recovery have their advantages and disadvantages. Surgical recovery allows younger (prior to 5 days) and, therefore, more robust embryos to be collected, but at a much greater risk to the mare and limited possibilities of repeat collections. Non-surgical recovery results in embryos that are older (day 6 onwards) and, therefore, less robust, but with less risk to the mare and with potential for multiple recoveries. The robustness of embryos is particularly important if freezing is to be considered. The ideal scenario would be one in which early embryos, those prior to day 5, could be collected non-surgically. This is now possible with the topical laparoscopic application of

prostaglandin E (PGE) to the external surface of the utero-tubular junction (Robinson *et al.*, 2000) ipsilateral to the ovary that has ovulated 4 days previously. Work by Weber *et al.* (1991) demonstrated that the selective passage of fertilized ova through the utero-tubular junction is due to their ability to secrete PGE. Hence, its application to the utero-tubular junction allows premature passage of embryos (day 4) into the uterus and so their possible collection via non-surgical means. In reality, however, the need to starve a mare for 36 h (a general requirement prior to laparoscopy) means it is not a popular option with competition mares, although use of endoscopic application of PGE and even the oral progestogen misoprostol may prove more viable (Checura and Momont, 2017). In non-surgical recovery the next oestrous cycle can be advanced by administering PG-F2α at the time of collection, which induces the mare to return to oestrus about 4 days later, and hence allows another crop of embryos to be collected from that mare within 10–12 days (McCue *et al.*, 2010). As such, non-surgical recovery of embryos at days 7–8 is normally the commercial method of choice.

22.2.4. Embryo evaluation

Once collected, the flushings are then examined microscopically for embryos; a filter system may be used to aid the search. Their relative weight means that viable embryos older than day 6 will sink to the bottom of the collecting vessel, allowing a significant amount of the flushing medium to be decanted off and so easing identification. Throughout the evaluation process embryos and all equipment used should be kept warm (35–38°C). Embryos are evaluated to assess their viability prior to transfer. They are measured and their stage of development matched to their age. Morphological features such as shape, colour, and number and compactness of cells are noted. Using this information, embryos are graded 1–5, 1 being excellent and 5 dead. Embryos graded 3 or better are normally selected for transfer (McCue *et al.*, 2009; Mortensen *et al.*, 2009; Campbell, 2014). Using grade 1 embryos, 15-day pregnancy rates of 70–85% have been reported (Squires *et al.*, 2003; McCue *et al.*, 2009; Hartman, 2011). The number of grade 1 embryos yielded (75–80%) in a flush in the mare is much higher than that seen in other animals. This is because unfertilized ova and compromised embryos are retained within the Fallopian tube, owing to their inability to produce PGE and so drive their passage to the uterus (McCue *et al.*, 2009, 2010). Once identified and considered appropriate for transfer, embryos are washed to remove any microorganisms and debris (Bielanski, 2007).

22.2.5. Embryo storage

Recovered embryos are either immediately transferred as fresh embryos, or cooled or occasionally frozen for use at a later date.

22.2.5.1. Fresh embryo storage

For fresh storage and transfer, equine embryos can be stored for up to 24 h at 35–38°C, allowing some limited transportation. During initial research embryos were successfully transported in ligated rabbit oviducts, and transferred into recipients within 48 h (Allen *et al.*, 1976). Alternatively, and more normally, embryos can be stored in Ham F10 medium with or without fetal calf serum which has been previously gassed with 5% CO_2, 5% O_2 and 90% N, Ringer's solution or modified Dulbecco's PBS. Ham F10 medium, in particular, is challenging to prepare and so several commercial complete holding media have been developed, which incorporate nutrients, buffers, growth factors, amino acids, etc. Two widely used examples are EmCare® (ICPBio, Auckland, New Zealand) and Vigro Holding Plus® (A-B Technology, Pullman, Washington, USA) and are used with good success (Carney *et al.*, 1991; Moussa *et al.*, 2003; Squires *et al.*, 2003). Varying pregnancy rates have been reported for fresh transfer but seem to be similar or slightly better compared to transfer

after chilling (65–80%) (Carney *et al.*, 1991; McCue *et al.*, 2011b).

22.2.5.2. Chilled embryo storage

More recently it has been possible to chill embryos and, as such, they can be successfully stored for 24–48 h at 4–5°C, allowing reasonable transportation (Carney *et al.*, 1991; Martin *et al.*, 1991; Moussa *et al.*, 2004; McCue *et al.*, 2011b). Storage mediums include: modified Ham F10 medium Ringer's solution or modified Dulbecco's PBS but, as indicated previously, these have largely been replaced in commercial practice by pre-prepared holding media, all of which are reported to be equally effective (Moussa *et al.*, 2002, 2003). Commercially, embryos can then be cooled and stored, as described for semen, in an Equitainer® (Hamilton Research Inc., Ipswich, Massachusetts, USA) (Fig. 21.7; Section 21.6.5.5) which acts like a cool box, cooling embryos by −0.3°C min[-1] down to 5°C, and maintains them at this temperature for 24–48 h (Moussa *et al.*, 2002, 2003; McCue *et al.*, 2007a, 2011b). Pregnancy rates with cooled embryos stored for 24 h are equivalent or slightly poorer than those with fresh transfer and vary between 40% and 65% (Carney *et al.*, 1991; Hudson *et al.*, 2006; McCue *et al.*, 2011b). Any poorer success rates seem to be correlated with a lower percentage of grade 1 embryos being evident after chilled storage. Embryo size is also reported to have an effect, small-for-age embryos being less able to survive the cooling process (Carney *et al.*, 1991; Moussa *et al.*, 2002, 2003, 2006). More recently, in common with semen storage (Section 21.6.4), cooling and storing at ambient temperature (15–18°C) in Ham's F10 with HEPES buffer and 0.4% bovine serum albumin (BSA) has been investigated with some success (Fleury *et al.*, 2002).

22.2.5.3. Frozen embryo storage

The only means of long-term storage is by cryopreservation (freezing) with or without vitrification. Cryopreservation is the term given to cooling embryos (and also sperm, Section 21.6.6) or oocytes (Section 23.11) to −196°C. One of the biggest risks of such treatment is the formation of ice crystals within the embryo during the freezing process; this causes physical damage in a similar way to that described for sperm (Section 21.6.6.1). This damage has traditionally been reduced by the use of a cryoprotectant (or antifreeze) which spreads the formation of ice crystals over a wider temperature range, so ensuring an opportunity for equilibration of osmotic pressure and therefore water movement, and more widely open inter-crystal water channels in which embryos can survive. This allows more time for water to pass out of the embryo into the surrounding fluid and so reduces intercellular ice crystal formation and associated damage (Bruyas, 2011). Unfortunately, cryopreservation is currently not very successful in horses, although it is quite successful and commercially viable in sheep, cattle and goats. The first successful birth of a foal from a frozen embryo was not achieved until 1982, with only one live foal from 14 embryos (Yamamoto *et al.*, 1982). Success rates since then have been very variable with some commercial practitioners reporting success rates of up to 70% (Lascombes and Pashen, 2000; Vullers, 2004), but in controlled experimental work much lower success rates are reported, in the region of 20–50% (Skidmore *et al.*, 1990; Huhtinen *et al.*, 2000; Maclellan *et al.*, 2002a; Squires *et al.*, 2003; Duchamp *et al.*, 2006; Bruyas, 2011; Sanchez *et al.*, 2017). Poor success rates have been postulated to be due to a variation in embryo size at freezing. Most of the embryos recovered from mares are via the non-surgical technique, hence are 6–7 days old and so 500–1000 μm in diameter and at the blastocyst stage (Fig. 3.4). Experiments have shown that cryopreservation of equine embryos larger than 250 μm in diameter (early blastocysts, approximately day 5) gives relatively poor results (Skidmore *et al.*, 1990; Bruyas, 2011). The poorer success of using older embryos may be because the equine conceptus is unique in developing, at around days 4–5 of pregnancy, an acellular glycoprotein capsule (Section 3.2.2.1). It appears that this may impede the passage of cryoprotectants into the conceptus and so reduces success rates (Tharasanit *et al.*, 2005; Bruyas, 2011; Stout, 2012b). Indeed Legrand *et al.* (2002) and Maclellan *et al.* (2002a) reported that the success of freezing was related to the thickness of the capsule and that, if embryos greater than 500 μm in diameter were treated with 0.2% weight to volume trypsin for 15 min (to enzymatically destroy the capsule prior to addition of glycerol, and freezing), then 75% of the embryos (three out of four) were viable post-thaw and went on to produce pregnancies. The success rates for the transfer of equine morula and early blastocysts which do not as yet have a fully formed capsule are much better. However, recovering such young embryos (prior to day 5) from the mare via the non-surgical technique is challenging (Section 22.2.3.1) as they have not yet passed into the uterus and so need to be collected surgically. However, as discussed previously, this may in part be overcome by the use of PGE. On the other hand, older and larger 6–7-day-old blastocysts can be collected more easily non-surgically, but do not freeze well (Stout, 2012b). There is the added practical challenge that equine embryos at a specific age vary considerably in their size and in the number of cells (Colchen *et al.*, 2000). Hence, selecting embryos for freezing by age does not necessarily guarantee they are at the correct stage to freeze successfully. Apart from the peculiarities of the capsule, equine embryos develop very rapidly compared to ruminant embryos for example, so contain many more cells at a specific age. For example, at day 6.5 an equine embryo will contain up to 600 cells, whereas a ruminant embryo will only contain 100 cells. It is possible that the greater the number of cells within the embryo the less effective and the poorer the interaction between the blastocyst and the cryoprotectant, and the greater the blastocyst's sensitivity to the cryoprotectant (Colchen *et al.*, 2000; Dobrinsky, 2002; Tharasanit *et al.*, 2005; Stout, 2012b). Larger blastocysts also have larger volumes of fluid (blastocoel) which are again greater than those found in ruminants, presenting the opportunity for more ice crystal formation and, therefore, damage at freezing (Choi *et al.*, 2011; Pérez-Marín *et al.*, 2018). Finally, it has been suggested that failure of cryopreservation in older embryos may not be owing to the capsule, which is permeable to large molecules, but to the unusual change in the blastocoel from hypertonic to hypotonic when the embryo is approximately 500 μm in diameter (day 6). Penetrating cryoprotectants such as glycerol and ethylene glycol in most mammalian embryos and equine embryos < 500 μm causes initial shrinkage (within 1 min) to 40–60% of their original size, followed by expansion back to normal as cryoprotectant enters the embryo. However, in equine embryos > 500 μm, there is a slow and very minimal initial shrinkage and no subsequent expansion or recovery indicating a change in the blastocoel at 500 μm (Hochi *et al.*, 1994a, 1995; Hinrichs, 2018).

To cryopreserve embryos a cryoprotectant (Section 21.6.6.1), traditionally glycerol, is required. Other cryoprotectants (1,2 propandiol, ethylene glycol, dimethyl sulfoxide (DMSO), sucrose, galactose) have been tried with some success (Hochi *et al.*, 1994a; Ferreira *et al.*, 1997; Huhtinen *et al.*, 1997; Bruyas *et al.*, 2000; Bruyas, 2011; Pérez-Marín *et al.*, 2018). Not only does the presence of the capsule and the number of embryonic cells provide an explanation for poor freezing success but, in addition, cryoprotectants such as glycerol are known to be toxic to equine embryos, affecting their micro-ultrastructure (and particularly that of mitochondria) (Tharasanit *et al.*, 2005). There are two methods by which equine embryos can be cryopreserved: slow freezing and vitrification.

Slow freezing

Slow freezing is the traditional method used and, as with sperm (Section 21.6.6.5), embryos need to be frozen in a slow, stepwise fashion. The temperature is initially dropped down quite rapidly to –6° or –7°C and then more gradually dropped through the period of formation of ice crystals down to –33°C and to –35°C. This is followed by a rapid temperature drop by plunging into liquid nitrogen for storage at –196°C, at which temperature storage is presumed to be indefinite (Skidmore *et al.*, 1990; Lascombes and Pashan, 2000; Arav, 2014; Squires and McCue, 2016). Prior to transfer they need to be thawed out by a gradual stepwise increase in temperature, with the possible addition of a thawing extender (see Section 21.6.6.6) such as a sucrose solution to aid rehydration and help prevent excessive alterations in osmotic pressure (Hochi *et al.*, 1996; Young *et al.*, 1997). This slow freezing protocol gives equivalent success to transfer of frozen bovine embryos (Squires and McCue, 2016). However, the inaccessibility of such young embryos is a problem, and the use of PGE (Section 22.2.3.2) to allow early transit of the embryo into the uterus (although possible) is not without its challenges for commercial use, hence a more successful method of cryopreserving older and more easily accessible embryos is required.

22.2.5.4. Vitrification

More recently, vitrification (Section 21.6.6.3; Hochi *et al.*, 1994b, 1995; Young *et al.*, 1997; Oberstein *et al.*, 2001; Carnevale, 2004; Squires and McCue, 2016; Pérez-Marín *et al.*, 2018) has been tried. Vitrification is the ultra-rapid cooling of the embryo that prevents ice crystals by cooling so fast that any liquid changes to a solid, glass-like phase without ice formation (Saragusty and Arav, 2011; Stout, 2012b; Arav, 2014; Hendriks *et al.*, 2014). This bypasses any deleterious effects of ice formation and water movement into or out of the conceptus. The other advantage of vitrification is it is a very fast and easy technique, but it does require high concentrations of cryoprotectants. So the issues of cryoprotectant toxicity remain and may be even more crucial. Thus, the type of cryoprotectants and the timing of exposure to these agents is very important. Numerous cryoprotectants have been used, with varied success

(Hochi *et al.*, 1995; Elderidge-Panuska, 2005; Hudson *et al.*, 2006; Squires and McCue, 2016). However, in common with slow freezing, older and larger embryos > 300 μm in diameter do not survive vitrification well and post-thaw pregnancy rates are no better than in slow cooling (Saragusty and Arav, 2011).

The main issue still appears to be the amount, and freezing, of fluid within the conceptus. More recent work has looked at treatment of large embryos prior to vitrification. Maclellan *et al.* (2002a) and others (Hochi *et al.*, 1994b; Eldridge-Panuska *et al.*, 2005) have used enzymes such as trypsin to remove the embryonic capsule and so allow the cryopreservative to penetrate the embryo more easily, but with limited success. Alternatively, the intracellular fluid can be removed prior to vitrification. This can be done by physical penetration of the capsule by micromanipulation, piezo drill or laser, possibly along with aspiration (Choi *et al.*, 2010; Scherzer *et al.*, 2011; Diaz *et al.*, 2016). This showed some encouraging results with the larger embryos. Finally, fluid can be removed by desiccation of the embryo by developing a strong osmotic pressure gradient between the embryo and its surrounding fluid. This can be achieved, for example, by placing the embryo for a short time into a highly concentrated solution of sugars (often sucrose or galactose) which draws the water out of the embryo and so dehydrating it before it is immediately plunged into liquid nitrogen (Oberstein *et al.*, 2001; Squires and McCue, 2016). Although these techniques have had some success with larger embryos they are still less successful than when used with smaller embryos, presumably due to the protective nature of the capsule, making the conceptus less impermeable and so dehydration difficult.

22.2.6. Transfer of embryos

The transfer of embryos can, as with collection, be done either surgically or non-surgically.

22.2.6.1. Surgical embryo transfer

Surgical transfer is not popular today. As with surgical embryo collection, it initially required a general anaesthetic and ventral midline incision into the abdomen. The preferred method is now flank incision (laparotomy) in a standing, sedated mare. The mare is prepared as for surgical collection and a similar, but smaller, ventral midline or flank incision is made. Just the uterine horn/Fallopian tube are exteriorized through this incision and a small hole is made at the top of the horn/into the Fallopian tube with a blunt needle. A Pasteur pipette or equivalent, containing the embryo held between two bubbles of air, is introduced through this hole into the uterus and the embryo expelled into the lumen of the uterine horn/Fallopian tube (Allen, 1982; Squires *et al.*, 1985a).

Surgical transfer has the advantage that younger embryos of 2–4 days old may be replaced into the Fallopian tubes, as access to the Fallopian tube (as well as to the top of the uterine horns) is possible. The success rates are very variable, 50–90%, but were initially reported to be higher than those in non-surgical transfer. With experience and more widespread use the success rates of surgical and non-surgical transfers are now very similar. Pregnancy rates with cooled embryos are equivalent to fresh transfer; although, as discussed previously, success with cryopreserved embryos is still poor (Imel *et al.*, 1981; Allen, 1982; Sertich *et al.*, 1988; Carney *et al.*, 1991). In the light of newer laparoscopic and ultrasound-guided deep intrauterine and hysteroscopic transfer techniques, surgical transfer of embryos is not done commercially and rarely used in research.

22.2.6.2. Laparoscopic embryo transfer

Laparoscopic ET is successful in a number of animals and has been attempted with some success in the mare. A laparoscope, inserted in the flank of a mare sedated and held in stocks, is used to guide a long needle containing the embryo(s) through the abdominal wall and into the top of the uterine horn. Similarly, a long, flexible catheter can be passed down a wide-bore needle passed through the anterior wall of the vagina, and inserted blind into the uterine horn, which is manipulated per rectal palpation. Although success rates are reported to be good, both techniques require considerable skill and dexterity (Muller and Cunat, 1993).

22.2.6.3. Non-surgical embryo transfer

Owing to the complications of surgical and laparoscopic ET, the most popular technique currently widely used is transcervical ET, very similar to that used in cattle and in AI (Fig. 22.7; Section 21.10.1; Meira and Henry, 1991; Hartman, 2011). The mare is restrained within stocks; the perineal area is thoroughly washed; and the transfer gun or catheter with attached syringe – containing the embryo held between two bubbles of air – is passed in through the mare's cervix and into the uterine body. Once in place, the embryo and the associated fluids are expelled into the uterus by slowly depressing the plunger of the syringe (Fig. 22.7; Jasko, 2002).

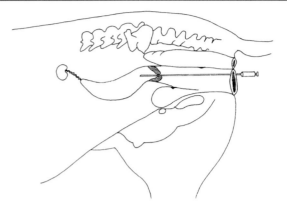

Fig. 22.7. Non-surgical transfer of embryos into a recipient mare.

Non-surgical transfer is a relatively easy and quick procedure with good pregnancy rates, although these do very much depend on the donor mare and quality of embryos transferred (Allen, 2005). Some reports suggest poorer pregnancy rates with non-surgical versus surgical transfer. This may be due to the increased risk of introducing low-grade infections into the reproductive tract (Wilsher and Allen, 2004) and also possibly to induced release of PGF2α and/or oxytocin by manual manipulation of the cervix when trying to pass through the catheter, causing early luteolysis (Kask *et al.*, 1997; Handler *et al.*, 2002), plus a localized uterine inflammatory response to the technique (Squires *et al.*, 1999). However, as the technique becomes more widespread, and the importance of hygiene and minimal insult to the cervix is appreciated, pregnancy rates have improved significantly (Hartman, 2011). In an attempt to reduce uterine infection and excessive cervical manipulation in particular, Wilsher and Allen (2004) developed a new technique for the placement of the embryo into the recipient's uterus. Mares are sedated and, following a strict hygiene regime, a duck-billed vaginal speculum is inserted into the vagina and opened to allow the cervix to be viewed clearly. A pair of elongated, smooth-ended grasping forceps is inserted and the cervical external os grasped and pulled caudally. This straightens the cervical canal, elevates the uterus within the abdomen and straightens the uterine lumen, making insertion of the catheter easier and much less traumatic on the reproductive tract. Pregnancy rates of up to 85% have been reported using this technique (Wilsher and Allen, 2004; Cuervo-Arango *et al.*, 2018c).

Conventional non-surgical transfer only allows the deposition of embryos into the uterine body or the lower part of the uterine horns and is, therefore, of limited use with embryos less than 5 days old. Ultrasound-guided deep intrauterine and hysteroscopic transfer techniques, identical to the deep intrauterine and hysteroscopic low-dose techniques used in AI (Section 21.10.2), have been advocated for younger embryos, allowing them to be placed higher up into the tract, nearer to where they would naturally be located. Placing embryos actually into the Fallopian tube, however, is only possible using surgical transfer.

The site of embryo deposition in relation to the functional CL seems to be less crucial in the mare than in the ewe and the cow. This is presumably due to the natural transuterine migration of equine embryos. The medium in which the embryos are transferred is reported to have an effect on pregnancy rates. However, reports are conflicting, and the new commercially available embryo holding media give good results (Carney *et al.*, 1991; Moussa *et al.*, 2003; Squires *et al.*, 2003).

22.3. Conclusion

Equine ET has developed considerably over the last 15 years and the use of fresh or chilled embryos to allow competition mares to breed, without interrupting their careers, is now a commercial reality and widely used. However, the inability to effectively super-ovulate mares, the poor success with cryopreservation and the continuing reluctance of some breed societies to accept progeny conceived via ET (or the limits they place on the number that can be registered each year), remain major stumbling blocks to the continued development of equine ET and realization of its full potential.

Study Questions

'Embryo transfer is the future for breeding mares'. Discuss this statement with reference to the techniques used, the types of mares most likely to benefit from the techniques and the various procedures involved.

Discuss the challenges faced when cryopreserving equine embryos and how these may be overcome. Why is success poorer than that reported when freezing bovine embryos? Detail the current and potential uses of, and the procedures involved in, equine embryo transfer.

You have valuable 10-year-old Warmblood mare that is competing at Grand Prix level dressage and is doing really well. You wish to breed this mare before she gets too old but you are reluctant to retire her from competition. Detail how you could do this without interrupting her dressage career, along with the procedures involved.

Suggested Reading

Squires, E.L., Carnevale, E.M., McCue, J.E. and Bruemmer, J.E. (2003) Embryo technologies in the horse. *Theriogenology* 59, 151–170.

Stout, T.A. (2006) Equine embryo transfer: review of developing potential. *Equine Veterinary Journal* 38(5), 467–478.

McCue, P.M. Ferris, R.A., Lindholm, A. and DeLuca, C.A. (2010) Embryo Recovery Procedures and Collection Success: Results of 492 Embryo-Flush Attempts. *Proceedings of the American Association of Equine Practionners* 56, 318–321.

Hartman, D.L. (2011) Embryo transfer. In: McKinnon, A.O., Squires, E.L., Vaala, E. and Varner, D.D. (eds) *Equine Reproduction*, 2nd edn. Wiley-Blackwell, Philadelphia, London, pp. 2871–2879.

Campbell, M.L. (2014) Embryo transfer in competition horses : managing mares and expectations, *Equine Veterinary Education* 26(6), 322–327.

McCue, P.M. and Squires, E.L. (2015) *Embryo Transfer*, Teton New Media Jackson, WY, pp 169.

Squires, E.L. and McCue, P.M. (2016) Cryopreservation of equine embryos. *Journal of Equine Veterinary Science* 41, 7–12.

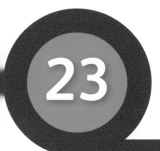

23 Advanced Reproductive Techniques

The Objectives of this Chapter are:

To detail the various advanced reproductive techniques (ART) that are available to assist reproduction in the horse.

To enable you to make an informed decision about whether ART is appropriate for any breeding scenario or requirement.

To provide you with the knowledge to enable you to have an informed discussion with an ART practitioner on the procedures available, their advantages and disadvantages, the challenges they present and the appropriateness of their use.

To enable you to appreciate both the limitations and future use of various ART within the equine industry.

23.1. Introduction

Artificial insemination (AI) and embryo transfer (ET) are commercially viable techniques in many parts of the world and, as such, are viable options for breeding horses. However, there are also many associated advanced reproductive techniques (ART) that have been developed in other species – for example human, cattle, sheep and pigs – to assist reproduction. Although the horse in many ways lags behind the sophistication of ART in these species, many of the techniques are now being attempted in horses, and may present opportunities for future breeding practice (Squires, 2019).

23.2. *In Vitro* Fertilization

In vitro fertilization (IVF) is the fertilization of a collected oocyte by a sperm within the laboratory rather than within the mare's tract. Oocytes are collected by aspiration from: pre-ovulatory follicles in mares in oestrus (mature oocytes); immature follicles from mares in dioestrus (immature oocytes in need of *in vitro* maturation); or, occasionally, at post-mortem (both mature and immature oocytes, depending on stage of oestrus at death) (Sections 23.3 and 23.4). Sperm is collected as per AI at any time (Chapter 21). Once fertilization and initial development has taken place the embryo is placed into the uterus of a recipient mare as described for ET (Section 22.2.6). The technique is used quite commonly in humans but is rarely practised in horses, largely because of poor success rates, and to date only two foals have been born from IVF (Palmer *et al.*, 1991; Bezard, 1992). The poor success rates appear to be due to the failure of stallion sperm to capacitate and/or an inability of stallion sperm to penetrate the cumulus oophorous cells surrounding the ovum *in vitro* (Leemans *et al.*, 2019; Moros-Nicolás *et al.*, 2019). If IVF does become successful it would be of advantage to subfertile mares that have had problems in producing viable embryos for conventional ET, or in the case of stallions with poor semen quality or quantity.

23.2.1. *In vitro* sperm capacitation

Capacitation of sperm is a prerequisite for fertilization (Section 3.2.1). The two foals reported some 30 years ago were obtained using mature ova and sperm pre-treated with calcium (Ca) ionophore as a capacitation agent. The results, however, have not been repeatable and, despite the successful use of a range of other potential capacitation agents (such as caffeine, heparin, procaine, pre-ovulatory fluid and progesterone) to produce 8–16-cell embryos (Leemans *et al.*, 2015, 2016b, 2019), their subsequent survival is very poor and no live foals have been born (Alm *et al.*, 2001; McPartlin *et al.*, 2009; Mugnier *et al.*, 2009; Lange-Consiglio *et al.*, 2016; Moros-Nicolás *et al.*, 2019). After such capacitation, sperm penetration of the oocyte can then be facilitated by exposing the ovum cumulous oophorous and zona pellucida to acid but, again, success is very poor beyond the 8–16-cell stage (Li *et al.*, 1995). Work by Sessions-Bresnahan *et al.* (2014) suggests that problems with IVF do not lie solely with the sperm.

23.3. Oocyte Collection

Oocytes are essential for many ART. In addition to IVF these include intra-cytoplasmic sperm injection (ICSI), gamete intra-Fallopian tube transfer (GIFT), oocyte transfer and cloning. Oocyte collection was initially from slaughterhouse material. Ovaries were collected and returned to the laboratory, where the follicles were aspirated using a needle or catheter and syringe, and the fluid was then filtered to isolate the oocyte(s) (Carnevale, 2011a). Additional scraping of the internal follicle wall was also advocated by some (Carnevale *et al.*, 2004; Ribeiro *et al.*, 2008; Hinrichs, 2011b). This is not commonly practised today as a commercial procedure, but is occasionally required if a valuable mare dies or has to be euthanized suddenly (Dell'Aquila *et al.*, 2000; Hinrichs *et al.*, 2012). Alternatively, and more commonly, oocytes are aspirated from follicles in the ovary of the live mare either at oestrus, in which case the follicles will be pre-ovulatory follicles (> 30 mm in diameter), and so the oocyte will have matured *in vivo* before collection and can – in theory – be fertilized immediately (Carnevale and Ginther, 1995). These are the oocytes that have been used to produce the few successful IVF foals. Alternatively, oocytes can be collected from smaller follicles (varying sizes up to 25 mm in diameter) during dioestrus and then matured *in vitro*. This allows many more oocytes to be gained per collection but they require maturation before use, which currently presents a challenge (Hinrichs *et al.*, 2002; Carnevale, 2011a; Hinrichs, 2018). The timing of the collection of pre-ovulatory oocytes is often achieved by administration of ovulation-inducing agents such as human chorionic gonadotrophin (hCG) or gonadotrophin-releasing hormone (GnRH), ensuring pre-ovulatory follicles are aspirated, and so mature oocytes are collected (Riera *et al.*, 2016; Hinrichs, 2018). Whatever the size of the follicle, pre-ovulatory or immature, aspiration is relatively standard and involves transvaginal, ultrasound-guided follicle aspiration plus possible flushing. A long needle and catheter is passed through the anterior vaginal wall and guided via ultrasound to the follicle to be aspirated. Once the follicle has been located it is punctured with the needle, the catheter is then pushed into the follicle, and the fluid and (it is hoped) the oocyte is withdrawn (Hinrichs, 2010, 2018). Dislodging the attachment of the oocyte to the cumulus oophorus upon which it sits can be challenging, and one advantage of pre-ovulatory follicle collection is the natural loosening of this attachment due to exposure to increasing gonadotrophin (follicle-stimulating hormone (FSH) and luteinizing hormone (LH)) levels (Bruck *et al.*, 1999; Hinrichs, 2018). Some workers, therefore, flush the follicle with a small amount of fluid (50–100 ml) after aspiration in an attempt to improve recovery rates, especially in immature oocyte collection. A major disadvantage of collecting from pre-ovulatory follicles is the failure of super-ovulation in the mare (Section 22.2.2.1) and so the availability of only one or, occasionally, two oocytes at collection; however, those collected will be mature and so bypass the challenge of *in vitro* maturation (Section 23.4). On the other hand, the advantage of collecting immature oocytes is their greater availability owing to the presence of numerous developing follicles, as opposed to a single or occasionally two pre-ovulatory follicles. As any follicles over 2–5 mm are normally aspirated it also means that, during the non-breeding season, follicles can also be aspirated with equally good success rates (Galli *et al.*, 2014; Choi *et al.*, 2016; Hinrichs, 2018). The varying stages of development of oocytes at collection give more flexibility in when they need to be used, allowing storage overnight, etc., prior to use. The two main disadvantages are the more difficult procedure to aspirate very small follicles effectively and, once aspirated, the challenge of maturing the oocytes *in vitro* (Section 23.4). Repeated aspirations and/or flushings are not reported to be detrimental to future oocyte collection or to any subsequent pregnancy (Mari *et al.*, 2005). Once collected, oocytes are kept in Dulbecco PBS or M199 with 10% fetal bovine serum or in one of the commercial preparations such as EmCare Complete Ultra® (ICPbio, Auckland, New Zealand). Oocytes are usually 150–170 µm in diameter, and invariably have a clump of cumulous oophorus cells attached to them, making them easier to identify. Once collected, immature oocytes can be kept at room temperature (22°C) for up to 24 h before processing; mature oocytes, however, must be fertilized as soon as possible (Hinrichs *et al.*, 2000a; Carnevale, 2011a; Hinrichs, 2018).

23.4. Oocyte Maturation

Oocyte maturation, along with sperm capacitation, is a prerequisite for IVF and other ART (Hinrichs, 2011b). Unfortunately, *in vitro* maturation of oocytes collected from small, immature follicles is problematic in the mare. *In vitro* oocyte maturation, both nuclear (resumption of meiosis) and cytoplasmic (changes in preparation for embryo development), does occur in some aspirated oocytes stored for 24–30 h, especially those that are from follicles > 20 mm in diameter. Hence oocytes are incubated to either complete maturation (mature oocytes from pre-ovulatory follicles) or to initiate and complete maturation (immature oocytes from immature follicles). A variety of success has been reported in *in vitro* oocyte maturation by culturing oocytes in a range of media including TCM-199; follicular fluid from pre-ovulatory follicles; M199 with 10% PBS or 10% fetal bovine serum and FSH; blood serum from an oestrous mare; ionomycin; ethanol; thimerosal; inositol; oviductal epithelial cells; and fetal fibroblast cells (Dell'Aquila *et al.*, 1997a,b; Li *et al.*, 2000, 2001; Choi *et al.*, 2002; Galli *et al.*, 2007, 2014; Hinrichs, 2011b). Once matured the oocytes are fertilized by IVF or ICSI (Section 23.8) and the resulting embryos are developed *in vitro* to the blastocyst stage, at which time they can be placed into the uterus of a recipient mare as per ET or used for GIFT; Section 23.10) oocyte transfer, cloning, etc. Despite all the work, conventional IVF in horses is largely unsuccessful. ICSI in particular, plus other ART, have been developed in an attempt to overcome some of the problems of IVF, especially those associated with sperm capacitation.

23.5. Embryo Splitting

Embryo splitting involves the bisection of an undifferentiated embryo (young morula; Section 3.2.2) into a number of potential new individuals that can then be transferred into a number of recipient mares. Commercially, such a procedure could compensate for the significant difficulties encountered in super-ovulating mares, allowing an increase in the number of embryos per mare (Skidmore *et al.*, 1989). The first two sets of identical twin foals (one set of colts, the other fillies) resulting from embryo splitting were reported by Allen and Pashan (1984). The original embryo was collected surgically on days 2–3 post-fertilization and pairs of blastomeres from an 8-cell morula were separated. Each pair was injected into empty pig zona pellucida,

embedded in agar and transferred to sheep oviducts for 3–4 days until the blastocyst stage, when each conceptus was then transferred to a recipient mare. More recently, success has been achieved by collecting morula (6–6.5 days post-fertilization) before capsule formation and bisecting them into two demi-embryos. Each embryo was then transferred into a recipient mare. Work with embryo bisection and the formation of identical twins which are subsequently transferred into different uteri has underlined the importance played by uterine and placental competence and size in fetal development. Despite identical genotype, transfer of one embryo into a mare with a smaller or compromised uterus limits placental size and hence foal birth weight, which may not necessarily be compensated for by accelerated growth before mature size is achieved (Allen, 2005). Although quite a lot of work was done on bisecting horse embryos in the 1980s and 1990s, success rates have not been good enough for it to be widely available commercially. However, several of the techniques developed when bisecting embryos are now applied to embryo biopsy, and allow for preimplantation genetic analysis.

23.6. Embryo Biopsy

Embryos collected from live mares, as well as embryos produced *in vitro* can be biopsied for genetic analysis. Biopsy removes a small number of trophoblast cells and can be performed by micromanipulation or by using a microblade. This can be done with no detrimental effect on embryo survival, providing (in the case of microblade) that embryos are young (< 300 μm) (Choi *et al.*, 2010; Troedsson *et al.*, 2010; Herrera *et al.*, 2014; Guignot *et al.*, 2015). Subsequent genetic analysis of the trophoblast cells allows embryos to be selected on the basis of gender, and enables selection against those with genetic abnormalities or genetic-related mutations. Expanded blastocysts can also be used, but the capsule makes the process more difficult. Simplification of the technique by aspirating blastocoel fluid for analysis, as opposed to trophoblast cells, has been attempted but with limited success (Herrera *et al.*, 2015).

23.7. Embryonic Stem Cells

Related to embryo biopsy is the potential use of embryonic stem cells (ESC) for genetic engineering/introducing advantageous genes. ESC are derived from undifferentiated morula cells, so are collected from the early, pre-blastocyst embryo. As they are undifferentiated they still have the potential to develop into either of the three germ cell layers and so into any body part (Section 3.2.2). In other animals, including farm livestock, these ESC have provided a valuable genetic engineering tool to improve selection for disease resistance, including the introduction of resistant traits and for the study of functional genomics. They may also be used as systems for xenotransplantation, and for the development of new pharmaceutical drugs and pharmacokinetic studies, as well as for regenerative studies (Blomberg and Telugu, 2012). Although not currently practised in horses, ESC may provide future opportunities.

23.8. Intra-cytoplasmic Sperm Injection

ICSI involves the injection of a single sperm into the cytoplasm of a collected oocyte, which is usually at metaphase II stage, in order to achieve fertilization (Choi and Hinrichs, 2011; Salamone et al., 2017). It therefore bypasses the need for sperm capacitation, acrosome reaction, binding to and then penetration of the zona pellucida and sperm–ovum fusion, so overcoming the challenges seen with equine IVF. For this reason it can be used with immotile sperm from post-mortem epididymis or testis cells, freeze-dried sperm and even isolated sperm nuclei (Choi et al., 2006; Hinrichs et al., 2010; Choi and Hinrichs, 2011). ICSI also avoids the need for the mare to be mated or inseminated, so assisting mares with acute persistent post-coital endometritis. Following fertilization the conceptus is allowed to develop in vitro for 4–6 days to the morula or early blastocyst stage before transfer into a recipient mare by standard ET technique. ICSI has also been successfully used to produce foals from in vitro-matured oocytes (Cochran et al., 1998; McKinnon et al., 2000). In vitro maturation still remains a challenge (Section 23.4). The culture of ova after ICSI is also important and some of the best results were initially obtained by placing the embryos into the oviducts of mares, rabbits or sheep (Galli et al., 2002; Lazzari et al., 2002; Choi et al., 2004). The first ICSI foal was born in 1996 (Squires et al., 1996) and until 2002 results remained unimpressive with blastocyst formation rates of less than 15%. In 2001 the development of the Piezo drill, which produced minute vibrations of the injection pipette, enhanced penetration of the oocyte and so reduced the damage previously caused by conventional injection pipettes. The media used both prior to and post-ICSI have been known for a long time to have a significant effect on survival, and numerous types have been used (see Section 23.4; Cuervo-Arango et al., 2019). However, the most successful now appears to be DMEM/F-12 plus 10% fetal calf serum which, when combined with the Piezo drill method, results in significantly increased blastocyst formation rates of 25–42%, with post-transfer pregnancy rates of 80–85% (Choi et al., 2002; Galli et al., 2007; Garcia-Rosello et al., 2009; Hinrichs, 2010, 2018). Further new techniques, including laser-assisted ICSI have been used with some success (Smits et al., 2012). ICSI has been used with a variety of sources of sperm and with both in vitro- and in vivo-matured oocytes, but results can be poor and inconsistent (McKinnon et al., 2000; Choi et al., 2006; Alonso et al., 2007). There has been much commercial interest in ICSI, particularly as a means of breeding stallions with poor semen quality, and with sex-sorted sperm (Colleoni et al., 2007). However, before the process can reach its full commercial potential the challenge of oocyte maturation has to be overcome (Galli et al., 2014). No detrimental effect on foal, weight and height or on placental development is reported with the use of ICSI, or indeed with several other ART (Valenzuela et al., 2017; Hinrichs, 2018).

ICISI can also be used to genetically manipulate embryos by the introduction of beneficial nuclear material. DNA is introduced into the sperm, which is then used to fertilize the oocyte by ICSI, so introducing that DNA to the embryo. The process is called ICSI-mediated gene transfer (ICSI-MGT) (Zaniboni et al., 2013).

23.9. Oocyte Transfer

Oocyte transfer is the collection of oocytes, rather than an embryo, from a donor mare (Carnevale 2011b; Hinrichs, 2018). As with ICSI, oocytes at metaphase II are required and – as discussed in Sections 23.3 and 23.4 – oocytes are either matured in vivo (i.e. collected from pre-ovulatory follicles) or matured in vitro. Once maturation has been achieved the oocyte is transferred on to the fimbrae of the infundibulum or 2–3 cm into the Fallopian tube of the recipient mare, usually by sedated, standing, flank laparotomy to exteriorize and access the Fallopian tube (Carnevale et al., 2004; Riera et al., 2016). The recipient mare needs to be synchronized with the donor mare, and so in oestrus at the same time, allowing her to be mated either naturally or by AI between 12 h before and 2 h after oocyte transfer (Scott et al., 2001). Prior to mating the recipient mare has her own pre-ovulatory follicle aspirated to prevent her becoming pregnant with her own foal. Preventing the recipient mare conceiving to her own ovum is the biggest challenge. Use of cyclic mares and aspiration of the dominant follicle is often successful (Coutinho da Silva *et al.*, 2002b), but asynchronous multiple ovulation in mares is not uncommon (Davies Morel and Newcombe, 2008; Davies Morel *et al.*, 2015), and so late development and ovulation of a second follicle may occur. Hormonally manipulated dioestrous mares have been used in an attempt to overcome this, as dioestrous follicles are smaller and so less likely to ovulate (Hinrichs *et al.*, 2000a). Non-cyclic mares, either in the non-breeding season or hormonally induced in the breeding season, have also successfully been used (Carnevale, 2011b). Despite this, the potential for fertilization of the recipient's own ova remains a major drawback, so monitoring for multiple pregnancies along with genetic identification of offspring must be conducted. Oocyte transfer is of particular use in mares that are also good candidates for IVF, and this is where the likely commercial application will lie. These are frequently older donor mares and those that have problems in ovulating, or have incompetent Fallopian tubes or uterus, often owing to persistent infections (Hinrichs *et al.*, 2000a; Carnevale *et al.*, 2001, 2005a). The advantage of oocyte transfer over IVF is that fertilization takes place *in vivo* and so the problems associated with sperm capacitation are avoided. The first successful oocyte transfer was reported by McKinnon *et al.* (1988b) but recently has been used more commercially with pre-ovulatory oocytes; that is, those collected from mares 24–36 h after treatment with hCG in the presence of a > 35 mm follicle (Carnevale *et al.*, 2000a,b; Hinrichs *et al.*, 2000a). Success rates are much higher at 60–80% with oocytes collected from pre-ovulatory follicles (i.e. *in vivo*-maturated oocytes from young fertile donors); however, commercial application is likely to use oocytes from subfertile, older mares and so lower conception rates can be expected (Carnevale *et al.*, 2000a, 2001, 2005a; Galli *et al.*, 2014, 2016; Riera *et al.*, 2016).

23.10. Gamete Intra-Fallopian Tube Transfer

Oocyte transfer relies upon a natural covering or AI for fertilization. Occasionally sperm numbers or the semen quality is so low, due to stallion subfertility or after semen sexing, that the chances of natural conception are very poor. In this case GIFT is an option as it involves placing a low number of sperm (between $5 \times 10^{4-5} \times 10^{5}$) plus the oocyte (usually at metaphase II

stage) into the Fallopian tube or onto the fimbrae of the infundibulum of the Fallopian tube of a recipient mare (McCue *et al.*, 2000; Carnevale, 2004; Coutinho da Silva *et al.*, 2004; Coutinho da Silva, 2011). The same issues with *in vivo* and *in vitro* maturation of oocytes exist and so the best results have been obtained with oocytes collected from pre-ovulatory follicles. Similarly, the challenge remains of ensuring the conceptus is the result of the transfer and not from the mare's own ovum. However, one advantage of GIFT over IVF is that fertilization takes place within the most suitable environment (i.e. the Fallopian tube), and the need to induce sperm capacitation evident in IVF is overcome, as sperm naturally undergo capacitation in the Fallopian tube (Carnevale *et al.*, 2000a; Carnevale, 2011b; Leemans *et al.*, 2016). The first successful GIFT foal was reported by Carnevale *et al.* (1999) using *in vivo*-matured oocytes and fresh sperm. Success rates up to 80% are currently reported (Hinrichs *et al.*, 2000b, 2002; Scott *et al.*, 2001); however, success with frozen semen is poor, as low as 8% (Coutinho da Silva *et al.*, 2002a; Squires *et al.*, 2003). Overcoming relatively poor success rates with chilled and frozen semen is essential before widespread commercial use is viable.

A similar process to both GIFT and IVF is zygote intra-Fallopian tube transfer (ZIFT), in which fertilization takes place *in vitro* as per IVF but the fertilized ova (now a zygote) is transferred immediately to the Fallopian tube of the recipient mare, instead of allowing initial development to take place *in vitro*. This has not been investigated to date in the mare, largely due to the challenges of IVF in the horse, but is successful in other mammals and so may warrant further consideration.

23.11. Oocyte Freezing

Much work has been carried out into the freezing of stallion sperm, with some success (Section 21.6.6). Embryo freezing (Section 22.2.5.3) has also been investigated, again with some success when freezing young embryos. However, success is variable and so a feasible alternative may be to freeze oocytes; these could then be available for fertilization by IVF, GIFT, ZIFT or ICSI at a later date (Maclellan, 2011). This would be particularly useful for valuable mares that die or have to be euthanized unexpectedly. Some success in oocyte freezing has been reported in other livestock, but work in horses is limited and the results poor (Maclellan *et al.*, 2002b, 2010). The same challenges as those discussed for embryo freezing (Section 22.2.5.3) apply to oocyte cryopreservation. In particular the challenges of identifying the best cryoprotectant, and balancing the concentration of cryoprotectant with potential cellular damage and rate of cooling, remain. Several cryoprotectants have been used and currently ethylene glycol appears the best for cryopreservation (Hochi *et al.*, 1994a). Vitrification (Section 21.6.6.3) may require combinations such as ethylene glycol, propylene glycol and dimethyl sulfoxide (DMSO), possibly plus sugars such as sucrose or trehalose (Maclellan *et al.*, 2001). Both cryopreservation and vitrification have been attempted, with some success (Hochi *et al.*, 1994a,b; Hurtt *et al.*, 2000; Arav *et al.*, 2002; Maclellan *et al.*, 2010; Canesin *et al.*, 2017, 2018; Ortiz-Escribano *et al.*, 2018). From the limited work reported to date it appears that cryopreservation or vitrification of mature oocytes and immature oocytes is equally successful, but pregnancy rates with both are still poor (20–40%) (Maclellan *et al.*, 2002b; Squires *et al.*, 2003; Tharasanit *et al.*, 2006, De Leon *et al.*, 2012).

23.12. Cloning (Nuclear Transfer)

Since the successful cloning (nuclear transfer) and birth of Dolly the sheep, cloning has become a hot topic in reproductive technology work. The horse has not escaped, and in 2002 Woods reported the first successfully cloned equid, a mule (Woods *et al.*, 2002, 2003). This was followed shortly by the first cloned horse (Galli *et al.*, 2003). Cloning or somatic cell nuclear transfer involves the collection of donor metaphase II oocytes (Section 23.3) from the recipient mare or produced *in vitro*. These are then enucleated (the nucleus removed so as to remove their own genetic material) and the nuclear material from the animal to be cloned is then introduced into these enucleated cells by direct injection of the donor cell nucleus into the recipient's oocyte cytoplasm. The cells used are often somatic cells, but skin cells, fetal cells, cumulus cells, fetal and adult fibroblast cells, and bone marrow cells have also been used (Galli *et al.*, 2003; Vanderwall *et al.*, 2004; Hinrichs, 2010, 2011a; Olivera *et al.*, 2016, 2018). Tissue frozen with and without the use of cryoprotectant has also been successful (Hoshino and Saeki, 2010). Once nuclear material transfer has occurred, the oocyte – plus new nuclear material (karyoplast) – needs to be activated to simulate fertilization, and the production of an undifferentiated embryonic stem cell. This is normally achieved by triggering the Ca oscillations mimicking those that occur at natural fertilization (Section 3.2.1). This can be done by inducing Ca to enter the oocyte from the surrounding medium by electrical stimulation;

Ca ionophore treatment; or by injecting sperm cytoplasm, which contains the sperm factors responsible for naturally inducing the Ca oscillations seen at fertilization (Bedford *et al.*, 2004). This increase in cytoplasmic Ca (and subsequent Ca oscillations) mimics natural fertilization, causing the oocyte to complete meiosis and undergo cell division to form a zygote (Wen *et al.*, 2014). The oocyte then multiplies up like a conventional fertilized oocyte to form an embryo of identical genotype to the animal from which the original diploid cell was taken (Fig. 23.1).

The resulting embryo is then placed immediately into the lumen of the Fallopian tube or cultured to blastocyst stage and placed into the uterus of the recipient mare. As mentioned previously the first cloned equine was a mule; in fact three clones were created from cultured fetal cells (Woods *et al.*, 2002, 2003). This was followed very shortly by the first cloned horse (Galli *et al.*, 2003) which was a clone of an adult skin cell taken from the mare into which the clone was subsequently placed. This means that the mare was both the donor of the cell and the recipient of the resulting clone and so, in essence, gave birth to itself. In 2006 the commercial company ViaGen was developed and started to provide cloning commercially. Since then cloning has become commercially available, although at a cost, with numerous cloned foals reported in both the scientific and popular press (Olivera *et al.*, 2016; Hinrichs, 2018). In 2012 Hinrichs estimated that there were 100–200 cloned horses worldwide (Hinrichs, 2012); it has also been suggested that 20 viable clones were born in 2000–2014 in South America (Herrera, 2015) and 2–5 cloned foals per year in Europe (Reis, 2015). Gambini and Maserati (2017) reported 370 clones worldwide. The technique has gained particular popularity in Argentina for the production of polo horses. In 2016 the renowned polo player Adolfo Cambiaso won the Palermo Open polo match, riding six clones of one of his best mares. In the USA, Australia, New Zealand and Europe production is largely for performance sports horses, with the reproduction of geldings having the greatest potential. The majority of top performance horses are geldings and so their superior genetic material is largely lost to subsequent generations; however, if entire (stallion) clones of the gelding can be produced they can then breed 'on behalf of' the original gelding. Most recently, cloned horses have reached sexual maturity and have bred successfully, making this aim of breeding geldings a reality. Cloning is also used to preserve the genetics of rare, aged or deceased horses.

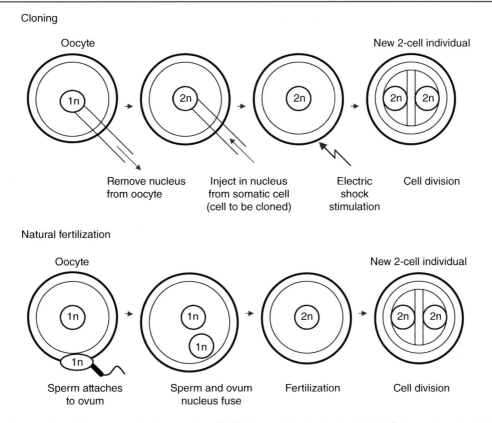

Fig. 23.1. A comparison of the early events in conventional fertilization and cloning. 1n, haploid (half the genetic material; 2n diploid (full complement of genetic material).

Despite this potential use and increasing commercial availability, the success rates of cloning are not high, 20–30% of cloned blastocysts actually resulting in a live foal (Hinrichs *et al.*, 2007; Choi *et al.*, 2009; Hinrichs, 2011a; Campbell, 2016). However, many cloned oocytes do not make it to blastocyst stage to enable transfer. Johnson *et al.* (2010) reported that over a 4-year period (2004–2008) 81% of cloned oocytes cleaved (began cell division), but of those only 5% developed into blastocysts. After transfer to recipient mares 51% of these blastocysts resulted in pregnancy at days 11–16, and 45% of these resulted in a live foal, giving an overall live foal rate per oocyte starting the cloning process of 0.95%. Olivera *et al.* (2018) reported similar poor success rates (0.5%) using nearly 8000 cloned oocytes, although more than one blastocyst was transferred into the recipient mare on many occasions. Despite the inevitable improvements in cloning techniques success rates have not improved that much. Cloning may also generate ethical concerns,

which need to be considered, as well as concerns over the health and longevity of clones. Little is reported on the health issues of equine clones but Hinrichs (2010, 2011a) and Campbell (2016) reported that many equine clones (around 50%) are lost during pregnancy; of those that are born most survive but have an increased incidence of contracted or crooked front legs, large umbilical remnants and varying degrees of neonatal maladjustment, although all of these respond successfully to treatment (Johnson *et al.*, 2008, 2010). There is also the concern as to whether clones will age prematurely. As yet there is no definitive evidence to support or refute this in horses (Campbell, 2016). Finally, there is the question of how similar the clone will be to the original animal. There are three aspects to this: epigenetic factors, environmental influence and mitochondrial DNA. Epigenetic factors (random changes to DNA that occur during development) may result in subtle changes in proteins sequenced and relative amounts produced, which are then evident in subtle phenotypical changes in the clone. Mitochondrial DNA is a very minor portion of the cellular DNA; however, mitochondrial DNA will be present within the enucleated oocyte and so becomes the mitochondrial DNA of the clone, and so different from the mitochondrial DNA of the original animal. It is unknown whether this will have any significant effect on the phenotype of the clone. It is interesting to note, however, that the mitochondrial DNA of female clones will be passed to subsequent generations through natural breeding, and so will remain different from the original female animal cloned. In the case of stallions the mitochondrial DNA, although present in sperm, is eliminated at fertilization and so a clone of a male (such as a gelding) will produce offspring genetically identical to that which the original male would have produced. Finally, environmental factors will have an effect, as they do in all animals, and will range from the pre-partum uterine environment to post-partum exposure to factors such as disease, feeding, environmental conditions and training. Cloning allows a near-genetically identical individual to be produced, but the way in which (and the extent to which) that genetic potential is realized is affected by environment.

Despite the challenges to cloning, and the ethical concerns, its acceptance within the industry continues to increase. Most international studbooks will register clones, including the majority of Warmblood stud books; and the World Breeding Federation for Sport Horses, the Fédération Équestre Internationale (FEI), will also allow clones and their offspring to compete. Some stud books do not allow the registration of clones, the most notable being the Thoroughbreds and the American Quarter Horse Association. However, EU legislation awaiting approval proposes banning the use of cloning in farm livestock, which will include equids (Campbell, 2016).

There is no doubt that cloning is possible, is becoming commercially available and is accepted by some breed societies; however, along with this and other existing ART comes an ethical responsibility that may govern the extent of their use.

Conclusion

ART in horses have a significant potential for development, both in their success and use. However this is not without its challenges, including concern over the ethics of the use of some ART and the continuing reluctance of some breed societies, most notably the Thoroughbred, to accept for registration progeny conceived by

any form of ART. The expansion of ART within the equine industry is dependent not only on breed society acceptance but also on the value of horses; the performance of foals; the cost of the procedures; refinement of techniques; and the attitude of the equine industry to their application. However, even within these constraints, ART in horses are valuable experimental tools and present exciting opportunities for horse breeding in the future.

Study Questions

'ART in the equine are the way forward for stud management'. Discuss this statement with reference to the ART techniques available and their current and potential use.

Discuss the ethical concerns related to the use of ART in horses and how these may be addressed.

You are the owner of a valuable gelding competing at the elite level of dressage and you wish to use his genetics in future generations. Discuss the options available to you to achieve this, and the techniques involved, plus the challenges these techniques may present to achieving your goal.

You are the owner of an elite but aged mare that has habitually suffered from endometritis and so is unable to conceive naturally or carry a foal to term. Discuss how ART may be used to produce a foal from this mare.

Suggested Reading

Hinrichs, K. (2010) Application of assisted reproductive technologies (ART) to clinical practice. *Proceedings of the American Association of Equine Practitioners* 56, 195–206.

Hinrichs, K. (2011) Immature oocyte collection and maturation. In: McKinnon, A.O., Squires, E.L., Vaala, E. and Varner, D.D. (eds) *Equine Reproduction*, 2nd edn. Wiley-Blackwell, Philadelphia, London, pp. 2931–2935.

Hinrichs, K. (2012) Assisted reproduction techniques in the horse. *Reproduction Fertility and Development* 25, 80–93.

Hinrichs, K. (2018) Assisted reproductive techniques in mares. *Reproduction in Domestic Animals* 53, Supplement 2, 4–13.

Carnevale, E.M. (2011) Mature oocyte collection. In: McKinnon, A.O., Squires, E.L., Vaala, E. and Varner, D.D. (eds) *Equine Reproduction*, 2nd edn. Wiley-Blackwell, Philadelphia, London, pp. 2936–2940.

Carnevale, E.M. (2011) Oocyte transfer. In: McKinnon, A.O., Squires, E.L., Vaala, E. and Varner, D.D. (eds) *Equine Reproduction*, 2nd edn. Wiley-Blackwell, Philadelphia, London, pp. 294–2944.

Choi, Y.H. and Hinrichs, K. (2011) Intracytoplasmic sperm injection (ICSI) In: McKinnon, A.O., Squires, E.L., Vaala, E. and Varner, D.D. (eds) *Equine Reproduction*, 2nd edn. Wiley-Blackwell, Philadelphia, London, pp. 2948–2952.

Coutinho da Silva, M.A. (2011) Gamete Intrafallopian Transfer (GIFT) In: McKinnon, A.O., Squires, E.L., Vaala, E. and Varner, D.D. (eds) *Equine Reproduction*, 2nd edn. Wiley-Blackwell, Philadelphia, London, pp. 2945–2947.

Maclellan, L.J. (2011) Oocyte cryopreservation In: McKinnon, A.O., Squires, E.L., Vaala, E. and Varner, D.D. (eds) *Equine Reproduction*, 2nd edn. Wiley-Blackwell, Philadelphia, London, pp. 2953–2956.

Leemans, B., Gadella, B.M., Stout, T.A., De Schauwer, C., Nelis, H., Hoogewijs, M., Va Soom, A. (2016) Why doesn't conventional IVF work in the horse? The equine oviduct as a micro-environment for capacitation/fertilization. *Reproduction* 152(6), R233–R245.

Campbell, M.L.H. (2016) Is cloning horses ethical? *Equine Veterinary Education* 30(5), 268–273.

Squires, E.L. (2019) Perspectives on the development and incorporation of assisted reproduction in the equine industry. *Reproduction and Fertility* 31(12), 1753–1757.

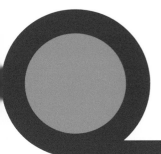

Glossary

Term	Explanation in the context of reproductive physiology and stud management
Abortion	Fetal death after day 40
Acute	Sudden, severe
Adenohypophysis	Anterior pituitary
Allometric growth	Grows at a different rate (more or less) from main body growth
Amplitude	Measure of change over a set period of time – amount of hormone release
Analogue	Similar or comparable to something else/artificially produced – many commercially produced hormones
Asphyxia	Lower circulating oxygen due to physical inhibition of breathing/inability to breathe
Barren	Lack of a pregnancy at the end of the season, but perfectly capable of producing a foal, as demonstrated in previous years
Bactericidal	Kills bacteria
Bilateral	Both sides
Caput	Head end
Cauda	Tail
Caudal	Tail end/direction
Circadian	Occurring daily, 24-h cycle
Chronic	Long term, ongoing
Circannual	Occurring annually, 12 months
Corpus	Body
Cranial	Head end/direction
Diurnal	Daytime
Dorsal	Upper side, back
Early embryo death (EED)	Embryo loss prior to day 15
Embryo mortality (EM)	Embryo loss prior to day 40, often evident between scanning on days 15 and 40
Endogenous	Made/synthesized within the organ/body – naturally produced hormones
Episodic	A regular or irregular event (similar to pulsatile) – release of a hormone
Exogenous	Made/synthesized outside the organ/body – artificial hormones/analogues used as treatments
Fertile	Able to produce a live foal
Fertilization rate	Number of ova fertilized per ovulation
Gametogenic	Produces gametes – ova or sperm

Term	Explanation in the context of reproductive physiology and stud management
Genotype	Individual's collection of genes
Gonadotrophic	Drives the development/function of the gonads (testis or ovaries)
Gravid	Previously pregnant
Hyperflexion	Overflexion (of limbs)
Hyper-	Greater than
Hypercapnic	High level of carbon dioxide
Hypermetric	Exaggerated gait
Hypertonic	More concentrated
Hypo-	Less than
Hypotonic	More diluted
Hypoxaemia	Low circulating blood oxygen levels
Hypoxia	Low oxygen supply to an organ, etc.
Infertility	A temporary inability to reproduce
Isometric growth	Grows at the same rate as/in line with main body growth
…itis	Inflammation – often, but not always, caused by infection
Lateral	Side
Live foal rate	Number of mares foaling per number of mares bred over the season
Medial	Middle
Multiparous	Given birth previously to a number of foals
Neurohypophysis	Posterior pituitary
Nocturnal	Night time
Non-gravid	Not previously pregnant
Oedema	Fluid accumulation
Parous	Been pregnant before
Phenotype	Physical characteristics/appearance
Photoperiod	Day length
Photophase	Period of light
Pregnancy rate	Number of mares pregnant on a specified day, expressed per oestrous cycle or per breeding season
Primiparous	First pregnancy
Pulsatile	A regular or irregular event (similar to episodic) – release of a hormone
Scotophase	Period of dark
Spermicidal	Kills sperm
Sterile	A permanent inability to reproduce
Steroidogenic	Produces steroid hormones
Stillborn	Fetal death after day 300
Subfertile	Inability to reproduce at full potential, may be temporary or permanent
Tonic	Background secretion of hormones, superimposed upon which are pulses of release
Tonin	Drives activity

Term	Explanation in the context of reproductive physiology and stud management
Trophic	Drives development/growth
Unilateral	One side
Uterotonin	Driver of uterine activity – PGF2α, oxytocin
Uterotrophic	Drives/facilitates uterine development/activity – oestrogen
Ventral	Lower side, abdomen

Bibliography

Aanes, W.A. (1993) Cervical lacerations. In: McKinnon, A.O. and Voss, J.L. (eds) *Equine Reproduction*. Lea and Febiger, Philadelphia, Pennsylvania, pp. 444–449.

Abbott, J.B., Mellor, D.J., Barrett, E.J., Proudman, C.J. and Love, S. (2008) Serological changes observed in horses infected with *Anoplocephata perfoilata* after treatment with praziquantel and natural re-infection *Veterinary Record* 162, 50–53.

Abernathy-Young, K.K., LeBlanc, M.M., Embertson, R.M., Pierce, S.W. and Stromberg, A.J. (2014) Survival rates of mares and foals and postoperative complications and fertility of mares after cesarean section: 95 cases (1986–2000). *Journal of the American Veterinary Medical Association* 241(7), 927–934.

AboEl-Maaty, A.M. (2011) Stress and its effect on horse's reproduction *Veterinary Science and Development* 1(3), 54–57.

Acland, H.M. (1993) Abortion in mares. In: McKinnon, A.O. and Voss, J.L. (eds) *Equine Reproduction*. Lea and Febiger, Philadelphia, Pennsylvania, pp. 554–562.

Acworth, N.R.L. (2003) The healthly neonatal foal: routine examinations and preventative medicine. *Equine Vet Journal* 15(6), 45–49.

Adams, R. (1993a) Identification of mare and foal at high risk for perinatal problems. In: McKinnon, A.O. and Voss, J.L. (eds) *Equine Reproduction*. Lea and Febiger, Philadelphia, Pennsylvania, pp. 985–996.

Adams, R. (1993b) Neonatal disease: an overview. In: McKinnon, A.O. and Voss, J.L. (eds) *Equine Reproduction*. Lea and Febiger, Philadelphia, Pennsylvania, pp. 997–1002.

Adams, W.M. and Wagner, W.C. (1970) Role of corticosteroids in parturition. *Biology of Reproduction* 3, 223–226.

Adams-Brendemuehl, C. and Pipers, F.S. (1987) Antepartum evaluations of the equine fetus. *Journal of Reproduction and Fertility, Supplement* 35, 565–573.

Aerts, J.M. and Bols, P.E. (2010a) Ovarian follicular dynamics: a review with emphasis on the bovine species. Part I: Folliculogenesis and pre-antral follicle development. *Reproduction in Domestic Animals* 45, 171–179.

Aerts, J.M. and Bols, P.E. (2010b) Ovarian follicular dynamics. A review with emphasis on the bovine species. Part II: Antral development, exogenous influence and future prospects. *Reproduction in Domestic Animals* 45, 180–187.

Ainsworth, C.G.V. and Hyland, J.H. (1991) Continuous infusion of gonadotrophin releasing hormone (GnRH) advances the onset of oestrous cycles in Thoroughbred mares on Australian stud farms. *Journal of Reproduction and Fertility, Supplement* 44, 235–240.

Aitken, J.R., Lambourne, S. and Gibb, Z. (2014) The John Hughes Memorial Lecture: Aspects of sperm physiology – oxidative stress and functionality of stallion spermatozoa. *Journal of Equine Veterinary Science* 34, 17–27.

Akcay, E., Reilas, T., Andersson, M. and Katilla, T. (2006) Effect of seminal plasma fractions on stallion sperm survival after cooled storage. *Journal of Veterinary Medicine* 53, 481–485.

Al-Essawe, E.M., Johannisson, A., Wulf, M., Aurich, C. and Morrell, J.M. (2018) Addition of seminal plasma to thawed stallion spermatozoa did not repair cryoinjuries. *Animal Reproduction Science* 196, 48–58.

Alexander, S.L. and Irvine, C.H.G. (1991) Control of onset of breeding season in the mare and its artificial regulation by progesterone treatment. *Journal of Reproduction and Fertility, Supplement* 44, 307–318.

Alexander, S.L. and Irvine, C.H.G (1998) The effect of social stress on adrenal axis activity in horses: the importance of monitoring corticosteroid-binding globulin capacity. *Journal of Endocrinology* 157, 425–432.

Alexander, S.L. and Irvine, C.H.G. (2011a) GnRH. In: McKinnon, A.O., Squires, E.L., Vaala, E. and Varner, D.D. (eds) *Equine Reproduction*, 2nd edn. Wiley-Blackwell, Philadelphia, London, pp. 1608–1618.

Alexander, S.L. and Irvine, C.H.G. (2011b) FSH and LH. In: McKinnon, A.O., Squires, E.L., Vaala, E. and Varner, D.D. (eds) *Equine Reproduction*, 2nd edn. Wiley-Blackwell, Philadelphia, London, pp. 1619–1630.

Alghamdi, A., Troedsson, M.H., Laschkewitsch, T. and Xue, J.L. (2001) Uterine secretion from mares with post-breeding endometritis alters sperm motion characteristics *in vitro*. *Theriogenology* 55(4), 1019–1028.

Alghamdi, A.S., Foster, D.N. and Troedsson, M.H.T. (2004) Equine seminal plasma reduces sperm binding to polymorphonuclear neutrophils (PMNs) and improves the fertility of fresh semen inseminated into inflamed uteri. *Reproduction* 127, 593–600.

Al-Kass, Z., Spergser, J., Aurich, C., Kuhl, J., Schmidt, K. and Morrell, J. (2018) Effect of presence or absence of antibiotics and use of modified single layer centrifugation on bacteria in pony stallion semen. *Reproduction in Domestic Animals* 54(2), 342–349.

Al-Kass, Z., Eriksson, E., Bagge, E., Wallgren, M. and Morrell, J. M. (2019) Bacteria detected in the genital tract, semen or pre-ejaculatory fluid of Swedish stallions from 2007 to 2017. *Acta Veterinaria Scandinavica* 61, 25.

Allen, W.R. (1974) Palpable development of the conceptus and fetus in Welsh pony mares. *Equine Veterinary Journal* 6, 69–73.

Allen, W.R. (1979) Evaluation of uterine tube function in pony mares. *Veterinary Record* 105, 364–366.

Allen, W.R. (1982) Embryo transfer in the horse. In: Adams, C.E. (ed.) *Mammalian Egg Transfer*. CRC Press, Boca Raton, Florida, pp. 135–154.

Allen, W.R. (1991) Investigations into the use of exogenous oxytocin for promoting uterine drainage in mares susceptible to endometritis. *Veterinary Record* 128, 593–594.

Allen, W.R. (1992) The diagnosis and handling of early gestational abnormalities in the mare. *Animal Reproduction Science* 28, 31–38.

Allen, W.R. (2001a) Fetomaternal interactions and influences during equine pregnancy. *Reproduction* 121, 513–527.

Allen, W.R. (2001b) Luteal deficiency and embryo mortality in the mare. *Reproduction in Domestic Animals* 36, 121–131.

Allen, W.R. (2005) The development and application of modern reproductive technologies to horse breeding. *Reproduction in Domestic Animals* 40, 310–329.

Allen, W.R. and Bracher, V. (1992) Videoendoscopic evaluation of the mare's uterus; III Findings in the pregnant mare. *Equine Veterinary Journal* 24, 285–291.

Allen, W.R. and Goddard, P.J. (1984) Serial investigations of early pregnancy in pony mares using a real time ultrasound scanning. *Equine Veterinary Journal* 15, 509–514.

Allen, W.R. and Pashan, R.L. (1984) Production of monozygotic (identical) horse twins by embryo micromanipulation. *Journal of Reproduction and Fertility* 71, 607–613.

Allen, W.R. and Rowson, L.E.A. (1972) Transfer of ova between horses and donkeys. In: *Proceedings of the 7th International Congress on Animal Reproduction and AI*. Munich, Germany, pp. 484–487.

Allen, W.R. and Rowson, L.E.A. (1975) Surgical and non-surgical egg transfer in horses. *Journal of Reproduction and Fertility, Supplement* 23, 525–530.

Allen, W.R. and Stewart, F. (1993) eCG. In: McKinnon, A.O. and Voss, J.R. (eds) *Equine Reproduction*. Lea and Febiger, Philadelphia, Pennsylvania, pp. 81–86.

Allen, W.R. and Stewart, F. (2001) Equine placentation. *Reproduction, Fertility and Development* 13, 623–634.

Allen, W.R. and Wilsher, S. (2009) A review of implantation and early placentation in the mare. *Placenta* 30, 1005–1015.

Allen, W.R. and Wilsher, S. (2018) Review Article: Celebrating 50 years of Equine Veterinary Journal. Half a century of equine reproduction research and application: A veterinary tour de force. *Equine Veterinary Journal* 50, 10–12.

Allen, W.R., Stewart, F., Trounson, A.O., Tischner, M. and Bielanski, W. (1976) Viability of horse embryos after storage and long distance transport in the rabbit. *Journal of Reproduction and Fertility, Supplement* 47, 387–390.

Allen, W.R., Bielanski, W., Cholewinski, G., Tischner, M. and Zwolinski, J. (1977) Blood groups in horses born after double transplantation of embryos.

Bulletin of the Acadamy of the Polish Scientific Service of Science and Biology 25(11), 757.

Allen, W.R., Kydd, J.H., Boyle, M.S. and Antczak, D.F. (1987) Extra-specific donkey-in-horse pregnancy as a model of early fetal death. *Journal of Reproduction and Fertility, Supplement* 35, 197–209.

Allen, W.R., Mathias, S., Lennard, S.N. and Greenwood, R.E.S. (1995) Serial measurement of periferal oestrogen and progesterone concentrations in oestrus mares to determine optimum mating time and diagnose ovulation. *Equine Veterinary Journal* 27(6), 460–464.

Allen, W.R., Wilsher, S., Stewart, F., Ousey, J. and Fowden, A. (2002a) The influence of maternal size and placental, fetal and postnatal growth in the horse. II Endocrinology of pregnancy. *Journal of Endocrinology* 172, 237–246.

Allen, W.R., Wilsher, S., Turnbull, C., Stewart, F., Ousey, J.C., Rossdale, P.D. and Fowden, A.L. (2002b) Influence of maternal size on placental, fetal and postnatal growth in the horse. I. Development in utero. *Reproduction* 123(3), 445–453.

Allen, W.R., Wilsher, S., Tiplady, C. and Butterfield, R.M. (2004) The influence of maternal size on pre-and postnatal growth in the horse: III Postnatal growth. *Reproduction* 127(1), 67–77.

Allen, W.R., Wilsher, S., Morris, L., Crowhurst, J.S., Hillyer, M.H. and Neal, H.N. (2006) Laparoscopic application of PGE2 to re-establish oviducal patency and fertility in infertile mares: a preliminary study. *Equine Veterinary Journal* 38(5), 454–459.

Allen, W.R., Gower, S. and Wilsher, S. (2007a) Imunohistochemical localization of vascular endothelial growth factor (VEGF) and its two receptors (Flt-1 and KDR) in the endometrium and placenta of the mare during the oestrous cycle and pregnancy. *Reproduction in Domestic Animals* 42, 516–526.

Allen, W.R., Bowen, L., Wright, M. and Wilsher, S. (2007b) Reproductive efficiency of Flat race and National Hunt Thoroughbred mares and stallions in England. *Equine Veterinary Journal* 39, 438–445.

Allen, W.R., Gower, S. and Wilsher, S. (2011) Fetal membrane differentiation, implantation and early placentation. In: McKinnon, A.O., Squires, E.L., Vaala, E. and Varner, D.D. (eds) *Equine Reproduction*, 2nd edn. Wiley-Blackwell, Philadelphia, London, pp. 2187–2199.

Alm, C.C., Sullivan, J.J. and First, N.L. (1974) Induction of premature parturition by parenteral administration of dexamethasone in the mare. *Journal of the American Veterinary Medical Association* 165, 721–722.

Alm, C.C., Sullivan, J.J. and First, N.L. (1975) The effect of corticosteroid (Dexamethasone) progesterone, estrogen and prostaglandin F2α on gestation length in normal and ovariectomised mares. *Journal of Reproduction and Fertility, Supplement* 23, 637–640.

Alm, H., Torner, H., Blottner, S., Nurnberg, G. and Kanitz, W. (2001) Effect of sperm cryopreservation and treatment with calcium ionophore or heparin on *in vitro* fertilisation of horse oocytes. *Theriogenology* 58, 817–829.

Almeida, J., Conley, A.J. and Ball, B.A. (2013) Expression of anti-Müllerian hormone, CDKN1 B, connexin 43, androgen receptor and steroidogenic enzymes in the equine cryp torchid testis. *Equine Veterinary Journal* 45(5), 538–545.

Alonso, A., Miragaya, M., Losinno, L. and Herrera, C. (2007) Intracytoplasmic sperm injection of equine oocytes using air-dried sperm or sperm stored in a high osmolarity medium. *Reproduction, Fertility and Development* 19, 301.

Althouse, G.C. and Hopkins, S.M. (1995) Assessment of boar sperm viability using a combination of two flurophores. *Theriogenology* 43, 595–603.

Alvarenga, M., McCue, P., Squires, E. and Neves Neto, J. (2000) Improvement of ovarian superstimulatory response and embryo production in mares treated with equine pituitary extract. In: Katila, T., Wade, J.F. (eds) *Havemeyer Foundation Monograph Series No. 3*. R. and W. Publications Ltd, Newmarket, pp. 79–80.

Alvarenga, M.A. and Leao, K.M. (2002) Hysteroscopic insemination of mares with low number of frozen-thawed spermatozoa selected by Percoll gradient. *Theriogenology* 58, 651.

Alvarenga, M.A., McCue, P.M., Bruemmer, J., Neves Neto, J.R. and Squires, E.L. (2001) Ovarian superstimulatory response and embryo production in mares treated with equine pituitary extract twice daily. *Theriogenology* 56, 879–887.

Alvarenga, M.A., Papa, F.O., Landim-Alvarenga, F.C. and Medeiros, A.S.L. (2005) Amides as cryoprotectant for freezing stallion semen. A review. *Animal Reproduction Science* 89, 105–113.

Álvarez, C., Luño, V., González, N., Guerra, P. and Gil, L. (2019) Effect of mare colostrum in extenders for freezing stallion semen. *Journal of Equine Veterinary Science* 77, 23–27.

Amann, R.P. (1981a) A review of the anatomy and physiology of the stallion. *Equine Veterinary Science* 1(3), 83–105.

Amann, R.P. (1981b) Spermatogenesis in the stallion, a review. *Equine Veterinary Science* 1(4), 131–139.

Amann, R.P. (1984) Effects of extender, storage temperature and centrifugation on stallion spermatozoal motility and fertility. In: *Proceedings of the 10th International Congress on Animal Reproduction and Artificial Insemination*. Paper No. 186. Urbana, Illinois.

Amann, R.P. (1989) Treatment of sperm to predetermine sex. *Theriogenology* 31, 49–60.

Amann, R.P. (1993a) Functional anatomy of the adult male. In: McKinnon, A.O. and Voss, J.L. (eds) *Equine Reproduction*. Lea and Febiger, Philadelphia, Pennsylvania, pp. 645–657.

Amann, R.P. (1993b) Physiology and endocrinology. In: McKinnon, A.O. and Voss, J.L. (eds) *Equine Reproduction*. Lea and Febiger, Philadelphia, Pennsylvania, pp. 658–685.

Amann, R.P. (2011a) Functional anatomy of the adult male. In: McKinnon, A.O., Squires, E.L., Vaala, E. and Varner, D.D. (eds) *Equine Reproduction*, 2nd edn. Wiley-Blackwell, Philadelphia, London, pp. 867–880.

Amann, R.P. (2011b) Physiology and endocrinology. In: McKinnon, A.O., Squires, E.L., Vaala, E. and Varner, D.D. (eds) *Equine Reproduction*, 2nd edn. Wiley-Blackwell, Philadelphia, London, pp. 881–908.

Amann, R.P. (2011c) Drugs that adversely affect spermatogenesis In: McKinnon, A.O., Squires, E.L., Vaala, E. and Varner, D.D. (eds) *Equine Reproduction*, 2nd edn. Wiley-Blackwell, Philadelphia, London, pp. 1175–1183.

Amann, R.P. and Graham, J.K. (1993) Spermatozoal function. In: McKinnon, A.O. and Voss, J.L. (eds) *Equine Reproduction*. Lea and Febiger, Philadelphia, Pennsylvania, pp. 715–745.

Amann, R.P. and Graham, J.K. (2011) Spermatozoal function. In: McKinnon, A.O., Squires, E.L., Vaala, E. and Varner, D.D. (eds) *Equine Reproduction*, 2nd edn. Wiley-Blackwell, Philadelphia, London, pp. 1053–1084.

Amann, R.P. and Pickett, B.W. (1987) Principles of cryopreservation and a review of cryopreservation of stallion spermatozoa. *Equine Veterinary Science* 7, 145–173.

Anand, A. and Singh, S.S. (2015) Inside-out continuous suturing technique for the repair of third-degree perineal laceration in mares. *Journal of Equine Veterinary Science* 35(2), 147–152.

Anaya, G., Moreno-Millán, M., Bugno-Poniewierska, M., Pawlina, K., Membrillo, A., Molina, A. and Demyda-Peyrás, S. (2014) Sex reversal syndrome in the horse: four new cases of feminization in individuals carrying a 64, XY SRY negative chromosomal complement. *Animal Reproduction Science* 151(1/2), 22–27.

Antczak, D.F., de Mestre, A.M., Wilsher, S. and Allen, W.R. (2013) The equine endometrial cup reaction: a fetomaternal signal of significance. *Annual Review of Animal Biosciences* 1, 419–442.

Aoki, T., Yamakawa, K. and Ishii, M. (2013) Factors affecting gestation length in heavy draft mare. *Journal of Equine Veterinary Science* 33, 437–440.

Aoki, T., Yamakawa, K. and Ishii, M. (2014) Factors affecting the incidence of postpartum fever in heavy draft mares. *Journal of Equine Veterinary Science* 34(5), 719–721.

Apter, R.C. and Householder, D.D. (1996) Weaning and weaning management of foals: a review and some recommendations. *Journal of Equine Veterinary Science* 16(10), 428–435.

Arav, A. (2014) Cryopreservation of oocytes and embryos. *Theriogenology* 81, 96–102.

Arav, A., Yavin, S., Zeron, Y., Natan, D., Dekel, I. and Gacitua, H. (2002) New trends in gamete's cryopreservation. *Molecular and Cell Endocrinology* 187(1–2), 77–81.

Arbeiter, K., Barth, U. and Jochle, W. (1994) Observations on the use of progesterone intravaginally and of desorelin in acyclic mares for induction of ovulation. *Journal of Equine Veterinary Science* 14(1), 21–25.

Aresu, L., Benali, S., Giannuzzi, D., Mantovani, R., Castagnaro, M., Falomo, M.E. (2012) The role of inflammation and matrix metalloproteinases in equine endometriosis *Journal of Veterinary Science* 13(2), 171–177.

Argo, C.M., Cox, J.E. and Gray, J.L. (1991) Effect of oral melatonin treatment on the seasonal physiology of pony stallions. *Journal of Reproduction and Fertility, Supplement* 44, 115–125.

Arighi, M. (2011a) Testicular descent. In: McKinnon, A.O., Squires, E.L., Vaala, E. and Varner, D.D. (eds) *Equine Reproduction*, 2nd edn. Wiley-Blackwell, Philadelphia, London, pp. 1099–1108.

Arighi, M. (2011b) Developmental abnormalities of the male reproductive tract. In: McKinnon, A.O., Squires, E.L., Vaala, E. and Varner, D.D. (eds) *Equine Reproduction*, 2nd edn. Wiley-Blackwell, Philadelphia, London, pp. 1109–1112.

Armstrong, D.T (2001) Effects of maternal age on oocyte developmental competence. *Theriogenology* 55, 1303–1322.

Arns, M.J., Webb, G.W., Kreider, J.L., Potter, G.D. and Evans, J.W. (1987) Use of diluent glycolysable sugars to maintain stallion sperm viability when frozen or stored at 37°C and 5°C in bovine serum albumin. *Journal of Reproduction and Fertility, Supplement* 35, 135–141.

Asbury, A.C. (1984) Uterine defense mechanisms in the mare. The use of intrauterine plasma in the management of endometritis. *Theriogenology* 21, 387–393.

Asbury, A.C. (1990) Large volume uterine lavage in the management of endometritis and acute metritis in the mare. *Compendium of Continuing Education for Practising Veterinary Surgeons* 12, 1477–1479.

Asbury, A.C. (1991) Diseases of the reproductive system. The mare. Examination of the mare. In: Colahan, P.T., Mayhew, I.G., Merritt, A.M. and Moore, J.N. (eds) *Equine Medicine and Surgery*. Vol. 2, 4th edn. American Veterinary Publications, Goleta, California, pp. 949–963.

Asbury, A.C. (1993) Care of the mare after foaling. In: McKinnon, A.O. and Voss, J.L. (eds) *Equine Reproduction*. Lea and Febiger, Philadelphia, Pennsylvania, pp. 976–980.

Asbury, A.C. and LeBlanc, M.M. (1993) The placenta. In: McKinnon, A.O. and Voss, J.L. (eds) *Equine Reproduction*. Lea and Febiger, Philadelphia, Pennsylvania, pp. 509–516.

Asbury, A.C. and Lyle, S.K. (1993) Infectious causes of infertility. In: McKinnon, A.O. and Voss, J.L. (eds) *Equine Reproduction*. Lea and Febiger, Philadelphia, Pennsylvania, pp. 381–391.

Assad, N.I. and Pandey, A.K. (2015) Different approaches to diagnose uterine pathology in mares : A review. *Theriogenology Insights* 5(3), 157–182.

Astudillo, C.R., Hajek, G.E. and Diaz, O.H. (1960) Influencia de algunos factores climaticos sobre la duracion de la gestacion de yeguas fina sangre de carrera: estudio preliminary (the influence of some climate factors on pregnancy duration in Thoroughbred mares: preliminary account). *Zoolatria* 2, 35/38, 37 (*Animal Breeding Abstracts* (1962) 30, 2348).

Aurich, C. (2005) Factors affecting the plasma membrane function of cooled-stored stallion spermatozoa. *Animal Reproduction Science* 89, 65–75.

Aurich, C. (2011a) Reproductive cycles of horses. *Animal Reproduction Science* 124, 220–228.

Aurich, C. (2011b) Semen extenders for colled semen (Europe). In: McKinnon, A.O., Squires, E.L., Vaala, E. and Varner, D.D. (eds) *Equine Reproduction*, 2nd edn. Wiley-Blackwell, Philadelphia, London, pp. 1336–1340.

Aurich, C. and Budik, S. (2015) Early pregnancy in the horse revisited – does exception prove the rule? *Journal of Animal Science and Biotechnology* 6, 50.

Aurich, C. and Spergser, J. (2006) Influence of genitally pathogenic bacteria and gentamicin on motility and membrane integrity of cooled-stored stallion spermatozoa. *Animal Reproduction Science* 94, 117–120.

Aurich, C. and Spergser, J. (2007) Influence of bacteria and gentamicin on cooled-stored stallion spermatozoa. *Theriogenology* 67, 912–918.

Aurich, C., Schlote, S., Hoppen, H.-O., Klug, E., Hope, H. and Aurich, J.E. (1994) Effects of opioid antagonist naloxane on release of LH in mares during the anovulatory season. *Journal of Endocrinology* 142, 139–144.

Aurich, C., Hoppe, H. and Aurich, J.E. (1995) Role of endogenous opioids for regulation of the oestrous cycle in the horse. *Reproduction in Domestic Animals* 30(4), 188–192.

Aurich, C., Gerlach, T., Aurich, J.E., Hoppen, H.O., Lange, J. and Parvizi, N. (2002) Dopaminergic and opiodergic regulation of gonadotrophin and prolactin release in stallion. *Reproduction in Domestic Animals* 37, 335–340.

Aurich, C., Königm, N. and Budik, S. (2011) Effects of repeated embryo collection on embryo recovery rate in fertile mares. *Reproduction in Domestic Animals* 46(3), 419–422.

Aurich, C., Seeber, P. and Muller-Schlosser, F. (2007) Comparison of different extenders with defined protein composition for storage of stallion spermatozoa at 5°C. *Reproduction in Domestic Animals* 42(4), 445–448.

Aurich, J.E., Kuhne, A., Hoppe, H. and Aurich, C. (1996) Seminal plasma affects membrane integrity and motility of equine spermatozoa after cryopreservation. *Theriogenology* 46(5), 791–797.

Avdatek, F., Gundogan, M. and Yeni, D. (2010) Functional tests in semen quality determination. *Journal of Animal and Veterinarian Advances* 9(5), 862–871.

Axon, J.F. and Palmer, J.E. (2008) Clinical pathology of the foal. *Veterinary Clinics of North America : Equine Practice* 24, 357–385.

Bachelot, A. and Binart, N. (2007) Reproductive role of prolactin. *Reproduction* 133, 361–369.

Back, W., Smit, L.D., Schamhardt, H.C. and Barneveld, A. (1999) The influence of different exercise regimens on the development of locomotion in the foal. *Equine Veterinary Journal, Supplement* 31, 106–111.

Bacus, K.L., Ralston, S.L., Noekels, C.F. and McKinnon, A.O. (1990) Effects of transport on early embryonic death in mares. *Journal of Animal Science* 68, 345–351.

Baemgartl, C., Bader, H., Drommer, W. and Luning, I. (1980) Ultrastructural alterations of stallion spermatozoa due to semen conservation. In: *Proceedings of the International Congress of Animal Reproduction and Artificial Insemination* 5, 134–137.

Bailey, J.H. (2007) Cell signalling during capacitation and the acrosome reaction. In : *Proceedings of the Havemeyer Foundation Workshop on Stallion Reproduction, 22–25 September 2006,* Bandera, Texas.

Bailey, A.M., Troedsson, M.H.T. and Wheaton, J.E. (2002) Inhibin concentrations in mares with granulose cell tumours. *Theriogenology* 57, 1885–1895.

Bailey, M.T., Bott, R.M. and Gimenez, T. (1995) Breed registries regulations on artificial insemination and embryo transfer. *Journal of Equine Veterinary Science* 15(2), 60–61.

Baker, C.B., Little, T.V. and McDowell, K.J. (1993) The live foaling rate per cycle in mares. *Equine Veterinary Journal, Supplement* 15, 28–30.

Balasuriya, U.B.R., Carossino, M. and Timoney, P.J. (2018) Equine viral arteritis: a respiatory and reproductive disease of significant economic importance to the equine industry. *Equine Veterinary Education* 30(9), 497–512.

Baldwin, D.M. Roser, J.F., Muyan, M., Lasley, B. and Dybdal, N. (1991) Direct effects of free and conjugated steroids on GnRH stimulated LH release in cultured equine pituitary cells. *Journal of Reproduction and Fertility, Suppl* 44, 327–332.

Ball, B.A. (1993a) Embryonic death in mares. In: McKinnon, A.O. and Voss, J.L. (eds) *Equine Reproduction.* Lea and Febiger, Philadelphia, Pennsylvania, pp. 517–530.

Ball, B.A. (1993b) Management of twin embryos and foetuses in the mare. In: McKinnon, A.O. and Voss, J.L. (eds) *Equine Reproduction.* Lea and Febiger, Philadelphia, Pennsylvania, pp. 532–536.

Ball, B.A. (2011a) Sperm-oviduct interations. In: McKinnon, A.O., Squires, E.L., Vaala, E. and Varner, D.D. (eds) *Equine Reproduction,* 2nd edn. Wiley-Blackwell, Philadelphia, London, pp. 1085–1091.

Ball, B.A. (2011b) Embryonic loss. In: McKinnon, A.O., Squires, E.L., Vaala, E. and Varner, D.D. (eds) *Equine Reproduction,* 2nd edn. Wiley-Blackwell, Philadelphia, London, pp. 2327–2338.

Ball, B.A. (2014) Applied andrology in horses In: Chenoweth, P.J. and Lorton, S.P. (eds) *Animal Andrology: Theories and Applications.* CABI, Wallingford, Oxfordshire, UK, pp 254–296.

Ball, B.A. and Brinsko, S.P. (1992) Early embryonic loss. A research update. *Modern Horse Breeding* 9(1), 8–9.

Ball, B.A., Little, T.V., Weber, J.A. and Woods, G.L. (1989) Survivability of day 4 embryos from young normal mares and aged subfertile mares after transfer to normal recipient mares. *Journal of Reproduction and Fertility* 85, 187–194.

Ball, B.A., Altschul, M., McDowell, K.J., Ignotz, G. and Currie, W.B. (1991) Trophoblastic vessicles and maternal recognition of pregnancy in mares. *Journal of Reproduction and Fertility, Supplement* 44, 445–454.

Ball, B.A., Fagnan, M.S. and Dobrinski, V. (1997) Determination of acrosin amidase activity in equine spermatozoa. *Theriogenology* 48(7), 1191–1198.

Ball, B.A., Medina, V., Gravance, C.G. and Baumber, J. (2001) Effect of antioxidants on preservation of motility, viability and acrosomal integrity of equine spermatozoa during storage at 5°C. *Theriogenology* 56, 577–589.

Barbacini, S. (2011) Breeding with frozen semen In: McKinnon, A.O., Squires, E.L., Vaala, E. and

Varner, D.D. (eds) *Equine Reproduction*, 2nd edn. Wiley-Blackwell, Philadelphia, London, pp. 2985–2993.

Barbacini, S., Gulden, P., Marchi, V. and Zavaglin, G. (1999) Incidence of embryo loss in mares inseminated before or after ovulation. *Equine Veterinary Education* 11(5), 251–254.

Barbacini, S., Zavaglia, G., Gulden, P., Marchi, V. and Necchi, D. (2000) Retrospective study on the efficacy of hCG in equine artificial insemination programme using frozen semen. *Equine Veterinary Education* 12, 312–317.

Barbary, H.A., Abo-ghonema, I.I., El-Bawab, I.E. and Fadel, M.S. (2016) Diagnosis and treatment of bacterial endometritis in Arabian mares. *Alexandria Journal of Veterinary Sciences* 49, 116–125.

Barker, C., Echeverria, K., Davis, M., Whisnant, C.S. and Pinto, C.R.F. (2006) Effects of different doses of PGF2α on luteal function and the subsequent oestrous cycle *Animal Reproduction Science* 94, 207–209.

Barnea, E.R., Kirk, D. and Paidas, M.J. (2012) Preimplantation factor (PIF) promoting role in embryo implantation: increases endometrial integrin-α2β3, amphiregulin and epiregulin while reducing betacellulin expression via MAPK in decidua. *Reproductive Biology Endocrinology* 12(10), 50.

Barnes, R.J., Nathanielsz, P.W., Rossdale, P.D., Comline, R.S. and Silver, M. (1975) Plasma progestagens and oestrogens in fetus and mother in late pregnancy. *Journal of Reproduction and Fertility, Supplement* 23, 617–623.

Barnisco, M.J.V. and Potes, N.M. (1987) The effects of teasing on the reproductive cycle in Portugese mares. *Revista Porteguesa Ciencias Veterinarias* 82, 37–43.

Barr, B. (2011) Gastrodudenal ulcer complex of the older foal. In: McKinnon, A.O., Squires, E.L., Vaala, E. and Varner, D.D. (eds) *Equine Reproduction*, 2nd edn. Wiley-Blackwell, Philadelphia, London, pp. 683–688.

Barrandeguy, M. and Thiry, E. (2012) Equine coital exanthema and its potential economic implications for the equine industry. *Veterinary Journal* 191(1), 35–40.

Barrandeguy, M., Vissani, A., Olguin, C., Beccerra, L., Mino, S., Pereda, A., Oriol, J. and Thiry, E. (2008) Experimental reactivation of equine herpes virus-3

following corticosteroid treatment. *Equine Veterinary Journal* 40, 593–595.

Barrier-Battut, I., Kempfer, A., Becker, J., Lebailly, L., Camugli, S. and Chevrier, L. (2016) Development of a new fertility prediction model for stallion semen, including flow cytometry. *Theriogenology* 86(4), 1111–1131.

Barrier-Battut, I., Kempfer, A., Lemasson, L.N., Chevrier, L. and.Camugli, S. (2017) Predition of the fertility of stallion frozen-thawed semen using a combination of computer-a sisted motility analysis, microscopical observation and flow cytometry. *Theriogenology* 97, 186–200.

Bataille, B., Magistrini, M. and Palmer, E. (1990) Objective determination of sperm motility in frozen-thawed stallion semen. Correlation with fertility. *Quoi de neuf en matiere d'etudes et de recherches de le cheval? 16eme journee d'etude, Paris, 7 Mars 1990.* CEREOPA, Paris, pp. 138–141.

Batellier, F., Duchamp, G., Vidament, M., Arnaud, G., Palmer, E. and Magistrini, M. (1998) Delayed insemination is successful with a new extender for storing fresh equine semen at 15°C under aerobic conditions. *Theriogenology* 50, 229–236.

Batellier, F., Gerard, N., Courtens, J.L., Palmer, E. and Magistrini, M. (2000) Preservation of stallion sperm by native phosphocaseinate: a direct or indirect effect. *Journal of Reproduction and Fertility, Supplement* 56, 69–77.

Batellier, F., Vidament, M., Fauquant, J., Duchamp, G., Arnaud, G., Yvon, J.M. and Magistrini, M. (2001) Advances in cooled semen technology. *Animal Reproduction Science* 68, 181–190.

Baucus, K.L., Squires, E.L., Ralston, S.L. and McKinnon, A.O. (1990) Effect of transportation on the oestrus cycle and concentrations of hormones in mares. *Journal of Animal Science* 68, 419–426.

Bauer, J.E. (1990) Normal blood chemistry. In: Koterba, A.M., Drummond, W.H., Kosch, P.C. (ed.) *Equine Clinical Neonatology.* Lea & Febiger, Philadelphia, Pennsylvania, pp. 602–614.

Baumber-Skaife, J. (2011) Evaluation of semen. In: McKinnon, A.O., Squires, E.L., Vaala, E. and Varner, D.D. (eds) *Equine Reproduction*, 2nd edn. Wiley-Blackwell, Philadelphia, London, pp. 1278–1291.

Bazer, F.W., Vallet, J.L., Harney, J.P., Gross, T.S. and Thatcher, W.W. (1989) Comparative aspects of maternal recognition of pregnancy between sheep and pigs. *Journal of Reproduction and Fertility Supplement* 37, 85–89.

Bazer, F.W., Ott, T.L. and Spencer, T.C. (1994) Pregnancy recognition in ruminants, pigs and horses, signals from the trophoblast. *Theriogenology* 41, 79–94.

Bazer, F.W., Spencer, T.E., Johnson, G.A. and Burghardt, R.C. (2009) *Comparative aspects of implantation Reproduction* 138, 195–209.

Bazer, F.W., Song, G., Kim, J., Dunlap, K.A., Satterfield, M.C., Johnson, G.A., Burghardt, R.C. and Wu, G. (2012) Uterine biology in pigs and sheep. *Journal of Animal Science and Biotechnology* 3, 23.

Bazer, F.W., Wu, G. and Johnson, G.A. (2017) Pregnancy recognition signals in mammals: the roles of interferons and estrogens. *Animal Reproduction* 14(1), 7–29.

Beard, T. and Knight, F. (1992) Developmental orthopaedic disease. In: Robinson, N.E. (ed.) *Current Therapy in Equine Medicine 3*. W.B. Saunders, Philadelphia, Pennsylvania, pp. 105–166.

Beard, W. (2011) Abnormalities of the testicles. In: McKinnon, A.O., Squires, E.L., Vaala, E. and Varner, D.D. (eds) *Equine Reproduction*, 2nd edn. Wiley-Blackwell, Philadelphia, London, pp. 1161–1165.

Beavers, K.N., Burden, C.A. and McKinnon, A.O. (2017) Management of twin pregnancies by umbilical and fetal oscillation in the mare. *Clinical Theriogenology* 9(3), 468.

Beck, C., Charles, J.A. and Maclean, A.A. (2001) Ultrasound appearance of an equine testicular seminoma. *Veterinary Radiology Ultrasound* 42, 355–357.

Bedford, S.J., Kurokawa, M., Hinrichs, K. and Fissore, R.A. (2004) Patterns of intracellular calcium oscillations in horse oocytes fertilized by intracytoplasmic sperm injection: possible explanations for the low success of this assisted reproduction technique in the horse. *Biology of Reproduction* 70(4), 936–944

Bedford, S.J., Jasko, D.J., Graham, J.K., Amann, R.P., Squires, E.L. and Pickett, B.W. (1995a) Use of two freezing extenders to cool stallion spermatozoa to 5°C with and without seminal plasma. *Theriogenology* 43(5), 939–953.

Bedford, S.J., Jasko, D.J., Graham, J.K., Amann, R.P., Squires, E.L. and Pickett, B.W. (1995b) Effect of seminal extenders containing egg yolk and glycerol on motion characteristics and fertility of stallion spermatozoa. *Theriogenology* 43(5), 955–967.

Beech, D.J., Sibbons, P.D., Rossdale, P.D., Ousey, J.C., Holdstock, N.B., Chavatte, P. and Ansari, T. (2001) Organogenesis of lung and kidney in Thoroughbreds and ponies. *Equine Veterinary Journal* 33, 438–445.

Beg, M.A. and Bergfeldt, D.R. (2011) Folliculogenesis. In: McKinnon, A.O., Squires, E.L., Vaala, E. and Varner, D.D. (eds) *Equine Reproduction*, 2nd edn. Wiley-Blackwell, Philadelphia, London, pp. 2009–2019.

Beg, M.A. and Ginther, O.J. (2006) Follicle selection in cattle and horses: role of intrafollicular factors. *Reproduction* 132, 365–377.

Behrendt-Adam, C.Y., Adams, M.H., Simpson, K.S. and McDowell, K.J. (2000) The effect of steroids on endometrial oxytocin mRNA production. *Journal of Reproduction and Fertility, Supplement* 56, 297–304.

Belin, F., Goudet, G., Duchamp, G. and Gerard, N. (2000) Intrfollicular concentrations of steroids and steroidogenic enzymes in relation to follicular development in the mare. *Biology of Reproduction* 62, 1335–1343.

Bell, R.J. and Bristol, F.M. (1991) Equine chorionic gonadotrophin in mares that conceive at foal oestrus. *Journal of Reproduction and Fertility, Supplement* 44, 719–721.

Belonje, C.W.A. (1965) Operation of retroversion of the penis in the stallion. *Journal of the South African Veterinary Medicine Association* 27, 53.

Beltaire, K.A., Cheong, S.H. and Coutinho da Silva, M.A. (2012) Retrospective study on equine uterine fungal isolates and antifungal susceptibility patterns (1999–2011). *Equine Veterinary Journal* 44(s43), 84–87.

Bemis, L.T., McCue, P.M., Hatzel, J.N., Bemis, J. and Ferris, R.A. (2012) Evidence for production of early pregnancy factor (Hsp10), microRNAs and exosomes by day 8 equine embryos *Journal of Equine Veterinary Science* 32(7), 398.

Benhajali, H., Ezzaouia, M., Lunel, C., Charfi, F. and Hausberger, M. (2014) Stereotypic behaviours and mating success in domestic mares. *Applied Animal Behaviour Science* 153, 36–42.

Bennett, W.K., Loch, W.E., Plata-Madrid, H. and Evans, T. (1998) The effects of perphenazine and bromocriptine on follicular dynamics and endocrine profiles in anoestrus pony mares. *Theriogenology* 49, 717–733.

Berezowski, C.J., Stitch, K.L., Wendt, K.M. and Vest, D.G. (2004) Clinical Comparison of 3 Products

Available to Hasten Ovulation in Cyclic Mares. *Veterinary Review* 24(6), 231–233.

Berger, J.M., Spier, S.J., Davies, R. Gardner, I.A., Leutenegger, C.M. and Bain, M. (2013) Behavioural and physiological responses of weaned foals treated with equine appeasing pheromone : A double blinded, placebo controlled, randomised trial. *Journal of Veterinary Behaviour* 8, 265–277.

Bergeron, A. and Manjunath, P. (2006) New insights towards understanding the mechanisms of sperm protection by egg yolk and milk. *Molecular Reproduction and Development* 73, 1338–1344.

Bergfeldt, D.R. (2000) Anatomy and physiology of the mare. In: Samper, J.C. (ed.) *Equine Breeding Management and Artificial Insemination*. W.B. Saunders, Philadelphia, Pennsylvania, pp. 141–164.

Bergfeldt, D.R. and Adams, G.P. (2011a) Luteal development. In: McKinnon, A.O., Squires, E.L., Vaala, E. and Varner, D.D. (eds) *Equine Reproduction*, 2nd edn. Wiley-Blackwell, Philadelphia, London, pp. 2055–2064.

Bergfeldt, D.R. and Adams, G.P. (2011b) Pregnancy. In: McKinnon, A.O., Squires, E.L., Vaala, E. and Varner, D.D. (eds) *Equine Reproduction*, 2nd edn. Wiley-Blackwell, Philadelphia, London, pp. 2065–2079.

Bergfeldt, D.R. and Ginther, O.J. (1992) Relationship between circulating concentrations of FSH and follicular waves during early pregnancy in mares. *Journal of Equine Veterinary Science* 12, 274–279.

Bergfeldt, D.R. and Ginther, O.J. (1993) Relationship between FSH surges and follicular waves during the oestrous cycles in mares. *Theriogenology* 39, 781–796.

Bergfeldt, D.R., Pierson, R.A. and Ginther. O.J. (2006) Regression and resurgence of the CL following PGF2α. Theriogenology 65, 1605–1619.

Bergfeldt, D.R., Meira, C., Fleury, J.J., Fleury, P.D., Dell'Aqua, J.A. and Adams, G.P. (2007) Ovulation synchronization following commercial application of ultrasound-guided follicle ablation during the estrous cycle in mares. *Theriogenology* 68(8), 1183–1191.

Berghold, P., Mostl, E. and Aurich, C. (2007) Effects of reproductive staus and management on cortisol secretion and fertility of oestrous horse mares. *Animal Reproduction Science* 102, 276–285.

Berndston, W.E. and Jones, L.S. (1989) Relationship of intratesticular testosterone content to age,

spermatogenesis, sertoli cell distribution and germ cell:sertoli cell ratio. *Journal of Reproduction and Fertility* 85, 511–518.

Berndston, W.E., Pickett, B.W. and Nett, T.H. (1974) Reproductive physiology of the stallion and seasonal changes in the testosterone concentrations of peripheral plasma. *Journal of Reproduction and Fertility, Supplement* 39, 115–118.

Bertone, J.J. and Jones, R.L. (1988) Evaluation of a field test kit for determination of serum IgG concentrations in foals. *Journal of Veterinary Internal Medicine* 2, 181–183.

Besognek, B., Hansen, B.S. and Daels, P.F. (1995) Prolactin secretion during the transitional phase and relationships to onset of reproductive season in mares. *Biology of Reproduction, Monograph series* 1, 459–467.

Betsch, J.M., Hunt, P.R., Spalart, M., Evenson, D. and Kenney, R.M. (1991) Effects of chlorhexidene penile washing on stallion semen parameters and sperm chromatin structure assay. *Journal of Reproduction and Fertility, Supplement* 44, 655–656.

Betteridge, K.J. (2007) Equine embryology: an inventory of unanswered questions. *Theriogenology* 68 Supplement 1, S9–S21.

Betteridge, K.J. (2011) Embryo morphology, growth and development. In: McKinnon, A.O., Squires, E.L., Vaala, E. and Varner, D.D. (eds) *Equine Reproduction*, 2nd edn. Wiley-Blackwell, Philadelphia, London, pp. 2168–2186.

Betteridge, K.J., Eaglesome, M.D., Mitchell, D., Flood, P.F. and Beriault, R. (1982) Development of horse embryos up to twenty two days after ovulation: observations on fresh specimens. *Journal of Anatomy* 135, 191–209.

Beythien, E., Aurich, C., Wulf, M. and Aurich, L. (2017) Effects of season on placental, foetal and neonatal development in horses *Theriogenology* 97, 98–103.

Bezard, J. (1992) In vitro fertilization in the mare. *Proceedings of the Science Conference of Biotechnology and Horse Reproduction*, Agricultural University of Krakow, Poland, 12.

Bezard, J., Magistrini, M., Duchamo, G. and Palmer, E. (1989) Chronology of equine fertilisation and embryonic development in vivo and in vitro. *Equine Veterinary Journal, Supplement* 8, 105–110.

Bhattacharya, B.C., Shome, P. and Gunther, A.H. (1977) Successful separation of X and Y spermatozoa in human and bull semen. *International Journal of Fertility* 22, 30–35.

Bidstrup, L.A., Dean, D.J., Pommer, A.C. and Roser, J.F. (2002) Transferrin production in cultured Sertoli cells during testicular maturation in the stallion. *Biology of Reproduction (Suppl)* 66, 493.

Bielanski, A. (2007) Disinfection procedures for controlling microorganisms in the semen and embryos of humans and farm animals. *Theriogenology* 68, 1–22.

Binor, Z., Sokoloski, J.E. and Wolf, P.P. (1980) Penetration of the zona free hamster egg by human sperm. *Fertility and Sterility* 33, 321–327.

Bishop, M.W.H., David, J.S.E. and Messervey, A. (1964) Some observations on cryptorchidism in the horse. *Veterinary Record* 76, 1041–1048.

Blach, E.L., Amann, R.P., Bowen, R.A., Sawyer, H.R. and Hermenet, M.J. (1988) Use of a monoclonal antibody to evaluate integrity of the plasma membrane of stallion sperm. *Gamete Research* 21(3), 233–241.

Blanchard, T.L. (1995) Dystocia and post parturient disease. In: Kobluk, C.N., Ames, T.R. and Giver, R.J. (eds) *The Horse, Diseases and Clinical Management*. W.B. Saunders, Philadelphia, Pennsylvania, pp. 1021–1027.

Blanchard, T.L. (2011) Postpartum metritis. In: McKinnon, A.O., Squires, E.L., Vaala, E. and Varner, D.D. (eds) *Equine Reproduction*, 2nd edn. Wiley-Blackwell, Philadelphia, London, pp. 2530–2536.

Blanchard, T.L. and Macpherson, M.L. (2007) Postparturient abnormalities. In: Samper, J.S., Pycock, J.P. and McKinnon, A.O. (eds.) *Current Therapy in Equine Reproduction*. Elsevier, St. Louis, Missouri, pp. 465–475.

Blanchard, T.L. and Macpherson, M.L. (2011) Breeding mares on foal heat. In: McKinnon, A.O., Squires, E.L., Vaala, E. and Varner, D.D. (eds) *Equine Reproduction*, 2nd edn. Wiley-Blackwell, Philadelphia, London, pp. 2294–2301.

Blanchard, T.L. and Varner, D.D. (1993a) Uterine involution and post partum breeding. In: McKinnon, A.O. and Voss, J.L. (eds) *Equine Reproduction*. Lea and Febiger, Philadelphia, Pennsylvania, pp. 622–625.

Blanchard, T.L. and Varner, D.D. (1993b) Testicular degeneration. In: McKinnon, A.O. and Voss, J.L. (eds) *Equine Reproduction*. Lea and Febiger, Philadelphia, Pennsylvania, pp. 855–860.

Blanchard, T.L., Cummings, M.R., Garcia, M.C., Hurtgen, J.P. and Kenney, R.M. (1981) Comparison of two techniques for obtaining endometrial bacteriologic cultures in the mare. *Theriogenology* 16, 85–93.

Blanchard, T.L., Elmore, R.G., Youngquist, R.S., Loch, W.E., Hardin, D.K., Bierschwal, C.J., Ganjam, V.K., Balke, J.M., Ellersiek, M.R., Dawson, L.J. and Miner, W.S. (1983) The effects of stanozolol and boldenone undecylenate on scrotal width, testis weight and sperm production in pony stallions. *Theriogenology* 20, 121–131.

Blanchard, T.L., Varner, D.D., Love, C.C., Hurtgen, J.P., Cummings, M.R. and Kenney, R.M. (1987) Use of semen extender containing antibiotic to improve the fertility of a stallion with seminal vesiculitis due to *Pseudomonas aeroginosa*. *Theriogenology* 28, 541–546.

Blanchard, T.L., Bretzlaff, K.N. and Varner, D.D. (1990) Identifying testicular hypoplasia in large animals. *Veterinary Medicine* 85(4), 404–408.

Blanchard, T.L., Varner, D.D., Burns, P.J., Everett, S.P., Brinsko, L. and Boehnke, L. (1992) Regulation of oestrus and ovulation in mares with progesterone or progesterone and estradiol biodegradable microsphere with or without PGF2α. *Theriogenology* 38, 6, 1091–1106.

Blanchard, T.L., Johnson, L. and Roser, A.J. (2000) Increased germ cell loss rates and poor semen quality in stallions with idiopathic testicular degeneration *Journal of Equine Veterinary Science* 20, 263–265.

Blanchard, T.L., Thompson, J.A., Brinsko, S.P., Stich, K.L., Wendt, K.M., Varner, D.D. and Rigby, S.L. (2004) Mating mares on foal heat: a 5 year retrospective study. In: Palmer, S.E. (ed.) In: *Proceedings of the 50th Annual Convention of the American Association of Equine Practitioners, Denver, Colorado*, pp. 1496–1504.

Blanchard, T.L., Thompson, J.A., Love, C.C., Brinsko, S.P., Ramsey, J., O'Meara, A. and Varner, D.D. (2012) Influence of day of postpartum breeding on pregnancy rate, pregnancy loss rate, and foaling rate in Thoroughbred mares. *Theriogenology* 77, 1290–1296.

Bleul, U., Theiss, F., Rütten, M. and Kähn, W. (2007) Clinical, cytogenetic and hormonal findings in a stallion with hypospadias – a case report. *Veterinary Journal* 173(3), 679–682.

Blomberg, L.A. and Telugu, B.P.V.L. (2012) Twenty Years of Embryonic Stem Cell Research in Farm Animals. *Reproduction in Domestic Animals* 47, Suppl 4, 80–85.

Boerboom, D., Brown, K.A., Vaillancourt, D., Poitras, P., Goff, A.K., Watanabe, K., Dore, M. and Sirois, J. (2004) Expression of key prostaglandin sythases in equine endometrium during late dioestrus and early pregnancy. *Biology of Reproduction* 70, 391–399.

Bollwein, H., Mayer, R., Weber, F. and Stolla, R. (2002) Luteal blood flow during the estrous cycle in mares. *Theriogenology* 57, 2043–2051.

Bollwein, H., Mayer, R. and Stolla, R. (2003) Transrectal Doppler sonography of uterine blood flow during early pregnancy in mares. *Theriogenology* 60, 597–605.

Bollwein, H., Weber, F., Woschee, I. and Stolla, R. (2004) Transrectal Doppler sonography of uterine and umbilical blood flow during pregnancy in mares. *Theriogenology* 61(2–3), 499–509.

Bone, J.F. (1998) *Animal Anatomy and Physiology*, 3rd edn. Prentice-Hall, New Jersey.

Borg, K., Colenbrander, B., Fazeli, A., Parlevliet, J. and Malmgren, L. (1997) Influence of thawing method on motility, plasma membrane integrity and morphology of frozen-thawed stallion spermatozoa. *Theriogenology* 48(4), 531–536.

Bos, H. and Van der May, G.J.W. (1980) Length of gestation periods for horses and ponies belonging to different breeds. *Livestock Production Science* 7, 181–187.

Bosh, K.A., Powell, D., Neibergs, J.S., Shelton B. and Zent W. (2009a) Impact of reproductive efficiency over time and mare financial value on economic returns among Thoroughbred mares in central Kentucky. *Equine Veterinary Journal* 41, 889–894.

Bosh, K.A., Powell, D., Shelton, B. and Zent, W. (2009b) Reproductive performance measures among Thoroughbred mares in central Kentucky, during the 2004 mating season. *Equine Veterinary Journal* 41, 883–888.

Bosu, W.T.K. and Smith, C.A. (1993) Ovarian abnormalities. In: McKinnon, A.O. and Voss, J.L. (eds) *Equine Reproduction*. Lea and Febiger, Philadelphia, Pennsylvania, pp. 397–403.

Bosu, W.T.K., Van Camp, S.D., Miller, R.B. and Owen, R. (1982) Ovarian disorders: clinical and morphological observations in 30 mares. *Canadian Veterinary Journal* 23, 6–14.

Bowen, J.M., Tobin, N. and Simpson, R.B. (1982) Effect of washing on the bacterial flora of the stallion's penis. *Journal of Reproduction and Fertility, Supplement* 32, 41–45.

Bowling, A.T. (1996) *Horse Genetics*. CAB International, Wallingford, UK, pp. 200.

Bowling, A.T. and Hughes, J.P. (1993) Cytogenic abnormalities. In: McKinnon, A.O. and Voss, J.L. (eds) *Equine Reproduction*. Lea and Febiger, Philadelphia, Pennsylvania, pp. 258–265.

Bowling, A.T., Milton, L. and Hughes, J.P. (1987) An update of chromosomal abnormalities in mares. *Journal of Reproduction and Fertility, Supplement* 35, 149–155.

Bowman, T.R. (2011) Direct rectal palpation. In: McKinnon, A.O., Squires, E.L., Vaala, E. and Varner, D.D. (eds) *Equine Reproduction*, 2nd edn. Wiley-Blackwell, Philadelphia, London, pp. 1904–1913.

Boyle, M.S. (1992) Artificial insemination in the horse. *Annales de Zootechnie* 41(3–4), 311–318.

Boyle, M.S., Skidmore, J., Zhange, J. and Cox, J.E. (1991) The effects of continuous treatment of stallions with high levels of a potent GnRH analogue. *Journal of Reproduction and Fertility, Supplement* 44, 169–182.

Boyle, A.G., Magdesian, K.G. and Ruby, R.E (2005) Neonatal isoerythrolysis in horse foals and a mule foal: 18 cases (1988–2003) *Journal of the American Veterinary Medical Association* 227(8), 1276–1283.

Brachen, F.K. and Wagner, P.C. (1983) Cosmetic surgery for equine pseudohermaphrodism. *Veterinary Medicine of Small Animal Clinics* 78, 879–884.

Bracher, V. (1992) Equine endometritis. PhD thesis. University of Cambridge, Cambridge.

Bracher, V., Neuschaefer, A. and Allen, W.R. (1991) The effect of intra-uterine infusion of kerosene on the endometrium of mares. *Journal of Reproduction and Fertility* 44, 706–707.

Bracher, V., Mathias, S. and Allen, W.R. (1992) Videoendoscope evaluation of the mare's uterus : II Findings in subfertile mares. *Equine Veterinary Journal* 24(4), 279–284.

Bracher, V., Mathias, S. and Allen, W.R. (1996) Influence of chronic degenerative endometritis (endometriosis) on placental development in the mare. *Equine Veterinary Journal* 28(3), 180–188.

Bradecamp, E.A. (2007) Estrous synchronisation. In: Samper, J.C., Pycock, J.F. and McKinnon, A.O. (eds) *Current Therapy in Equine Reproduction.* Saunders Elsevier, St Louis, Missouri, pp. 22–25.

Bradecamp, E.A. (2011a) Synchronisation of ovulation. In: McKinnon, A.O., Squires, E.L., Vaala, W.E. and Varner, D.D. (eds) *Equine Reproduction*, 2nd edn. Wiley-Blackwell, Philadelphia, London, pp. 1870–1878.

Bradecamp, E.A. (2011b) Pneumovagina. In: McKinnon, A.O., Squires, E.L., Vaala, W.E. and Varner, D.D. (eds) *Equine Reproduction*, 2nd edn. Wiley-Blackwell, Philadelphia, London, pp. 2537–2544.

Bradecamp, E.A., Woodie, B., Wornall, P., Schnobrich, M.R. and Scoggin, C.F. (2017) Diagnosis and surgical removal of uteine masses in two mares. *Clinical Theriogenology* 9(3), 481.

Bragg Weber, N.D., Pierson, R.A. and Card, C.E. (2002) Relationship between estradiol 17-ß and endometrial echotexture during natural and hormonally manipulated estrus in mares. *Proceedings American Association of Equine Practitionners* 41–47.

Brainard, G.C., Sliney, D., Hanifin, J.P., Glickman, G., Byrne, B., Greeson, J.M., Jasser, S., Gerner, E. and Rollag M.D. (2008) Sensitivity of human circadian systems to short wavelength (420-nm) light. *Journal of Biological Rhythms* 23, 379–86.

Braun, J., Oka, A., Sato, K. and Oguri, N. (1993) Effect of extender, seminal plasma and storage temperature on spermatozoal motility in equine semen. *Japanese Journal of Equine Science* 4(1), 25–30.

Braun, J., Torres-Boggino, F., Hochi, S. and Oguri, N. (1994) Effect of seminal plasma on motion characteristics of epididymal and ejaculated stallion spermatozoa during storage at 5°C. *Deutsche Tierarztliche Wochenschrift* 101(8), 319–322.

Breen, K.M. and Karsch, F.J. (2006) New insights regarding glucocorticoids, stress and gonadotrophin suppression. *Frontiers in Neuroendocrinology* 27, 233–245.

Breen, V.B. and Bowman, R.T. (1994) Retained placenta: solving a sticky situation. *Modern Horse Breeding* March, 18–20.

Brendemuehl, P.J. and Cross, D.L. (2000) Influence of the dopamine antagonist domperidone on the vernal transition in seasonally anoestrous mares. *Reproduction and Fertility, Supplement* 56, 185–193.

Brewer, B.D., Clement, S.F., Lotz, W.S. and Gronwall, R. (1991) Renal clearance, urinary excretion of endogenous substances, and urinary diagnostic indices in healthy neonatal foals. *Journal of Veterinary Internal Medicine* 5(1), 28–33.

Briant, C., Ottogalli, M. and Guillaume, D. (2004) Attempt to control the day pf ovulation in cycling mares by associating a GnRH antagonist with hCG. *Domestic Animal Endocrionology* 27, 165–178.

Brinsko, S.P. (1996) GnRH therapy for subfertile stallions. *Veterinary Clinics of North America: Equine Practice* 12, 149–160.

Brinsko, S.P. (2006) Insemination doses: how low can we go? *Theriogenology* 66, 543–550.

Brinsko, S.P. (2011a) Semen collection techniques and insemination procedures. In: McKinnon, A.O., Squires, E.L., Vaala, E. and Varner, D.D. (eds) *Equine Reproduction*, 2nd edn. Wiley-Blackwell, Philadelphia, London, pp. 1268–1277.

Brinsko, S.P. (2011b) Semen extenders for cooled semen (North America) In: McKinnon, A.O., Squires, E.L., Vaala, E. and Varner, D.D. (eds) *Equine Reproduction*, 2nd edn. Wiley-Blackwell, Philadelphia, London, pp. 1341–1343.

Brinsko, S.P. and Varner, D.D. (1992) Artificial insemination and preservation of semen. *Veterinary Clinical Equine Practice* 8, 205–218.

Brinsko, S.P. and Varner, D.D. (1993) Artificial insemination. In: McKinnon, A.O. and Voss, J.L. (eds) *Equine Reproduction*. Lea and Febiger, Philadelphia, PA, pp. 790–797.

Brinsko, S.P., Varner, D.D., Blanchard, T.L. and Meyers, S.A. (1990) The effect of postbreeding uterine lavage on pregnancy rate in mares. *Theriogenology* 33(2), 465–475.

Brinsko, S.P., Varner, D.D., Blanchard, T.L., Relford, R.L. and Johnson, L. (1992) Bilateral infectious epididymitis in a stallion equine. *Veterinary Journal* 24, 325–328.

Brinsko, S.P., Ball, B.A., Miller, P.G., Thomas, P.G. and Ellington, J.E. (1994) In vitro development of day 2 embryos obtained from young, fertile mares and aged, subfertile mares. *Journal of Reproduction and Fertility* 102(2), 371–378.

Brinsko, S.P., Rowan, K.R., Varner, D.D. and Blanchard, T.L. (2000) Effects of transport container and ambient storage temperature on motion characteristics of equine spermatozoa. *Theriogenology* 53(8), 1641–1655.

Brinsko, S.P., Rigby, S.L., Lindsey, A.C., Blanchard, T.L., Love, C.C. and Varner, D.D. (2003) Pregnancy rates in mares following hysteroscopic or transrectally-guided insemination with low sperm numbers at the utero-tubal papilla. *Theriogenology* 59(3–4), 1001–1009.

Brinsko, S.P., Blanchard, T.L., Varner, D.D., Schumacher, J., Love, D.D., Hinrichs, K. and Hartman D.L. (2011) Semen Preservation. In: *Manual of Equine Reproduction*, 3rd edn. pp. 207–227, Elsevier, Missouri.

Bristol, F. (1982) Breeding behaviour of a stallion at pasture with 20 mares in synchronised oestrus. *Journal of Reproductive Fertility, Supplement* 32, 71–77.

Bristol, F. (1986) Estrus synchronisation in mares. In: Morrow, D.A. (ed.) *Current Therapy in Theriogenology*. W.B. Saunders, Philadelphia, Pennsylvania, pp. 661–664.

Bristol, F. (1987) Fertility of pasture bred mares in synchronised oestrus. *Journal of Reproduction and Fertility, Supplement* 35, 39–43.

Bristol, F. (1993) Synchronization of ovulation. In: McKinnon, A.O. and Voss, J.L. (eds) *Equine Reproduction*. Lea and Febiger, Philadelphia, Pennsylvania, pp. 348–352.

Bristol, F., Jacobs, K.A. and Pawlyshyn, V. (1983) Synchronisation of estrus in post-partum mares with progesterone and estradiol 17β. *Theriogenology* 19, 779–785.

British Equine Veterinary Association (1991) *Codes of Practice for 1) Veterinary Surgeons and 2) Breed Societies In the United Kingdom and Ireland using AI for breeding Equids*. British Equine Veterinary Association, London, pp. 24.

British Equine Veterinary Association (1997) *Equine AI: Course for Technicians*. British Equine Veterinary Association, London.

Brito, L.F.C. (2007) Evaluation of stallion semen morphology. *Clinical Techniques in Equine Practice* 6, 249–264.

Brito, L.F.C., Sertich, P.L., Durkin, K., Chowdary, B.P., Turner, R.M. and McDonnell, S. (2008) Autosomic 27 trisomy in a standardbred colt. *Journal of Equine Veterinary Science* 28, 431–436.

Brito, L., Engiles, J., Turner, R.M., Getman, L. and Ebling, A. (2009) Bilateral testicular mixed germ cell-sex cord-stromal tumours in a stallion. *Reproduction in Domestic Animals* 44, 846–851.

Britton, J.W. and Howell, C.E. (1943) Physiological and pathological significance of the duration of gestation in the mare. *Journal of the American Veterinary Medical Association* 102, 427–430.

Brommer, H. and van Oldruitenborgh-Oosterbaan, M.M. (2001) Iron deficiency in stabled Dutch warmblood foals. *Journal of Veterinary Internal Medicine* 15(5), 482–485.

Brook, D. (1993) Uterine cytology. In: McKinnon, A.O. and Voss, J.L. (eds) *Equine Reproduction*. Lea and Febiger, Philadelphia, Pennsylvania, pp. 246–254.

Broussard, J.R., Roussel, J.D., Hibbard, M., Thibodeaux, J.K., Moreau, J.D., Goodeaux, S.D. and Goodeaux, L.L. (1990) The effect of Monoject and Rir-Tite syringes on equine spermatozoa. *Theriogenology* 33, 200.

Brown, C. (1999) Diseases affecting multiple sites. Dourine. In: Colahan, P.T., Merritt, A.M., Moore, J.N. and Mayhew, I.G. (eds) *Equine Medicine and Surgery*, 5th edn. Mosby, St. Louis, Missouri, pp. 2012–2013.

Brown, C.A., MacKay, R.J, Chandra, S., Davenport, D. and Lyons, E.T. (1997) Over whelming strongyloidosis in a foal. *Journal of American Veterinary Medicine Association* 211, 333.

Brown, J.S. (1984) Surgical repair of the lacerated cervix in the mare. *Theriogenology* 22, 351–359.

Brown-Douglas, C.G., Firth, E.C., Parkinson, T.J. and Fennessy, P.F. (2004) Onset of puberty in pasture-raised Thoroughbreds born in the southern hemisphere spring and autumn. *Equine Veterinary Journal* 36, 499–504.

Brown-Douglas, C.G., Parkinson, T.J., Firth, E.C. and Fennessy, P.F. (2005) Body weights and growth rates of spring- and autumn-born Thoroughbred horses raised on pasture. *New Zealand Veterinary Journal* 53(5), 326–331.

Brown-Douglas, C.G., Huntington, P. and Pagan, J. (2011) Growth of horses. In: McKinnon, A.O., Squires, E.L., Vaala, E. and Varner, D.D. (eds) *Equine Reproduction*, 2nd edn. Wiley-Blackwell, Philadelphia, London, pp. 280–291.

Bruck, I., Greve, T. and Hyttel, P. (1999) Morphology of the oocyte-follicular connection in the mare. *Anatomy and Embryology* 199, 21–28.

Bruemmer, J.E., Coy, R.C., Squires, E.L. and Graham, J.K. (2002) Efect of pyruvate on the function of stallion spermatozoa stored for 48 hours. *Journal of Animal Science* 80, 12–18.

Brum, A.M., Thomas, A.D., Sabeur, K. and Ball, B.A. (2006) Evaluation of Coomassie blue staining of the acrosome of equine and canine spermatozoa. *American Journal of Veterinary Research* 67, 358–362.

Brun, R., Hecker, H. and Lun, Z.-R. (1998) *Trypanosoma evansi* and *T. equiperdum:* distribution, biology, treatment and phylogenetic relationship. *Veterinary Parasitology* 79, 95–107.

Bruns, K. and Casillas, E.R. (1990) Partial purification and characterization of an acetylcarnitine hydrolase from bovine epididymal spermatozoa. *Archives of Biochemistry and Physiology* 277(1), 1–7.

Bruyas, J.F. (2011) Freezing of embryos. In: McKinnon, A.O., Squires, E.L., Vaala, W.E. and Varner, D.D. (eds) *Equine Reproduction*, 2nd edn. Wiley-Blackwell, Philadelphia, London, pp. 2887–2920.

Bruyas, J.F., Sanson, J.P., Battut, I., Fieni, F. and Tainturier, D. (2000) Comparison of the cryoprotectant properties of glycerol and ethylene glycol for early day 6 equine embryos. *Journal of Reproduction and Fertility, Supplement* 56, 549–560.

Bryant-Greenwood, G.D. (1982) Relaxin a new hormone. *Endocrinology Review* 3, 62–90.

Bucca, S. and Carli, A. (2011) Efficacy of human chorionic gonadotropin to induce ovulation in the mare, when associated with a single dose of dexamethasone administered at breeding time. *Equine Veterinary Journal Supplement* 40, 32–34.

Buchanan, B.R., Seidel Jr, G.E., McCue, P.M., Schenk, J.L., Herickhoff, L.A. and Squires, E.L. (2000) Insemination of mares with low numbers of either unsexed or sexed spermatozoa. *Theriogenology* 53, 1333–1344.

Buchanan, B.R., Sommardahl, C.S., Rohrbach, B.W. and Andrews, F.M. (2005) Effect of a 24hr infusion of an isotonic electrolyte replacement fluid on the renal clearance of electrolytes in healthy neonatal foals. *Journal of the American Veterinary Association* 227, 1123–1129.

Budik, S., Walter, I., Tschulenk, W., Helmreich, M., Deichsel, K., Pitner, F. and Aurich, C. (2008) Significance of aquaporinsand sodium potassium ATPase subunits for the expansion of early equine conceptuses. *Reproduction* 135, 497–508.

Bugno, M., Slota, E. and Koscielny, M. (2007) Karyotype examination among young horse populations in Poland. *Schweizer Archiv für Tierheilkunde* 149, 227–232.

Bugno-Poniewierska, M., Kozub, D., Pawlina, K., Tischner, M. Jr., Tischner, M., Słota, E. and Wnuk, M. (2011) Determination of the correlation between stallion's age and number of sex chromosome aberrations in spermatozoa. *Reproduction in Domestic Animals* 46(5), 787–792.

Bunning, M.L., Bowen, R.A., Cropp, C.B., Sullivan, K.G., Davis, B.S., Komar, N., Godsey, M.S., Baker, D., Hettler, D.L., Holmes, D.A., Biggerstaff, B.J. and Mitchell, C.J. (2002) Experimental infection of horses with West Nile virus. *Emerging Infectious Diseases* 8(4), 380–386.

Burger, D., Dolivo, G., Marti, E., Sieme, H. and Wedekind, C. (2015) Female major histo compatibility complex type affects male testosterone levels and sperm number in the horse (*Equus caballus*). *Proceedings of the Royal Society of Biology* 282, 20150407.

Burger, L.L., Haisenleder, D.J., Dalkin, A.C. and Marshall, J.C. (2004) Regulation of gonadotrophin subunit gene transcription. *Journal of Molecular Endocrinology* 33, 559–584.

Burkhardt, T. (1947) Transition from anoestrus in the mare and the effects of artificial lighting. *Journal of Agricultural Science Cambridge* 37, 64–68.

Burns, P.J. and Douglas, R.H. (1985) Reproductive hormone concentrations in stallions with breeding problems: case studies. *Journal of Equine Veterinary Science* 5, 40–42.

Burns, P.J. and Reasner, D.S. (1995) Computerized analysis of sperm motion: effects of glycerol concentration on cryopreservation of equine spermatozoa. *Journal of Equine Veterinary Science* 15(9), 377–380.

Burns, P.J., Morrow, C. and Abraham, J. (2008) P4LA 300 in the mare. In: *Proceedings of the 7th Equine Embryo Transfer Symposium, Cambridge*. R & W Publications, Newmarket, Cambridgeshire.

Burns, T.A. (2016). Effects of common equine endocrine diseases on reproduction. *Veterinary Clinics of North America. Equine Practice* 32(3), 435–449.

Buss, D.B., Asbury, A.C. and Chevalier, L. (1980) Limitations in equine fetal electrocardiography. *Journal of the American Veterinary Medical Association* 177, 174–176.

Buss, T., Aurich, J. and Aurich, C. (2019) Evaluation of a portable device for assessment of motility in stallion semen. *Reproduction in Domestic Animals* 54(3), 514–519.

Button, C. (1987) Congenital disorders of cardiac blood flow. In: Robinson, N.E. (ed.) *Current Therapy in Equine Medicine*. W.B. Saunders, Philadelphia, Pennsylvania, pp. 167–170.

Byers, T.D. and Divers, T.J. (2011) Periparturient hemorrhage. In: McKinnon, A.O., Squires, E.L., Vaala, E. and Varner, D.D. (eds) *Equine Reproduction*, 2nd edn. Wiley-Blackwell, Philadelphia, London, pp. 2517–2520.

Caballeros, J.E., Camacho, C., Cazales, N., Estradé, M.J., Fiala-Rechsteiner, S., Jobim, M.I.M. and Mattos, R.C. (2019) Ultrastructural and histological characteristics of the equine endometrium at day 5 post ovulation. *Theriogenology* 132, 106–112.

Cadario, M.E. (2014) Revisiting the diagnosis and the treatment options for an old problem: Chronic and post-breeding endometritis in the mare. *The Practitioner* 1, 21–25.

Camargo, C.E., Macan, R., Munhoz, M.L., Kozicki, L.E., Ollhoff, R.D., Segui, M.S., Tlini, R. Weiss, R.R., Steinberg-Galan, T.G. and Felicio, L.C.S. (2018) Effect of different types of artificial insemination and semen dose on reproductive efficiency in mares. *Pfer deheilkunde* 34(1), 57–60.

Camillo, F., Marmorini, P., Romagnoli, S., Vannozzi, J. and Bagliacca, M. (1997) Fertility in the first oestrus compared with fertility at following oestrous cycles in foaling mares and with fertility in non foaling mares. *Journal of Equine Veterinary Science* 17(11), 612–615.

Camillo, F., Marmorini, P., Romagnoli, S., Cela, M., Duchamp, G. and Palmer, E. (2000) Clinical studies on daily low dose oxytocin in mares at term. *Equine Veterinary Journal* 32(4), 307–310.

Camillo, F., Pacini, M., Panzani, D., Vanozzi, I., Rota, A. and Aria, G. (2004) Clinical use of twice daily injections of buserelin acetate to induce ovulation in the mare. *Veterinary Research Communications* 28, 169–172.

Camozzato, G.C., Martinez, M.N., Bastos, H.B.A., Fiala-Rechsteiner, S., Meikle, A., Jobim, M.I.M., Gregory, R.M. and Mattos, R.C. (2019) Ultrastructural and histological characteristics of the endometrium during early embryo development in mares. *Therogenology* 123, 1–10.

Campbell, M.L. (2014) Embryo transfer in competition horses : managing mares and expectations. *Equine Veterinary Education* 26(6), 322–327.

Campbell, M.L.H. (2016) Is cloning horses ethical? *Equine Veterinary Education* 30(5), 268–273.

Campbell, M.H.L. and England, G.C.W. (2002) A comparison of the ecbolic efficacy of intravenous and intrauterine oxytocin treatments. *Theriogenology* 58, 473–477.

Campbell, M.L. and England, G.C. (2004) Effect of teasing, mechanical stimulation and the intrauterine infusion of saline on uterine contractions in mares. *Veterinary Record* 155(4), 103–110.

Campbell, M.L. and England, G.C. (2006) Effects of coitus and the artificial insemination of different volumes of fresh semen on uterine contractions in mares. *Veterinary Record* 159(25), 843–849.

Canesin, H.S., Brom-de-Luna, J.G., Choi, Y.H., Ortiz, I., Diaw, M. and Hinrichs, K. (2017). Blastocyst development after intracytoplasmic sperm injection of equine oocytes vitrified at the germinal- vesicle stage. *Cryobiology* 75, 52–59.

Canesin, H.S., Brom-de-Luna, J.G., Choi, Y.H., Pereira, A.M., Macedo, G.G., and Hinrichs, K. (2018) Vitrification of germinal-vesicle stage equine oocytes: Effect of cryoprotectant exposure time on in- vitro embryo production. *Cryobiology*, 81, 185–191.

Canisso, I.F., Ball, B.A., Troedsson, M.H., Silva, E.S.M. and Davolli, G.M. (2013a) Decreasing pH of mammary gland secretions is associated with parturition and is correlated with electrolyte concentrations in prefoaling mares. *Veterinary Record* 173, 218.

Canisso, I.F., Beltaire, K.A., and Bedford-Guaus, S.J. (2013b) Premature luteal regression in a pregnant mare and subsequent pregnancy maintenance with the use of oral altrenogest. *Equine Veterinary Journal* 45(1), 97–100.

Canisso, I.F., Stewart, J. and Silva, M.A.C. da (2016) Endometritis: managing persistent post-breeding endometritis. *Veterinary Clinics of North America, Equine Practice* 32(3), 465–480.

Card, C.E. (2000) Management of pregnant mares. In: Samper, J.C. (ed.) *Equine Breeding Management and Artificial Insemination*. W.B. Saunders, Philadelphia, Pennsylvania, pp. 247–266.

Card, C. (2005) Post-breeding inflammation and endometrial cytology in mares. *Theriogenology* 64(3), 580–588.

Card, C.E. (2011a) Endoscopic examination. In: McKinnon, A.O., Squires, E.L., Vaala, E. and Varner, D.D.

(eds) *Equine Reproduction*, 2nd edn. Wiley-Blackwell, Philadelphia, London, pp. 1940–1950.

Card, C.E. (2011b) Ovarian neoplasia. In: McKinnon, A.O., Squires, E.L., Vaala, E. and Varner, D.D. (eds) *Equine Reproduction*, 2nd edn. Wiley-Blackwell, Philadelphia, London, pp. 2707–2718.

Card, C.E. (2012) Congental abnormalities of the cervix in mares. *Equine Veterinary Education* 24(7), 347–350.

Card, C.E. and Hillman, R.D. (1993) Parturition. In: McKinnon, A.O. and Voss, J.L. (eds) *Equine Reproduction*. Lea and Febiger, Philadelphia, Pennsylvania, pp. 567–574.

Card, C.E., Bruemmer, J., Moffett, P., Helvight, U., Pledger, A., Jamison, S., Longson, G., Loomis, P. and Squires, E.L. (2003) Comparison of oestrus synchronisation in mares treated with CIDR-B, estradiol-17β, estradiol cypionate, and prostaglandin F2α. In: *Proceedings of the Annual Confenerence for the Society for Theriogenology, 11–13 January 2003, Aukland, New Zealand*. Elsevier Inc. p39.

Carleton, C.L. (2011) Endoscopy of the internal reproductive tract. In: McKinnon, A.O., Squires, E.L., Vaala, E. and Varner, D.D. (eds) *Equine Reproduction*, 2nd edn. Wiley-Blackwell, Philadelphia, London, pp. 1448–1457.

Carluccio, A., Gloria, A., Mariotti, F., Petrizzi, L., Varasano, V., Robbe, D. and Contri, A. (2018) Ethanol sclerotherapy for the treatment of uterine cysts in the mare. *Journal of Equine Veterinary Science* 63, 27–29.

Carnevale, E.M. (1998) Folliculogenesis and ovulation. In: Rantanen, N.W. and McKinnon, A.O. (eds) *Equine Diagnostic Ultrasonography*. Williams and Wilkins, Baltimore, Maryland, pp. 201–212.

Carnevale, E.M. (2004) Oocyte transfer and gamete intrafallopian transfer in the mare. *Animal Reproduction Science* 82–83, 617–624.

Carnevale, E.M. (2011a) Mature oocyte collection. In: McKinnon, A.O., Squires, E.L., Vaala, E. and Varner, D.D. (eds) *Equine Reproduction*, 2nd edn. Wiley-Blackwell, Philadelphia, London, pp. 2936–2940.

Carnevale, E.M. (2011b) Oocyte transfer. In: McKinnon, A.O., Squires, E.L., Vaala, E. and Varner, D.D. (eds) *Equine Reproduction*, 2nd edn. Wiley-Blackwell, Philadelphia, London, pp. 294–2944.

Carnevale, E.M. and Ginther, O.J. (1992) Relationship of age to uterine function and reproductive efficiency in mares. *Theriogenology* 37, 1101–1105.

Carnevale, E.M. and Ginther, O.J. (1995) Defective oocytes as a cause of subfertility in old mares. *Biology of Reproduction, Monograph* 1, 209–214.

Carnevale, E.M. and Ginther, O.J. (1997) Age and pasture effects on vernal transition in mares. *Theriogenology* 47, 1009–1018.

Carnevale, E.M., Griffin, P.G. and Ginther, O.J. (1993) Age associated subfertility before entry of embryos into the uterus in mares. *Equine Veterinary Journal, Supplement* 15, 31–35.

Carnevale, E.M., Bergeildt, D.R. and Ginther, O.J. (1994) Follicular activity and concentrations of FSH and LH associated with senescence in mares. *Animal Reproduction Science* 35, 231–246.

Carnevale, E.M., Alvarenga, M.A., Squires, E.L. and Choi, Y.H. (1999) Use of non cycling mares as recipients for oocyte transfer and GIFT. In: *Proceedings of the Annual Conference of the Society of Theriogenology, 1–5 September 1999, Nashville, Tennessee. USA*. Elsevier Inc. p. 44.

Carnevale, E.M., Maclellan, L.J., Coutinho da Silva, M., Scott, T.J. and Squires, E.L. (2000a) Comparison of culture and insemination techniques for equine oocyte transfer. *Theriogenology* 54, 981–987.

Carnevale, E.M., Ramirez, R.J., Squires, E.L., Alvarenga, M.A. and McCue, P.M. (2000b) Factors affecting pregnancy rates and early embryonic death after equine embryo transfer. *Theriogenology* 54, 965–979.

Carnevale, E.M., Ramirez, R.J., Squires, E.L., Alvarenga, M.A., Vanderwall, D.K. and McVue, P.M. (2000c) Factors affecting pregnancy rates and early embryonic death after equine embryo transfer. *Theriogenology* 54, 965–979.

Carnevale, E.M., Squires, E.L., Maclellan, L.J., Alvarenga, M.A. and Scott, T.J. (2001) Use of oocyte transfer in a commercial breeding program for mares with various abnormalities. *Journal of the American Veterinary Medicine Association* 218, 87–91.

Carnevale, E.M., Coutinho da Silva, M.A., Preis, K.A., Stokes, J.E., and Squires, E.L. (2004) Establishment of pregnancies from oocytes collected from the ovaries of euthanized mares. *Proceedings of the American Association of Equine Practitioners* 50, 531–533.

Carnevale, E.M., Coutinho da Silva, M.A., Panzani, D., Stokes, J.F. and Squires, E.L. (2005a) Factors affecting the success of oocyte transfer in a clinical program for subfertile mares. *Theriogenology* 64, 519–527.

Carnevale, E.M., Beisner, A.E., McCue, P.M., Bass, L.D. and Squires, E.L. (2005b) Uterine changes associated with repeated inseminations and embryo collections in mares. *Proceedings of the American Association of Equine Practionners* 51, 202–203.

Carney, N.J., Squires, E.L., Cook, V.M., Seidel, G.E. and Jasko, D.L. (1991) Comparison of pregnancy rates from transfer of fresh versus cooled transported equine embryos. *Theriogenology* 36(1), 23–32.

Caron, J., Barber, S. and Bailey, J. (1985) Equine testicular neoplasia. *Compendium of Continuing Education for Practising Vets* 6, 5296.

Carossino, M., Wagner, B., Loynachan, A.T., Cook, R.F., Canisso, I.F., Chelvarajan, L., Edwards, C.L., Nam, B., Timoney, J.F., Timoney, P.J. and Balasuriya, U.B.R. (2017) Equine arteritis virus elicits a mucosal antibody response in the reproductive tract of persistently infected stallions. *Clinical and Vaccine Immunology* 24(10), e00215–17.

Carson, K. and Wood-Gush, D.E.M. (1983a) Behaviour of Thoroughbred foals during nursing. *Equine Veterinary Journal* 15, 257–262.

Carson, K. and Wood-Gush, D.E.M. (1983b) Equine behaviour: I. A review of the literature on social and dam-foal behaviour. II. A review of the literature on feeding, eliminative and resting behaviour. *Applied Animal Ethology* 10(3), 165–190.

Carter, A.M. and Enders, A.C. (2013) The evolution of epitheliochorial placentation. *Annual Review of Animal Biosciences* 1, 443–467.

Carver, D.A. and Ball, B.A. (2002) Lipase activity in stallion seminal plasma and the effect of lipase on stallion spermatozoa during storage at 5 degrees C. *Theriogenology* 58(8), 1587–1595.

Casey, P.J., Robertson, K.R., Lui, I.K.M., Botta, E.S. and Drobnis, E. (1991) Separation of motile spermatozoa from stallion semen. In: Milne, F.J. (ed.) *Proceedings of the 17th Annual Convention of American Association of Equine Practitioners, Chicago, Illinois.* American Association of Equine Practitioners, pp. 203–210.

Casey, P.J., Hillman, R.B., Robertson, K.R., Yudin, A.I., Lui, I.K. and Drobonis, E. (1993) Validation of an acrosomal stain for equine sperm that differentiates between living and dead sperm. *Journal of Andrology* 14, 282–297.

Cash, R.S.G. (1999) Colostral quality determined by refractometry. *Equine Veterinary Education* 11, 36–38.

Caslick, E.A. (1937) The vulva and vulvo-vaginal orifice and its relation to genital tracts of the Thoroughbred mare. *Cornell Veterinarian* 27, 178–187.

Caspo, J., Stefler, J., Martin, T.G., Makray, S. and Cspo-Kiss, Z. (1995) Composition of mare's colostrum and milk. Fat content, fatty acid composition and vitamin content. *International Dairy Journal* 5, 393–402.

Castagnetti, C., Pirrone, A., Mariella, J. and Mari, G. (2010) Venous blood lactate evaluation in equine neonatal intensive care. *Theriogenology* 73(3), 343–357.

Castillo-Olivares, J., Tearle, J.P., Montesso, F., Westcott, D., Kydd, J.H., Davis-Poynter, N.J. and Hannant, D. (2003) Detection of equine arteritis virus (EAV)-specific cytotoxic CD8+ T lymphocyte precursors from EAV-infected ponies. *Journal of General Virology* 84, 1–9.

Castle-Miller, J., Bates, D.O. and Tortonese, D.J. (2017) Mechanisms regulating angiogensis underlie seasonal control of pituitary function. *Proceedings of the National Academy Sciences USA* 21, 114.

Castleberry, R.S., Schneider Jr, H.J. and Griffin, J.L. (1980) Recovery and transfer of equine embryos. *Theriogenology* 13, 90–94.

Castro, T.A.M., Gastal, E.L., Castro Jr, F.G. and Augusto, C. (1991) Physical, chemical and biochemical traits of stallion semen. *Anais, IX Congresso Brasileiro de Reproducao Animal,* Belo Horizonte, Brazil, 22 a 26 de Junho de 1991. Vol. II. Colegio Brasileiro de Reproducao Animal, Belo Horizonte, Brazil, p. 443.

Causey, R.C. (2006) Making sense of equine uterine infections: The many faces of physical clearance. *The Veterinary Journal* 172(3), 405–421.

Causey, R.C. (2007) Mucus and the mare: how little we know. *Theriogenology* 68(3) 386–394.

Causey, R.C., Lehnhard, R.A., Finucane, K.A., Oliver, T.M. (2005) Effects of exercise on maternal and foetal heart rate in pregnant mares. *Equine and Comparative Exercise Physiolgy* 2(4), 225–228.

Cavinder, C.A., Vogelsang, M.M., Gibbs, P.G., Forrest, D.W. and Schmitz, D.G. (2007) Endocrine profile comparisons of fat versus moderately conditioned mares following parturition. *Jounal of Equine Veterinary Science* 27(2), 72–79.

Cebulj-Kadunc, N., Cestnik, V. and Kosec, M. (2006) Onset of puberty and duration of seasonal cyclicity in Lipizzan fillies. *Equine Veterinary Journal* 38, 350–353.

Celebi, M. and Demirel, M. (2003) Pregnancy diagnosis in mares by determination of oestradiol-17-β levels in faeces. *Turkish Journal of Veterinary and Animal Sciences* 27, 373–375.

Challis, J.R., Sloboda, D.M., Alfraidy, N., Lye, S.J., Gibb, W., Patel, F.A., Whittle, W.L. and Newnham, J.P. (2002) Prostaglandins and mechanisms of preterm birth. *Reproduction* 124, 1–17.

Chan, J.P.W., Huang, T.H., Chuang, S.T., Cheng, F.P., Fung, H.P., Chen, C.L. and Mao, C.L. (2003) Quantitative echotexture analysis for prediction of ovulation in mares. *Journal of Equine Veterinary Science* 23(9), 397–402.

Chaney, K.P., Holcombe, S.J., LeBlanc, M.M., Hauptman, J.G., Embertson, R.M., Mueller, P.O.E. and Beard, W.L. (2007) The effect of uterine torsion on mare and foal survival: a retrospective study, 1985–2005. *Equine Veterinary Journal* 39, 33–36.

Charneco, R., Pool, K.C. and Arns, M.J. (1993) Influence of vesicular gland rich and vesicular gland poor seminal plasma on the freezability of stallion spermatozoa. In: *Proceedings of the 13th Conference of the Equine Nutrition and Physiology Symposium, University of Florida, Gainesville, Florida*. Equine and Physiology Society, pp. 385–386.

Chavatte, P. (1991) Maternal behaviour in the horse: theory and practical applications to foal rejection and fostering. *Equine Veterinary Education* 3(4), 215–220.

Chavatte, P. (1997a) Twinning in the mare. *Equine Veterinary Education* 9(6), 286–292.

Chavatte, P. (1997b) Lactation in the mare. *Equine Veterinary Education* 9, 62–67.

Chavatte, P., Brown, G., Ousey, J.C., Silver, M., Cotrill, C., Fowden, A.L., McGladdery, A.J. and Rossdale, P.D. (1991) Studies of bone marrow and leucocyte counts in peripheral blood in fetal and newborn foals. *Journal of Reproduction and Fertility, Supplement* 44, 603–608.

Chavatte, P., Holton, D., Ousey, J.C. and Rossdale, P.D. (1997a) Biosynthesis and possible roles of progestogens during equine pregnancy and in the new born foal. *Equine Veterinary Journal, Supplement* 24, 89–95.

Chavatte, P., Rossdale, P.D. and Tait, A.D. (1997b) Corticosteroid synthesis by the equine fetal adrenal. *Biology of Reproduction, Monograph* 1, 13–20.

Chavatte, P., Duchamp, G., Palmer, E., Ousey, J.C., Rossdale, P.D. and Lombes, M. (2000) Progesterone, oestrogen and glucocorticoid receptors in the uterus and mammary glands of mares from mid-to late-gestation. *Journal of Reproduction and Fertility, Supplement* 56, 661–672.

Chavatte-Palmer, P. (2002) Lactation in the mare. *Equine Veterinary Education* 5, 88–93.

Chavatte-Palmer, P., Arnaud, G., Duvaux-Ponter, C., Zanazi, C., Gerard, M., Kindahl, H. and Clement, F. (2002) The use of microdoses of oxytocin in mares to induce parturition. *Theriogenology* 58, 837–840.

Checura, C.M. and Momont, H.W. (2017) Use of the prostaglandin E1 analog misoprostol to hasten oviductal transport of equine embryos. *Clinical Theriogenology* 9(3), 484.

Chenier, T.S. (2000) Anatomy and physical examination of the stallion. In: Samper, J.C. (ed.) *Equine Breeding Management and Artificial Insemination*. W.B. Saunders, Philadelphia, Pennsylvania, pp. 1–26.

Chenier, T.S. (2008) Anatomy and physical examination of the stallion. In: Samper, J.C. (ed.) 2nd ed. *Equine Breeding Management and Artificial Insemination*. W.B. Saunders, Philadelphia, Pennsylvania, pp. 336.

Choi, S.J., Anderson, G.B. and Roser, J.F. (1995) Production of estrogen conjugates and free estrogens by the pre-implantation equine embryo. *Biology of Reproduction* 52, Supplement, 179.

Choi, Y.H. and Hinrichs, K. (2011) Intracytoplasmic sperm injection (ICSI) In: McKinnon, A.O., Squires, E.L., Vaala, E. and Varner, D.D. (eds) *Equine Reproduction*, 2nd edn. Wiley-Blackwell, Philadelphia, London, pp. 2948–2952.

Choi, Y.H., Love, C.C., Love, L.B., Varner, D.D., Brinsko, S. and Hinrichs, K. (2002) Developmental in vitro matured oocytes fertilised by intracytoplasmic sperm injection with fresh or frozen-thawed spermatozoa. *Reproduction* 123, 455–465.

Choi, Y.H., Roasa, L.M., Love, C.C., Varner, D.D., Brinsko, S.P. and Hinrichs, K. (2004) Blastocyst formation rates in vivo and in vitro of in vitro-matured equine oocytes fertilised by intracytoplasmic sperm injection. *Biology of Reproduction* 70(5), 1231–1238.

Choi, Y.H., Varner, D.D., Hartman, D.L. and Hinrichs, K. (2006) Blastocyst prosuction from equine oocytes fertilized by intracytoplasmic sperm injection of lyophilized sperm. *Animal Reproduction Science* 94, 307–308.

Choi, Y.H., Hartman, D.L., Fissore, R.A. and Hinrichs, K. (2009) Effect of sperm extract injection volume, injection of PLC, cRNA, and tissue cell line on efficiency of equine nuclear transfer. *Cloning Stem Cells* 11, 301–308.

Choi, Y.H., Gustafson-Seabury, A., Velez, J.C., Hartman, D.L., Bliss, S., Riera, F.L. Roldan, J.E., Chowdary, B. and Hinrichs, K. (2010) Viability of equine embryos after puncture of the capsule and biopsy for preimplantation genetic diagnosis. *Reproduction* 140, 893–902.

Choi, Y.H., Velez, I.C., Riera, F.L., Roldan, J.E., Hartman, D.L., Bliss, S.B., Blanchard, T.L., Hayden, S.S. and Hinrichs, K. (2011) Successful cryopreservation of expanded equine blastocysts. *Theriogenology* 76, 143–152.

Choi, Y.H., Velez, I.C., Macias-Garcia, B., Riera, F.L., Ballard, C.S. and Hinrichs, K. (2016) Effect of clinically related factors on in vitro blastocyt development after ICSI. *Therogenology* 85, 1289–1296.

Chopin, J.B. (2011) Preventative medicine for broodmare farms. In: McKinnon, A.O., Squires, E.L, Vaala, W.E. and Varner, D.D. (eds) *Equine Reproduction*, 2nd edn. Wiley-Blackwell, Philadelphia, London, pp. 2747–2752.

Christanelli, M.J., Amann, R.P., Squires, E.L. and Pickett, B.W. (1985) Effects of egg yolk and glycerol levels in lactose-EDTA-egg yolk extender and of freezing rate on the motility of frozen-thawed stallion spermatozoa. *Theriogenology* 24(6), 681–686.

Christensen, B., (2008) Managing dystocia in the mare. Proceedings of the Central Veterinary Conference, Baltimore, Maryland, pp. 1–5.

Christensen, B.W. (2011a) Estrogens. In: McKinnon, A.O., Squires, E.L., Vaala, W.E. and Varner, D.D. (eds) *Equine Reproduction*, 2nd edn. Wiley-Blackwell, Philadelphia, London, pp. 1631–1636.

Christensen, B.W. (2011b) Parturition. In: McKinnon, A.O., Squires, E.L., Vaala, W.E. and Varner, D.D. (eds)

Equine Reproduction, 2nd edn. Wiley-Blackwell, Philadelphia, London, pp. 2268–2276.

Christensen, B.W., Troedsson, M.H., Murchie, T.A., Pozor, M.A., Macpherson, M.L., Etrada, A.H., Carrillo, N.A., Mackay, R.J., Roberts, G.D. and Langlois, J. (2006) Management of hydrops amnion in a mare resulting in birth of a live foal. *Journal of American Veterinary Medicine Association* 228(8), 1228–233.

Christensen, J., Ladewig, J., Sondergaard, E. and Malmkvist, J. (2002a) Effects of individual versus group stabling on social behaviour in domestic stallions. *Applied Animal Behaviour Science* 75, 233–248.

Christensen, J.W., Zharkikh, T., Ladewig, J. and Yasinetskaya, N. (2002b) Social behaviour in stallion groups (*Equus prezewalskii* and *Equus caballus*) kept under natural and domestic conditions. *Applied Animal Behaviour Science* 76, 11–20.

Christoffersen, M. and Troedsson, M.H.T. (2017) Inflammation and fertility in the mare. *Reproduction in Domestic Animals* 52, (Suppl 3) 14–20.

Christoffersen, M., Söderlind, M., Rudefalk, S.R., Pedersen, H.G., Allen, J. and Krekeler, N. (2015) Risk factors associated with uterine fluid after breeding caused by *Streptococcus zooepidemicus*. *Theriogenology* 84(8), 1283–1290.

Claes, A., Ball, B.A., Scoggin, K.E.A., Esteller-Vico, J.J., Kalmar, A.J., Conley, Squires, E.L. and Troedsson, M.H. (2015) The iterrelationship between anti-Mullerian hormone, ovarian follicular populations and age in mares. *Equine Veterinary Journal* 47, 537–541.

Claes, F., Agbo, E.C., Radwanska, M., Te Pas, M.F.W., Baltz, T., De Waal, D.T., Goddeeris, B.M., Claassen, E. and Buscher, P. (2003) How does *Trypanosoma equiperdum* fit into the Trypanozoon group? A cluster analysis by RAPD and multiplex-endonuclease genotyping approach. *Parasitology* 126, 425–431.

Clark, K.E., Squires, E.L., Takeda, T. and Seidel Jr, G.E. (1985) Effects of culture media on viability of equine embryos in vitro. *Equine Veterinary Journal, Supplement* 3, 35.

Clarke, I.J. and Pompolo, S. (2005) Synthesis and secretion of GnRH. *Animal Reproduction Science* 88, 29–55.

Clay, C.M. and Clay, J.N. (1992) Endocrine and testicular changes with season, artificial photoperiod and peri-pubertal period in stallions. *Veterinary Clinics of North America, Equine Practice* 8(1), 31–56.

Cleaver, B.D., Grubaugh, W.R., Davis, S.D., Sheerin, P.C., Franklin, K.J. and Sharp, D.C. (1991) Effect of constant light exposure on circulating gonadotrophin levels and hypothalamic gonadotrophin-releasing hormone (GnRH) content in the ovariectomized pony mare. *Journal of Reproduction and Fertility, Supplement* 44, 259–266.

Clement, F., Guerin, B., Vidament, M., Diemert, S. and Palmer, E. (1993) Microbial quality of stallion semen. *Pratique Veterinaire Equine* 25(1), 37–43.

Clement, F., Vidament, M. and Guerin, B. (1995) Microbial contamination of stallion semen. *Biology of Reproduction Monograph Equine Reproduction VI* 1, 779–786.

Clulow, J.R., Buss, H., Sieme, H., Rodger, J.A., Cawdell-Smith, A.J., Evans, G., Rath, D., Morris, L.H. and Maxwell, W.M. (2007) Field fertility of sex-sorted and non-sorted frozen-thawed stallion spermatozoa. *Animal Reproduction Science* 108, 287–297.

Cocchia, N., Paciello, O., Auletta, L., Uccello, V., Silvestro, L., Mallardo, K., Paraggio, G. and Pasolini, M.P. (2012) Comparison of the cytobrush, cottonswab, and low-volume uterine flush techniques to evaluate endometrial cytology for diagnosing endometritis in chronically infertile mares. *Theriogenology* 7, 89–98.

Cochran, J.D., Amann, R.P., Froman, D.P. and Pickett, G.W. (1984) Effects of centrifugation, glycerol level, cooling to 5°C, freezing rate and thawing rate on the post thaw motility of equine spermatozoa. *Theriogenology* 22, 25–38.

Cochran, R., Meintjes, M., Reggio, B., Hyland, D., Carter, J., Pinto, C., Paccamonti, D. and Godke, R.A. (1998) Live foals produced from sperm-injected oocytes derived from pregnant mares. *Journal of Equine Veterinary Science* 18, 736–740.

Coffman, E.A. and Pinto, C.R. (2016) A review on the use of Prostaglandin F2α for controling the estrus cycle in mares. *Journal Equine Vet Science* 40, 34–40.

Colchen, S., Battut, I., Fieni, F., Tainturier, D., Silart, S. and Bruyas, J.-F. (2000) Quantitive histological analysis of equine embryos at exactly 156 and 168h after ovulation. *Journal of Reproduction and Fertility, Supplement* 56, 527–537.

Coleman, R.J., Mathison, G.W. and Burwash, L. (1999) Growth and condition at weaning of extensively creep fed foals. *Journal of Equine Veterinary Science* 19(1), 45–49.

Colenbrander, B., Puyk, H., Zandee, A.R. and Parlevliet, J. (1992) Evaluation of the stallion for breeding. *Acta Veterinaria Scandinavica, Supplement* 88, 29–37.

Colenbrander, B., Gadella, B.M. and Stout, T.A.E. (2003) The predictive value of semen analysis in the evaluation of stallion fertility. *Reproduction in Domestic Animals* 38(4), 305–311.

Colleoni, S., Barbacini, S., Necchi, D., Duchi, R., Lazzari, G. and Galli, C. (2007). Application of ovum pick-up, intracytoplasmic sperm injection and embryo culture in equine practice. *Proceedings of the American Association of Equine Practitioners* 53, 554–559.

Collingsworth, M.G., Fuller, Z., Cox, J.E. and Argo, C.M. (2001) Changes in plasma gonadotrophin and prolactin concentrations following castration of the pony stallion. *Theriogenology* 55(5), 1171–1180.

Collins, A.M. and Buckley, T.C. (1993) Comparison of methods for early pregnancy detection. *Journal of Equine Veterinary Science* 13, 627–630.

Collins, C.W., Songsasen, N., Monfort, S.L., Bush, M., Wolfe, B., James, S.B., Wildt, D.E. and Pukashenthi, B.S. (2006) Seminal traits in the Przewalski's horse (*Equus ferus przewalski*) following electroejaculation. *Animal Reproduction Science* 94, 46–49.

Combs, G.B., LeBlanc, M.M., Neuwirth, L. and Tran, T.Q. (1996) Effects of prostaglandin F2 α, cloprostenol and fenprostenolene on uterine clearance of radiocoloid in the mare. *Theriogenology* 45, 1449–1455.

Conboy, H.S. (2011a) Management of stallions in artificial insemination. In: McKinnon, A.O., Squires, E.L., Vaala, W.E. and Varner, D.D. (eds) *Equine Reproduction*, 2nd edn. Wiley-Blackwell, Philadelphia, London, pp. 1197–1207.

Conboy, H.S. (2011b) The novice breeding stallion. In: McKinnon, A.O., Squires, E.L., Vaala, W.E. and Varner, D.D. (eds) *Equine Reproduction*, 2nd edn. Wiley-Blackwell, Philadelphia, London, pp. 1396–1401.

Conley, A.J. (2016) Review of reproductive endocrinology of the pregnant and parturient mare. *Theriogenology* 86, 355–365.

Conn, M. and Crowley, W.F. (1994) Gonadotropin-releasing hormone and its analogues. *Annual Reviews in Medicine* 45, 391–405.

Consuegra, C., Crespo, F., Dorado, J., Ortiz, I., Diaz-Jimenez, M., Pereira, B. and Hidalgo, M. (2018a) Comparison of different sucrose-based extenders for stallion sperm vitrification in straws. *Reproduction in Domestic Animals* 53(s2), 59–61.

Consuegra, C., Crespo, F., Dorado, J., Diaz-Jimenez, M., Pereira, B. and Hidalgo, M. (2018b) Low-density lipoproteins and milk serum proteins improve the quality of stallion sperm after vitrification in straws. *Reproduction in Domestic Animals* 54(s4), 86–89.

Consuegra, C., Crespo, F., Dorado, J., Diaz-Jimenez, M., Pereira, B., Ortiz, I. and Hidalgo, M. (2019) Vitrification of stallion sperm using 0.25 ml straws: effect of volume, concentration and carbohydrates (sucrose/trehalose/raffinose). *Animal Reproduction Science* 206, 69–77.

Cooke, C.D. (2015) Prophylactic intra-uterine antibacterial therapy. *Equine Veterinary Education* 27(10), 554–555.

Coomer, R.P.C., Gorvy, D.A., McKane, S.A. and Wilderjans, H. (2016) Inguinal percutaneous ultrasound to locate cryptorchid testes. *Equine Veterinary Education* 28(3), 150–154.

Cooper, J.J., Mcdonald, L. and Mills, D.S. (2000) The effect of increasing visual horizons on stereotypic weaving: implications for the social housing of stabled horses. *Applied Animal Behaviour Science* 69, 67–83.

Copetti, M.V., Santurio, J.M., Boeck, A.A.P., Silva, R.B., Bergermaier, L.A., Lubeck, I., Leal, A.B.M., Alves, J.H. and Ferreiro, L. (2001) Agalactia in mares fed with grass contaminated with *Claviceps purpurea*. *Mycopahologia* 154, 199–200.

Correa, J.R. and Zavos, P.M. (1994) The hypoosmotic swelling test: its employment as an assay to evaluate the functional integrity of frozen-thawed bovine spermatozoa. *Theriogenology* 42, 351–360.

Correa, J.R., Heersche Jr, G. and Zavos, P.M. (1997) Sperm membrane functional integrity and response of frozen-thawed bovine spermatozoa during the hypoosmotic swelling test incubation at varying temperatures. *Theriogenology* 47, 715–721.

Cottrill, C.M., Yenho, S. and O'Connor, W.N. (1997) Embryological development of the embryonic heart. *Equine Veterinary Journal, Supplement* 24, 14–18.

Coutinho da Silva, M.A. (2011) Gamete Intrafallopian Trasfer (GIFT) In: McKinnon, A.O., Squires, E.L., Vaala, E. and Varner, D.D. (eds) *Equine Reproduction*, 2nd edn. Wiley-Blackwell, Philadelphia, London, pp. 2945–2947.

Coutinho da Silva, M.A. and Alvarenga, M.A. (2011) Fungal endometritis. In: McKinnon, A.O., Squires, E.L., Vaala, E. and Varner, D.D. (eds) *Equine Reproduction*, 2nd edn. Wiley-Blackwell, Philadelphia, London, pp. 2643–2651.

Coutinho da Silva, M.A., Carnevale, E.M., Maclellan, K.A., Leao, K.M. and Squires, E.L. (2002a) Use of cooled and frozen semen during gamete intrafallopian transfer in mares. *Theriogenology* 58, 763–766.

Coutinho da Silva, M.A., Carnevale, E.M., Maclellan, L.J. and Scoggin, C.F. (2002b) Injection of blood into preovulatory follicles of equine oocyte transfer recipients does not prevent fertilisation of the recipient's oocyte. *Theriogenology* 57, 538.

Coutinho da Silva, M.A., Carnevale, E.M., Maclellan, I.J., Preis, K.A., Seidel, G.E. and Squires, E.L. (2004) Oocyte transfer in mares with intrauterine or intraoviductal insemination using fresh, cooled and frozen stallion semen. *Theriogenology* 61, 705–713.

Coutinho da Silva, M.A., Seidel Jr, G.E., Squires, E.L., Graham, J.K. and Carnevale, E.M. (2012) Effects of components of semen extenders on the binding of stallion spermatozoa to bovine or equine zonae pellucidae *Reproduction* 143, 577–585.

Couto, M.A. and Hughes, J.P. (1993) Sexually transmitted (venereal) diseases of horses. In: McKinnon, A.O. and Voss, J.L. (eds) *Equine Reproduction*. Lea and Febiger, Philadelphia, Pennsylvania, pp. 845–854.

Cox, J.E. (1975) Oestrone and equilin in the plasma of the pregnant mare. *Journal of Reproduction and Fertility Supplement* 23, 463–468.

Cox, J.E. (1982) Factors affecting testis' weight in normal and cryptorchid horses. *Journal of Reproduction and Fertility* 32, 129–134.

Cox, J.E. (1988) Hernias and ruptures: words to the heat of deeds. *Equine Veterinary Journal* 20, 155–156.

Cox, J.E. (1993a) Developmental abnormalities of the male reproductive tract. In: McKinnon, A.O. and

Voss, J.L. (eds) *Equine Reproduction*. Lea and Febiger, Philadelphia, Pennsylvania, pp. 895–906.

Cox, J.E. (1993b) Cryptorchid castration. In: McKinnon, A.O. and Voss, J.L. (eds) *Equine Reproduction*. Lea and Febiger, Philadelphia, Pennsylvania, pp. 915–920.

Cox, J.E., Williams, J.H., Rowe, P.H. and Smith, J.A. (1973) Testosterone in normal, cryptorchid and castrated male horses. *Equine Veterinary Journal* 5(2), 85–90.

Cox, J.E., Redhead, P.H. and Dawson, F.E. (1986) Comparison of the measurement of plasma testosterone and plasma estrogens for the diagnosis of cryptorchidism in the horse. *Equine Veterinary Journal* 18, 179–182.

Cox, L., Vanderwall, D.K., Parkinson, K.C., Sweat, A. and Isom, S.C. (2015) Expression profiles of select genes in cumulus-oocyte complexes from young and aged mares. *Reproduction, Fertility and Development* 27(6), 914–924.

Crabtree, J.R., Mateu-Sanchez, S., Cooke, C.D., Rogers, I.G., Rendle, D.I. and Wilsher, S. (2018) Investigation into the safety and clinical effects of a new progesterone releasing intra-vaginal device (PRID®Delta) in mares. *Journal of Equine Veterinary Science* 66, 123–133.

Craig, T.M., Scrutchfield, W.L. and Martin, M.T. (1993) Comparison of prophylactic pyrantel and suppressive invermectin anthelmintic programs in young horses. *Equine Practice* 15(3), 24–29.

Cran, D.G., Johnson, L.A. and Polge, C. (1995) Sex preselection in cattle: a field trial. *Veterinary Record* 136, 495–496.

Crews, L.J., Waelchi, R.O., Huang, C.X., Canny, M.J., McCully, M.E. and Betteridge, K.J. (2007) Electrolyte distribution and yolk sac morphology in frozen hydrated equine conceptuses during the second week of pregnancy. *Reproduction, Fertility and Development* 19, 804–814.

Cross, D.L., Redmond, L.M. Strickland, J.R. (1995) Equine fescue toxicosis: signs and solutions. *Journal of Animal Science* 73(3), 899–908.

Crossett, B., Stewart, F. and Allen, W.R. (1995) A unique progesterone dependant equine endometrial protein that associates strongly with embryonic capsule. *Journal of Reproduction and Fertility Abstract Series* 15, 11.

Crossett, B., Suire, E., Herrler, A., Allen, W.R. and Stewart, F. (1998) Transfer of a uterine lipocalin from the endometrium of the mare to the developing equine conceptus. *Biology of Reproduction* 59(3), 483–490.

Crowell-Davis, S.L. (2007) Sexual behavior of mares. *Hormones and Behaviour* 52, 12–17.

Crowhurst, R.C. (1977) Genital infection in mares. *Veterinary Record* 100, 476–478.

Crowhurst, R.C., Simpson, D.Y., Greenwood, R.E.S. and Ellis, D.R. (1979) Contagious equine metritis. *Veterinary Record* 104, 465.

Crozet, N. (1993) Fertilisation in vivo and in vitro. In: Thibault, C., Levasseur, M.C. and Hunter, R.H.F. (eds) *Reproduction in Mammals and Man*. Ellipses, Paris, pp. 327–347.

Cuervo-Arango, J. and Clark, A. (2010) The first ovulation of the breeding season in the mare: the effect of progesterone priming on pregnancy rate and breeding management (hCG response rate and number of services per cycle and mare). *Animal Reproduction Science* 118(2), 265–269.

Cuervo-Arango, J. and Newcombe, J.R. (2008) Repeatability of preovulatory follicular diameter and uterine edema pattern in two consecutive cycles in the mare and how they are in fluenced by ovulation inductors. *Theriogenology* 69(6), 681–687.

Cuervo-Arango, J. and Newcombe, J.R. (2009) The effect of manual removal of placenta immediately after foaling on subsequent fertility parameters in the mare. *Journal of Equine Veterinary Science* 29, 771–774.

Cuervo-Arango, J., Claes, A.N., Ruijter-Villani, M., Stout, T.A. (2018a) Likelihood of pregnancy after embryo transfer is reduced in recipient mares with a short preceding oestrus. *Equine Veterinary Journal* 50(3), 386–390.

Cuervo-Arango, J., Claes, A.N. and Stout, T.A.E. (2018b) Horse embryo diameter is influenced by the embryonic age but not by the type of semen used to inseminate donor mares. *Theriogenology* 115, 90–93.

Cuervo-Arango, J., Claes, A.N. and Stout, T.A. (2018c) Effect of embryo transfer technique on the likelihood of pregnancy in the mare: a comparison of conventional and Wilsher's forceps-assisted transfer. *Veterinary Record* 183(10), 323–328.

Cuervo-Arango, J., Claes, A.N., Beitsma, M. and Stout, T.A.E. (2019) The effect of different flushing media used to aspirate follicles on the outcome of a commercial ovum pickup-ICSI program in mares. *Journal of Equine Veterinary Science* 75, 74–77.

Cullinane, A., Weld, J., Osborne, M., Nelly, M., Mcbride, C. and Walsh, C. (2001) Field studies on equine influenza vaccination regimes in thoroughbred foals and yearlings. *Veterinary Journal* 161(2), 174–185.

Cupps, P.T. (1991) *Reproduction in Domestic Animals*, 4th edn. Academic Press, New York.

Curcio, B.R. and Nogueira, C.E.W. (2012) Newborn adaptations and healthcare throughout the first age of the foal. *Animal Reproduction* 9(3), 182–187.

Curnow, E.M. (1991) Ultrasonography of the mare's uterus. *Equine Veterinary Education* 3(4), 190–193.

Curry, M.R., Eady, P.E. and Mills, D.S. (2007) Reflections on mare behavior: social and sexual perspectives. *Journal of Veterinary Behaviour* 2, 149–157.

Daels, P.F. and Hughes, J.P. (1993a) The normal estrous cycle. In: McKinnon, A.O. and Voss, J.L. (eds) *Equine Reproduction*. Lea and Febiger, Philadelphia, Pennsylvania, pp. 121–132.

Daels, P.F. and Hughes, J.P. (1993b) The abnormal cycle. In: McKinnon, A.O. and Voss, J.L. (eds) *Equine Reproduction*. Lea and Febiger, Philadelphia, Pennsylvania, pp. 144–160.

Daels, P.F., Stabenfeldt, G.H., Hughes, J.P., Odensvik, K. and Kindahl, H. (1990) The source of oestrogen in early pregnancy in the mare. *Journal of Reproduction and Fertility, Supplement* 90(1), 55–61.

Daels, P.F., Ammon, D.C., Stabenfeldt, G.H., Liu, I.K., Hughes, J.P. and Lasley, B.L. (1991a) Urinary and plasma oestrogen conjugates, estradiol, and estrone concentrations in nonpregnant and early pregnant mares. *Theriogenology* 35, 1001–1017.

Daels, P.F., Jorge De Moraes, M., Stabenfeldt, G.H., Hughes, H. and Lesley, B. (1991b) The corpus luteum a major source of oestrogen in early pregnancy in the mare. *Journal of Reproduction and Fertility, Supplement* 44, 502–508.

Daels, P.F., Albrecht, B.A. and Mohammed, H.O. (1995) In vitro regulation of luteal function in mares. *Reproduction in Domestic Animals* 30, 211–217.

Daels, P.F., Besognet, B., Hansen, B., Mohammed, H., Odensvik, K. and Kindahl, H. (1996) Effect of progesterone on prostaglandin F 2 alpha secretion and outcome of pregnancy during chloprostenol induced abortion in mares *American Journal of Veterinary Research* 57, 1331–1337.

Daels, P.F., Fatone, B.S., Hansen, B.S. and Concannon, P.W. (2000) Dopamine antagonist-induced reproductive function in anoestrous mares; gonadotrophin secretion and the effects of environmental cues. *Journal of Reproduction and Fertility, Supplement* 56, 173–183.

Dalin, A.M.O., Andresen, O. and Malmgren (2002) Immunization against GnRH in mature mares: antibody titers, ovarian function, hormonal levels and estrous behavior. *Journal of Veterinary Medicine A: Physiology Pathology Clinical Medicine* 49, 125–131.

Darenius, K., Kindahl, H. and Madej, A. (1988) Clinical and endocrine studies in mares with a known history of repeated conceptus losses. *Theriogenology* 29, 1215–1232.

Darr, C.R., Moraes, L.E., Scanlan, T.N., Baumber-Skaife, J., Loomis, P.R., Cortopassi, G. A., and Meyers, S.A. (2017) Sperm Mitochondrial Function is Affected by Stallion Age and Predicts Post-Thaw Motility. *Journal of Equine Veterinary Science* 50, 52–61.

Dascanio, J. (2000) How to diagnose and treat fungal endometritis. In: *Proceedings of the 46th Annual American Association of Equine Practitioners*, pp. 316–319.

Dascanio, J. (2011a) External reproductive anatomy. In: McKinnon, A.O., Squires, E.L., Vaala, W.E., Varner, D.D. (eds) *Equine Reproduction*, 2nd edn. Wiley-Blackwell, Philadelphia, London, pp. 1577–1582.

Dascanio, J.J. (2011b) How and when to treat endometritis with systemic or local antibiotics. *Proceedings of the 57th Annual Convention of the American Association of Equine Practionners* 18–22 November 2011, San Antonio, Texas, pp. 24–31.

Dascanio, J. (2014a) Twins reduction: Transabdominal fetal cardiac puncture. In: Dascanio, J. and McCue, P.M. (eds) *Equine Reproductive Proceedures*, Wiley-Blackwell, Hoboken, New Jersey.

Dascanio, J. (2014b) Removal of persistent hymen. In: Dascanio, J. and McCue, P.M. (eds) *Equine Reproductive Proceedures*, Wiley-Blackwell, Hoboken, New Jersey.

Dascanio, J.J., Schweizer, C. and Ley, W.B. (2001) Equine fungal endometritis. *Equine Veterinary Education* 13, 324–329.

Davies Morel, M.C.G. (1999) *Equine Artificial Insemination*. CAB International, Wallingford, UK, pp. 406.

Davies Morel, M.C.G. and Gunnarsson, V. (2000) A survey of the fertility of Icelandic stallions. *Animal Reproduction Science* 64, 49–64.

Davies Morel, M.C.G. and Newcombe, J.R. (2008) The efficacy of different hCG dose rates and the effect of hCG treatment on ovarian activity: ovulation, multiple ovulation, pregnancy, multiple pregnancy, synchrony of multiple ovulation in the mare. *Animal Reproduction Science* 109 1–4), 189–199.

Davies Morel, M.C.G. and O'Sullivan, J.A.M. (2001) Ovulation rate and distribution in the thoroughbred mare, as determined by ultrasonic scanning: the effect of age. *Animal Reproduction Science* 66, 59–70.

Davies Morel, M.C.G., Newcombe, J.R. and Holland, S.J. (2002) Factors affecting gestation length in the Thoroughbred mare. *Animal Reproduction Science* 74, 175–185.

Davies Morel, M.C.G., Newcombe, J. and Swindlehurst, J. (2005) The effect of age on mutiple ovulation rates, multiple pregnancy rates and embryonic vesicle diameter in the mare. *Theriogenology* 63(9), 2482–2493.

Davies Morel, M.C.G., Newcombe, J.R. and Hinchliffe, J. (2009) The relationship between consecutive pregnancies in Thoroughbred mares. Does the location of one pregnancy affect the location of the next, is this affected by mare age and foal heat to conception interval or related to pregnancy success. *Theriogenology* 7, 1072–1078.

Davies Morel, M.C.G., Newcombe, J.R. and Lauber, M. (2012) Manual reduction of multiple embryos in the mare. The effect on subsequent pregnancy outcome. *The Veterinary Journal* 192, 322–324.

Davies Morel, M.C.G., Lawlor, O. and Nash, D.M. (2013) Equine endometrial cytology and bacteriology: effectiveness for predicting live foaling rates. *Veterinary Journal* 198(1), 206–211.

Davies Morel, M.C.G., Newcombe, J. and Reynolds, N. (2015) Asynchronous ovulations in the mare: different frequency with season. *Veterinary Record* 176(12), 310–311.

Davies, T.J. (1995) Turner's syndrome (karyotype 63 XO) in a Thoroughbred mare. *Equine Veterinary Education* 7(1), 15–17.

Day, F.T. (1940) The stallion and fertility. The technique of sperm collection and insemination. *Veterinary Record* 52, 597–602.

Day, W.E., Evans, J.W., Vogelsang, M.M. and Westhusin, M.E. (1995) Characterisation of the cervix in cycling mares using ultrasound. *Biology of Reproduction, Monograph 1 Equine Reproduction VI*, Society for the Study of Fertility, pp. 519–526.

De Amorim, M.D., Chenier, T., Nairn, D., Green, J., Manning, S. and Card, C.J. (2016) Complications associated with intrauterine glass marbles in five mares. *American Veterinary Medicine Assocociation* 249(10), 1196–1201.

De Coster, R., Cambiaso, C.L. and Masson, P.L. (1980) Immunological diagnosis of pregnancy in the mare by agglutination of latex particles. *Theriogenology* 13, 433.

Deichsel, K., Schrammel, N., Aurich, J. and Aurich, C. (2016) Effects of a long-day light programme on the motility and membrane integrity of cooled-stored and cyropreserved semen in Shetland pony stallions. *Animal Reproduction Science* 167, 68–73.

De la Cueva, F.I., Pujol, M.R., Rigau, T., Bonet, S., Briz, M. and Rodriguez-Gill, J.E. (1997) Resistance to osmotic stress of horse spermatozoa: the role of ionic pumps and their relationship to cryopreservation success. *Theriogenology* 48, 947–968.

Del Campo, M.R., Donoso, M.X., Parrish, J.J. and Ginther, O.J. (1990) In vitro fertilisation of in vitro-matured equine oocytes. *Journal of Equine Veterinary Science* 10, 18–22.

De Leon, P.M., Campos, V.F., Corcini, C.D., Santos, E.C., Rambo, G., Lucia, T. Jr., Dechamps, J.C. and Collares, T. (2012) Cryopreservation of immature equine oocytes, coparing a solid surface vitrification process with open pulled straws and the use of a sythetic ice blocker. *Theriogenology* 77 (1), 21–27.

Dell'Aquila, M.E., Cho, Y.S., Minoia, P., Triana, V., Fusco, S., Lacalandra, G.M. and Maritato, F. (1997a) Effects of follicular fluid supplementation of in-vitro maturation medium on the fertilization and development of equine oocytes after in-vitro fertilization or intracytoplasmic sperm injection. *Human Reproduction* 12, 2766–2772.

Dell'Aquila, M.E., Cho, Y.S., Minoia, P., Traina, V., Fusco, S., Lacalandra, G.M. and Maritato, F. (1997b) Intracytoplasmic sperm injection (ICSI) versus conventional IVF on abattoir-derived and in vitro-matured equine oocytes. *Theriogenology* 47, 1139–1156.

Dell'Aquila, M.E., Masterson, M., Maritato, F. and Hinrichs, J. (2000) Chromatin configuration meiotic competence and success of intra-cytoplasmic sperm injection in horse oocytes collected by follicular aspiration or scaping. In: Katila, T. and Wade, J.F. (eds) *Proceedings of the 5th International Symposium on Equine Embryo Transfer*, Havemeyer Foundation Monograph Series 3. Saari, Finland, pp. 37–38.

Del Piero, F., Wilkins, P.A., Lopez, J.W., Glaser, A.L., Dubovi, E.J., Schlafer, D.H. and Lein, D.H. (1997) Equine viral arteritis in new-born foals: clinical, pathological, serological, microbiological and immunohistochemical observations *Equine Veterinary Journal* 29, 178–185.

De Mestre, A.M., Hanlon, D., Adams, A.P., Runcan, E., Leadbeater, J.C., Tallmadge, R., Erb, H.N., Costa, C.C., Miller, D., Allen, W.R. and Antczak, D.F. (2010) Prolonged estrus suppression by ectopic transplantation of invasive equine trophoblast. *Animal Reproduction Science* 121(1–2 Supplement), 60–61.

De Mestre, A.M., Antczak, D.F. and Allen, W.R. (2011) Equine chorionic gonadotrophin (eCG) In: McKinnon, A.O., Squires, E.L., Vaala, E. and Varner, D.D. (eds) *Equine Reproduction*, 2nd edn. Wiley-Blackwell, Philadelphia, London, pp. 1648–1664.

De Mestre, A.M., Rose, B.V., Chang, Y.M., Wathes, D.C. and Verheyen, K.L.P. (2019) Multivariable analysis to determine risk factors associated with early pregnancy loss in thoroughbred broodmares. *Theriogenology* 124, 18–23.

Demick, D.S., Voss, J.L. and Pickett, B.W. (1976) Effect of cooling, storage, glycerolization and spermatozoal numbers on equine fertility. *Journal of Animal Science* 43, 633–637.

Deng, I., Duan, H., Zhang, X., Zeng, S., Wu, C. and Han, G. (2014) Advances in the research and application of artificial insemination to equids in China. *Journal of Equine Veterinary Science* 34(3), 351–359.

Denker, H.W., Betteridge, K.J. and Sirois, J. (1987) Shedding of the capsule and proteinase activity in the horse. *Journal of Reproduction and Fertility Supplement* 35, 708.

Denniston, D.J., Graham, J.K., Squires, E.L. and Brinsko, S.P. (1997) The effect of liposomes composed of phosphatidylserine and cholesterol on fertility rates using thawed equine spermatozoa. *Journal of Equine Veterinary Science* 17(12), 675–676.

De Ribeaux, M.B. (1994) Weaning wisdom. *Modern Horse Breeding* 11(7), 28–31.

Devireddy, R.V., Swanlund, D.J., Alghamdi, A.S., Duoos, L.A., Troedsson, M.H., Bischof, J.C. and Roberts, K.P. (2002a) Measured effect of collection and cooling conditions on the motility and the water transport parameters at subzero temperatures of equine spermatozoa. *Reproduction* 124(5), 643–648.

Devireddy, R.V., Swandlund, D.J., Olin, T., Vincente, W., Troedsson, M.H.T., Bischof, J.C. and Roberts, K.P. (2002b) Cryopreservation of equine sperm: optimal cooling rates in the presence and absence of cryoprotective agents determined using differential scanning calorimetry. *Biology Reproduction* 66, 222–231.

De Vries, P.J. (1987) Evaluation of the use of fresh, extended, transported stallion semen in the Netherlands. *Journal of Reproduction and Fertility, Supplement* 35, 641.

De Vries, P.J. (1993) Diseases of the testes, penis and related structures. In: McKinnon, A.O. and Voss, J.L. (eds) *Equine Reproduction*. Lea and Febiger, Philadelphia, Pennsylvania, pp. 878–884.

Dias, E.H., Mezalira, T.S., Pinto Neto, A., Silva, L.S. da, Tironi, S.M.T., Almeida, A.R.G. and Martinez, A.C. (2018) Deslorelin acetate to induce ovulation in mares. *Pubvet* 12(5), 88, 1–4.

Diaz, F., Bondiolli, K., Paccamonti, D. and Gentry, G. (2016) Cryopreservation of day 8 embryos after blastocyst micromanipulation and vitrification. *Theriogenology* 85, 894–903.

Didelot, X., Bowden, R., Wilson, D.J., Peto, T.E.A. and Crook, D.W. (2012) Transforming clinical microbiology with bacterial genome sequencing. *Nature Reviews Genetics* 13, 601–612.

Diekman, M.A., Braun, W., Peter, D. and Cook, D. (2002) Seasonal serum concentrations of melatonin in cycling and non-cycling mares. *Journal of Animal Science* 80, 2949–2952.

Diemer, T., Huwe, P., Ludwig, M., Hauck, E.W. and Weidner, W. (2003) Urogenital infection and sperm motility. *Andrologia* 35(5), 283–287.

Digby, J. (1996) The likely impact of dual hemisphere serving (shuttle) stallions on the stalion population and on covering patterns in Australia. *Australian Equine Veterinaian* 14(3), 109–111.

Digrassie, W.A. and Slusher, S.H. (2002) Quality. In: Cowell, R.L. and Tyler, D. (eds) *Diagnostic Cytology and Hematology of the Horse*, 2nd edn. Mosby, St Louis, Missouri, pp.185–199.

Dimmick, M.A., Gimenez, T. and Schalager, R.L. (1993) Ovarian follicular dynamics and duration of estrus and diestrus in Arabian vs Quarter horse mares. *Animal Reproduction Science* 31, 123–129.

Dinger, J.E., Noiles, E.E. and Bates, M.L. (1981) Effect of progesterone impregnated vaginal sponges and PMS administration on oestrous synchronisation in mares. *Theriogenology* 16, 231–237.

Dippert, K.D., Hofferer, S., Palmer, E., Jasko, D.J. and Squires, E.L. (1992) Initiation of superovulation in mares 5 or 12 days after ovulation using equine pituitary extract with or without GnRH analogue. *Theriogenology* 38, 695–710.

Dixon, P.A. (2017) The Evolution of Horses and the Evolution of Equine Dentistry. In: *Proceedings of the 63rd Annual Convention of the American Association of Equine Practitioners* San Antonio, Texas November 17–21, pp. 79–116.

Doarn, R.T., Threlfall, W.R. and Kline, R. (1985) Umbilical blood flow and effects of premature severance in the neonatal horse. In: *Proceedings of the 1985 Annual Society of Theriogenology*. Society of Theriogenology, Hastings, Nebraska, pp. 175–178.

Doarn, R.T., Threlfall, W.R. and Kline, R. (1987) Umbilical blood flow and the effects of premature severance in the neonatal horse. *Theriogenology* 28, 789–800.

Dobrinski, I., Thomas, P.G.A. and Ball, B.A. (1995) Cryopreservation reduces the ability of equine spermatozoa to attach to oviductal epithelial cells and zonae pellucdiae in vitro. *Journal of Andrology* 16, 536–542.

Dobrinsky, J.R. (2002) Advancements in cryopreservation of domestic animal embryos. *Theriogenology* 57, 285–302.

Dobson, H. and Smith, R.F. (2000) What is stress and how does it affect reproduction. *Animal Reproduction Science* 60, 743–752.

Doig, P.A. and Waelchi, R.O. (1993) Endometrial biopsy. In: McKinnon, A.O. and Voss, J.L. (eds) *Equine Reproduction*. Lea and Febiger, Philadelphia, Pennsylvania, pp. 225–233.

Doig, P.A., McKnight, J.D. and Miller R.B. (1981) The use of endometrial biopsy in the infertile mare. *Canadian Veteerinary Journal* 22, 72–76.

Donadeu, F.X. and Pedersen, H.G. (2008) Follicle development in mares. *Reproduction in Domestic Animals* 43 Supplement 2, 224–231.

Doreau, M. and Boulet, S. (1989) Recent knowledge on mare's milk production. A review. *Livestock Production Science* 22, 213–235.

Doreau, M., Martin-Rosset, W. and Boulet, S. (1988) Energy requirements and the feeding of mares during lactation: a review. *Livestock Production Science* 20(1), 53–68.

Doreau, M., Boulet, S., Bauchart, D., Barlet, J. and Patureau-Mirand, P. (1990) Yield and composition of milk from lactating mares: effect of lactation stage and individual differences. *Journal of Diary Research* 57, 449–454.

Dott, H.M. (1975) Morphology of stallion spermatozoa. *Journal of Reproduction and Fertility, Supplement* 23, 41–46.

Dott, H.M. and Foster, G.C. (1972) A technique for studying the morphology of mammalian spermatozoa which are eosinophilic in differential "live/dead" stain. *Journal of Reproduction and Fertility* 29, 443–445.

Douglas, R.H. (1979) Review of induction of superovulation and embryo transfer in the equine. *Theriogenology* 11(1), 33–46.

Douglas, R.H. (1980) Pregnancy rates following non-surgical embryo transfer in the equine. *Journal and Animal Science* 51(Suppl 1), 272.

Douglas, R.H. (2004) Endocrine diagnostics in the broodmare: what you need to know about progestins and estrogens. *Proceedings of society of Theriogenology* pp. 1–10.

Douglas, R.H. and Ginther, O.J. (1975) Development of the equine fetus and placenta. *Journal of Reproduction and Fertility, Supplement* 23, 503–505.

Douglas, R.H., Nuti, L. and Ginther, O.J. (1974) Induction of ovulation and multiple ovulation in seasonally anovulatory mares with equine pituitary fractions. *Theriogenology* 2(6), 133–141.

Douglas, R.H. and Umphenour, N. (1992) Endocrine abnormalities and hormonal therapy. In: Blanchard, T.L., Varner, D.D. and Turner, A.S. (eds) *Stallion Management. The Veterinary Clinics of*

North America, Equine Practice. W.B. Saunders, Philadelphia, Pennsylvania, pp. 237–249.

Douglas-Hamilton, D.H., Osol, R., Osol, G., Driscoll, D. and Noble, H. (1984) A field study of the fertility of transported equine semen. *Theriogenology* 22(3), 291–304.

Dowsett, K.F. and Knott, L.M. (1996) The influence of age and breed on stallion semen. *Therogenology*, 46(3), 397–412.

Dowsett, K.F., Knott, C.M., Woodward, R.A. and Bodero, D.A.V. (1993) Seasonal variation in the oestrus cycle of mares in the subtropics. *Theriogenology* 39, 631–653.

Draincourt, M.A., Paris, A., Roux, C., Mariana, J.C. and Palmer, E. (1982) Ovarian follicular populations in pony and saddle-type mares. *Reproduction Nutrition and Development* 22, 1035–1047.

Dubcová, J., Bartošová, J. and Komárková, M. (2015) Effects of prompt versus stepwise relcation to a novel environment on foals' responses to weaning in domestic horses (*Equus caballus*). *Journal of Veterinary Behavior: Clinical Applications and Research* 10(4), 346–352.

Duchamp, G., Allard, A., Grizelj, J., Plotto, A., Bruneau, B., Mermillod, P., Meriaux, J.C., Bruyas, J-F. and Vidament, M. (2006) Effect of condition of incorporation and concentration of cryoprotectants on equine embryo viability after freezing. *Animal Reproduction Science* 94, 374–377.

Duggan, V.E., Holyoak, G.R., MaCallister, C.G. and Confer, A.W. (2007) Influence of induction of parturition on the neonatal acute phase response in foals. *Theriogenology* 67(2), 372–381.

Dunn, H.O., Smiley, D. and Mcentee, K. (1981) Two equine true hermaphrodites with 64XX/64XY and 63X/63XY chimerism. *Cornell Veterinarian* 71, 123–135.

Duranthan, V., Watson, A.J. and Lonergan, P. (2008) Preimplantation embryo programming, transcription, epigenetics and cutural environment. *Reproduction* 135, 141–150.

Duren, S.E. and Crandell, K. (2001) The role of vitamins in the growth of horses. In: Pagan, J.O. and Geor, R.J. (eds) *Advances in Equine Nutrition II*. Nottingham University Press, Nottingham, UK, pp. 169–178.

Durkin, K.W., Raudsepp, T. and Chowdhary, B.P. (2011) Cytogenic evaluation. In: McKinnon, A.O., Squires, E.L., Vaala, E. and Varner, D.D. (eds) *Equine Reproduction*, 2nd edn. Wiley-Blackwell, Philadelphia, London, pp. 1462–1468.

Dybdal, N.O., Hargreaves, K.H., Madigan, J.E., Gribble, D.H., Kennedy, D.C. and Stabendfeldt, G.H. (1994) Diagnostic testing for pituitary pars intermedia dysfunction in horses. *Journal of the American Veterinary Association* 204, 627–632.

Dyce, K.M., Sack, W.O. and Wensing, C.J.G. (1996) *Textbook of Veterinary Anatomy*, 2nd edn. W.B. Saunders, Philadelphia, Pennsylvania.

Eagle, R.C. and Tortonese, D.J. (2000) Characterisation and distribution of gonadotrophs in the pars distalis and pars tuberalis of the equine pituitary gland during the oestrus cycle and seasonal anoestrus. *Biology of Reproduction* 63(3), 826–832.

Easley, J. (1993) External perineal conformation. In: Mckinnon, A.O. and Voss, J.L. (eds) *Equine Reproduction*. Lea and Febiger, Philadelphia, Pennsylvania, pp. 19–26.

East, L.M., Van Saun, R.J. and Vanderwall, D.K. (1999a) A review of the technique and 1997 practitioner-based survey, equine embryo transfer: Part 1: donor recipient selection and preparation. *Equine Practice* 20(8), 16–20.

East, L.M., Van Saun, R.J. and Vanderwall, D.K. (1999b) A review of the technique and 1997 practitioner based survey, equine embryo transfer. Part 2: embryo recovery and transfer techniques. *Equine Practice* 21(1), 8–12.

East, L.M., Van Saun, R.J. and Vanderwall, D.K. (1999c) A review of the technique and 1997 practitioner-based survey, equine embryo transfer: Part 3: client and veterinary economics. *Equine Practice* 21, 16–19.

Edwards, D.J., Brownlow, M.A. and Hutchins, D.R. (1990) Indices of renal function: values in eight normal foals from birth to 56 days. *Australian Veterinary Journal* 67, 251–254.

Edwards, J. (2008). Pathologic conditions of the stallion reproductive tract. *Animal Reproduction Science*, 107(3–4), 197–207.

El-Badry, D.A., El-Maaty, A.M.A. and El-Sisy, G.A. (2017) The effect of trehalose supplmentation of INRA-82 extender on quality and fertility of cooled and frozen-thawed stalion spermatozoa. *Journal of Equine Veterinary Science* 48, 86–92.

Eilts, B.E. (2011) Puberty. In: McKinnon, A.O., Squires, E.L, Vaala, W.E. and Varner, D.D. (eds)

Equine Reproduction, 2nd edn. Wiley-Blackwell, Pennsylvania, London, pp. 1689–1695.

Eilts, B.E., Scholl, D.T., Paccamonti, D.C., Causey, R., Klimczak, J.C. and Corley, J.R. (1995) Prevalance of endometrial cysts and their effect of fertility. *Biological Reproductive Monographs* 1, 527–532.

Elderidge-Panuska, W.D., Caracciolo di Brienza, V., Seidel, G.E., Squires, E.L. and Carnevale, E.M. (2005) Establishment of pregnancies after serial dilution or direct transfer by vitrified equine embryos. *Theriogenology* 63, 1308–1319.

Elhay, M., Newbold, A., Britton, A., Turley, P., Dowsett, K. and Walker, J. (2007) Supression of behaviour and physiological oestrus in the mare by vaccination against GnRH. *Australian Veterinary Journal* 85(1–2), 39–45.

Elkasapy, A.H. and Ibrahim, I.M. (2015) Contribution to reconstruction of third degree retovestibular lacerations in mares. *Open Veterinary Journal* 5(1), 23–26.

Ellenberger, C., Wilsher, S., Allen, W.R., Hoffmann, C., Kölling, M., Bazer, F.W., Klug, J., Schoon, D. and Schoon, H.A. (2008) Immunolocalisation of the uterine secretory proteins uterocalin, uteroferrin and uteroglobin in the mare's uterus and placenta throughout pregnancy. *Theriogenology* 70(5), 746–757.

Ellerbrock, R., Canisso, I., Feijo, L., Lima, F., Shipley, C. and Kline, K. (2016) Diagnosis and effects of urine contamination in cooled-extended stallion semen. *Theriogenology* 85(7), 1219–1224.

Ellendorff, F. and Schams, D. (1988) Characteristics of milk ejection, associated intramammary pressure changes and oxytocin release in the mare. *Journal of Endocrinology* 119, 219–227.

Elliott, C., Morton, J. and Chopin, J. (2009) Factors affecting foal birth weight in Thorough bred horses. *Theriogenology* 71, 683–689.

Embertson, R.M. (1992) The indications and surgical techniques for Caesarean section in the mare. *Equine Veterinary Education* 4, 31–36.

Embertson, R. (1999) Dystocia and caesarean section: the importance of duration and good judgement. *Equine Veterinary Journal* 31(3), 179–180.

Enders, A.C. and Carter, A.M. (2006) Comparative placentation: some interesting modifications for histotrophic nutrition—A review. *Placenta* 27, Supplement A, S11–16.

Enders, A.C. and Lui, I.K.M. (1991) Lodgement of the equine blastocyst in the uterus from fixation through endometrial cup formation. *Journal of Reproduction and Fertility, Supplement* 44, 427.

Enders, A.C., Lantz, K.C., Lui, I.K.M. and Schlafke, S. (1988) Loss of polar trophoblast during differentiation of the blastocyst of the horse. *Journal of Reproduction and Fertility* 83, 447–460.

Enders, A.C., Schlafke, S., Lantz, K.C. and Lui, I.K.M. (1993) Endoderm cells of the yolk sac from day 7 until formation of the definitive yolk sac placenta. *Equine Veterinary Journal, Supplement* 15, 3–9.

Enzerink, E. (1998) The menace response and papillary light reflex in neonatal foals. *Equine Veterinary Journal* 30, 546–548.

Eppig, J.J. (2001) Oocyte control of ovarian follicular development and function in mammals. *Reproduction* 122, 829–838.

Erber, R., Wulf, M., Rose-Meierhöfer, S., Becker-Birck, M., Möstl, E., Aurich, J., Hoffmann, G. and Aurich, C. (2012) Behavioral and physiological responses of young horses to different weaning protocols: a pilot study. *Stress* 15(2), 184–194.

Erhard, M.H., Luft, C., Remler, H.P. and Stangassinger, M. (2001) Assessment of colostrum stransffer and systemic availability of immunoglobulin G in new bornn foals using a newly developed enzyme-linked immunosorbent assay (ELISA) system. *Journal of Animal Physiology and Nutrition* 85, 164–173.

Ericsson, R.J. and Glass, R.H. (1982) Functional differences between sperm bearing the X-and Y-chromosome. In: Amann, R.P. and Seidel, G.E. (eds) *Prospects for Sexing Mammalian Sperm*. Colorado Association University Press, Boulder, Colorado, pp. 201–211.

Esteller-Vico, A., Ball, B.A., Troedsson, M.H.T. and Squires, E.L. (2017) Endocrine changes, fetal growth, and uterine artery hemodynamics after chronic estrogen suppression during the last trimester of equine pregnancy *Biology of Reproduction* 96(2), 414–423.

Estepa, J.C., Aguilera-Tejero, E., Zafra, R., Mayer-Valor, R., Rodriguez, M. and Perez, J. (2006a) An unusual case of generalized soft tissue mineralization in a suckling foal. *Veterinary Pathology* 43, 64–67.

Estepa, J.C., Mayer-Valor, R., Lopez, I., Santisteban, J.M., Ruiz, I. and Aguilera-Tejero, E. (2006b)

What is your diagnosis? Abscess developed as a result of a scrotal and testicular lesions. *Journal of the American Veterinary Medicine Association* 228, 515–516.

Eustace, A.R. (1992) *Explaining Laminitis and Its Prevention*. Laminitis Clinic, Chippenham, UK, pp. 96.

Evans, H.E. and Sack, W.O. (1973) Prenatal development of domestic and laboratory mammals: growth curves, external features and selected references. *Anatomy, Histology and Embryology* 2, 11–45.

Evans, M.J., Alexander, S.L., Irvine, C.H.G., Livesey, J.H. and Donald, R.A.S. (1991) *In vitro* and *in vivo* studies of equine prolactin secretion throughout the year. *Journal of Reproduction and Fertility, Supplement* 44, 27–35.

Evans, M.J., Alexaner, S.L., Irvine, C.H.G., Taylor, T.B., Kitson, N.E. and Livesey, J.H. (2002) Administration of the GnRH antagonist cetrorelix during the luteal phase in the mare. *Theriogenology* 58, 527–532.

Evans, M.J., Gastal, E.L., Silva, L.A., Gastal, M.O., Kitson, N.E., Alexander, S.L. and Irvine, C.H.G. (2006) Plasma LH concentrations after administration of human chorionic gonadotrophin to oestrous mares *Animal Reproduction Science* 94, 191–194.

Evenson, D.P., Sailer, B.L. and Josh, L.K. (1995) Relationship between stallion sperm deoxyribonucleic acid (DNA), susceptibility to denaturation *in situ* and presence of DNA strand breaks: implications for fertility and embryo viability. *Biology of Reproduction, Monograph Equine Reproduction VI* 1, 655–659.

Evenson, D.P., Larson, K.L. and Jost, L.K. (2002) Sperm chromatin structure assay: its clinical use for detecting sperm DNA fragmentation in male infertility and comparisons with other techniques *Journal of Andrology* 23, 25–43.

Fahy, G.M. (1986) The relevance of cryoprotectant 'toxicity' to cryobiology. *Cryobiology* 23, 1–13.

Fair, T. (2003) Follicular oocyte growth and acquisition of developmental competence. *Animal Reproduction Science* 78, 203–216.

Farjanikish, G., Sayari, M., Raisi, A. and Shirian, S. (2016) Diffuse type testicular seminoma in a stallion. *Compendium of Clinical Pathology* 25(6), 1133–1136.

Farquhar, V.J., McCue, P.M., Vanderwall, D.K. and Squires, E.L. (2000) Efficiency of the GnRH agonist deslorelin acetate for inducing ovulation in mares relative to age of mare and season. *Journal of Equine Veterinary Science* 20, 722–725.

Farquhar, V.J., McCue, P.M., Nett, T.M. and Squires, E.L. (2001) Effect of deslorelin acetate on gonadotrophin secretion and ovarian follicle development in cycling mares. *Journal of American Veterinary Medicine Association* 218, 749–752.

Fay, J.E. and Douglas, R.H. (1987) Changes in thecal and granulosa cell LH and FSH receptor content associated with follicular fluid and peripheral plasma gonadotrophin and steroid hormone concentrations in pre-ovulatory follicles of mares. *Journal of Reproduction and Fertility, Supplement* 37, 169–181.

Fazeli, A.R., Steenweg, W., Bevers, M.M., Bracher, V., Parlevliet, J.M. and Collenbrander, B. (1993) Use of sperm binding to homologous hemizona pellucida to predict stallion fertility. *Equine Veterinary Jounrnal* 15 (Suppl), 57–59.

Fazeli, A.R., Steenweg, W., Bevers, M.M., Broek van den, J., Bracher, V., Parlevliet, J.M. and Collenbrander, B. (1995) Relationships between stallion sperm binding to homologous hemizonae and fertility. *Theriogenology* 44, 751–760.

Fena, F.J., Ball, B.A. and Squires, E.L. (2018) A new method for evaluating stallion sperm viability and mitochondrial membrane potential in fixed semen samples. *Cytometry Part B Clinical Cytometry* 94(2), 302–311.

Ferreira, J.C.P., Meira, C., Papa, F.O., Landin, E., Alvarenga, F.C., Alveranga, M.A. and Buratini, J. (1997) Cryopreservation of equine embryos with glycerol plus sucrose and glycerol plus 1,2-propanediol. *Equine Veterinary Journal, Supplement* 25, 88–93.

Ferreira, J.C., Gastal, E.L. and Ginther, O.J. (2008) Uterine blood flow and perfusion in mares with uterine cysts: effect of the size of the cystic area and age. *Reproduction* 135, 541–550.

Ferris, R.A. and McCue, P.M. (2010) The effects of dexamethasone and prednisolone on pituitary and ovarian function in the mare. *Equine Veterinary Journal* 42(5), 438–443.

Ferris, R.A., McCue, P.M., Borlee, G.I., Glapa, K.E., Martin, K.H., Mangalea, M.R., Hennet, M.L., Wolfe, L.M., Broeckling, C.D. and Borleeb, B.R. (2017) Model of Chronic Equine Endometritis

Involving a Pseudomonas aeruginosa Biofilm. *Infection and Immunity* 25(12), 1–14.

First, N.L. and Alm, C. (1977) Dexamethosone induced parturition in pony mares. *Journal of Animal Science* 44, 1072–1075.

Fiser, P.S., Hansen, C., Underhill, K.L. and Shrestha, J.N.B. (1991) The effect of induced ice nucleation (seeding) on the post thaw motility and acrosomal integrity of boar spermatozoa. *Animal Reproduction Science* 24, 293–304.

Fischer, A.T. (1991) Standing lapaoscopic surgery. *Veterinary Clinics of North America, Equine* 7(3), 641–647.

Fitzgerald, B.P. and McManus, C.J. (2000) Photoperiodic signals as determinants of seasonal anestrus in the mare. *Biology of Reproduction* 63, 335–340.

Fitzgerald, B.P., Reedy, S.E., Sessions, D.R., Pwell, D.M. and McManus, C.J. (2002) Potential signals mediating the maintenance of reproductive activity during the non-breeding season of the mare. *Reproduction, Supplement* 59, 115–129.

Fletcher, M.S., Topliff, D.R., Cooper, S.R., Freeman, D.W. and Geisert, R.D. (2000) Influence of age and sex on serum osteocalcin concentrations in horses at weaning and during physical conditioning. *Journal of Equine Veterinary Science* 20(2), 125–126.

Fleury, J.J., Fleury, P.D.C. and Landim-Alvarenge, F.C. (2002) Effect of embryo diameter and storage period on pregnancy rates obtained with embryos stored in Ham's F-10 with Hepes buffer at a temperatire of 15–18°C – preliminary results. *Theriogenology* 58, 749–750.

Flood, P.F. (1993) Fertilisation, early embryo development and establishment of the placenta. In: McKinnon, A.O. and Voss, J.L. (eds) *Equine Reproduction*. Lea and Febiger, Philadelphia, Pennsylvania, pp. 473–485.

Flood, P.F., Betteridge, K.J. and Diocee, M.S. (1982) Transmission electron microscopy of horse embryos 3–16 days after ovulation. *Journal of Reproduction and Fertility, Supplement* 32, 319–327.

Flores, R.S., Byron, C.R. and Kline, K.H. (2011) Effect of Feed Processing Method on Average Daily Gain and Gastric Ulcer Development in Weanling Horses. *Journal of Equine Veterinary Science* 31(3), 124–128.

Flores-Flores, G., Velazquez-Canton, E., Boeta, M. and Zarco, L. (2014) Luteoprotective role of equine chorionic gonadotropin (eCG) during pregnancy in the mare. *Reprod Domest Anim* 49, 420–426.

Forsyth, I.A., Rossdale, P.D. and Thomas, C.R. (1975) Studies on milk composition and lactogenic hormones in the mare. *Journal of Reproduction and Fertility, Supplement* 23, 631–635.

Fortier, G., Vidament, M., DeCraene, F., Ferry, B. and Daels, P.F. (2002) The effect of GnRH antagonist on testosterone secretion, spermatogenesis and viral excretion in EVA-virus excreting stallions. *Theriogenology* 58, 425–427.

Fortune, J.E. and Kimmich, T.L. (1993) Purified pig FSH increases the rate of double ovulations in mares. *Equine Veterinary Journal, Supplement* 15, 95–98.

Foster, M.L., Love, C.C., Varner, D.D., Brinsko, S.P., Hinrichs, K., Teague, S., LaCaze, K. and Blanchard, T.L. (2011) Comparison of methods for assessing integrity of equine sperm membranes. *Theriogenology* 76(2), 334–341.

Fowden, A.L., Mundy, L., Ousey, J.C., McGladdery, A. and Silver, M. (1991) Tissue glycogen and glucose-6-phosphatase levels in fetal and newborn foals. *Journal of Reproduction and Fertility, Supplement* 44, 537–542.

Fowden, A.L., Ralph, M.M. and Silver, M. (1994) Nutritional regulation of uteroplacental prostaglandin production and metabolism in pregnant ewes and mares during late gestation. *Experimental Clinical Endocrinology* 102, 212–221.

Fowden, A.L., Forhead, A.J., White, K.L. and Taylor, P.M. (2000) Equine uteroplacental metabolism at mid and late gestation. *Experimental Physiology* 85(5), 539–545.

Fowden, A.L., Forehead, A.J., and Ousey, J.C. (2008) The endocrinology of equine parturition *Experimental Clinical Endocrinology and Diabetes* 116(7), 393–403.

Fradinho, M.J., Correia, M.J., Gracio, V., Bliebernicht, M., Farrim, A., Lateus, L., Martin Rosset, W., Bessa, R.J.B., Caldeira, R.M. and Ferreira-Dias, G. (2014) Effects of body condition and leptin on the reproductive performance of Lusitano mares on extensive systems. *Theriogenology* 81, 1214–1222.

Francavilla, S., Gabriele, A., Romano, R., Ginaroli, L., Ferraretti, A.P. and Francavilla, F. (1994) Sperm–zona pellucida binding of human sperm is correlated with immunocytochemical presence of proacrosin and acrosin in the sperm heads but not with proteolytic activity of acrosin. *Fertility and Sterility* 62(6), 1226–1233.

Frandson, R.D., Wilke, W.L. and Fails, A.D. (2009) *Anatomy and Physiology of Farm Animals*, 7th edn. Wiley-Blackwell.

Franklin, R.P. (2007) Identification and treatment of the high-risk foal. *Proceedings of the 53th Annual Convention of the American Association of Equine Practitioners*, Orlando, Florida, pp. 320–328.

Frape, D. (1998) *Equine Nutrition and Feeding*, 2nd edn. Blackwell Science, Oxford, pp. 564.

Frape, D. (2004) *Equine Nutrition and Feeding*, 3rd edn. Blackwell, Oxford, pp. 650.

Fraser, A.F., Keith, N.W. and Hastie, H. (1973) Summarised observations on the ultrasonic detection of pregnancy and foetal life in the mare. *Veterinary Record* 92(1), 20–21.

Frazer, G. (2007) Dystocia and Fetotomy. In: Samper, J.C., Pycock, J.F. and McKinnon, A.O. (eds) *Current Therapy in Equine Reproduction*. Saunders, Elsevier, St. Louis, Missouri, pp. 417–434.

Frazer, G.S. (2008) Stallion reproductive emergencies Large animal. *Proceedings of the North American Veterinary Conference*, Orlando, Florida, pp. 106–109.

Frazer, G. (2011a) Dystocia management. In: McKinnon, A.O., Squires, E.L., Vaala, E. and Varner, D.D. (eds) *Equine Reproduction*, 2nd edn. Wiley-Blackwell, Philadelphia, London, pp. 2479–2496.

Frazer, G. (2011b) Fetotomy. In: McKinnon, A.O., Squires, E.L., Vaala, E. and Varner, D.D. (eds) *Equine Reproduction*, 2nd edn. Wiley-Blackwell, Philadelphia, London, pp. 2497–2504.

Frazer, G.S., Perkins, N.R. and Embertson, R.M. (1999a) Normal parturition and evaluation of the mare in dystocia. *Equine Veterinary Education* 11(1), 41–46.

Frazer, G.S., Perkins, N.R. and Embertson, R.M. (1999b) Correction of Equine dystocia. *Equine Veterinary Education* 11(1), 48–53.

Freccero, F., Toaldo, M.B., Castagnetti, C., Cipone, M. and Diana, A. (2018) Contrast enhanced ultrasonography of the uterus during normal equine pregnancy: preliminary report in two mares. *Journal of Equine Veterinary Science* 54, 42–49.

Fredriksson, G., Kindahl, H. and Stabenfeldt, G.H. (1986) Endotxin-induced and prostaglandin-mediated effectson corpus luteum function in the mare *Theriogenology* 25, 309–316.

Freeman, D.A., Butler, J.E., Weber, J.A., Geary, R.T. and Woods, G.L. (1991) Coculture of day 5 to day 7 equine embryos in medium with oviductual tissue. *Theriogenology* 36, 815–822.

Freeman, D.E., Hungerford, L.L., Schaeffer, D., Lock, T.F., Sertich, P.L., Baker, G.J., Vaala, W.E. and Johnston, J.K. (1999) Caesarean section and other methods for assisted delivery: comparison of effects on mare mortality and complications. *Equine Veterinary Journal* 31(3), 203–207.

Freeman, D.E. (2011) Cesarean Section. In: McKinnon, A.O., Squires, E.L., Vaala, E. and Varner, D.D. (eds) *Equine Reproduction*, 2nd edn. Wiley-Blackwell, Philadelphia, London, pp. 2505–2510.

Freeman, K.P. and Johnston, J.M. (1987) Collaboration of a cytopathologist and practitioner using equine endometrial cytology in a private broodmare practice. In: Milne, F.J. (ed.) *Proceedings of the 33rd Annual Convention of the American Association of Equine Practitioners, New Orleans, Louisiana*. American Association of Equine Practitioners, pp. 629–639.

Freymond, S.B., Briefer, E.F., Von Niederhausern, R. and Bachmann, I. (2013) Pattern of social interactions after group integration: A possibility to keep stallions as a group. *Plos One* 8(1), e54688.

Friedman, R., Scott, M., Heath, S.E., Hughes, J.P., Daels, P.F. and Tran, T.Q. (1991) The effects of increased testicular temperature on spermatogenesis in the stallion. *Journal of Reproduction and Fertility, Supplement* 44, 127–134.

Fuchs, A.R., Periyasamy, S., Alexandrova, M. and Soloff, M.S. (1983) Correlation between oxytocin receptor concentration and responsiveness to oxytocin in pregnant rat myometrium. Effects of ovarian steroids. *Endocrinology* 113, 742–749.

Fuchs, A.R., Behrens, O. and Lire, H.C. (1992). Correlation of nocturnal increase in plasma oxytocin with a decrease in plasma estradiol/progesterone ratio in late pregnancy. *American Journal of Obstetrics and Gynaecology* 167, 1559–1563.

Fukuda, T., Kikuchi, M., Kurotaki, T., Oyomada, T., Yoshikawa, W. and Yoshikawa, T. (2001) Age related changes in the testes of horses. *Equine Veterinary Journal* 33(1), 20–25.

Gadella, B.M., Rathi, R., Brouwers, J.F., Stout, T.A. and Colenbrander, B. (2001) Capacitation and the acrosome reaction in equine sperm. *Animal Reproduction Science* 68(3–4), 249–265.

Gaivao, M.M.F., Rambags, B.P.B. and Stout, T.A.E. (2014) Gastrulation and the establishment of the three germ layers in the early horse conceptus. *Theriogenology* 82, 354–365.

Galli, A., Basetti, M., Balduzzi, D., Martignoni, M., Bornaghi, V. and Maffii, M. (1991) Frozen bovine semen quality and bovine cervical-mucus penetration test. *Theriogenology* 35(4), 837–844.

Galli, C., Crotti, G., Turini, P., Duchi, R., Mari, G., Zavaglia, G., Duchamp, G., Daels, P. and Lazzari, G. (2002) Frozen thawed embryos produced by ovum pick-up of immature oocytes and ICSI are capable to establish pregnancies in the horse. *Theriogenology* 58, 705–708.

Galli, C., Lagutina, I., Crotti, G., Colleoni, S., Turini, P., Ponderato, N., Duchi, R. and Lazzari, G. (2003) Pregnancy: a cloned horse born to its dam twin. *Nature* 424(6949), 635. Erratum in *Nature* (2003) 425(6959), 680.

Galli, C., Colleoni, S., Duchi, R., Lagutina, I. and Lazzari, G. (2007) Developmental competence of equine oocytes and embryos obtained by in vitro procedures ranging from in vitro maturation and ICSI to embryo culture, cryopreservation and somatic cell nuclear transfer. *Animal Reproduction Science* 98(1–2), 39–55.

Galli, C., Duchi, R., Colleoni, S., Lagutina, I. and Lazzari, G. (2014) Ovum pickup, intracyto plasmic sperm injection and somatic cell nuclear transfer in cattle, buffalo and horses: from the research laboratory to clinical practice. *Theriogenology* 81, 138–151.

Galli, C., Colleoni, S., Ducchi, R. and Lazzari, G. (2016) Male factors affecting the success of equine in vitro embryo production by ovum pick up intracytoplasmic sperm injection in a clinical setting. *Journal of Equine Veterinary Science* 43(S1), 6–10.

Gamba, M. and Pralong, F.P. (2006) Control of GnRH neuronal activity by metabolic factors. The role of leptin and insulin. *Molecular and Cellular Endocrinology* 254–255, 133–139.

Gambini, A. and Maserati, M. (2017) A journey through horse cloning. *Reproduction, Fertility and Development* 30(1), 8–17.

Gamo, S., Tozaki, T., Kakoi, H., Hirota, K., Nakamura, K., Nishii, N., Alumunia, J., and Tkasu, M. (2019) X monosomy in the endangered Kiso horse breed detected by a parentage test using sex chromosome linked genes and microsatellites. *Journal of Veterinary Medical Science* 81(1), 91–94.

Ganowiczow, A.M. and Ganowicz, M. (1966) Preliminary observations on the duration of pregnancy in English Thoroughbred mares. *Zeszyty Problemowe Postepow Nauk Roiniczych* 67, 99–102 (*Animal Breeding Abstracts* 39, 2209).

Garcia, M.C., Freedman, L.H. and Ginther, O.J. (1979) Interaction of seasonal and ovarian factors in the regulation of LH and FSH secretion in the mare. *Journal of Reproduction and Fertility, Supplement* 27, 103–111.

Garcia-Rosello, E., Garcia-Mengual, E., Coy, P., Alfonso, J. and Silvestre, M. (2009) Intracytoplasmic sperm injection in livestock species: an update. *Reproduction in Domestic Animals* 44(1), 143–151.

Garner, D.L., Pinkel, D., Johnson, L.A. and Pace, M.M. (1986) Assessment of spermatozoal function using dual fluorescent staining and flow-cytometric analyses. *Biology of Reproduction* 34, 127–138.

Gasser, R.B., Williamson, R.M.C. and Beveridge, I. (2005) Anoplocephala perfoliate of horses – significant scope for further research, improved diagnosis and control. *Parasitology* 131, 1–13.

Gastal, E.L. (2009) Recent advances and new concepts on follicle and endocrine dynamics during the equine periovulatory period. *Animal Reproduction* 6, 144–158.

Gastal, E.L., Augusto, C., Castro, T.A.M.G. and Gastal, M.O. (1991) Relationship between the quality of stallion semen and fertility. *Anais, IX Congresso Brasileiro de Reproducao Animal*, Belo Horizonte, Brazil, 22 a 26 de Junho de 1991. Vol. II. Colegio Brasileiro de Reproducao Animal, Belo Horizonte, Brazil, p. 446.

Gastal, E.L., Gastal, M.O., Bergfeldt, D.R. and Ginther, O.J. (1997) Role of diameter differences among follicles in selection of future dominant follicles in mares. *Biology of Reproduction* 57, 1320–1327.

Gastal, E.L., Bergfeldt, D.R., Nogueira, G.P., Gastal, M.O. and Ginther, O.J. (1999) Role of luteinising hormone in follicle deviation based on manipulating progesterone concentrations in the mare. *Biology of Reproduction* 61, 1492–1498.

Gastal, E.L., Gastal, M.O., Beg, M.A. and Ginther, O.J. (2004) Interrelationships among follicles during the common-growth phase of a follicular wave and capacity of individual follicles for dominance in mares. *Reproduction* 128(4), 417–422.

Gastal, E.L., Gastal, M.O. and Ginther, O.J. (2006) Serrated granulosa and other discrete ultrasound indicators of impending ovulation in mares. *Journal of Equine Veterinary Science* 26, 67–73.

Gastal, M.O., Gastal, E.L., Kot, K. and Ginther, O.J. (1996) Factors related to the time of fixation of the conceptus in mares. *Theriogenology* 46(7), 1171–1180.

Gastal, M.O., Gastal, E.L., Spinelli, V. and Ginther, O.J. (2004) Relationships between body condition and follicle development in mares. *Animal Reproduction* 1, 115–121.

Gatti, J.L., Castella, S., Dacheux, F., Ecroyd, H., Metayer, S., Thimon, V. and Dacheus, J.L. (2004) Post-testicular sperm environment and fertility. *Animal Reproduction Science* 82–83, 321–339.

Gee, E.K. and McCue, P.M. (2011) Mastitis. In: McKinnon, A.O., Squires, E.L., Vaala, E. and Varner, D.D. (eds) *Equine Reproduction*, 2nd edn. Wiley-Blackwell, Philadelphia, London, pp. 2738–2741.

Gee, E.K., Firth, E.C., Mrrel, P.C.H., Fennessy, P.F., Grace, N.D. and Mogg, T.D. (2005) Articular/epiphyseal osteochondrosis in Thoroughbred foals at 5 months of age: influences of growth of foal and prenatal copper supplementation of the dam. *New Zealand Veterinary Journal* 53, 448–456.

Gentry, L.R., Thompson Jr, D.L., Gentry Jr, G.T., Davis, K.A. and Godke, R.A. (2002a) High versus low body condition in mares: interactions with responses to somatotropin, GnRH analog, and dexamethasone. *Journal of Animal Science* 80(12), 3277–3285.

Gentry, L.R., Thompson Jr, D.L., Gentry Jr, G.T., Davis, K.A., Godke, R.A. and Cartmill, J.A. (2002b) The relationship between body condition, leptin, and reproductive and hormonal characteristics of mares during the seasonal anovulatory period. *Journal of Animal Science* 80(10), 2695–2703.

Georges, K.C., Ezeokoli, C.D., Sparagano, O., Pargass, I., Campbell, M., D'Abadie, R., and Yabsley, M. J. (2011) A case of transplacental transmission of *Theileria equi* in a foal in Trinidad. *Veterinary Parasitology* 175(3/4), 363–366.

Gerlach, T., and Aurich, J.E. (2000) Regulation of seasonal reproductive activity in the stallion, ram and hamster. *Animal Reproduction Science* 58, 197–213.

Ghei, J.C., Uppal, P.K. and Yaday, M.P. (1994) Prospects of AI in equines. *Cataur* XI, July, 1.

Ghosh, S., Das, P.J., Avila, F., Thwaits, B.K., Chowdhary, B.P. and Raudsepp, T. (2016) A non-reciprocal autosomal translocation 64,XX, t(4;10)(q21;p15) in an Arabian mare with repeated early embryonic loss. *Reproduction in Domestic Animals* 51(1), 171–174.

Giaretta, E., Munerato, M., Yeste, M., Galeati, G., Spinaci, M., Tamanini, C., Mari, G. and Bucci, D. (2017) Implementing an open-access CASA software for the assessment of stallion sperm motility: relationship with other sperm quality parameters. *Animal Reprduction Science* 176, 11–19.

Gibb, Z., Lambourne, S.R. and Aitkin, R.J. (2014) The paradoxical relationship between stallion fertility and oxidative stress. *Biology of Reproduction* 91(3), 77.

Gibb, Z., Grupen, C.G., Maxwell, W.M.C. and Morris, L.H.A. (2017) Field fertility of liquid stored and cryopreserved flow cytometrically sex-sorted stallion sperm. *Equine Veterinary Journal* 49, 160–166.

Gibb, Z., Clulow, J.R., Aitken, R.J. and Swegen, A. (2018) First publication to describe a protocol for the liquid storage of stallion spermatozoa for 7 days. *Journal of Equine Veterinary Science* 66, 37–40.

Gibbs, P.G., Potter, G.D., Blake, R.W. and McMullan, W.C. (1982) Milk production of Quarter Horse mares during 150 days of lactation. *Journal of Animal Science* 54, 496–499.

Ginther, O.J. (1982) Twinning in mares: a review of recent studies. *Journal of Equine Veterinary Science* 2, 127–135.

Ginther, O.J. (1983) Sexual behaviour following introduction of a stallion into a group of mares. *Theriogenology* 19, 877.

Ginther, O.J. (1988) Ultrasonic imaging of ovarian follicles and corpora lutea. *Veterinary Clinics of North America Equine Practitioners* 4, 197–213.

Ginther, O.J. (1989a) Twin embryos in mares: II. Post fixation embryo reduction. *Equine Veterinary Journal* 21, 171–174.

Ginther, O.J. (1989b) Twin embryos in mares: I. From ovulation to fixation. *Equine Veterinary Journal* 21, 166–170.

Ginther, O.J. (1990a) Prolonged luteal activity in mares–a semantic quagmire. *Equine Veterinary Journal* 22(3), 152–156.

Ginther, O.J. (1990b) Folliculogenesis during the transition period and early ovulatory season in mares *Journal of Reproduction and Fertility* 90, 311–320.

Ginther, O.J. (1992) *Reproductive Biology of the Mare, Basic and Applied Aspects*, 2nd edn. Equiservices, Cross Plains, Wisconsin, pp. 642.

Ginther, O.J. (1993) Equine foal kinetics: allantoic fluid shifts and uterine horn closures. *Theriogenology* 40, 241–256.

Ginther, O.J. (1995) *Ultrasonic Imaging and Animal Reproduction: Horses*. Book 2. Equiservices, Cross Plains, Wisconsin.

Ginther, O.J. (2008) *Ultrasonic imaging and animal reproduction: Color dopplor ultrasonography*. Book 4. Equiservices, Cross Plains, Wisconsin.

Ginther, O.J. (2012) The end of the tour de force of the corpus luteum in mares. *Theriogenology* 77, 1042–1049.

Ginther, O.J. and Beg, M.A. (2012) Dynamics of circulating progesterone concentrations before and during luteolysis: a comparison between cattle and horses *Equine Veterinary Journal* 9(1), 4–12.

Ginther, O.J. and Bergfeldt, D.R. (1988) Embryo reduction before day 11: in mares with twin conceptuses. *Journal of Animal Science* 66(7), 1727–1731.

Ginther, O.J. and Bergfeldt, D.R. (1993) Growth of small follicles and concentrations of FSH during the equine oestrous cycle. *Journal of Reproduction and Fertility* 99, 105–111.

Ginther, O.J. and First, N.L. (1971) Maintenance of the corpus luteum in hysterectomised mares. *American Journal of Veterinary Research* 32(11), 1687–1691.

Ginther, O.J. and Griffin, P.G. (1994) Natural outcome and ultrasonic identification of equine fetal twins. *Theriogenology* 41, 1193–1199.

Ginther, O.J. and Utt, M.D. (2004) Doppler ultrasound in equine reproduction: principles, techniques and potential. *Journal of Equine Veterinary Science* 24, 516–526.

Ginther, O.J. and Williams, D. (1996) On-the-farm incidence and nature of equine dystocia. *Journal of Equine Veterinary Science* 16, 159–164.

Ginther, O.J., Scraba, S.T. and Nuti, R.C. (1983) Pregnancy rates and sexual behaviour under pasture breeding conditions in mares. *Theriogenology* 20, 333–345.

Ginther, O.J., Beg, M.A., Bergfeldt, D.R., Donadeu, F.X. and Kot, K. (2001) Follicle selection in monovular species. *Biology of Reproduction* 65, 638–647.

Ginther, O.J., Meira, C., Beg, M.A. and Bergfeldt, D.R. (2002) Follicle and endocrine dynamics during experimental follicle deviation in mares. *Biology of Reproduction* 67(3), 862–867.

Ginther, O.J., Beg, M.A., Donadeu, F.X. and Bergfeldt, D.R. (2003) Mechanism of follicle deviation in monovular farm species. *Animal Reproduction Science* 78, 239–257.

Ginther, O.J., Gastel, E., Gastel, M. and Beg, M. (2004a) Seasonal influence on equine follicle dynamics. *The Journal of Animal Reproduction* 1(1), 31–44.

Ginther, O.J., Gastal, E.L., Gastal, M.O., Bergfeldt, D.R., Baerwald, A.R. and Pierson, R.A. (2004b) Comparative study of dynamics of follicular waves in mares and women. *Biology of Reproduction* 71, 1195–1201.

Ginther, O.J., Gastal, E.L., Gastal, M.O., and Beg, M.A. (2005) Regulation of circulating gonadotrophins by the negative effects of ovarian hormones in the mare. *Biology of Reproduction* 73, 315–323.

Ginther, O.J., Utt, M.D., Bergfeldt, D.R. and Beg, M.A. (2006) Controlling interrelationships of progesterone/LH and estradiol/LH in mares. *Animal Reproduction Science* 95, 144–150.

Ginther, O.J., Gastal, E.L. and Gastal, M.O. (2007a) Spatial relationships between serrated granulosa and vascularity of the preovulatory follicle and developing corpus luteum. *Journal Equine Veterinary Science* 27, 20–27.

Ginther, O.J., Utt, M.D. and Beg, M.A. (2007b) Follicle deviation and diurnal variation in circulating hormone concentrations in mares. *Animal Reproduction Science* 100, 197–203.

Ginther, O.J., Gastal, E.L., Gastal, M.O. and Beg, M.A. (2008) Intrafollicular effect of IGF1 on development of follicle dominance in mares. *Animal Reproduction Science* 105, 417–423.

Ginther, O.J., Gastal, M.O., Gastal, E.L., Jacob, J.C. and Beg, M.A. (2009a) Age related dynamics of follicles and hormones during an induced ovulatory follicular wave in mares. *Theriogenology* 71, 780–788.

Ginther, O.J., Jacob, J.C., Gastal, M.O., Gastal, E.L. and Beg, M.A. (2009b) Development of one versus multiple ovulatory follicles and associated systemic hormone concentrations in mares. *Reproduction in Domestic Animals* 44, 441–449.

Ginther, O.J., Baldrighi, J.M., Castro, T., Wolf, C.A., Santos, V.G. (2016a) Defective secretion of prostaglandin F2 during development of idiopathic persistent corpus luteum in mares. *Domestic Animal Endocrinology* 55, 60–65.

Ginther, O.J., Baldrighi, J.M., Castro, T., Wolf, C.A., Santos, V.G. (2016b) Concentrations of progesterone, a metabolite of PGF2α, prolactin, luteinizing hormone during development of idiopathic persistent corpus luteum in mares *Domestic Animal Endocrinology* 55, 114–122.

Glade, M.J. (1993) Effects of gestation, lactation and maternal calcium intake on mechanical strength of equine bone. *Journal of the American College of Nutrition* 12, 372–377.

Glaser, A.L., Chimside, E.D., Horzinek, M.C. and DeVries, A.A.F. (1997) Equine viral arteritis. *Theriogenology* 47, 1275–1295.

Godoi, D.B., Gastal, E.L. and Gastal, M.O. (2002) A comparative study of follicular dynamics between lactating and non-lactating mares: effect of body condition. *Theriogenology* 58, 553–556.

Goff, A.K., Panbrin, D. and Sirois, J. (1987) Oxytocin stimulation of plasma 15-keto-13, 14-dihydro prostaglandin F2 α release during the oestrus cycle and early pregnancy in the mare. *Journal of Reproduction and Fertility, Supplement* 35, 253–260.

Goff, A.K., Sirois, J. and Pontbriand, D. (1993) Effect of oestradiol on oxytocin-stimulated prostaglandin F2α release in mares. *Journal of Reproduction and Fertility* 98, 107–112.

Gold, J.R., Divers, T.J., Barton, M.H., Lamb, S.V., Place, N.J., Mohammed, H.O. and Bain, F.T. (2007) Plasma adrenocorticotrophin, cortisol and adrenocorticotrophin/cortisol ratios in septic and normal-term foals. *Journal of Veterinary Internal Medicine* 21, 791–796.

Golnik, W. (1992) Viruses isolated from fetuses and still born foals. In: Plowright, W. (ed.) *Equine Infectious Diseases VI: Proceedings of the Sixth International Conference*. RW Publications, Newmarket, UK, p. 314.

Gonzalez-Castro, R.A. and Carnevale, E.M. (2019) Use of microfluidics to sort stallion sperm for intracytoplasmic sperm injection. *Animal Reproduction Science* 202, 1–9.

Gores-Lindholm, A.R., LeBlanc, M.M., Causey, R., Hitchborn, A., Fayrer-Hosken, R.A., Kruger, M., Vandenplas, M.L., Flores, P. and Ahlschwede, S. (2013) Relationships between intrauterine infusion of N-acetylcysteine, equine endometrial pathology, neutrophil function, post-breeding therapy, and reproductive performance *Theriogenology* 80, 218–227.

Gould, J.C., Rossano, M.G., Lawrence, L.M., Burk, S.V., Ennis, R.B. and Lyons, E.T. (2012) The effects of windrow composting on the viability of *Parascaris equorum* eggs. *Veterinary Parasitology* 191, 73–80.

Govaere, J.L., Hoogewijs, M.K., de Schauwer, C., Dewulf, J. and de Kruif, A. (2008) Transvaginal ultrasound-guided aspiration of unilateral twin gestation in the mare. *Equine Veterinary Journal* 40(5), 521–522.

Govaere, J., Hoogewijs, M., De Schauwer, C., Van Zeveren, A., Smits, K., Cornillie, P. and De Kruif, A. (2009) An abortion of monozygotic twins in a warmblood mare. *Reproduction in Domestic Animals* 44(5), 852–854.

Gracia-Calvo, L.A., Duque, J., Silva, C.B. da , Ezquerra, J. and Ortega-Ferrusola, C. (2015) Testicular perfusion after standing laparoscopic peritoneal flap hernioplasty in stallions. *Theriogenology* 84(5), 797–804.

Gradil, C., Yoon, S.Y., Brown, J., He, C., Visconti, P. and Fissore, R. (2006) PLCζ: a marker of fertility for stallions? *Animal Reproduction Science* 94, 23–25.

Graham, E.F. (1996) Cryopreservation of stallion sperm. *Veterinary Clinics of North America Equine Practionner* 12(1), 131–147.

Graham, J.K. (2011a) Principles of cooled semen. In: McKinnon, A.O., Squires, E.L., Vaala, E. and Varner, D.D. (eds) *Equine Reproduction*, 2nd edn. Wiley-Blackwell, Philadelphia, London, pp. 1308–1315.

Graham, J.K. (2011b) Principles of cryopreservation. In: McKinnon, A.O., Squires, E.L., Vaala, E. and Varner, D.D. (eds) *Equine Reproduction*, 2nd edn. Wiley-Blackwell, Philadelphia, London, pp. 2959–2963.

Graham, J.K. and Card, C. (2007) Preservation of genetics from dead or dying stallions. In: Samper, J.C., Pycock, J.F. and McKinnon, A.O. (eds)

Current Therapy in Equine Reproduction. Saunders Elsevier, St Louis, Missouri, pp. 281–285.

Gravance, C.G., Liu, I.K.M., Davis, R.O., Hughes, J.P. and Casey, P.J. (1996) Quantification of normal morphometry of stallion spermatozoa. *Journal of Reproduction and Fertility* 108(1), 41–46.

Greaves, H.E., Porter, M.B. and Sharp, D.C. (2000) Effect of oestradiol on LH secretion and pituitary responsiveness to GnRH in ovarectomised mares. *Journal of Reproduction and Fertility, Supplement* 56, 227–237.

Greco, G.M., Burlamaqui, P.G., Pinna, A.E., Queiroz, F.R., Cunha, M.S. and Brandão, F.Z. (2012) Use of long-acting progesterone to acyclic embryo recipient mares. *Revista Brasileira de Zootecnia* 41(3), 607–611.

Greco, G.M., Fioratti, E.G., Segabinazzi, L.G., Dell'Aqua Jr., J.A., Crespilho, A.M., Castro Chaves, M.B. and Alvarenga, M.A. (2016) Novel long-acting progesterone protocols used to successfully synchronize donor and recipient mares with satisfactory pregnancy and pregnancy loss rate. *Journal of Equine Veterinary Science* 39, 58–61.

Green, J. (1993) Feeding the orphan or sick foal. *Equine Veterinary Education* 5(5), 274–275.

Green, J.M., Raz, T., Epp, T., Carley, S.D. and Card, C.E. (2007) Relationships between utero-ovarian parameters and ovulatory response to human chorionic gonadotrophin (hCG) in mares. In: *Proceedings of the 53rd Annual Convention of Equine Practicers, Orlando*, USA 563–567.

Greiwe-Crandell, K., Kronfeld, D.S., Gay, L.S., Sklan, D., Tiegs, W. and Harris, P. (1997) Vitamin A repletion in thoroughbred mares with retinylpalmitate of beta-carotene. *Journal of Animal Science* 75, 2684–2690.

Griffin, P.G. (2000) The breeding soundness examination in the stallion. *Journal of Equine Veterinary Science* 20(3), 168–171.

Griffin, P.G. and Ginther, O.J. (1990) Uterine contractile activity in mares during the estrous cycle and early pregnancy. *Theriogenology* 34(1), 47–56.

Griggers, S., Paccamonti, D.L., Thompson, R.A. and Eilts, B.E. (2001) The effects of pH, osmolarity and urine contamination on equine spermatozoal motility. *Theriogenology* 56(4), 613–622.

Grimmett, J.B., Hanlon, D.W., Duirs, G.F. and Jochle, W. (2002) A new intra-vaginal progesterone releasing device (Cue-Mare) for controlling the estrous cycle in mares. *Theriogenology* 16(2) 231–237.

Grogan, E.H. and McDonnell, S.M. (2005) Mare and Foal Bonding and Problems. *Clinical and Technical Equine Practice* 4, 228–237.

Grondahl, C., Grondahl Nielsen, C., Eriksen, T. Greve, T. and Hyttel, P. (2011) In vivo fertilisation and initial embryogenesis in the mare. *Equine Veterinary Journal* 15(Suppl), 79–83.

Guice, S.E., Kass, P.H. and Christensen, B.W. (2017) Equine cooled-semen shipping container effectiveness comparison. *Clinical Theriogenology* 9(3), 48.

Guignot, F., Reigner, F., Perreau, C., Tartarin, P., Babilliot, J. M., Bed'hom, B., Vidament, M, Mermillod P and Duchamp, G. (2015) Preimplantation genetic diagnosis in Welsh pony embryos after biopsy and cryopreservation. *Journal of Animal Science*, 93, 522–523

Guillaume, D., Duchamp, G., Nagy, P. and Palmer, E. (2000) Determination of minimum light treatment required for photostimulation od winter anoestrous mares. *Journal of Reproduction and Fertility* 56(Suppl), 205–216

Guillaume, D., Breneau, B and Briant, C.C. (2002) Ccomparison of the effects of two GnRH antagonists on LH and FSH secretion, follicular growth and ovulation in the mare. *Reproduction and Nutrition Development* 42, 251–264.

Guerin, M.U. and Wang, X.J. (1994) Environmental temperature has an influence on timing of the first ovulation of seasonal estrus in the mare. *Theriogenology* 42, 1053–1060.

Haard, M.C. and Haard, M.G.H. (1991) Successful commercial use of frozen stallion semen abroad. *Journal Reproduction and Fertility* 44(Suppl), 647–648.

Hafez, E.S.E. and Hafez, B. (2000) *Reproduction in Farm Animals*, 7th edn. Williams and Wilkins, Baltimore, Maryland, pp. 509.

Haffner, J.C., Fecteau, K.A., Held, J.P. and Eiler, H. (1998) Equine retained placenta: technique for and tolerance to umbilical injections of collagenase. *Theriogenology* 49, 711–716.

Hall, J.L. (1981) Relationship between semen quality and human sperm penetration of zona free hamster ova. *Fertility and Sterility* 35, 457–463.

Hallowell, A.L. (1989) The use of ultrasonography in equine reproduction on the breeding farm. In: *2nd Annual Conference Society of Theriogenology, Coeur D'Alene*, Idaho. Society of Theriogenology, pp. 202–205.

Halnan, C.R.E. (1985) Sex chromosome mosaicism and infertility in mares. *Veterinary Record* 116, 542–543.

Halnan, C.R.E. and Watson, J.I. (1982) Detection of G and C band karyotyping of genome anomalies in horses of different breeds. *Journal of Reproduction and Fertility, Supplement* 32, 626.

Haluska, G.J. and Currie, W.B. (1988) Variation in plasma concentrations of oestradiol 17 Beta and their relationship to those of progesterone. 13,14-dihydro-15-ketoprostaglandin F2 a and oxytocin across pregnancy and at parturition in pony mares. *Journal of Reproduction and Fertility* 84, 635–646.

Haluska, G.J. and Wilkins, K. (1989) Predictive utility of the pre-partum temperature changes in the mare. *Equine Veterinary Journal* 21, 116–118.

Haluska, G.J., Lowe, J.E. and Currie, W.B. (1987a) Electromyographic properties of the myometrium correlated with the endocrinology of the pre-partum and post partum periods and parturition in pony mares. *Journal of Reproduction and Fertility* 35(Suppl), 553–564.

Haluska, G.J., Lowe, J.E. and Currie, W.B. (1987b) Electromyographic properties of the myometrium of the pony mare during pregnancy. *Journal of Reproduction and Fertility* 81, 471–478.

Hamann, H., Jude, R.V., Sieme, H., Mertens, U., Töpfer-Petersen, E., Distl, O. and Leeb, T. (2007) A polymorphism within the equine CRISP3 gene is associated with stallion fertility in Hanoverian warmblood horses. *Animal genetics* 38(3), 259–264.

Hammerstedt, R.H., Graham, J.K. and Nolan, J.P. (1990) Cryopreservation of mammalian sperm: what we ask them to survive. *Journal of Andrology* 11(1), 73–88.

Hanada, M., Maeda, Y. and Oikawa, M. (2014) Histopathological characteristics of endomtrosis in Thoroughbred mares in Japan: results from 50 necropsy cases *Journal of Equine Science* 25 (2), 45–52

Handler, J., Gomes, T., Waelchli, R.O., Betteridge, K.J. and Raeside, J.I. (2002) Influence of cervical dilation on pregnancy rates and embryonic development in inseminated mares. In: Evans, M. (ed.) *Equine Reproduction VIII*. Elsevier, New York, pp. 671–674.

Handler, J., Schonlieb, S., Hoppen, H.O. and Aurich, C. (2006) Seasonal effects on attempts to synchronize estrus and ovulation by intrvaginal application of progesterone releasing device (PRID) in mares. *Theriogenology* 65, 1145–1158.

Hanlon, D.W. and Firth E.C. (2012) The reproductive performance of Thoroughbred mares treated with intravaginal progesterone at the start of the breeding season *Theriogenology* 77 (5) 952–958.

Hanlon, D.W., Stevenson, M., Evans, M.J. and Firth, E.C. (2012a) Reproductive performance of Thoroughbred mares in the Waikato region of New Zealand: Descriptove analysis New Zealand Veterinary Journal 60 (6) 329–334

Hanlon, D.W., Stevenson, M., Evans, M.J. and Firth, E.C. (2012b) Reproductive performance of Thoroughbred mares in the Waikato region of New Zealand: 2. Multivarable analyses and sources of variation at the mare, stallion and stud farm level. *New Zealand Veterinary Journal* 60 (6) 335–343.

Hansen, C., Vermeiden, T., Vermeiden, J.P.W., Simmet, C., Day, B.C. and Feitsma, H. (2006) Comparison of FACSCount AF system, Improved Neubauer hemocytometer, Corning 254 photometer, SpermVision, UltiMate and NucleoCounter SP-100 for determination of sperm concentration of boar semen. *Theriogenology* 66, 2188–2194.

Harold, C.S. (2011) Review of azotemia in foals. *Proceedings of the 57th Annual Convention of the American Association of Equine Practitioners*, San Antonio, Texas, pp. 328–334.

Harris, P.A. (2003) Feeding the pregnant and lactating mare. *Equine Veterinary Education* 6, 38–44.

Harrison, L.A., Squires, E.L., Nett, T.M. and McKinnon, A.O. (1990) Use of gonadotrophin releasing hormone for hastening ovulation in transitional mares. *Journal of Animal Science* 68, 690–699.

Harrison, R.A.P. and Vickers, S.E. (1990) Use of fluorescent probes to assess membrane integrity in mammalian spermatozoa. *Journal of Reproduction and Fertility* 88, 343–352.

Harrison, L.A., Squires, E.L. and McKinnon, A.O. (1991) Comparison of hCg, buserelin and luprostiol for induction of ovulation in cycling mares. *Journal of Equine Veterinary Science* 11, 163–166.

Hartman, D.L. (2011) Embryo transfer. In: McKinnon, A.O., Squires, E.L., Vaala, E. and Varner, D.D. (eds) *Equine Reproduction*, 2nd edn. Wiley-Blackwell, Philadelphia, London, pp. 2871–2879.

Hartman, D.L. and Bliss, S. (2011) Laboratory methods for isolation and evaluation of bacteria, fungi and yeast. In: McKinnon, A.O., Squires, E.L., Vaala, E. and Varner, D.D. (eds) *Equine Reproduction*, 2nd edn. Wiley-Blackwell, Philadelphia, London, pp. 2674–2684.

Hartmann, C., Lidauer, L., Aurich, J., Aurich, C. and Nagel, C. (2018) Detection of the time of foaling by accelerometer technique in horses (*Equus caballus*)-a pilot study. *Reproduction in Domestic Animals* 53(6), 1279–1286.

Hayes, H.M. (1986) Epidemiological features of 5009 cases of equine cryptorchidism. *Equine Veterinary Journal* 18, 467–471.

Hayes, K.E.N. and Ginther, O.J. (1989) Relationship between estrous behavior in pregnant mares and the presence of a female conceptus. *Journal of Equine Veterinary Science* 9, 316–318.

Hayes, M.A., Quinn, B.A., Kierstead, N.D., Katvolos, P., Waelchi, R.O. and Betteridge, K.J. (2008) Proteins associated with the early intrauterine equine conceptus. *Reproduction in Domestic Animals* 43, Supplement 2, 1–6.

Heap, R.B., Hamon, M. and Allen, W.R. (1982) Studies on oestrogen synthesis by pre-implantation equine conceptus. *Journal of Reproduction and Fertility, Supplement* 32, 343–352.

Heape, W. (1897) The artificial insemination of mammals and subsequent fertility on impregnation of their ova. *Proceedings of the Royal Society of London* 61, 52.

Heeseman, C.P., Squires, E.L., Webel, S.K., Shideler, R.K. and Pickett, B.W. (1980) The effect of ovarian activity and allyl trenbolone on the oestrous cycle and fertility in mares. *Journal of Animal Science, Supplement* 1(51), 284.

Heidler, B., Parvizi, N., Sauerwein, H., Bruckmaier, R.M., Heintges, U., Aurich, J.E. and Aurich, C. (2003) Effects of lactation on metabolic and reproductive hormones in Lipizzaner mares. *Domestic Animal Endocrinology* 25(1), 47–59.

Heidler, B., Aurich, J.E., Pohl, W., Aurich, C. (2004) Body weight of mares and foals, estrous cycles and plasma glucose concentration in lactating and non-lactating Lipizzaner mares. *Theriogenology* 61, 883–893.

Heiskanen, M.L., Hilden, L., Hyyppa, S., Kangasniemi, A., Pirhonen, A. and Maenpaa, P.H. (1994a) Freezability and fertility results with centrifuged stallion semen. *Acta Veterinaria Scandinavia* 35(4), 377–382.

Heiskanen, M.L., Huhtinen, M., Pirhonen, A. and Maepaa, P.H. (1994b) Insemination results with slow cooled stallion semen stored for approximately 40 hours. *Acta Veterinarian Scandinavia* 35(3), 257–262.

Heitland, A.V., Jasko, D.J., Graham, J.K., Squires, E.L., Amann, R.P. and Pickett, B.W. (1995) Motility and fertility of stallion spermatozoa cooled and frozen in a modified skim milk extender containing egg yolk and liposome. *Biology of Reproduction Monograph Equine Reproduction VI* 1, 753–759.

Heitland, A.V., Jasko, D.J., Squires, E.L., Graham, J.K., Pickett, B.W. and Hamilton, C. (1996) Factors affecting motion characteristics of frozen-thawed stallion spermatozoa. *Equine Veterinary Journal* 28(1), 47–53.

Heleski, C.R., Shelle, A.C., Neilsen, B.D. and Zanella, A.J. (2002) Influence of housing on weanling horse behaviour and subsequent welfare. *Applied Animal Behaviour Science* 78, 291–302.

Hellsten, T.E., Jorjania, H. and Philipsson, J. (2009) Genetic correlations between similar traits in the Danish and Swedish Warmblood sport horse populations. *Livestock Science* 124, 15–20.

Hemberg, E., Lundeheim, N. and Einarsson, S. (2004) Reproductive performance of Thoroughbred mares in Sweden. *Reproduction in Domestic Animals* 39(2), 81–85.

Hemberg, E., Lundeheim, N. and Einarsson, S. (2005) Retrospective study on vulvar conformation in relation to endometrial cytology and fertility in Thoroughbred mares. *Journal of Veterinary Medicine* 52, 474–477.

Henderson, K. and Stewart, J. (2000) A dipstick immunoassay to rapidly measure serum oestrone sulphate concentrations in horses. *Reproduction and Fertility Development* 12, 183–189.

Henderson, K. and Stewart, J. (2002) Factors influencing the measurement of oestrone sulphate by dipstick particle capture immunoassay. *Journal of Immunological Methods* 270, 77–84.

Henderson, K., Stevens, S., Bailey, C., Hall, G., Stewart, J. and Wards, R. (1998) Comparison of the merits of measuring equine chorionic gonadotrophin (eCG) and blood and faecal concentrations of oestrone sulphate for determining pregnancy status of miniature horses. *Reproduction, Fertility and Development* 10(5), 441–444.

Hendrikson, D.A. and Wilson, D.G. (2011) Laparoscopy. In: McKinnon, A.O., Squires, E.L., Vaala, E. and Varner, D.D. (eds) *Equine Reproduction*, 2nd edn. Wiley-Blackwell, Philadelphia, London, pp. 1991–2002.

Hendriks, W.K., Roelen, B.A.J., Colenbrander, B. and Stout, T.A.E. (2014) Cellular damage suffered by equine embryos after exposure to cryoprotectants or cryopreservation by slow freezing or vitrification. *Equine Veterinary Journal*, 47(6), 701–707.

Heninger, N.L. (2011) Puberty. In: McKinnon, A.O., Squires, E.L., Vaala, E. and Varner, D.D. (eds) *Equine Reproduction*, 2nd edn. Wiley-Blackwell, Philadelphia, London, pp. 1015–1025.

Henneke, D.R., Potter, G.D. and Kreider, J.L. (1984) Body condition during pregnancy and lactation and reproductive efficiency of mares. *Theriogenology* 21, 897–909.

Henry, S., Zanella, A.J., Sankey, C., Richard-Yris, M-A., Marko, A. and Hausberger, M. (2012) Adults may be used to alleviate weaning stress in domestic foals (*Equus caballus*). *Physiology and Behaviour* 106, 428–438.

Herfen, K., Jager, C. and Wehrend, A. (1999) Genital infection in mares and their clinical significance. *Reproduction in Domestic Animals* 34, 20–21.

Hermenet, M.J., Sawyer, H.R., Pickett, B.W., Amann, R.P., Squires, E.L. and Long, P.L. (1993) Effect of stain, technician, number of spermatozoa evaluated and slide preparation on assessment of spermatozoal viability by light microscopy. *Journal of Equine Veterinary Science* 13(8), 449–455.

Hernandez-Aviles, C., Zambrano-Varon, J. and Jimenez, C. (2019) Current trends on stallion evauation: What other methids can be used to improve our capacity for semen quality assessment? *Journal of Veterinary Andrology* 4(1), 1–19.

Herrara, C (2015) Social acceptance of equine ARTs: situation in South Aneerica. *Proceedings of the IETS Equine Reproduction Symposium, Paris*. pp. 30–31.

Herrera, C., Morikawa, M.I., Bello, M.B., von Meyeren, M., Centeno, J.E., Dufourq, P., Martinez, M.M. and Llorente, J. (2014). Setting up equine embryo gender determination by preimplantation genetic diagnosis in a commercial embryo transfer program. *Theriogenology* (81), 758–763.

Herrera, C., Morikawa, M.I., Castex, C.B., Pinto, M.R., Ortega, N., Fanti, T., Garaguso, R., Franco, M.J., Castanares, M., Casterira, C., Losinno, L., Miragaya, M.H. and Mutto, A.A. (2015) Blastocele fluid from in vitro- and in vivo- produced equine embryos contains nuclear DNA. *Theriogenology* 83, 415–420.

Hess, M.B., Parker, N.A., Purswell, B.J. and Dascanio, D.J. (2002) Use of lufenuron as a treatment for fungal endometritis in four mares. *Journal of the American Veterinary Medicine Association* 221(2), 266–267.

Hevia, M.L., Quiles, A.J., Fuentes, F. and Gonzalo, C. (1994) Reproductive performance of Thoroughbred mares in Spain. *Journal of Equine Veterinary Science* 14(2), 89–92.

Hidalgo, M., Consuegra, C., Dorado, J., Diaz-Jimenez, M., Ortiz, I., Pereira, B., Sanchez, R. and Crespo, F. (2018) Concentrations of non-permeable cryoprotectants and equilibration temperatures are key factors for stallion sperm vitrification success. *Animal Reproduction Science* 196, 91–98.

Higgins, A.J. and Wright, I.M. (1999) *The Equine Manual*. Saunders, Oval Road, London.

Hillman, R.B. and Ganjam, V.K. (1979) Hormonal changes in the mare and foal associated with oxytocin induction of parturition. *Journal of Reproduction and Fertility, Supplement* 27, 541–546.

Hillman, R.B., Olar, T.T. and Squires, E.L. (1980) Temperature of the artificial vagina and its effect on seminal quality and behavioural characteristics of stallions. *Journal of the American Veterinary Medical Association* 177(8), 720–722.

Hines, K.K., Hodge, S.L., Kreider, J.L., Potter, G.D. and Harms, P.G. (1987) Relationship between body condition and levels of serum luteinising hormone in post partum mares. *Theriogenology* 28, 815–825.

Hinrichs, K. (2010) Application of assisted reproductive technologies (ART) to clinical practice. *Proceedings of the American Association of Equine Practitioners* (56), 195–206.

Hinrichs, K. (2011a) Nuclear Transfer. In: McKinnon, A.O., Squires, E.L., Vaala, E. and Varner, D.D. (eds) *Equine Reproduction*, 2nd edn. Wiley-Blackwell, Philadelphia, London, pp. 2924–2927.

Hinrichs, K. (2011b) Immature oocyte collection and maturation. In: McKinnon, A.O., Squires, E.L., Vaala, E. and Varner, D.D. (eds) *Equine Reproduction*, 2nd edn. Wiley-Blackwell, Philadelphia, London, pp. 2931–2935.

Hinrichs, K. (2012) Assisted reproduction techniques in the horse. *Reproduction Fertility and Development* 25, 80–93.

Hinrichs, K. (2018) Assisted reproductive techniques in mares. *Reproduction in Domestic Animals* 53, Supplement 2, 4–13.

Hinrichs, K. and Hunt, P.R. (1990) Ultrasound as an aid to diagnosis of granulosa cell tumour in the mare. *Equine Veterinary Journal* 22, 99–103.

Hinrichs, K. and Kenney, R.M. (1988) Effect of timing of progesterone administration on pregnancy rate after embryo transfer in ovarectomised mares. *Journal of Reproduction and Fertility, Supplement* 35, 439–443.

Hinrichs, K., Betschart, R.W., McCue, P.M. and Squires, E.L. (2000a) Effect of timing of follicle aspiration on pregnancy rate after oocyte transfer in mares. *Journal of Reproduction and Fertility, Supplement* 56, 493–498.

Hinrichs, K., Provost, P.J. and Torello, E.M. (2000b) Treatments resulting in pregnancy to nonovulating, hormone-treated oocyte recipient mares. *Theriogenology* 54, 1285–1293.

Hinrichs, K., Love, C.C., Brinsko, S.P., Choi, Y.H. and Varner, D.D. (2002) *In vitro* fertilisation of *in vitro* matured equine oocytes: effect of maturation medium, duration of maturation and sperm calcium ionophore treatment, and comparison with rates of fertilisation *in vivo* after oviductal transfer. *Biology of Reproduction* 67, 256–262.

Hinrichs, K., Choi, Y.H., Varner, D.D. and Hartman, D.L. (2007) Production of cloned horse foals using roscovitine-treated donor cells and activation with sperm extract and/or ionomycin. *Reproduction* 134, 319–325.

Hinrichs, K., Choi, Y.H., Norris, J.D., Love, L.B., Bedford-Guaus, S.J., Hartman, D.L. and Velez, J.C. (2010) Use of intracytoplasmic sperm injection and in vitro culture to the blastocyst stage for clinical production of foals post mortem. *Animal Reproduction Science* 121, 239–240.

Hinrichs, K., Choi, Y.H., Norris, J.D., Love, L.B., Bedford-Guaus, G.J., Hartman, D.L. and Velez, I.C. (2012) Evaluation of foal production following intracytoplasmic sperm injection and blastocyst culture of oocytes from ovaries collected immediately before euthanasia or after death of mares under field conditions. *Journal of the American Veterinary Medical Association* 241, 1070–1074.

Hintz, H.F. (1993a) Nutrition of the broodmare. In: McKinnon, A.O. and Voss, J.L. (eds) *Equine Reproduction*. Lea and Febiger, Philadelphia, Pennsylvania, London, pp. 631–639.

Hintz, H.F. (1993b) Feeding the stallion. In: McKinnon, A.O. and Voss, J.L. (eds) *Equine Reproduction*. Lea and Febiger, Philadelphia, Pennsylvania, London, pp. 840–842.

Hochereau-de Riviers, M.T., Courtens, J.-L., Courot, M. and De Rivers, M. (1990) Spermatogenesis in mammals and birds. In: Laming, G.E. (ed.) *Marshall's Physiology of Reproduction, Volume 2, Reproduction in the Male*, 4th edn. Churchill Livingstone, London, pp. 106–182.

Hochi, S., Fujimato, T., Choi, Y., Braun, J. and Oguri, N. (1994a) Cryopreservation of equine oocytes by 2-step freezing. *Theriogenology* 42(3), 1085–1094.

Hochi, S., Fujimato, T., Braun, J. and Oguri, N. (1994b) Pregnancies following transfer of equine embryos cryopreserved by vitrification. *Theriogenology* 42(3), 483–488.

Hochi, S., Fujimato, T. and Oguri, N. (1995) Large equine blastocysts are damaged by vitrification procedures. *Reproduction, Fertility and Development* 7, 113–117.

Hochi, S., Maruyana, A. and Oguri, N. (1996) Direct transfer of equine blastocysts frozen-thawed in the presence of ethylene glycol and sucrose. *Theriogenology* 46(7), 1217–1224.

Hodder, D.J., Liu, I.K.M. and Ball, B.A. (2008) Current methods for the diagnosis and maagement of twin pregnancy in the mare. *Equine Veterinary Education* 20(9), 493–502.

Hodge, S.L., Kieider, J.L., Potter, G.D., Harms, P.G. and Fleeger, J.L. (1982) Influence of photoperiod on the pregnant and post partum mare. *American Journal of Veterinary Research* 43, 1752–1755.

Hofferer, S., Duchamp, G. and Palmer, E. (1991) Ovarian response in mares to prolonged treatment with exogenous equine pituitary gonadotrophins. *Journal of Reproduction and Fertility, Supplement* 44, 341–349.

Hoffman, R.M., Konfeld, D.S., Holland, J.R. and Greiwe-Crandell, K.M. (1995) Pre-weaning diet and stall weaning influences on stress response in foals. *Journal of Animal Science* 73, 2922–2930.

Hoffman, R.M., Morgan, K.L., Lynch, M.P., Zinn, S.A., Fautsman, C. and Harris, P.A. (1999) Dietary vitamin E supplemented in the peri-parturient period influences immunologloglobulins in equine colostrum and passive transfer in foals. *Proceedings of the 16th Equine Nutrition and Physiology Symposium*, Raleigh, North Carolina, pp 96–97.

Hoffmann, B., Gentz, F. and Failing, K. (1996) Investigations into the course of progesterone, oestrogen and eCG concentrations in normal and impaired pregnancy in the mare *Reproduction in Domestic Animals* 31, 717–723.

Hoffmann, C., Ellenberger, C., Mattos, R.C., Aupperle, H., Dhein, S., Stief, B. and Schoon, H.A. (2009) The equine endometrosis: new insights into the pathogenesis. *Animal Reproduction Science* 111, 261–278.

Holder, R.D. (2011) Equine fetal sex determination between 55 and 150 days. In: McKinnon, A.O., Squires, E.L., Vaala, E. and Varner, D.D. (eds) *Equine Reproduction*, 2nd edn. Wiley-Blackwell, Philadelphia, London, pp. 2080–2093.

Holdstock, N.B., Ousey, J.C. and Rossdale, P.D. (1998) Glomerular filtration rate, effective renal plasma flow, blood pressure and pulse rate in equine neonate during the first 10 days post partum. *Equine Veterinary Journal* 30(4), 335–343.

Holland, J.L., Kronfeld, D.S., Hoffman, R.M., Greiwe-Crandell, K.M., Boyd, T.L., Cooper, W.L. and Harris, P.A. (1996). Weaning stress is affected by nutrition and weaning methods. *Pferdeheilkunde*, 3, 257–260.

Holland, J.L., Kronfeld, D.S., Hoffman, R.M. and Harris, P.A. (1997) Weaning stress assessment in mares. In: *Proceedings of the 15th Equine Nutrition and Physiology Symposium 14, Fort Worth, Texas*. Equine and Physiology Society pp. 219–221.

Holstein, A.F., Schulze, W. and Davidoff, M. (2003) Understanding spermatogenesis is a pre-requisite for treatment. *Reproductive Biology and Endocrinology* 1, 107.

Holtan, D. (1993) Progestin therapy in mares with pregnancy complication. Necessity and efficacy. In: *Proceedings of the 39th Annual Association of Equine Practitioners Convention, Fort Worth, Texas.* American Association of Equine Practitioners, pp. 165–166.

Holtan, D.W. and Silver, M. (1992) Readiness for birth; another piece of the puzzle. *Equine Veterinary Journal* 24(5), 336–337.

Holtan, D.W., Nett, T.M. and Estergreen, V.L. (1975a) Plasma progestins in pregnant, postpartum and cyclic mares. *Journal of Animal Science* 40, 251–260.

Holtan, D.W., Nett, T.M. and Estergreen, V.L. (1975b) Plasma progestagens in pregnant mares. *Journal of Reproduction and Fertility*, Supplement 23, 419–424.

Holtan, D.W., Squires, E.L., Lapin, D.R. and Ginther, O.J. (1979) Effect of ovariectomy on pregnancy in mares. *Journal of Reproduction and Fertility, Supplement* 27, 457–463.

Holtan, D.W., Houghton, E., Silver, M., Fowden, A.L., Ousey, J. and Rossdale, P.D. (1991) Plasma progestagens in the mare, fetus and newborn foal. *Journal of Reproduction and Fertility, Supplement* 44, 517–528.

Holyoak, G.R., Balasuriya, U.B.R., Broaddus, C.C. and Timoney, P.J. (2008) Equine viral arteritis: current status and prevention. *Theriogenology* 70, 403–414.

Honnas, C.M., Spensley, M.S., Laverty, S. and Blanchard, P.C. (1988) Hydramnios causing uterine rupture in a mare. *Journal of American Veterinary Medicine Association* 193, 332–336.

Hoshino, Y. and Saeki, K. (2010) Animal cloning by nuclear transfer using somatic cells recovered from organs frozen without cryoprotectant. *Journal of Mammalian Ova Research* 27(3), 93–100.

Horse Race Betting Levy Board (2019) *Codes of Practice 20118–19 on Contagious Equine Metritis, Klebsiella pneumoniae, Pseudomonas aeroginosa, Equine Viral Arteritis and Equine Herpes Virus 1.* Horse Race Betting Levy Board, London.

Hossain, A.M. and Osuamkpe, C.O. (2007) Sole use of sucrose in human sperm cryopreservation. *Archives in Andrology* 53(2), 99–103.

Hossain, M.S., Johannisson, A., Wallgren, M., Nagy, S., Siqueira, A.P. and Rodriguez-Matinez, H. (2011)

Flow cytometry for the assessment of animal sperm integrity and functionality: state of the art review. *Asian Journal of Andrology* 13(3), 406–419.

Houghton, E., Holton, D., Grainger, L., Voller, B.E., Rossdale, P.D. and Ousey, J.C. (1991) Plasma progestagen concentrations in the normal and dysmature newborn foal. *Journal of Reproduction and Fertility, Supplement* 44, 609–617.

Householder, D.D., Pickett, B.W., Voss, J.L. and Olar, T.T. (1981) Effect of extender, number of spermatozoa and hCG on equine fertility. *Equine Veterinary Science* 1, 9–13.

Howarth, S., Lucke, V.M. and Pearson, H. (1991) Squamous cell carcinoma of the equine external genitalia: A review and assessment of penile amputation and urethrostomy as a surgical treatment. *Equine Veterinary Journal* 23, 53–58.

Hudson, J.J. and McCue, P.M. (2004) How to increase recovery rates and transfer success. In: Palmer, S.E. (ed.) *Proceedings of the 50th Annual Convention of the American Association of Equine Practitioners, Denver, Colorado.* American Association of Equine Practitioners, pp. 406–408.

Hudson, J.J. McCue, P.M. Carnevale, E.M., Welsh, S. and Squires, E.L. (2006) The effects of cooling and vitrification of embryos from mares treated with equine follicle-stimulating hormone on pregnancy rates after nonsurgical transfer. *Journal of Equine Veterinary Science* 26, 51–54.

Huff, A.N., Meacham, T.N. and Wahlberg, M.L. (1985) Feeds and feeding: a review. *Journal of Equine Veterinary Science* 5, 96–108.

Hughes, J.P. (1993) Developmental anomalies of the female reproductive tract. In: McKinnon, A.O. and Voss, J.L. (eds) *Equine Reproduction.* Lea and Febiger, Philadelphia, Pennsylvania, London, pp. 408–416.

Hughes, J.P. and Loy, R.G. (1970) Artificial insemination in the equine. A comparison of natural breeding and AI of mares using semen from six stallions. *Cornell Veterinary* 60, 463–475.

Hughes, J.P., Stabenfeldt, G.H. and Evans, J.W. (1975a) The oestrous cycle of the mare. *Journal of Reproduction and Fertility*, Supplement 23, 161–166.

Hughes, J.P., Stabenfeldt, G.H., Kindhal, H., Kennedy, P.C., Edquist, L.E., Nealy, D.P. and Schalm, O.W. (1979) Pyrometra in the mare. *Journal of Reproduction and Fertility, Supplement* 27, 321–329.

Hughes, J.P., Marcelo, A.C. and Stabenfeldt, G.H. (1985) Luteal phase ovulations: what are the options? *Proceedings of Annual Meeting of the Society of Theriogenology*, 11–13 Setember, Sacramento pp. 123–125.

Huhtinen, M., Lagneaux, D., Koskinen, E. and Palmer, E. (1997) The effect of sucrose in the thawing solution on the morphology and mobility of frozen equine embryos. *Equine Veterinary Journal, Supplement* 25, 94–97.

Huhtinen, M., Sjoholm, A. and Panko, J. (2000) Comaprison of glycerol and ethylene glycol in equine embryo freezing using confocal microscopy, DAPI- staining and nonsurgical transfer. Proceedings of the 5th International Symposium on Equine Embryo Transfer. *Havemeyer Foundation Monograph Series* 3, 52–54.

Hunt, R.J., Hay, W., Collatos, C. and Welles, E. (1990) Testicular seminoma associated with torsion of the spermatic cord in two cryptorchid stallions. *Journal of the American Veterinary Medical Association* 197(11), 1484–1486.

Hunter, R.H.F. (1990) Gamete lifespan in the mare's genital tract. *Equine Veterinary Journal* 22(6), 378–379.

Hunter, R.H. (2008) Sperm release for oviductal epithelial binding is controlled hormonally by peri-ovulatory Graafian follicles *Molecular Reproduction Development* 75, 167–174.

Huppes, T., Stout, T.A.E. and Ensink, J.M. (2017) Decision making for cryptorchid castrtion; a retrospective analysis of 280 cases. *Journal of Equine Veterinary Science* 48, 73–81.

Hurtgen, J.P. (1987) Stallion genital abnormalities. In: Robinson, N.E. (ed.) *Current Therapy in Equine Medicine,* 2nd edn. W.B. Saunders, Philadelphia, Pennsylvania, pp. 558–562.

Hurtgen, J.P. (1997) Commercial freezing of stallion semen. In: *Proceedings of the 19th Bain-Fallon Memorial Lectures, Equine Reproduction.* Australian Equine Veterinary Association, Manly, New South Wales, Australia, pp. 17–23.

Hurtgen, J.P. (2000) Breeding management of the warmblood stallion. In: Samper, J.C. (ed.) *Equine Breeding Management and Artificial Insemination.* W.B. Saunders, Philadelphia, Pennsylvania, pp. 73–80.

Hurtgen, J.P. (2006) Pathogenesis and treatment of endometritis in the mare: a review. *Therogenology* 66(3), 560–566.

Hurtgen, J.P. (2011a) Uterine abnormalities. In: McKinnon, A.O., Squires, E.L., Vaala, E. and Varner, D.D. (eds) *Equine Reproduction*, 2nd edn. Wiley-Blackwell, Philadelphia, London, pp. 2669–2673.

Hurtgen, J.P. (2011b) Abnormalities of cervical and vaginal development. In: McKinnon, A.O., Squires, E.L., Vaala, E. and Varner, D.D. (eds) *Equine Reproduction*, 2nd edn. Wiley-Blackwell, Philadelphia, London, pp. 2719–2720.

Hurtt, A.E., Landin-Alvarenga, F., Seidel Jr, G.E. and Squires, E.L. (2000) Vitrification of immature and mature equine and bovine oocytes in an ethylene glycol, ficoll and sucrose solution using open-pulled straws. *Theriogenology* 54, 119–128.

Hyland, J.H. (1993) Uses of gonadotrophin releasing hormone (GnRH) and its analogues for advancing the breeding season in the mare. *Animal Reproduction Science* 33(1–4), 195–207.

Hyland, H.J. and Langsford, D.A. (1990) Changes in urinary and plasma oestrone sulphate concentrations after induction of foetal death in mares at 45 days of gestation. *Australian Veterinary Journal* 67, 349–351.

Ijaz, A. and Ducharme, R. (1995) Effects of various extenders and taurine on survival of stallion sperm cooled to 5°C. *Theriogenology* 44(7), 1039–1050.

Imel, K.J., Squires, E.L., Elsden, R.P. and Shideler, R.K. (1981) Collection and transfer of equine embryos. *Journal of the American Veterinary Medical Association* 179(10), 987–989.

Imboden, I., Janett, F., Burger, D., Crowe, M.A., Hässig, M., Thun, R. (2006) Influence of immunization against GnRH on reproductive cyclicity and estrous behavior in the mare. *Theriogenology* 66(8), 1866–1875.

Inoue, Y. and Sekiguchi, M. (2017) Vestibuloplasty for persistent pneumovagina in mares. *Journal of Equine Veterinary Science* 48, 9–14.

Irvine, C.H.G. (1984) Hypothyroidism in the foal. *Equine Veterinary Journal* 16, 302–305.

Irvine, C.H.G. and Alexander, S.L. (1991) Effect of sexual arousal on gonadotrophin releasing hormone, luteinising hormone and follicle stimulating hormone secretion in the stallion. *Journal of Reproduction and Fertility, Supplement* 44, 135–143.

Irvine, C.H.G. and Alexander, S.C. (1993a) Secretory patterns and rates of GnRH, FSH and LH revealed by intensive sampling of pituitary venous blood in the luteal phase mare. *Endocrinology* 132, 212–218.

Irvine, C.H.G. and Alexander, S.C. (1993b) GnRH. In: McKinnon, A.O. and Voss, J.L. (eds) *Equine Reproduction*. Lea and Febiger, Philadelphia, Pennsylvania, pp. 37–45.

Irvine, C.H.G. and Alexander, S.C. (1994) The dynamics of gonadotrophin releasing hormone, LH and FSH secretion during spontaneous ovulatory surge of the mare as revealed by intensive sampling of pituitary venous blood. *Journal of Endocrinology* 140, 283–295.

Irvine, C.H.G. and Alexander, S.L. (1997) Patterns of secretion of GnRH, LH and FSH during the postovulatory period in mares: mechanisms prolonging the LH surge *Journal of Reproduction and Fertility* 109, 263–271.

Irvine C.H., Sutton, P., Turner, J.E. and Mennick, P.E. (1990) Changes in plasma progesterone concentrations from day 17 to 42 of gestation in mares maintaining or losing pregnancy. *Equine Veterinary Journal* 22, 104–106.

Irvine, C.H.G., Turner, J.E., Alexander, S.L., Shand, N. and van Noordt, S. (1998) Gonadotrophin profiles and dioestrus pulsatile release patterns in mares as determined by collection of jugular vein blood at 4hr intervals throughout an oestrous cycle. *Journal of Reproduction and Fertility* 113, 315–322.

Irvine, C.H.G., McKeough, V.L., Turner, J.E., Alexander, S.L. and Taylor, T.B. (2002) Effectiveness of a two does regime of prostaglandin administration in inducing luteolysis without side effects in mares. *Equine Veterinary Journal* 34, 191–194.

Ishii, M., Shimamura, T., Utsumi, A., Jitsukawa, T., Endo, M., Fukuda, T. and Yamanoi, T. (2001) Reproductive performance and factors that decrease pregnancy rate in heavy draft horses bred at the Foal Heat. *Journal of Equine Veterinary Science* 21(3), 131–136.

Jackson, G., Carson, T., Heath, P. and Cooke, G. (2002) CEMO in a UK stallion. *Veterinary Record* 151, 582–583.

Jackson, P.G.G. (1982) Rupture of the prepubic tendon in a Shire mare. *Veterinary Record* 111(2), 38.

Jackson, P.G.G. (2004) *Handbook of Veterinary Obstetrics*, 2nd edn. Saunders Elsevier, Missouri.

Jackson, S.G. (2011) Nutrition and exercise for breeding stallions. In: McKinnon, A.O., Squires, E.L., Vaala, E. and Varner, D.D. (eds) *Equine Reproduction*, 2nd edn. Wiley-Blackwell, Philadelphia, London, pp. 1228–1239.

Jacob, J.C., Gastal, E.L., Gastal, M.O., Carvalho, G.R., Beg, M.A. and Ginther, O.J. (2009) Temporal relationships and repeatability of follicle diameters and hormone concentrations within individuals in mares. *Reproduction in Domestic Animals* 44, 92–99.

Jacobson, N.L. and McGillard, A.D. (1984) The mammary gland and lactation. In: Swenson, M.J. (ed.) *Duke's Physiology of Domestic Animals*, 10th edn. Canstock Publishing Associates, Cornell University Press, Ithaca, New York, pp. 871–891.

Jahromi, A.R., Salaran, M., Parizi, A.M. and Mogheiseh, A. (2015) Bilateral traumatic orchitis with unilateral inguinal hernia in a stallion. *Online Journal of Veterinary Research* 19(12), 813–816.

Jainudeen, M.R. and Hafez, E.S.E. (1993) Reproductive failure in males. In: Hafez, E.S.E. (ed.) *Reproduction in Farm Animals*, 6th edn. Lea and Febiger, Philadelphia, Pennsylvania, pp. 287–297.

Jalim, S.L. and McKinnon, A.O. (2010) Surgical results and fertility following correction of vesico-vaginal reflux in mares. *Australian Veterinary Journal* 88(5), 182–185.

Jasko, D.J. (1992) Evaluation of stallion semen. In: Blanchard, T.L. and Varner, D.D. (eds) *The Veterinary Clinics of North America, Equine Practitioners*. W.B. Saunders, Philadelphia, Pennsylvania, pp. 129–148.

Jasko, D.J. (2002) Comparison of pregnancy rates following non-surgical transfer of day 8 equine embryos using various transfer devices. In: Evans, M.J. (ed.) *Equine Reproduction VIII Theriogenology 58*. Elsevier, New York, pp. 713–716.

Jasko, D.J., Lein, D.H. and Foote, R.H. (1990a) Determination of the relationship between sperm morphologic classifications and fertility in stallions: 66 cases (1987–1988). *Journal of the American Veterinary Association* 197(3), 389–394.

Jasko, D.J., Lein, D.H. and Foote, R.H. (1990b) A comparison of two computer automated semen analysis instruments for the evaluation of sperm motion characteristics in the stallion. *Journal of Andrology* 11, 453–459.

Jasko, D.J., Lein, D.H. and Foote, R.H. (1991) Stallion spermatozoal morphology and its relationship to spermatozoal motility and fertility. In: Blake-Caddel, L. (ed.) *Proceedings of 37th Annual Convention of the American Association of Equine Practitioners, San Francisco, California*. American Association of Equine Practitioners, pp. 211–221.

Jasko, D.J., Hathaway, J.A., Schaltenbrand, V.L., Simper, W.D. and Squires, E.L. (1992a) Effect of seminal plasma and egg yolk on motion characteristics of cooled stallion spermatozoa. *Theriogenology* 37, 1241–1252.

Jasko, D.J., Little, T.V., Lein, D.H. and Foote, R.H. (1992b) Comparison of spermatozoal movement and semen characteristics with fertility in stallions: 64 cases (1987–1988). *Journal of the American Veterinary Association* 200(7), 979–985.

Jasko, D.J., Bedford, S.J., Cook, N.L., Mumford, E.C., Squires, E. and Pickett, B.W. (1993a) Effect of antibiotics on motion characteristics of a cooled stallion spermatozoa. *Theriogenology* 40, 885–893.

Jasko, D.J., Moran, D.M., Farlin, M.E., Squires, E.L., Amann, R.P. and Pickett, B.W. (1993b) Pregnancy rates utilising fresh, cooled and frozen-thawed stallion semen. In: Blake-Caddel, L. (ed.) *Proceedings of the 38th Annual Convention of the American Association of Equine Practitioners, Orlando, Florida*. American Association of Equine Practitioners, pp. 649–660.

Jeffcote, L. (2005) The growing horse: nutrition and prevention of growth disorders. *European Federation of Animal Science (EAAP) Publication No 114*, 243–255.

Jeffcote, L.B. and Rossdale, P.D. (1979) A radiographic study of the foetus in late pregnancy and during foaling. *Journal of Reproduction and Fertility, Supplement 27*, 563–569.

Jeffcote, L.B. and Whitwell, K.E. (1973) Twinning as a cause of foetal and neonatal loss in the Thoroughbred mare. *Journal of Comparative Pathology* 83, 91–106.

Jeffcote, L.B., Rossdale, P.D. and Leadon, D.P. (1982) Haematological changes in the neonatal period of normal and induced premature foals. *Journal of Reproduction and Fertility, Supplement 32*, 537–544.

Jennings, M.W., Boime, I., Daphna-Iken, D., Jablonka-Shariff, A., Conley, A.J., Colgin, M., Bidstrup,

L.A., Meyers-Brown, G.A., Famula, T.R. and Roser, J.F. (2009) The efficacy of recombinant equine follicle stimulating hormone (reFSH) to promote follicular growth in mares using a follicular suppression model. *Animal Reproduction Science* 116, 291–307.

Jennes, R. and Sloane, R.G. (1970) Review article. *Dairy Science Abstract* 32, 158–162.

Jeyendran, R.S., Van der Ven, H.H., Perez-Pelaez, M., Crabo, B.G. and Zanveld, L.J.D. (1984) Development of an assay to assess the functional integrity of the human sperm membrane and its relationship to other semen characteristics. *Journal of Reproduction and Fertility* 70, 219–228.

Jochle, W. and Trigg, T.E. (1994) Control of ovulation in the mare with ovuplant a short-term release implant (STI) containing GnRH analogue Deslorelin Acetate. Studies from 1990–1994. A review. *Journal of Equine Veterinary Science* 14(12), 632–644.

Jochle, W., Irvine, C.H.G., Alexander, S.L. and Newby, T.J. (1987) Release of LH, FSH and GnRH into pituitary venous blood in mares treated with PGF analogue, luprostiol, during the transition period. *Journal of Reproduction and Fertility, Supplement* 35, 261–267.

Johansson, C.S., Matsson, F.C., Lehn-Jensen, H., Nielsen, J.M. and Petersen, M.M. (2008) Equine spermatozoa viability comparing the Nucleo-Counter SP-100 and the eosin–nigrosin stain. *Animal Reproduction Science* 107, 325–326.

Johnson, A.K. (2011) Sperm chromatin structure assay. In: McKinnon, A.O., Squires, E.L., Vaala, E. and Varner, D.D. (eds) *Equine Reproduction*, 2nd edn. Wiley-Blackwell, Philadelphia, London, pp. 1506–1509.

Johnson, A.K., Clark-Price, S.C., Choi, Y.H., Hartman, D.L. and Hinrichs, K. (2010) Physical and clinicopathologic findings in foals derived by use of somatic cell nuclear transfer: 14 cases (2004–2008). *Journal of the American Veterinary Medical Association* 236, 983–990.

Johnson, J.R. (2011) Neonatal isoerythrolysis. In: McKinnon, A.O., Squires, E.L., Vaala, E. and Varner, D.D. (eds) *Equine Reproduction*, 2nd edn. Wiley-Blackwell, Philadelphia, London, pp. 353–360.

Johnson, L. (1991a) Spermatogenesis. In: Cupps, D.T. (ed.) *Reproduction in Domestic Animals*, 3rd edn. Academic Press, New York, pp. 173–219.

Johnson, L. (1991b) Seasonal differences in equine spermatogenesis. *Biology of Reproduction* 44, 284–291.

Johnson, L. and Tatum, M.E. (1989) Temporal appearance of seasonal changes in numbers of sertoli cells, leidig cells and germ cells in stallions. *Biology of Reproduction* 40, 994–999.

Johnson, L. and Thompson, D.L. (1983) Age related and seasonal variation in the sertoli cell population, daily sperm production and serum concentration of follicle stimulating hormone, luteinising hormone and testosterone in stallions. *Biology of Reproduction* 29, 777–789.

Johnson, L., Varner, D.D. and Thompson, D.L. (1991) Effect of age and season on the establishment of spermatogenesis in the horse. *Journal of Reproduction and Fertility, Supplement* 44, 87–97.

Johnson, L., Blanchard, T.L., Varner, D.D. and Scrutchfield, W.I. (1997) Factors affecting spermatogenesis in the stallion. *Theriogenology* 48(7), 1199–1216.

Johnson, L., Thompson, D.L and Varner, D.D. (2008) Role of sertoli cell number and function on regulation of spermatogenesis. *Animal Reproduction Science* 105, 23–51.

Johnson, L., Griffin, C.E. and Martin, M.T. (2011) Spermatogenesis. In: McKinnon, A.O., Squires, E.L., Vaala, E. and Varner, D.D. (eds) *Equine Reproduction*, 2nd edn. Wiley-Blackwell, Philadelphia, London, pp. 1026–1052.

Johnson, L.A. (2000) Sexing mammalian sperm for production of offspring: the state of the art. *Animal Reproduction Science* 60, 93–107.

Johnson, L.A., Flook, J.P. and Hawk, H.W. (1989) Sex preselection in rabbits: live birth from X and Y sperm separated by DNA and cell sorting. *Biology of Reproduction* 41, 199–203.

Johnson, L.A., Welch, G.R., Rens, W. and Dobrinsky, J.R. (1998) Enhanced cytometric sorting of mammalian X and Y sperm: high speed sorting and orientating nozzle for artificial insemination. *Theriogenology* 49(1), 361.

Jones, C.T. and Rolph, T.P. (1985) Metabolism during fetal life: a functional assessment of metabolic development. *Physiology Review* 65(2), 357–430.

Jordon, R.M. (1982) Effect of weight loss of gestating mares on subsequent production. *Journal of Animal Science* 55(Supplement 1), 208.

Jouanisson, E., Murcia, Y., Beauchamp, G. and Diaw, M. (2017) Morphological evaluation of the stallion spermatozoa through three staining methods. *Clinical Theriogenology* 9(3), 473.

Juhász, J., Nagy, P., Kulcsár, M. and Huszenicza, G. (2001) A review: factors influencing semen quality and endocrinological sex function in stallions – with emphasis on glucocorticoids. *Folia Veterinaria* 45(1), 3–8.

Jung, C., Hospes, R., Bostedt, H. and Litzke, L.F. (2008) Surgical treatment of uterine torsion using a ventral midline laparotomy in 19 mares. *Australian Veterinary Journal* 86, 272–276.

Juzawiak, J.J., Slone, D.E., Santschi, E.M. and Moll, H.D. (1990) Cesarean section in 19 mares. Results and postoperative fertility. *Veterinary Surgery* 19(1), 50–52.

Kabisch, J., Klose, K. and Schoon, H.A. (2019) Endometrial biopsies of old mares – what to expect? *Pferdeheilkunde* 35(3), 211–219.

Kainer, R.A. (1993) Reproductive organs of the mare. In: McKinnon, A.O. and Voss, J.L. (eds) *Equine Reproduction.* Lea and Febiger, Philadelphia, pp. 3–19.

Kainer, R.A. (2011) Internal reproductive anatomy. In: McKinnon, A.O., Squires, E.L., Vaala, W.E. and Varner, D.D. (eds) *Equine Reproduction*, 2nd edn. Wiley-Blackwell, Philadelphia, London, pp. 1582–1597.

Kakoi, H., Hirora, K., Gawahara, H., Kurosawa, M. and Kuwajima, M. (2005) Genetic diagnosis of sex chromosome aberrations in horses based on parentage test by microsatalite DNA and analysis of X- and Y- linked markers. *Equine Veterinary Journal* 37, 143–147.

Kalsbeck, A., Kreiner, F., Fliers, E., Sauerwein, H.P., Romijn, J.A., Buijs, R.M. (2007) Minireview: Circadian control of metabolism by the suprachiasmatic nuclei. *Endocrinology* 148, 5635–5639.

Kankofer, M., Kolm, G., Aurich, J. and Aurich, C. (2005) Activity of glutathione peroxidase, superoxide dismutase and catalase and lipid peroxidation intensity in stallion semen during storage at 5 degrees C. *Theriogenology* 15(63), 1354–1365.

Kaplan, R.M. and Nielsen, M.K. (2010) An evidence-based approach to equine parasite control: It ain't the 60s anymore. *Equine Veterinary Education* 22, 306–316.

Kaplan, R.M., Klei, T.R., Lyons, E.T., Lester, G.D., French, D.D., Tolliver, S.C., Courtney, C.H., Vidyanshankar, A.N. and Zhao, Y. (2004) Prevalence of anthelmintic resistance cathostomes in horse farms. *Journal of the American Veterinary Medicine Association* 225, 903–910.

Karasek, M. and Winczyk, K. (2006) Melatonin in humans. *Journal of Physiology and Pharmacology* 57 (Suppl 5), 19–39.

Kareskoski, A.M., Reilas, T., Andersson, M. and Katila, T. (2006) Motility and plasma membrane integrity of spermatozoa in fractionated stallion ejaculates after storage. *Reproduction in Domestic Animals* 41(1), 33–38.

Karouse, K. (2013) Testing mammary gland secretions to help predict when a mare will foal. *Veterinary Record* 173, 216–217.

Karouse, K., Murase, H., Sato, F., Ishimaru, M., Endo, Y. and Nambo, Y. (2012) Assessment for predicting parturition in mares based on prepartum temperature changes using a digital rectal thermometer and microchip transponder thermometry device. *Journal of Veterinary Medical Science* 74(7), 845–850.

Kaseda, Y., Khalil, A.M. and Ogawa, H. (1995) Harem stability and reprodictive success in Misaki feral mares. *Equine Veterinary Journal* 27, 368–372.

Kask, K., Odensvik, K. and Kindahl, H. (1997) Prostaglandin F release associated with an embryo transfer procedure in the mare. *Equine Veterinary Journal* 29, 286–289.

Katila, T. (1997) Procedures for handling fresh stallion semen. *Theriogenology* 48(7), 1217–1227.

Katila, T. (2005) Effect of inseminate and the site of insemination on the uterus and pregnancy rates of mares. *Animal Reproduction Science* 89(1), 31–38.

Katila, T. (2011) Sperm–uterine interactions. In: McKinnon, A.O., Squires, E.L., Vaala, E. and Varner, D.D. (eds) *Equine Reproduction*, 2nd edn. Wiley-Blackwell, Philadelphia, London, pp. 1092–1098.

Katila, T. (2012) The equine cervix. *Pferdeheilkunde* 28(1), 35–38.

Katila, T., Celebi, M. and Koskinen, E. (1996) Effect of timing of frozen semen insemination on pregnancy rate in mares. *Acta Veterinaria Scandinavica* 37(3), 361–365.

Katila, T., Combes, G.B., Varner, D.D. and Blanchard, T.L. (1997) Comparison of three containers used for the transport of cooled stallion semen. *Theriogenology* 48(7), 1085–1092.

Katila, T., Sankari, S. and Makela, O. (2000) Transport of spermatozoa in the genital tracts of mares. *Journal of Reproduction and Fertility Supplement* 56, 571–578.

Kavazis, A.N., Kivipelto, J. and Ott, E.A. (2002) Supplementation of broodmares with copper, zinc, iron, manganese, cobalt, iodine and selenium. *Journal of Equine Veterinary Science* 22, 460–464.

Kay, A.T., Spirito, M.A., Rodgerson, D.H. and Brown, S.E. (2008) Surgical technique to repair Grade IV rectal tears in post-parturient mares. *Veterinary Surgery* 37(4), 345–349.

Kayser, J.P., Amann, R.P., Sheideler, R.K., Squires, E.L., Jasko, D.J. and Pickett, B.W. (1992) Effects of linear cooling rates on motion characteristics of stallion spermatozoa. *Theriogenology* 38, 601–614.

Keifer, N.M. (1976) Male pseudohermaphroditism of the testicular, feminizing type in a horse. *Equine Veterinary Journal* 8, 38–41.

Kelley, D.E., Gibbons, J.R., Smith, R., Vernon, K.L., Pratt-Phillip, S.E. and Mortensen, C.J. (2011) Exercise affects both ovarian follicular dynamics and hormone concentrations in mares. *Theriogenology* 76, 615–622.

Kelly, G.M.M. and Newcombe, J.R. (2009) Uterus bicorpora bicollis as a possible cause of infertility in a mare. Short Communication. *Veterinary Record* 64, 20–21.

Kelly, S.M., Buckett, W.M., Abdul-Jalil, A.K. and Tan, S.L. (2003) The cryobiology of assisted reproduction. Review. *Minerva Gynecology* 55(5), 389–398.

Kenney, R.M. (1975) Clinical fertility evaluation of the stallion. In: Milne, J.F. (ed.) *Proceedings of the 21st American Association of Equine Practitioners, Boston, Massachusetts*. American Association of Equine Practitioners, pp. 336–355.

Kenney, R.M. (1977) Clinical aspects of endometrium biopsy in fertility evaluation of the mare. In: Milne, J.F. (ed.) *Proceedings of the 23rd Annual Meeting American Association of Equine Practitioners, Vancouver, British Columbia*. American Association of Equine Practitioners, pp. 355–362.

Kenney, R.M. (1978) Cyclic and pathological changes of the mare endometrium as detected by biopsy, with a note on early embryonic death. *Journal of*

the American Veterinary Medical Association 172(3), 241–262.

Kenney, R.M. (1990) Estimation of stallion fertility: the use of sperm cromatin structure assay, DNA Index and karyotype as adjuncts to traditional tests. In: Wade, J.F. (ed.) Proceedings of the 5th International Symposium on Equine Reproduction, Deauville, France. *Journal of Reproduction and Fertility* 42–43.

Kenney, R.M., Bergman, R.V., Cooper, W.L. and Morse, G.W. (1975a) Minimal contamination techniques for breeding mares: techniques and preliminary findings. In: Milne, J.F. (ed.) *Proceedings of 21st Annual Convention of the American Association of Equine Practitioners, Boston, Massachusetts*. American Association of Equine Practitioners, pp. 327–335.

Kenney, R.M., Evenson, D.P., Garcia, M.C. and Love, C.C. (1995) Relationships between sperm chromatin structure, motility and morphology of ejaculated sperm and seasonal pregnancy rate. *Biology of Reproduction Monograph Equine Reproduction VI*, 1, 647–653.

Kerschen, L. (2019) The Effect of Reproductive Status, Age, and Time of Year on the Incidence of Prolonged Dioestrus. MSc thesis, Aberystwyth University, UK.

Kershaw, C.M., Khalid, M., McGowan, M.R., Ingram, K., Leethongdee, S., Wax, G. and Scaramuzzi, R.J. (2005) The anatomy of the sheep cervix and its influence on the transcervical passage of an inseminating pipette into the uterine lumen. *Theriogenology* 64(5), 1225–1235.

Kiley-Worthington, M. and Wood-Gush, D. (1987) Stereotypic behavior. In: Robinson, N.E. (ed.) *Current Therapy in Equine Medicine*, 2nd edn. W.B. Saunders, Philadelphia, Pennsylvania, pp. 131–134.

Killian, B., Johnson, A., Wilborn, R., Jensen, R. and Barstow, C. (2017) A case of fescue toxicity in a broodmare. *Clinical Theriogenology* 9(3), 505.

Kilmer, D.N., Sharp, D.C., Berhund, L.A., Grubaugh, W., McDowell, K.J. and Peck, L.S. (1982) Melatonin rhythms in pony mares and foals. *Journal of Reproduction and Fertility, Supplement* 32, 303–307.

Kindahl, H., Knudsen, O., Madej, A. and Edquist, L.E. (1982) Progesterone, prostaglandin F2 alpha,

PMSG and oestrone sulphate during early pregnancy in the mare. *Journal of Reproduction and Fertility, Supplement* 32, 353–359.

King, S.S., Jones, K.L., Dille, E.A. and Roser, J.F. (2004) Prolactin receptors in the corpus luteum of mares. *Proceedings of the 15th International Congress on Animal Reproduction, Abstract 39, Potro Seguro, Brazil, 8–12 August 2004*, Elsevier.

King, S.S., Campbell, A.G., Dille, E.A., Roser, J.F., Murphy, L.L. and Jones, K.L. (2005) Dopamine receptors in equine ovarian tissues. *Domestic Animal Endocrinology* 28, 405–415.

King, S.S., Jones, K.L., Mullenix, B.A. and Heath, D.T. (2008) Seasonal relationships between dopmine D1 and D2 receptor and equine FSH receptor mRNA in equine ovarian eithelium. *Animal Reproduction Science* 108(1–2), 259–266.

Kirkpatrick, J.F., Vail, R., Devous, S., Schwend, S., Baker, C.B. and Weisner, L. (1976) Diurnal variation of plasma testosterone in wild stallions. *Biology of Reproduction* 15, 98–101.

Kiviniemi-Moore, J., Bradecamp, E.A., Schnobrich, M.R.and Scoggin, C.F. (2017) Clinical findings in a warmblood mare following intrauterine infusion of the commercial preperation of enrofloxacin (Baytril®). *Clinical Theriogenology* 9(3), 478.

Kjöllerström, H.J., Collares-Pereira, M.J. and Oom, M.M. (2011) First evidence of sex chromosome mosaicism in the endangered Sorraia Horse breed. *Livestock Science* 136(2/3), 273–276.

Kjöllerström, H.J., Oom, M. de M., Chowdhary, B.P. and Raudsepp, T. (2016) Fertility a sessment in Sorraia stallions by sperm-fish and Fkbp6 genotyping. *Reproduction in Domestic Animals* 51(3), 351–359.

Klein, C. (2016) Early pregnancy in the mare: old concepts revisited. *Domestic Animal Endocrinology* 56, S212–217.

Klein, C. and Troedsson, M.O.T. (2011) Maternal recognition of pregnancy in the horse: a mystery still to be solved. *Reproduction, Fertility and Development* 23(8), 952–963.

Klewitz, J., Krekeler, N., Ortgies, E., Heberling, A., Linke, C. and Sieme, H. (2013) Evaluation of pregnancy and foaling rates after trans-vaginal ultrasound guided aspiration in mares. *Journal of the American Veterinary Medical Association* 242(4), 527–532.

Klewitz, J., Stuebing, C., Rohn, K., Goergens, A., Martinsson, G., Orgies, F., Probst, J., Hollinshead, F., Bollwein, H. and Sieme, H. (2015) Effects of age, parity and pregnancy a normalities on foal birthweight and uterine blood flow in the mare. *Theriogenology* 83(4), 721–729.

Klonisch, T. and Hombach-Klonisch, S. (2000) Review: Relaxin expression at the feto-maternal interface. *Reproduction in Domestic Animals* 35, 149–152.

Klug, E. (1992) Routine artificial applications in the Hannovarian sport horse breeding association. *Animal Reproduction Science* 28, 39–44.

Knight, P.G. and Glister, C. (2001) Potential local regulatory functions for inhibins, activins and follistatin in the ovary. *Reproduction* 121(4), 503–512.

Knight, P.G. and Glister, C. (2006) TGF-B superfamily members and ovarian follicle development. *Society for Reproduction and Fertility* 132, 191–206.

Knopp, K., Hoffmann, N., Rath, D. and Sieme, H. (2005) Effects of cushioned centrifugation technique on sperm recovery and sperm quality in stallions with good and poor semen freezability. *Animal Reproduction Science* 89, 294–297.

Knottenbelt, D.C. (2003) The mammary gland. In: Knottenbelt, D.C., LeBlanc, M., Lopate, C.L. and Pascoe, R.R. (eds) *Equine Stud Farm Medicine and Surgery*. W.B. Saunders, Philadelphia, Pennsylvania, pp. 343–352.

Knottenbelt, D. and Pascoe, R. (2003) Routine stud management procedures. In: Knottenbelt, D.C., LeBlanc, M., Lopate, C.L. and Pascoe, R.R. (eds) *Equine Stud Farm Medicine and Surgery*. W.B. Saunders, Philadelphia, Pennsylvania, pp. 25–41.

Knottenbelt, D.C. and Holdstock, N. (2004a) The role of colostrum in immunity. In: Knottenbelt, D.C. (ed.) *Equine Neonatology and Surgery*. Saunders, Edinburgh, pp15–18.

Knottenbelt, D.C. and Holdstock, N. (2004b) Methods of assessing colotrum quality. In: Knottenbelt, D.C. (ed.) *Equine Neonatology and Surgery*. Saunders, Edinburgh, pp393–394.

Knottenbelt, D.C., Holdstock, N. and Madigan, J.E. (2004) *Equine Neonatology, Medicine and Surgery*. W.B. Saunders, Philadelphia, Pennsylvania, pp. 508.

Knutti, B., Pycock, J.F., Van Der Weijden, G.C. and Kupfer, U. (2000) The influences of early post breeding uterine lavage on pregnancy rates in mares with intrauterine fluid accumulations after breeding. *Equine Veterinary Education* 12(5), 267–276.

Ko, T.H. and Lee, S.E. (1993) Establishment of a biological assay for the fertilising ability of equine spermatozoa. *Korean Journal of Animal Science* 35(3), 175–179.

Kocher, A. and Staniar, W.B. (2013) The pattern of thoroughbred growth is affected by a foal's birthdate. *Livestock Science* 154(1–3), 204–214.

Koene, M.H., Boder, H. and Hoppen, H.O. (1990) Feasibility of using HMG as a superovulatory drug in a commercial embryo transfer programme. *Journal of Reproduction and Fertility, Supplement* 44, 710–711.

Koets, A.P. (1995) The equine endometrial cup reaction: a review. *Veterinary Quarterly* 17, 21–29.

Kohn, C.W., Knight, D., Hueston, W., Jacobs, R. and Reed, S.M. (1989) Cholesterol and serum IgG, IgA and IgM concentrations in Standardbred mares and their foals at parturition. *Journal of the American Veterinary Medical Association* 195, 64–68.

Köllmann, M., Probst, J., Baackmann, C., Klewitz, J., Squires, E.S. and Sieme, H. (2008) Embryo recovery rate following superovulation with equine pituitary extract (eFSH®) in mares. *Pferdeheilkunde* 24(3), 397–405.

Köllmann, M., Rötting, A., Heberling, A. and Sieme, H. (2011) Laparoscopic techniques for investigating the equine oviduct. *Equine Veterinary Journal* 43(1), 106–111.

Kooistra, L.H. and Ginther, O.J. (1975) Effects of photoperiod on reproduction activity and hair in mares. *American Journal of Veterinary Research* 36, 1413–1419.

Kooistra, L.H. and Loy, R.G. (1968) Effects of artificial lighting regimes on reproductive patterns in mares. In: Milne, J.F. (ed.) *Proceedings of the 14th Annual Convention of the Association of Equine Practitioners, Philadelphia, Pennsylvania*. American Association of Equine Practitioners, pp. 159–169.

Kosiniak, K. (1975) Characteristics of successive jets of ejaculated semen of stallions. *Journal of Reproduction and Fertility, Supplement* 23, 59–61.

Koskinen, E., Martila, P. and Katila, T. (1997) Effect of 19-norandrostenololylaurate on semen characteristics of colts. *Acta Veterinaria Scandinavica* 38(1), 41–50.

Koterba, A.M. (1990) Physical examination. In: Koterba, A.M., Drummond, W.H. and Kosch, P.C. (eds) *Equine Clinical Neonatology*. Lea and Febiger, Philadelphia, Pennsylvania, pp. 71–81.

Koterba, A.M. and Kosch, P.C. (1987) Respiratory mechanisms and breathing patterns in the neonatal foal. *Journal of Reproduction and Fertility* 35, 575–586.

Kotilainen, T., Huhtinen, M. and Katila, T. (1994) Sperm induced leukocytosis in the equine uterus. *Theriogenology* 41(3), 629–636.

Kowalczyk, A., Czerniawska-Piatkowska, E. and Kuczaj, M. (2019) Factors Influencing the Popularity of Artificial Insemination of Mares in Europe. *Animals* 9, 460.

Kreider, J.L., Tindall, W.C. and Potter, G.D. (1985) Inclusion of bovine serum albumin in semen extenders to enhance maintenance of stallion spermatozoa motility. *Theriogenology* 23, 399–408.

Krekeler, N., Hollinshead, F.K., Fortier, L.A., and Volkmann, D.H. (2006) Improved ovulation and embryo recovery rates in mares treated with porcine FSH. *Theriogenology* 66, 663–687.

Kristula, M.A. (2014) Contagious Equine Metritis. In: Seldon, D.C. and Long, M.T. (eds) *Equine Infectious Disease* (2nd edn.) Elsevier, pp 339–343.

Kristula, M.A. and Smith, B.I. (2004) Diagnosis and treatment of four stallions, carriers of contagious metritis organism: case report. *Theriogenology* 61, 595–601.

Kubiak, J.R., Crawford, B.H., Squires, E.L., Wrigley, R.H. and Ward, G.M. (1987) The influence of energy intake and percentage of body fat the reproductive performance of non pregnant mares. *Theriogenology* 28, 587–598.

Kubiak, J.R., Evans, J.W., Potter, G.D., Harms, P.G. and Jenkins, W.L. (1988) Parturition in the multiparous mare fed to obesity. *Journal of Equine Veterinary Science* 8(2), 135–140.

Kubien, E.M. and Tischner, M. (2002) Reproductive success of a mare with a mosaic karyotype: 64,XX /65,XX, +30. *Equine Veterinary Journal* 34(1), 99–100.

Kullander, S., Arvidson, G., Ekelung, L. and Astedt, B. (1975) A review of surfactant principles in the foetal physiology of man and animals. *Journal of Reproduction and Fertility, Supplement* 23, 659–661.

Kumi-Diaka, J. and Badtram, G. (1994) Effect of storage on sperm membrane integrity and other functional characteristics of canine spermatozoa: in vitro bio-assay for canine semen. *Theriogenology* 41, 1355–1366.

Kutvolgi, G., Stelfer, J. and Kovacs, A. (2006) Viability and acrosome staining of stallion spermatozoa by Chicago sky blue and Giemsa. *Biotechnology in Histochemistry* 81(4–6), 109–117.

Lagares, M.A., Petzoldt, R., Sieme, H. and Klug, E. (2000) Assessing equine sperm-membrane integrity. *Andrologia* 32(3), 163–167.

Łącka, K., Kondracki, S., Iwanina, M., and Wysokińska, A. (2016) Assessment of stallion semen morphology using two different staining methods, microscopic techniques, and sample sizes. *Journal of Veterinary Research* 60, 99–104.

Lamming, G.E. and Mann, G.E. (1995) Control of endometrial oxytocin receptors and prostaglandin F2∝ production in cows by progesterone and oestradiol. *Journal of Reproduction and Fertility* 103, 69–73.

Land, M., Hauser, L., Jun, S.R., Nookaew, I., Leuze, M.J., Ahn, T.H., Karpinets, T., Lund, O., Kora, G., Wassenaar, T., Poudel, S. and Ussery, D.W. (2015) Insights from 20 years of bacterial genomic sequencing. *Functional and Integrative Genomics* 15 (2), 141–161.

Lane, E., Bijnen, M. Osborne, M., More, S., Henderson, I., Duffy, F. and Crowe, M. (2016) Key factors affecting reproductive success of thoroughbred mares and stallions on a commercial stud farm *Reproduction in Domestic Animals* 51, 181–187.

Lange-Consiglio, A., Corradetti, B., Perrini, C., Bizzaro, D. and Cremonesi, F. (2016) Leptin and leptin receptor are detectable in equine spermatozoa but are not involved in in vitro fertilisation. *Reproduction, Fertility and Development.* 28, 574–585.

Langlois, B., Blouin, C. and Chaffaux, S. (2012) Analysis of several factors of variation of gestation loss in breeding mares. *Animal* 6(12), 1925–1930.

Lansade, L., Bertrand, M., Boivin, X. and Bouissou, M.F. (2004) Effects of handling at weaning on manageability and reactivity of foals. *Applied Animal Behaviour Science* 87, 131–149.

Lapin, D.R. and Ginther, O.J. (1977) Induction of ovulation and multiple ovulations in seasonally anovulatory and ovulatory mares with equine pituitary extract. *Journal of Animal Science* 44(5), 834–842.

Lascombes, F.A. and Pashen, R.L. (2000) Results from embryo freezing and post-ovulation breeding in a commercial embryo transfer programme. *Proceedings of the 5th International Symposium on Equine Embryo Transfer,* Havemeyer Foundation Monograph Series 3, pp. 95–96.

Lasley, B., Ammon, D., Daels, P., Hughes, J., Munro, C. and Stadenfeldt, G. (1990) Estrogen conjugate concentrations in plasma and urine reflect estrogen secretion in non-pregnant and pregnant mare: a review. *Journal of Equine Veterinary Science* 10, 444–448.

Laugier, C., Foucher, N., Sevin, C., Leon, A. and Tapprest, J. (2011) A 24-year retrospective study of equine abortion in Normandy (France). *Journal of Equine Veterinary Science* 31, 116–123.

Lawrence, L.M. (2011) Nutrition for the broodmare. In: McKinnon, A.O., Squires, E.L., Vaala, E. and Varner, D.D. (eds) *Equine Reproduction*, 2nd edn. Wiley-Blackwell, Philadelphia, London, pp. 2760–2770.

Lawson, K.A. (1996) Longevity of stallion semen in various extenders when chilled to 4°C. MSc thesis. University of Wales, Aberystwyth, UK.

Lawson, K.A. and Davies Morel, M.C.G. (1996) The use of mare's milk as a seminal extender for chilled stallion semen. In: *Warwick Horse Conference February 1996 New Developments in Equine Studies.* Royal Agricultural Society, Kenilworth, UK, pp. 26–39.

Lazić, S., Lupulović, D., Polaček, V., Valčić, M., Lazić, G., Pašagić, E. and Petrović, T. (2015) Detection of Equine Arteritis Virus in the semen of stallions in the Republic of Sebia. *Acta Veterinaria (Lawson, K.A. (1996) Longevity Beograd)* 65(4), 557–567.

Lazzari, G., Crotti, G., Turnin, P., Duchi, R., Mari, G. and Zavaglia, G. (2002) Equine embryos at the compacted morula and blastocyst stage can be obtained by intracytoplasmic sperm injection (ICSI) of in vitro matured oocytes with frozen-thawed spermatozoa from semen of different fertilities. *Theriogenology* 58, 709–712.

Leadon, D.P., Jeffcott, L.B. and Rossdale, P.D. (1984) Mammary secretions in normal spontaneous and induced premature parturition in the mare. *Equine Veterinary Journal* 16(4), 256–259.

Lear, T.L. and Layton, G. (2002) Use of zoo-FSH to characterize a reciprocal translocation in a thoroughbred mare t(1:16)(q16:q21.3). *Equine Veterinary Journal* 34, 207–209.

Lear, T.L. and Villagomez, D.A.F. (2011) Cytogenetic evaluation of mares and foals. In: McKinnon, A.O., Squires, E.L., Vaala, E. and Varner, D.D. (eds) *Equine Reproduction*, 2nd edn. Wiley-Blackwell, Philadelphia, London, pp. 1951–1962.

Leathwick, D.M., Sauermann, C.W. and Nielsen, M.K. (2019) Managing anthelmintic resistance in cyathostomin parasites: Investigating the benefits of refugia-based strategies. *International Journal of Parasitology Drugs and Drug Resistance* 10, 118–124.

LeBlanc, M.M. (1990) Immunologic considerations. In: Koterba, A.M., Drummond, W.H. and Kosch, P.C. (eds) *Equine Clinical Neonatology*. Lea and Febiger, Philadelphia, Pennsylvania, pp. 275–296.

LeBlanc, M.M. (1991) Reproductive system: the mare. In: Colahan, P.T., Mayhew, I.G., Merritt, A.M. and Moore, J.N. (eds) *Equine Medicine and Surgery*. Vol. II, 4th edn. American Veterinary Publications, Inc., Goleta, California, pp. 1148–1216.

LeBlanc, M.M. (1993a) Vaginal examination. In: McKinnon, A.O. and Voss, J.L. (eds) *Equine Reproduction*. Lea and Febiger, Philadelphia, Pennsylvania, pp. 221–224.

LeBlanc, M.M. (1993b) Endoscopy. In: McKinnon, A.O. and Voss, J.L. (eds) *Equine Reproduction*. Lea and Febiger, Philadelphia, Pennsylvania, London, pp. 255–257.

LeBlanc, M.M. (1994) Oxytocin. The new wonder drug for treatment of endometritis. *Equine Veterinary Education* 6, 39–43.

LeBlanc, M.M. (1995) Ultrasound of the reproductive tract. In: Kobluk, C.N., Ames, T.R. and Goer, R.J. (eds) *The Horse – Diseases and Clinical Management*. Vol. 2. W.B. Saunders, Philadelphia, Pennsylvania, pp. 926–935.

Leblanc, M.M., (1996) Equine perinatology: What we know and what we need to know. *Animal Reproduction Science* 42(1–4), 189–196.

LeBlanc, M.M. (1997) Identification and treatment of the compromised foetus. A clinical perspective. *Equine Veterinary Journal, Supplement* 24, 100–103.

LeBlanc, M.M. (2008) The chronically infertile mare. *Proceedings of the American Association of Equine Practitionners* 54, 39–407.

LeBlanc, M.M. (2010) Advances in the diagnosis and treatment of chronic infectious and post-mating-induced endometritis in the mare. *Reproduction in Domestic Animals* 45(s2), 21–27.

LeBlanc, M.M. (2011) Uterine cytology. In: McKinnon, A.O., Squires, E.L, Vaala, W.E. and Varner, D.D. (eds) *Equine Reproduction*. Wiley-Blackwell, pp. 1922–1928.

LeBlanc, M.M., (2010) Advances in the Diagnosis and Treatment of Chronic Infectious and Post-Mating-Induced Endometritis in the Mare. *Reproduction in Domestic Animals* 45 (Suppl. 2), 21–27.

LeBlanc, M.M. (2011) Uterine cytology. In: McKinnon, A.O., Squires, E.L., Vaala, E. and Varner, D.D. (eds) *Equine Reproduction*, 2nd edn. Wiley-Blackwell, Philadelphia, London, pp. 1922–1928.

LeBlanc, M.M. and Causey, R.C. (2009) Clinical and subclinical endometritis in the mare: both threats to fertility. *Reproduction in Domestic Animals* 44(3),10–22.

LeBlanc, M.M. and McKinnon, A.O. (2011) Breeding the problem mare. In: McKinnon, A.O., Squires, E.L., Vaala, E. and Varner, D.D. (eds) *Equine Reproduction*, 2nd edn. Wiley-Blackwell, Philadelphia, London, pp. 2620–2642.

LeBlanc, M.M. and Tran, T.Q. (1987) Relationships among colostral electrolytes, colostral IgG concentrations and absorption of colostral IgG by foals. *Journal of Reproduction and Fertility, Supplement.* 35, 735–736.

LeBlanc, M.M., Lawin, B.I. and Boswell, R. (1986) Relationships among serum immunoglobulin concentrations in foals, colostrol specific gravity and colostrol immunoglobulin concentrations. *Journal of the American Veterinary Medical Association* 186, 57–60.

LeBlanc, M.M., Tran, T. and Widders, P. (1991) Identification and opsonic activity of immunoglobulins recognising *Streptococcus zooepidemicus* antigens in uterine fluids of mares. *Journal of Reproduction and Fertility, Supplement* 44, 289–296.

LeBlanc, M.M., Tran, T., Baldwin, J.L. and Pritchard, E.L. (1992) Factors that influence passive transfer of immunoglobulins in foals. *Journal of the American Veterinary Medicine Association* 200, 179–183.

LeBlanc, M.M., Newrith, L., Maurag, D., Klapstein, E. and Tran, T. (1994) Oxytocin enhances clearance of radiocolloid from the uterine lumen of reproductively normal mares and mare susceptible to endometritis. *Equine Veterinary Journal* 26(4), 279–282.

LeBlanc, M.M., Lopate, C., Knottenbelt, D. and Pascoe, R. (2004) The mare. In: Knottenbelt, D., LeBlanc, M., Lopate, C. and Pascoe, R. (eds) *Equine Stud Farm Medicine and Surgery*. W.B. Saunders, Philadelphia, Pennsylvania, pp. 113–211.

LeBlanc, M.M., Magsig, J. and Stromberg, A.J. (2007). Use of low-volume uterine flush for diagnosing endometritis in chronically infertile mares. *Theriogenology* 68, 403–412.

Leboeuf, B., Guillouet, P., Batellier, F., Bernelas, D., Bonne, J.L., Forgerit, Y., Renaud, G. and Magistrini, M. (2003) Effect of native phophocaseinate on the in vitro preservation of fresh semen. *Theriogenology* 60, 867–877.

Lee, H.E. and Morris, L.H.A. (2005) Challenges facing sex preselection of stallion spermatozoa. *Animal Reproduction Science* 89(1–4), 147–157.

Leemans, B., Gadella, B.M., Stout, T.A., Heras, S., Smits, K., Ferrer-Buitrago, M., Claes, E., Heindryckx, B., De Vos, W.H., Nelis, H., Hoogewijs, M. and Van Soom, A. (2015) Procaine induces cytocines in horse oocytes via pH-dependent mechanism. *Biology of Reproduction* 93, 23.

Leemans, B., Gadella, B., Stout, T.A.E., De Schauwer, C., Nelis, H.M., Hoogewijs, M. and Van Soom, A. (2016a) The Role of Oviductal Cells in Activating Stallion Spermatozoa. *Journal of Equine Veterinary Science* 152(6), R233–R245.

Leemans, B., Gadella, B.M., Stout, T.A., De Schauwer, C., Nelis, H., Hoogewijs, M., Va-Soom, A. (2016b) Why doesn't conventional IVF work in the horse? The equine oviduct as a microenvironment for capacitation/fertilization. *Reproduction* 152(6), R233–R245.

Leemans, B., Stout, T.A.E., De Schauwer, C., Heras, S., Nelis, H. Hoogewijs, M., Van Soom, A. and Gadella, B. (2019) Update on mammalian sperm capacitation: How much does the horse differ from other species? *Reproduction*, 157(5), R181–R197. doi:10.1530/REP-18–0541.

Leendertse, I.P., Asbury, A.C., Boening, K.J. and von Saldern, F.C. (1990) Successful management of persistent urination during ejaculation in a Thoroughbred stallion. *Equine Veterinary Education* 2(2), 62–64.

Leese, H.J., Hugentobler, S.A., Gray, S.M., Morris, D.C., Sturney, R.G., Whitear, S.L. and Sreenan, J.M. (2008) Female reproductive tract fluids: composition, mechanism of formation and potential role in the developmental origins of health and disease. *Reproduction, Fertility and Development* 20, 1–8.

Legacki, E.L., Corbin, C.J., Ball, B.A., Wynn, M., Loux, S., Stanley, S.D. and Conley, A.J. (2016) Progestin withdrawal at parturition in the mare. *Reproduction* 152(4), 323–331.

Legrand, E., Bencharif, D., Barrier-Battut, I., Delajarraud, H. and Bruyas, J.-F. (2002) Comparison of pregnancy rates for days 7–8 equine embryos frozen in glycerol with or without previous enzymatic treatment of their capsule. *Theriogenology* 58, 721–723.

Legrand, L. and Bailly, A. (2019) Genetic tests available for horses. *Pratique Vétérinaire Equine* 51(202), 14–22.

Leipold, H.W. (1986) Cryptorchidism in the horse: genetic implications. In: Milne, F.J. (ed.) *Proceedings of the 32nd Annual Convention of the American Association of Equine Practitioners, Nashville, Tennessee* 31, 579–590.

Leipold, H.W. and Dennis, S.M. (1993) Congenital defects in foals. In: McKinnon, A.O. and Voss, J.L. (eds) *Equine Reproduction*. Lea and Febiger, Philadelphia, Pennsylvania, pp. 604–613.

Lemes K.M., Silva, D.F., Celeghini, E.C.C., Affonso, F.J., Pugliesi, G., Carvalho, H.F., Silva, L.A., Alonso, M.A., Paes de Arruda, R. and Leite, T.G. (2017) Uterine Vascular Perfusion and Involution During the Postpartum Period in Mares. *Journal Equine Vet Science* 51, 61–69.

Lennard, S.N., Stewart, F., Allen, W.R. and Heap, R.B. (1995) Growth factor production in the pregnant equine uterus. *Biology of Reproduction* 1, 161–170.

Lepeule, J., Bareille, N., Robert, C., Ezanno, P., Valette, J.P., Jacquet, S., Blanchard, G., Dnoix, J.M. and Seegers, H. (2009) Association of growth, feeding practices and exercise conditions with the prevelance of Developmental Orthopaedic Disease in limbs of French foals at weaning. *Preventative Veterinary Medicine* 89, 167–177.

Lester, G.D. (2005) Maturity of the neonatal foal. *Veterinary Clinics of North America Equine Practice* 21(2), 333–335.

Leung, S.T., Wathes, D.C., Young, I.R. and Jenkin, G. (1999) Effect of labour induction on the expression of oxytocin receptor, cytochrome P450 aromatase, and estradiol receptor in the reproductive tract of the late pregnant ewe. *Biology of Reproduction* 60, 814–820.

Ley, W.B. (1989) Daytime foaling management of the mare. 2. Induction of parturition. *Journal of Equine Veterinary Science* 9, 95–100.

Ley, W.B. (2011) Evaluation of uterine tubal patency In: McKinnon, A.O., Squires, E.L., Vaala, E. and Varner, D.D. (eds) *Equine Reproduction*, 2nd edn. Wiley-Blackwell, Philadelphia, London, pp. 1988–1990.

Ley, W.B., Hoffman, J.L., Crisman, M.V., Meacham, T.N., Kiracofe, R.L. and Sullivan, T.L. (1989) Daytime foaling management of the mare. 2. Induction of parturition. *Journal of Equine Veterinary Science* 9, 95–99.

Ley, W.B., Bowen, J.M., Purswell, B.J., Irby, M. and Greive-Candell, K. (1993) The sensitivity, specificity and predictive value of measuring calcium carbonate in mare's prepartum mammary secretions. *Theriogenology* 40, 189–198.

Ley, W.B., Bowen, J.M., Purswell, B.J., Dascanio, J.J., Parker, N.A., Bailey, T.L. and DiGrassie, W.A. (1998) Modified technique to evaluate uterine tubal patency in the mare. In: *Proceedings of the 44th Annual Convention of the American Association of Equine Practitioners, Baltimore, Maryland.* 44, 56–59.

Lezica, R.P., Filip, R., Gorzalczany, S., Ferraro, G., de Erausquin, G.A., Rivas, C. and Ladaga, G.J.B. (2009) Prevalence of ergot derivatives in nature ryegrass pastures: detection and pathogenicity in the horse *Theriogenology* 71, 422–431.

Li, L.Y., Meintjes, M., Graff, K.J., Paul, J.B., Denniston, R.S. and Godke, R.A. (1995) In vitro fertilisation and development of in vitro matured oocytes aspirated from pregnant mares. *Biology of Reproduction, Monographs Series* 1, 309–317.

Li, X., Morris, L.H. and Allen, W.R. (2000) Effects of different activation treatments on fertilization of horse oocytes by intracytoplasmic sperm injection. *Journal of Reproduction and Fertility* 119(2), 253–260.

Li, X., Morris, L.H. and Allen, W.R. (2001) Influence of co-culture during maturation on the developmental potential of equine oocytes fertilized by intracytoplasmic sperm injection (ICSI). *Reproduction* 121(6), 925–932.

Lieberman, R.J. and Bowman, T.R. (1994) Teasing naturally. Strategies to improve your mare's oestrus response. *Modern Horse Breeding* 11, 28–31.

Lieux, P. (1972) Reproductive and genital disease. In: Catcott, E.J. and Smithcors, J.F. (eds) *Equine Medicine and Surgery*, 2nd edn. American Veterinary Publications Book, Wheaton, Illinois, pp. 567–589.

Ligon, E.M., Love, C.C. and Varner, D.D. (2017) Validation of a fixable stain for assessing viability of stallion sperm. *Clinical Theriogenology* 9(3), 448.

Linden, L. de S. van der, Bustamante Filho, I. C., Schiavo, S.D., Maciel, M.A.P., Rodrigues, M.F., Santos, S.I. dos, Mattos, R.C. and Neves, A.P. (2014) *Use of Rhea americana* egg yolk in substitution to chicken egg yolk in equine semen extenders. Pferdheilkunde 30(1), 61–64.

Lindholm, A.R.G., Ferris, R.A., Scofield, D.B. and McCue, P.M. (2012) Comparison of deslorelin and 147 cystorelin for induction of ovulation in mares. *Journal of Equine Veterinary Science* 31, 230–231.

Lindsey, A.C., Bruemmer, J.E. and Squires, E.L. (2001) Low dose insemination of mares using non-sorted and sex-sorted sperm. *Animal Reproduction Science* 68(3–4), 279–289.

Lindsey, A.C., Schenk, J.L., Graham, J.K., Bruemmer, J.E. and Squires, E.L. (2002) Hysteroscopic insemination of low numbers of flow sorted fresh and frozen thawed spermatozoa. *Equine Veterinary Journal* 34, 121–127.

Lindsey, A.C., Varner, D.D., Seidel Jr, G.E., Bruemmer, J.E. and Squires, E.L. (2005) Hysteroscopic or rectally guided, deep uterine insemination of mares with spermatozoa stored 18 h at either 5°C or 15°C prior to flow cytometric sorting. *Animal Reproduction Science* 85, 125–130.

Linklater, W.L., Henderson, K.M., Cameron, E.Z., Stafford, K.J. and Minot, E.O. (2000) The robustness of faecal steroid determination for pregnancy testing Kaimanawa feral mares under field conditions. *New Zealand Veterinary Journal* 48 (4), 93–98.

Liptrap, R.M. (1993) Stress and reproduction in domestic animals *Annals of the New York Acadamy of Science* 697, 275–284.

Little, T.V. (1998) Accessory sex glands and internal reproductive tract evaluation. In: Rantanen, N.W.

and McKinnon, A.O. (eds) *Equine Diagnostic Ultrasonography*. Williams and Wilkins, Baltimore, Maryland, pp. 271–288.

Little, T.V. and Holyoak, R. (1992) Reproductive Anatomy and Physiology of the Stallion. *Veterinary Clinics of North America: Equine Practice* 8(1), 1–29.

Littlejohn, A. and Ritchie, J.D.S. (1975) Rupture of caecum at parturition. *Journal of the South African Veterinary Association* 46(1), 87.

Liu, I.K. and Troedsson, M.H. (2008) The diagnosis and treatment of endometritis in the mare: yesterday and today. *Theriogenology* 70(3), 415–420.

Liu, I.K.M. (2011) Disorders of the oviduct. In: McKinnon, A.O., Squires, E.L., Vaala, E. and Varner, D.D. (eds) *Equine Reproduction*, 2nd edn. Wiley-Blackwell, Philadelphia, London, pp. 2692–2696.

Liu, I.K.M., Lantz, K.C. and Schlafke, S. (1990) Clinical observations of oviductal masses. In: Royer, M.G. (ed.) *Proceedings of the 36th Annual Conference for the American Association of Equine Practitioners, Lexington, Kentucky* pp. 41–50.

Livsey, L.C., Marr, C.M., Boswood, A., Freeman, S., Bowen, I.M. and Corley, K.T.T. (1998) Auscillation and two dimensional, M mode, spectral and colour flow Doppler findings in pony foals from birth to seven weeks of age. *Journal of Veterinary Internal Medcine Lombard* 1990(12), 255–265.

Lofstedt, R.M. (1993) Miscellaneous diseases of pregnancy and parturition. In: McKinnon, A.O. and Voss, J.L. (eds) *Equine Reproduction*. Lea and Febiger, Philadelphia, Pennsylvania, pp. 596–603.

Lofstedt, R.M. (2011a) Diestrus. In: McKinnon, A.O., Squires, E.L., Vaala, E. and Varner, D.D. (eds) *Equine Reproduction*, 2nd edn. Wiley-Blackwell, Philadelphia, London, pp. 1728–1731.

Lofstedt, R.M. (2011b) Abnormalities of pregnancy. In: McKinnon, A.O., Squires, E.L., Vaala, E. and Varner, D.D. (eds) *Equine Reproduction*, 2nd edn. Wiley-Blackwell, Philadelphia, London, pp. 2442–2454.

Lofstedt, R. M. and Patel J.H. (1989) Evaluation of the ability of altrenogest to control the equine oestrous cycle. *Journal of the American Veterinary Association* 194, 361.

Lofstedt, R.M. and Newcombe, J.R. (1997) Pregnancy diagnosis and subsequent examinations in mares: when and why. *Equine Veterinary Education* 9(6), 293–294.

Logan, N.L., McCue, P.M., Alonso, M.A. and Squires, E.L. (2007) Evaluation of three equine FSH superovulation protocols in mares. *Animal Reproduction Science* 102(1–2), 48–55.

Lombard, C.W. (1990) Cardiovascular diseases. In: Koterba, A.M., Drummond, W.H. and Kosch, P.C. (eds) *Equine Clinical Neonatology*. Lea and Febiger, Philadelphia, Pennsylvania, pp. 240–261.

Long, M.T., Ostund, E.N., Porter, M.B. and Crom, R.L. (2002) Equine West Nile Encephalitis: epidemiological and clinical review for practitioners. *American Association of Equine Practitioners* 48, 1–6.

Loomis, P.R. (1993) Factors affecting the success of AI with cooled, transported semen. In: Blake-Caddel, L. (ed.) *Proceedings of 38th Annual Convention of American Association of Equine Practitioners 2, Orlando, Florida.* pp. 629–647.

Lopate, C., LeBlanc, M., Pascoe, R. and Knottenbelt, D. (2003) Parturition. In: Knottenbelt, D., LeBlanc, M., Lopate, C. and Pascoe, R.R. (eds) *Equine Stud Farm Medicine and Surgery*. W.B. Saunders, Philadelphia, Pennsylvania, pp. 269–324.

Lopez, C. and Carmona, J.U. (2010) Uterine torsion diagnosed in a mare at 515 days gestation. *Equine Veterinary Education* 22, 483–486.

Lopez-Bayghen, C., Zozaya, H., Ocampo, L., Brumbaugh, G.W. and Sumano, H. (2008) Melengestrol acetate as a tool for inducing early ovulation in transitional mares. *Acta Veterinaria Hungarica* 56(1), 125–131.

Love, C.C. (1992) Semen collection techniques. *Veterinary Clinics of North America, Equine Practice* 8(1), 111–128.

Love, C.C. (2003) Evaluation of breeding records In: Blanchard, T.L., Varner, D.D., Schumacher, J., Love, C.C., Brinsko, S.P., Rigby, S.L. (eds) *Manual of Equine Reproduction*, 2nd edn. Mosby, St Louis, Missouri, pp. 229–237.

Love, C.C. (2011a) Historical information. In: McKinnon, A.O., Squires, E.L., Vaala, E. and Varner, D.D. (eds) *Equine Reproduction*, 2nd edn. Wiley-Blackwell, Philadelphia, London, pp. 1429–1434.

Love, C.C. (2011b) Endometrial biopsy. In: McKinnon, A.O., Squires, E.L., Vaala, E. and Varner, D.D. (eds) *Equine Reproduction*, 2nd edn. Wiley-Blackwell, Philadelphia, London, pp. 1929–1939.

Love, C.C. (2011c) Relationship between sperm motility, morphology and the fertility of stallions. *Theriogenology* 76, 547–557.

Love, C.C., Garcia, M.C., Riera, F.R. and Kenney, R.M. (1991) Evaluation of measurements taken by ultrasonography and calipur to estimate testicular volume and predict daily sperm output in the stallion. *Journal of Reproduction and Fertility, Supplement* 44, 99–105.

Love, C.C., Thompson, J.A., Lowry, V.K. and Varner, D.D. (2002) Effect of storage time and temperature on stallion sperm DNA and fertility. *Theriogenology* 57, 1135–1142.

Love, C.C., Thompson, J.A., Brinsko, S.P., Rigby, S.L., Blanchard, T.L., Lowry, V.K. and Varner, D.D. (2003) Relationship between stallion sperm motility and viability as detected by two fluorescence staining techniques using flow cytometry. *Theriogenology* 60(6), 1127–1138.

Love, C.C., Brinsko, S.P., Rigby, S.L., Thompson, J.A., Blanchard, T.L. and Varner, D.D. (2005) Relationship of seminal plasma level and extender type to sperm motility and DNA integrity. *Theriogenology* 63(6), 1584–1591.

Love, C.C., Noble, J.K., Standridge, S.A., Bearden, C.T., Blanchard, T.L., Varner, D.D. and Cavinder, C.A. (2015) The relationship between sperm quality in cool-shipped semen and embryo recovery rate in horses. *Theriogenology* 84(9), 1587–1583.

Love, S. (1993) Equine Cushings disease. *British Veterinary Journal* 149, 139–153.

Love, S., Murphy, D., Mellor, D. (1999) Pathogenicity of cyathostome infection. *Veterinary Parasitology* 85, 113–121.

Lowe, J.N. (2001) Diagnosis and management of urospermia in a commercial Thoroughbred stallion. *Equine Veterinary Education* 13(1), 4–7.

Lowis, T.C. and Hyland, J.H. (1991) Analysis of post partum fertility in mares on a Thoroughbred stud in South Victoria. *Australian Veterinary Journal* 68(9), 304–306.

Lu, K.G. and Morrese, P.R. (2007) Infectious diseases in breeding stallions. *Clinical Techniques in Equine Practice* 6, 285–290.

Lu, K.G., Barr, B.S., Embertson, R. and Schaler, B.D. (2006) Dystocia – a true emergency. *Clinical and Technical Equine Practice* 5, 145–153.

Lubbeke, M., Klug, E., Hoppen, H.O. and Jochle, W. (1994) Attempts to synchronise estrus and ovulation in mares using progesterone (CIDR-B) and GnRH analogue deslorelin. *Reproduction in Domestic Animals* 29, 305–314.

Lucas, Z., Raeside, J.I and Betteridge, K.J. (1991) Non-invasive assessment of the incidences of pregnancy and pregnancy loss in the feral horses of Sable Island. *Journal of Reproduction and Fertility, Suppl.* 44, 479–488.

Luo, S.M., Schatten, H. and Sun, Q.Y. (2013) Sperm mitochondria in reproduction: good or bad and where do they go. *Journal of Genetics and Genomics* 40(11), 549–556.

Lyman, C. and Sertich, P.L. (2019) Oviduct (Uterine tube). In: Orsini, J.A., Grenager, N., de Lahunta, A. (eds) *Veterinary Clinical Anatomy*. Elsevier, St. Louis, Missouri.

Lyons, E.T. and Tolliver, S.C. (2004) Prevalence of parasite eggs (*Strongyloides westeri, Parascaris equorum* and strongtles) and oocytes (*Eimeria leukarti*) in the feces of Thoroughbred foals on 14 farms in central Kentucky in 2003. *Parasitology Research* 92, 4.

Lyons, E.T., Ionita, M. and Tolliver, S.C. (2011) Important gastrointestinal parasites. In: McKinnon, A.O., Squires, E.L., Vaala, E. and Varner, D.D. (eds) *Equine Reproduction*, 2nd edn. Wiley-Blackwell, Philadelphia, London, pp. 292–301.

Maaskant, A., de Brujin, C.M., Schutrups, A.H. and Stout, T.A.E. (2010) Dystocia in Fresian mares: Prevalence, causes and outcome following caesarean section. *Equine Veterinary Education* 22(4), 190–195.

MacDonald, A.A. and Fowden, A.L. (1997) Microscopic anatomy of the ungulate placenta. *Equine Veterinary Journal, Supplement* 24, 7–13.

MacDonald, A.A., Fowden, A.L., Silver, M., Ousey, J. and Rossdale, P.D. (1988) The foramen ovale of the foetal and neonatal foal. *Equine Veterinary Journal* 20, 255–260.

MacDonald, A. Chavatte, P. and Fowden, A. (2000) Scanning electron microscopy of the microcoteledonary placenta of the horse (*Equus caballus*) in the latter half of gestation. *Placenta* 21(5–6), 565–574.

Mach, N., Foury, A., Kittelmann, S., Reigner, F., Moroldo, M., Ballester, M., Esquerré, D., Rivière, J., Sallé, G., Gérard, P., Moisan, M.P. and Lansade, L. (2017) The Effects of Weaning Methods on Gut

Microbiota Composition and Horse Physiology. *Frontiers in Physiology* 25(8), 535.

Machida, N., Yasuda, J., Too, K. and Kudo, N. (1998) A morphological study on the obliteration of the ductus arteriosus in the horse. *Equine Veterinary Journal* 20(4), 249–254.

Mackie, E.J., Ahmed, Y.A., Tatarczuch, L., Chen, K-S. and Mirams, M. (2008) Endochondral ossification: How cartilage is converted into bone in the developing skeleton. *The International Journal of Biochemistry and Cell Biology* 40, 46–62.

Mackintosh, M.E. (1981) Bacteriological techniques in the diagnosis of equine genital infections *Veterinary Record* 108, 52–55.

MacLachlan, N. and Balasuriya, U. (2006) Equine viral arteritis. *Advances in Experimental Medical Biology* 581, 429–433.

MacLachlan, N., Balasuriya, U., Davis, N., Collier, M., Johnston, R., Ferraro, R. and Guthrie, A. (2007) Experiences with new generation vacinces against equine viral arteritis, West Nile disease and African horse sickness. *Vaccine* 25, 5577–5582.

Maclellan, L.J. (2011) Oocyte cryopreservation In: McKinnon, A.O., Squires, E.L., Vaala, E. and Varner, D.D. (eds) *Equine Reproduction*, 2nd edn. Wiley-Blackwell, Philadelphia, London, pp. 2953–2956.

Maclellan, L.J., Lane, M., Sims, M.M. and Squires, E.L. (2001) Effect of sucrose and trehalose on vitrification of equine oocytes 12 or 25 hours after onset of maturation. *Theriogenology* 55, 310.

Maclellan, L.J.M., Carnevale, E.M., Coutinho da Silva, M.A., McCue, P.M., Seidel, G.E. and Squires, E.L. (2002a) Cryopreservation of small and large equine embryos pretreated with cytochalasin-B and/or trypsin. *Theriogenology* 58, 717–720.

Maclellan, L.J.M., Carnevale, E.M., Coutinho da Silva, M.A., Scoggin, C.F., Bruemmer, J.E. and Squires, E.L. (2002b) Pregnancies from vitrified equine opocytes collected from superstimulated and non-stimulated mares. *Theriogenology* 5, 911–919.

Maclellan, L.J., Stokes, J.E., Preis, K.A., McCue, P.M., and Carnevale, E.M. (2010). Vitrification, warming, ICSI and transfer of equine oocytes matured in vivo. *Animal Reproduction Science* 121, 260–261.

Macpherson, M.L. and Blanchard, T.L. (2005) Breeding mares on the foal heat. *Equine Veterinary Education* 17(1), 44–52.

Macpherson, M.L. and Paccamonti, D.L. (2011) Induction of Parturition. In: McKinnon, A.O., Squires, E.L., Vaala, E. and Varner, D.D. (eds) *Equine Reproduction*, 2nd edn. Wiley-Blackwell, Philadelphia, London, pp. 2262–2267.

Macpherson, M.L. and Reimer, J.M. (2000) Twin reduction in the mare: current options. *Animal Reproduction Science* 60–61, 233–244.

Macpherson, M.L., Homco, L.D., Varner, D.D., Blanchard, T.L., Harms, P.G., Flanagan, M.N. and Forrest, D.F. (1995) Transvaginal Ultrasound-Guided Allocentesis for Pregnancy Elimination in the Mare. *Biology of Reproduction* 52, Monograph_series1, pp. 215–223.

Macpherson, M.L., Chaffin, M.K., Carroll, G.L., Jorgenson, J., Arrott, C., Varner, D.D. and Blanchard, T.L. (1997) Three methods of oxytocin-induced parturition and their effects on foals. *Journal of the American Veterinary Association* 210, 799–803.

Madigan, J.E. (1990) Management of the newborn foal. In: Royer, M.G. (ed.) *Proceedings of the 36th Annual Convention of the American Association of Equine Practitioners, Lexington, Kentucky*. American Association of Equine Practitioners, pp. 99–116.

Madill, S. (2002) Reproductive considerations: mare and stallion. Review. *Veterinary Clinics of North America Equine Practice* 18(3), 591–619.

Madill, S., Troedsson, M.H.T., Alexander, S.L., Shand, N., Santaschi, E.M. and Irvine, C.H.G. (2000) Simultaneous recording of pituitary oxytocin secretion and myometrial activity in oestrus mares exposed to various breeding stimuli. *Journal of Reproduction and Fertility, Supplement* 56, 351–361.

Madsen, M. and Christensen, P. (1995) Bacterial flora of semen collected from Danish warmblood stallions by artificial vagina. *Acta Veterinaria Scandinavia* 36(1), 1–7.

Magee, C., Foradori, C.D., Bruemmer, J.E., Arreguin-Arevalo, J.A., McCue, P.M., Handa, R.J., Squires, E.L. and Clay, C.M. (2009) Biological and anatomical evidence for kispeptin regulation of the hypothalamic-pituitary-gonadal axis of estrous horse mares. *Endocrinology* 150, 2813–2821.

Magistrini, M. and Vidamnet, M. (1992) Artificial insemination in horses. *Recueil de Medicine Veterinaire Special: Reproduction des Equides* 168(11–12), 959–967.

Magistrini, M., Couty, I. and Palmer, E. (1992) Interactions between sperm packaging, gas environment, temperature and diluent on fresh stallion sperm survival. *Acta Veterinaria Scandinavia, Supplement* 88, 97–110.

Magistrini, M., Guitton, E., Levern, Y., Nicolle, J.C., Vidament, M., Kerboeuf, D. and Palmer, E. (1997a) New staining methods for sperm evaluation estimated by microscopy and flow cytometry. *Theriogenology* 48, 1229–1235.

Magistrini, M., Sattler, M., Yvon, J.M. and Vidament, M. (1997) Freezability of stallion spermatozoa evaluated by motuility membrane integrity and ATP content. *Cryobiology* 35(4), 88.

Maher, J.K., Tresnan, D.B., Deacon, S., Hannah, L. and Antczak, D.F. (1996) Analysis of MHC class 1 expression in equine trophoblast cells usinh in situ hybridization. *Placenta* 17(5–6), 351–359.

Maher, J.M., Squires, E.L., Voss, J.L. and Shideler, R.K. (1983) Effect of anabolic steroids on reproductive function in young mares. *Journal of the American Veterinary Medical Association* 183, 519–524.

Mahon, G.A.T. and Cunningham, E.P. (1982) Inbreeding and the inheritance of fertility in the Thoroughbred mare. *Livestock Production Science* 9, 743–754.

Maischberger, E., Irwin, J.A., Carrington, S.D. and Duggan. V.E. (2008) Equine post-breeing endometritis: a review. *Irish Veterinary Journal* 61, 163–168.

Makinen, A., Katila, T., Anderson, M. and Gustavsson, I. (2000) Two sterile stallions with XXY syndrome. *Equine Veterinary Journal* 32(4), 358–360.

Malacarne, M., Martuzzi, F., Summer, A. and Mariani, P. (2002) Review: protein and fat composition of mare's milk: some nutritional remarks with reference to human and cow's milk. *International Dairy Journal* 12, 869–877.

Malinowski, K., Halquist, N.A., Heylar, L., Sherman, A.R. and Scanes, C.G. (1990) Effect of different separation protocols between mares and foals on plasma cortisol and cell mediated immune response. In: *Proceedings of the 11th Equine Nutrition and Physiology Symposium, Stillwater, Oklahoma.* 10(5), 363–368.

Malmgren, L. (1992a) Sperm morphology in stallions in relation to fertility. *Acta Veterinarian Scandinavia* 88 (Supplement) 52, 281–287.

Malmgren, L. (1992b) Ultrasonography: a new diagnostic tool in stallions with genital tract infection? *Acta Veterinaria Scandinavica, Supplement* 88, 91–94.

Malmgren, L. (1997) Assessing the quality of raw semen: a review. *Theriogenology* 48, 523–530.

Malmgren, L., Kamp, B., Wockener, A., Boyle, M. and Colenbrander, B. (1994) Motility, velocity and acrosome integrity of equine spermatozoa stored under different conditions. *Reproduction in Domestic Animals* 29(7), 469–476.

Malmgren, L., Andersen, O. and Dalin, A.M. (2001) Effect of GnRH immunization on hormonal levels, sexual behavior, semen quality and testicular morphology in mature stallions. *Equine Veterinary Science* 33, 1, 75–83.

Malpaux, B., Migaud, M., Tricoire, H. and Chemineau, P. (2001) Biology of mammalian photoperiodism and the critical role of the pineal gland and melatonin. *Journal of Biological Rhythms* 16, 336–347.

Malschitzky, E., Schilela, A., Mattos, A.L.G., Garbade, P., Gregory, R.M. and Mattos, R.C. (2002) Effect of intra-uterine fluid accumulation during and after foal-heat and of different management techniques on the post partum fertility of thoroughbred mares. *Theriogenology* 58, 495–498.

Malschitzky, E., Pimentel, A.M., Garbade, P., Joblin, M.I.M., Gregory, R.M. and Mortos, R.C. (2015) Management strategies aiming to improve horse welfare and reduce embryoic death rates in mares. *Reproduction in Domestic Animals* 50(4), 632–636.

Manning, S.T., Bowman, P.A., Fraser, L.M. and Card, C.E. (1998) Development of hysteroscopic insemination of the uterine tube in the mare. In: *Proceedings of Annual Meeting Society for Theriogenology, University of Wisconsin, Madigan.* Society of Theriogenology, pp. 84–85.

Manz, E., Vogel, T., Glatzel, P. and Schmidtke, J. (1998) Identification of equine Y chromosome specific to gene locus (ETSPY) with potential in preimplantation sex diagnosis. *Theriogenology* 49(1), 364–370.

Mari, G., Castagnetti, C. and Belluzzi, S. (2002) Equine fetal sex determination using a single ultrasonic examination under farm conditions. *Theriogenology* 58, 1237–1243.

Mari, G., Iancono, E., Merlo, B. and Castagnetti, C. (2005) Reduction of twin pregnancy in the mare by transvaginal ultrasound-guided aspiration. *Reproduction in Domestic Animals* 39(6), 434–439.

Mari, G., Barbara, M., Eleonora, I. and Stefano, B. (2005) Fertility in the mare after repeated transvaginal ultrasound-guided aspirations. *Animal Reproduction Science* 88(3–4), 299–308.

Martin, J.C., Klug, E. and Gunzel, A.R. (1979) Centrifugation of stallion semen and its storage in large volume straws. *Journal of Reproduction and Fertility* 27, 47–51.

Martin, R.G., McMeniman, N.P. and Dowsett, K.F. (1991) Effects of a protein deficient diet and urea supplementation on lactating mares. *Journal of Reproduction and Fertility, Supplement* 44, 543–550.

Martin, R.G., McMeniman, N.P. and Dowsett, K.F. (1992) Milk and water intakes of foals suckling grazing mares. *Equine Veterinary Journal* 24, 295–299.

Masko, M., Domino, M., Zdrojkowski, L., Jasinski, T., Matyba, P., Zabielski, R, Gajewski, Z. (2018) Breeding management of mares in late reproductive age considering improvement of welfare. A review *Journal of Animal and Feed Sciences* 27(4), 285–291.

Mason, G.J. and Latham, N.R. (2004) Can't stop, won't stop: is stereotypy a reliable animal welfare indicator? *Animal Welfare* 13, S57–S69.

Massey, R.E., LeBlanc, M.M. and Klapstein, E.F. (1991) Colostrum feeding of foals and colostrum banking. In: *Proceedings of the 37th Annual Convenstion of the American Asociation of Equine Practioners* pp. 1–8.

Mayhew, I.G. (1990) Neurological aspects of urospermia in the horse. *Equine Veterinary Education* 2(2), 68–69.

Maziero, R.R.D., de Freitas Guaitolini, C.R., Guasti, P.N., Monteiro, G.A., Martin, I., da Silva, J.P.M., Crespilho, A.M. and Papa, F.O. (2019) Effect of Using Two Cryopreservation Methods on Viability and Fertility of Frozen Stallion Sperm. *Journal of Equine Veterinary Science* 72, 37–40.

McAfee, L.M., Mills, D.S. and Cooper, J.J. (2002) The use of mirrors for the control of stereotypic weaning behaviour in the stabled horse. *Applied Animal Behaviour Science* 78(2), 159–173.

McAllister, R.A. and Sack, W.O. (1990) Identification of anatomical features of the equine clitoris as potential growth sites for *Taylorella equigenitalis*. *Journal of American Veterinary Medicine Association* 196(12), 1965–1966.

McBride, S.D. and Hemmings, A. (2005) Altered mesoaccumbens and nigro-striatal dopamine physiology is associated with stereotypy development in a non-rodent species. *Behaviour Brain Research* 159(1), 113–118.

McCall, C.A., Potter, G.D. and Kreidel, J.L. (1985) Locomotor, vocal and other behavioural responses to varying methods of weaning foals. *Applied Animal Behaviour Science* 14(1), 27–35.

McCall, C.A., Potter, G.D., Kreidel, J.L. and Jenkins, W.L. (1987) Physiological responses in foals weaned by abrupt and gradual methods. *Journal of Equine Veterinary Science* 7(6), 368–374.

McClure, C.C. (1993) The immune system. In: McKinnon, A.O. and Voss, J.L. (eds) *Equine Reproduction*. Lea and Febiger, Philadelphia, Pennsylvania, pp. 1003–1016.

McCue, P.M. (1992) Equine granulosa cell tumours. *Proceedings of the American Association of Equine Practictioners* 38, 587–593.

McCue, P.M. (1993) Lactation. In: McKinnon, A.O. and Voss, J.L. (eds) *Equine Reproduction*. Lea and Febiger, Philadelphia, Pennsylvania, pp. 588–595.

McCue, P.M. (1998) Review of ovarian abnormalities in the mare. *Proceedings of the Annual Convention of the American Association of Equine Practionners* 44, 125–133.

McCue, P.M. (2008) The Problem Mare: Management Philosophy, Diagnostic Procedures, and Therapeutic Options. *Journal of Equine Veterinary Science* 28(11), 619–626.

McCue, P.M. (2014) Evaluation of pH and osmolarity of semen In: Dascanio, J.J. and McCue, P.M. (eds) *Equine Reproductive Procedures*. Wiley, Chapter 122.

McCue, P.M. and Ferris, R.A. (2011) The abnormal estrous cycle. In: McKinnon, A.O., Squires, E.L., Vaala, E. and Varner, D.D. (eds) *Equine Reproduction*, 2nd edn. Wiley-Blackwell, Philadelphia, London, pp. 1754–1770.

McCue, P.M. and Ferris, R.A. (2012) Parturition, dystocia and foal survival: a retrospective study of 1047 births. *Equine Veterinary Journal* 41(2), 22–25.

McCue, P.M. and Ferris R.A. (2017) Review of ovarian abnormalities in the mare. *Proceedings of the American Association of Equine Practionners* 63, 61–68.

McCue, P.M. and McKinnon, A.O (2011a) Ovarian abnormalities. In: McKinnon, A.O., Squires, E.L., Vaala, E. and Varner, D.D. (eds) *Equine Reproduction*,

2nd edn. Wiley-Blackwell, Philadelphia, London, pp. 2123–2136.

McCue, P.M. and McKinnon, A.O (2011b) Pregnancy Examination. In: McKinnon, A.O., Squires, E.L., Vaala, E. and Varner, D.D. (eds) *Equine Reproduction*, 2nd edn. Wiley-Blackwell, Philadelphia, London, pp. 2245–2261.

McCue, P.M. and Sitters, S. (2011) Lactation. In: McKinnon, A.O., Squires, E.L., Vaala, E. and Varner, D.D. (eds) *Equine Reproduction*, 2nd edn. Wiley-Blackwell, Philadelphia, London, pp. 2277–2290.

McCue, P.M. and Squires, E.L. (2002) Persistent anovulatory follicles in the mare. *Theriogenology* 58, 541–543.

McCue, P.M. and Squires, E.L. (2015) *Embryo Transfer*. Teton New Media pp 169.

McCue, P.M. and Troedsson, M.H.T. (2003) Commercial embryo transfer in the United States. *Pfedeheilkunde* 19, 689–692.

McCue, P.M. and Wilson, W.D. (1989) Equine mastitis: a review of 28 cases. *Equine Veterinary Journal* 21, 351–353.

McCue, P.M., Fleury, J.J., Denniston, D.J., Graham, J.K. and Squires, E.L. (2000) Oviductal insemination of mares. *Journal of Reproduction and Fertility,* Supplememt 56, 499–502.

McCue, P.M., Farquhar, V.J., Carnevale, E.M. and Squires, E.L. (2002) Removal of deslorelin (Ovuplant) implant 48 h after administration results in normal interovulatory intervals in mares. *Theriogenology* 58(5), 865–870.

McCue, P.M., Niswender, K.D. and Macon, K.A. (2003) Modification of the flush procedure to enhance embryo recovery. *Journal of Equine Veterinary Science* 23, 1–2.

McCue, P.M., Hudson, J.J., Bruemmer, J.E. and Squires, E.L. (2004) Efficacy of hCG at inducing ovulation: a new look at an old issue. *Proceedings of the American Association of Equine Practioners* 50, 510–513.

McCue, P.M., Roser, J.F., Munro, C.J., Liu, I.K. and Lasley, B.L. (2006) Granulosa cell tumours of the equine ovary. *Veterinary Clinics of North American Equine Practionners* 22, 799–817.

McCue, P.M., LeBlanc, M.M. and Squires, E.L. (2007a) eFSH in clinical equine practice. Review. *Theriogenology* 68(3), 429–433.

McCue, P.M., Logan, N.I. and Magee, C. (2007b) Management of the transition period: hormone therapy. *Equine Veterinary Education* 19(4), 215–221.

McCue, P., Deluca, C., Patten, M. and Squires, E.L. (2008a) Effects of sham transvaginal embryo transfer and/or Altrenogest administration on plasma progesterone concentrations in recipient mares. *Proceedings of the International Symposium on Equine Embryo Transfer p. 73.*

McCue, P.M., Patten, M., Denniston, D.D., Bruemmer, J.E. and Squires, E.L. (2008b) Strategies for using eFSH for superovulating mares. *Journal of Veterinary Science* 28, 91–96.

McCue, P.M., DeLuca, C.A., Ferris, R.A. and Wall, J.J. (2009) How to evaluate equine embryos. *Proceedings of the 55th Annual American Association of Equine Practitioners Convention*, Las Vegas, Nevada. 5–9 December, 2009. American Association of Equine Practionners, pp. 252–256.

McCue, P.M. Ferris, R.A., Lindholm, A. and DeLuca, C.A. (2010) Embryo Recovery Procedures and Collection Success: Results of 492 Embryo-Flush Attempts. *Proceedings of the American Association of Equine Practionners* 56, 318–321.

McCue, P.M., Scoggin, C.F. and Lindholm, A.R.G. (2011a) Estrus. In: McKinnon, A.O., Squires, E.L, Vaala, W.E. and Varner, D.D. (eds) *Equine Reproduction* 2nd edn. Wiley-Blackwell, pp. 1716–1727.

McCue, P.M., Deluca, C.A. and Wall, J.J. (2011b) Cooled and transported embryo technology. In: McKinnon, A.O., Squires, E.L, Vaala, W.E. and Varner, D.D. (eds) *Equine Reproduction* 2nd edn. Wiley-Blackwell, pp. 2880–2886.

McDonnell, S.M. (1992) Normal and abnormal sexual behaviour. *Veterinary Clinics of North America Equine Practitioners* 8, 71–89.

McDonnell, S.M. (1995) Stallion behaviour and endocrinology: what do we really know? In: *Proceedings of the 41st Annual Meeting of the American Association of Equine Practitioners*, Lexington, Kentucky, December 1995, pp 18–19.

McDonnell, S.M. (2000a) Reproductive behaviour of stallion and mares: comparison of free-running and domestic in-hand breeding. *Animal Reproduction Science* 60–61, 211–219.

McDonnell, S.M. (2000b) Stallion sexual behaviour. In: Samper, J.C. (ed.) *Equine Breeding Management and Artificial Insemination*. W.B. Saunders, Philadelphia, Pennsylvania, pp. 53–61.

McDonnell, S.M. (2001) Oral imipramine and intravenous xylazine for pharmacologically-induced ex copula ejaculation in stallions. *Animal Reproduction Science* 68, 153–159.

McDonnell, S.M. (2005) Sexual Behaviour. In: Mills, D. and McDonnell, S.M. (eds) *The Domestic Horse, The origins, development and managemt of its behaviour*. Cambridge University Press, Cambridge, UK, pp. 110–125.

McDonnell, S.M. (2011a) Normal sexual behavior. In: McKinnon, A.O., Squires, E.L., Vaala, E. and Varner, D.D. (eds) *Equine Reproduction*, 2nd edn. Wiley-Blackwell, Philadelphia, London, pp. 1385–1390.

McDonnell, S.M. (2011b) Abnormal sexual behavior. In: McKinnon, A.O., Squires, E.L., Vaala, E. and Varner, D.D. (eds) *Equine Reproduction*, 2nd edn. Wiley-Blackwell, Philadelphia, London, pp. 1407–1412.

McDonnell, S.M. (2011c) Pharmacological manipulation of ejaculation. In: McKinnon, A.O., Squires, E.L., Vaala, E. and Varner, D.D. (eds) *Equine Reproduction*, 2nd edn. Wiley-Blackwell, Philadelphia, London, pp. 1413–1414.

McDonnell, S.M. (2011d) Pharmacological manipulation of stallion behaviour In: McKinnon, A.O., Squires, E.L., Vaala, E. and Varner, D.D. (eds) *Equine Reproduction*, 2nd edn. Wiley-Blackwell, Philadelphia, London, pp. 1415–1418.

McDonnell, S.M. and Love, C.C. (1990) Manual stimulated collection of semen from stallions. Training time, sexual behaviour and semen. *Theriogenology* 33, 1201–1210.

McDonnell, S.M. and Love, C.C. (1991) Xylazine induced ex-copulatory ejaculation in stallions. *Theriogenology* 36, 73–76.

McDonnell, S.M. and Murray, S.C. (1995) Bachelor and Harem stallion behaviour and endocrinology. *Biology of Reproduction Monographs* 1, 577–590.

McDonnell, S.M. and Turner, R.M.O. (1994) Post-thaw motility and longevity of motility of imipramine-induced ejaculate of pony stallions. *Theriogenology* 42(3), 475–481.

McDonnell, S.M., Garcia, M.C., Blanchard, T.L. and Kenney, R.M. (1986) Evaluation of androgenized mares as an estrus detection aid. *Theriogenology* 26, 261–266.

McDonnell, S.M., Hinrichs, K., Cooper, W.L. and Kenney, R.M. (1988) Use of an androgenised mare as an aid in detection of oestrus in mares. *Theriogenology* 30(3), 547–553.

McDonnell, S.M., Pozor, M.A., Beech, J. and Sweeney, R.W. (1991) Use of manual stimulation for the collection of semen from an atactic stallion unable to mount. *Journal of the American Veterinary Medical Association* 199(6), 753–754.

McDowell, K.J. and Sharp, D.C. (2011) Maternal recognition of pregnancy. In: McKinnon, A.O., Squires, E.L., Vaala, E. and Varner, D.D. (eds) *Equine Reproduction*, 2nd edn. Wiley-Blackwell, Philadelphia, London, pp. 2200–2210.

McDowell, K.J., Sharp, D.C., Grubaugh, W., Thatcher, W.W. and Wilcox, C.J. (1988) Restricted conceptus mobility results in failure of pregnancy maintenance in mares. *Biology of Reproduction* 39(2), 340–348.

McGee, S. and Smith, H.V. (2004) Accompanying pre-weaned Thoroughbred (*Equus caballus*) foals while separated from the mare during covering reduces behavioural signs of distress exhibited. *Applied Animal Behaviour* 88, 137–147.

McGlothlin, J.A., Lester, G.D., Hansen, P.J., Thomas, M., Pablo, L., Hawkins, D.L. and LeBlanc, M.M. (2004) Alteration in uterine contractility in mares with experimentally induced placentitis. *Reproduction* 127, 57–66.

McGreevey, P.D. (2011) Stereotypic behavior. In: McKinnon, A.O., Squires, E.L., Vaala, E. and Varner, D.D. (eds) *Equine Reproduction*, 2nd edn. Wiley-Blackwell, Philadelphia, London, pp. 2771–2775.

McGreevey, P.D., Cripps, P.J., French, N.P., Green, L.E. and Nicol, C.J. (1995) Management factors associated with stereotypic and redirected behavior in the thoroughbred horse. *Equine Veterinary Journal* 27(2), 86–91.

McIlwraith, C.W. (2011) Developmental orthopedic disease (DOD). In: McKinnon, A.O., Squires, E.L., Vaala, E. and Varner, D.D. (eds) *Equine Reproduction*, 2nd edn. Wiley-Blackwell, Philadelphia, London, pp. 772–782.

McKinnon, A.O. (1993) Pregnancy diagnosis. In: McKinnon, A.O. and Voss, J.L. (eds) *Equine Reproduction*. Lea and Febiger, Philadelphia, Pennsylvania, pp. 501–508.

McKinnon, A.O. (1998a) Uterine pathology. In: Rantanen, N.W. and McKinnon, A.O. (eds) *Equine*

Diagnostic Ultrasonography. Williams and Wilkins, Baltimore, Maryland, pp. 181–200.

McKinnon, A.O. (1998b) Ovarian abnormalities. In: Rantanen, N.W., McKinnon, A.O. (eds) *Equine diagnostic ultrasonography*. Williams & Wilkins, Baltimore, Maryland, pp. 233–251.

McKinnon, A.O. (2011) Orgin and outcome of twin pregnancies. In: McKinnon, A.O., Squires, E.L., Vaala, E. and Varner, D.D. (eds) *Equine Reproduction*, 2nd edn. Wiley-Blackwell, Philadelphia, London, pp. 2350–2358.

McKinnon, A.O. and Carnevale, E.M. (1993) Ultrasonography. In: McKinnon, A.O. and Voss, J.L. (eds) *Equine Reproduction*. Lea and Febiger, Philadelphia, Pennsylvania, London, pp. 211–220.

McKinnon, A.O. and Voss, J.L. (1993) Breeding the problem mare. In: McKinnon, A.O. and Voss, J.L. (eds) *Equine Reproduction*. Lea and Febiger, Philadelphia, Pennsylvania, pp. 369–378.

McKinnon, A.O. and Jalim, S.L. (2011) Surgery of the cudal reproductive tract. In: McKinnon, A.O., Squires, E.L., Vaala, E. and Varner, D.D. (eds) *Equine Reproduction*, 2nd edn. Wiley-Blackwell, Philadelphia, London, pp. 2545–2558.

McKinnon, A.O., Squires, E.L., Harrison, L.A., Blach, E.L. and Shideler, R.K. (1988a) Ultrasonic studies on the reproductive tracts of mares after parturition: Effect of involution and uterine fluid on pregnancy rates in mares with normal and delayed post partum ovulatory cycles. *Journal of the American Veterinary Medical Association* 192, 350–353.

McKinnon, A.O., Carnevale, E.M., Squires, E.L., Voss, J.L. and Seidel Jr, G.E. (1988b) Heterogenous and xenogenous fertilisation of in vitro matured equine oocytes. *Journal of Equine Veterinary Science* 8, 143–147.

McKinnon, A.O., Squires, E.L., Carnevale, E.M. and Hermenet, M.J. (1988c) Ovariectmized steroid-treated mares as embryo transfer recipients and as a model to study the role of progestins in pregnancy maintenance. *Theriogenology* 29(5), 1055–1063.

McKinnon, A.O., Voss, J.L., Squires, E.L. and Carnevale, E.M. (1993) Diagnostic ultrasonography. In: McKinnon, A.O. and Voss, J.L. (eds) *Equine Reproduction*. Lea and Febiger, Philadelphia, Pennsylvania, London, pp. 266–302.

McKinnon, A.O., Perriam, W.J., Lescun, T.B., Walker, J. and Vasey, J.P. (1997) Effect of a GnRH analog (Ovuplant), hCG and dexamethasone on time to ovulation in cycling mares. *World Equine Veterinary Research* 2, 16–18.

McKinnon, A.O., Lacham-Kaplan, O. and Trounson, A.O. (2000) Pregnancies produced from fertile and infertile stallions by intracytoplasmic sperm injection (ICSI) of single frozen/thawed spermatozoa into in-vivo matured oocytes. *Journal of Reproduction and Fertility, Supplement* 56, 513–517.

McKinnon, A.O., Squires, E.L., Vaala, E. and Varner, D.D. (2011) *Equine Reproduction*, 2nd edn. Wiley-Blackwell, Philadelphia, London, pp. 3057.

McLean, R.J. (2014) Incidence of Caslick vulvoplasty operations in a population of Thoroughbred mares. MSc Thesis. Aberystwyth University, UK.

McManus, C.J. and Fitzgerald, B.P. (2003) Effect of clenbuterol and exogenous melatonin treatment on body fat, serum leptin and the expression of seasonal anestrus in the mare. *Animal Reproduction Science* 76, 217–230.

McPartlin, L.A., Suarez, S.S., Czaya, C.A., Hinrichs, K. and Bedford-Guaus, S.J. (2009) Hyperactivation of stallion sperm is required for successful in vitro fertilization of equine oocytes. *Biology of Reproduction* 81, 199–206.

McTaggart, C., Penhale, J. and Raidal, S.L. (2005) Effect of plasma transfusion on neutrophil function in healthy and septic foals. *Australian Veterinary Journal* 83(8), 499–505.

Meager, D.M. (1978) Granulosa cell tumours in the mare. A review of 78 cases. In: Milne, F.J. (ed.) *Proceedings of the 23rd Annual Meeting of the American Association of Equine Practitioners, Vancouver, British Columbia*. American Association of Equine Practitioners, pp. 133–139.

Medan, M.S. (2014) Treatment of ovarian inactivity in mares during the breeding season with PMSG/hCG, PMSG or GnRH and the effect of treatment on estradiol and progesterone concentrations *American Journal of Animal and Veterinary Sciences* 9(4), 211–216.

Medica, P., Cravana, C., Bruschetta, G., Ferlazzo, A. and Fazio, E. (2018) Physiological and behavioral patterns of normal-term thoroughbred foals. *Journal of Veterinary Behavior: Clinical Applications and Research* 26, 38–42.

Meinert, C., Silva, J.F.S., Kroetz, I., Klug, E., Trigg, T.E., Hoppen, H.O. and Jochle, W. (1993) Advancing the time of ovulation in the mare with a short term implant releasing the GnRH analogue deslorelin. *Equine Veterinary Journal* 25, 65–68.

Meira, C. and Henry, M. (1991) Evaluation of two non-surgical equine embryo transfer methods. *Journal of Reproduction and Fertility, Supplement* 44, 712–713.

Melrose, P.A., Pickel, C., Cheramie, H.S., Henk, W.G., Littlefield-Chabaud, M.A. and French, D.D. (1994) Disribution and morphology of immunoreactive gonadotrophin-releasing hormone (GnRH) neurons in the basal forebrain of ponies. *Journal of Comparative Neurology* 339, 268–287.

Melrose, R.A., Walker, R.F. and Douglas, R.H. (1990) Dopamine in the cerebral spinal fluid of prepubertal and adult horses. *Brain and Behavioural Evolution* 5, 98–106.

Menzies-Gow, N. (2007) Diagnostic endoscopy of the urinary tract of the horse. *In Practice* 29(4), 208.

Mepham, B. (1987) *Physiology of Lactation*. Open University Press, Milton Keynes, UK, pp. 207.

Merkies, K., DuBois, C., Marshall, K., Parois, S., Graham, L. and Haley, D. (2016) A two stage approach to weaning horses using a physical barrier to prevent nursing *Applied Animal Behaviour Science* 183, 68–76.

Merkt, H., Klug, E. and Jochle, W. (2000) Reproduction management in the German Thoroughbred industry. *Journal of Equine Veterinary Science* 20(12), 822–868.

Metcalf, E.S. (1998) Pregnancy rates with cooled equine semen received in private practice. *Proceedings of the Annual Convention of the American Association of Equine Practionners*, p. 16–18.

Metcalf, E.S. (2001) The role of international transport of equine semen on disease transmission. *Animal Reproduction Science* 3(68), 229–237.

Metcalf, E.S. (2011) Venereal disease. In: McKinnon, A.O., Squires, E.L., Vaala, E. and Varner, D.D. (eds) *Equine Reproduction*, 2nd edn. Wiley-Blackwell, Philadelphia, London, pp. 1250–1260.

Meuten, D.J. and Rendano, V. (1978) Hypertrophic osteopathy in a mare with dysgerminoma. *Equine Medical Surgery* 2, 445–450.

Meyers, P.J. (1997) Control and synchronisation of oestrous cycles and ovulation. In: Youngquist, R.S. (ed.) *Current Therapy in Large Animal Theriogenology*. W.B. Saunders, Philadelphia, Pennsylvania, pp. 96–102.

Meyers, P.J. (2018) Equine endometritis : past, present and future Ontario Veterinary Medical Association Conference, Toronto, Ontario, Canada, 25–27 January 2018, pp. 308–312.

Meyers, P.J., Bonnett, B.N. and McKee, S.L. (1991) Quantifying the occurance of early embryonic mortality on three equine breeding farms. *Canadian Veterinary Journal* 32, 665–672.

Meyers, S.A. (2011) Acrosomal function. In: McKinnon, A.O., Squires, E.L, Vaala, W.E. and Varner, D.D. (eds) *Equine Reproduction* 2nd edn. Wiley-Blackwell, Philadelphia, London, pp. 1491–1497.

Meyers, S.A. and LeBlanc, M.M. (1991) Induction of parturition – clinical considerations for successful foalings. *Veterinary Medicine* 86, 1117–1121.

Meyers, S.A., Overstreet, J.W., Liu, I.K.M. and Drobnis, E.Z. (1995a) Capaciation in vitro of stallion spermatozoa: Comparison of progesterone-induced acrosome reactions in fertile and subfertile males. *Journal of Andrology* 16, 47–54.

Meyers, S.A., Liu, I.K.M., Overstreet, J.W. and Drobnis, E.Z. (1995b) Induction of acrosome reactions in stallion sperm by equine zona pellucida, porcine zona pellucida and progesterone. *Biology of Reproduction Monograph Equine Reproduction VI* 1, 739–744.

Meyers, S.A., Liu, I.K.M., Overstreet, J.W., Vadas, S. and Drobnis, E.Z. (1996) Zona pellucida binding and zona induced acrosome reactions in horse spermatozoa: comparisons between fertile and sub fertile stallions. *Theriogenology* 46(7), 1277–1288.

Meyers-Brown, G.A, McCue, P.M., Niswender, K.D., Squires, E.L., DeLuca, C.A., Bidstrup, L.A., Colgin, M., Famula, T.R. and Roser, J.F. (2010) Superovulation in mares usingrecombinant equine follicle stimulating hormone (reFSH): ovulation rates, embryo retrieval and hormone profiles. *Journal of Equine Veterinary Science* 30, 560–568.

Miki, W., Oniyama, H., Takeda, N., Kimura, Y., Haneda, S., Matsui, M., Taya, K. and Nambo, Y. (2016) Effects of a single use of GnRH analog buserelin on the induction of ovulation and endocrine profiles in heavy draft mares. *Journal of Equine Science* 27(4), 149–156.

Miller, C.D. (2008) Optimizing the use of frozen-thawed equine semen. *Theriogenology* 70(3), 463–468.

Miller, L.M.J. and Ferrer, S.M. (2014) Conception following endoscopic removal of edometrial cysts in a mare. *Clinical Theriogenology* 6(1), 41–45.

Millon, L. and Penedo, M. (2009). Chromosomal abnormalities and DNA genotyping in horses. *Fedequinas Journal* 57, 34–40.

Mills, D.S. (2005) Pheromonal therapy: theory and applications. *In Practice* 27, 368–377.

Mills, D. and McDonnell, S.M. (2005) *The Domestic Horse, The origins, development and management of its behaviour.* Cambridge University Press, Cambridge, UK, pp. 239.

Mills, D. and Nankervis, K. (1999) *Equine Behaviour, Principles and Practice.* Blackwell Science, Oxford, pp. 232.

Mills, D.S. and Riezebos, M. (2005) The role of the image of a conspecific in the regulation of stereotypic head movements in the horse. *Applied Animal Behaviour Science* 91, 155–165.

Mitchell, D. (1973) Detection of foetal circulation in the mare and cow by Doppler ultrasound. *Veterinary Record* 93, 365–368.

Mitchell, R.M., Scott, C.J., Cheong, S.H. and Collins, C.D. (2019) The Effect Of Routine Postpartum Uterine Lavage On Endometrial Cytology, Culture And Pregnancy Rates In Thoroughbred Broodmares. *Journal of Equine Veterinary Science* 80(8), p 5–9.

Miyakoshi, D., Shikichi, M., Ito, K., Iwata, K., Okai, K., Sato, F. and Nambo, Y. (2012) Factors affecting the frequency of pregnancy loss among Thoroughbred mares in Hidaka Japan. *Journal of Equine Veterinary Science* 32, 552–557.

Mizera, A. (2019) Insemination of Mares Versus Natural Mating in Europe in the 21st Century. In: *Agricultura, Alimentaria, Piscaria et Zootechnica.* Folia Pomeranae Universitatis Technologiae Stetinensis, Szczecin, Poland.

Moore, A.L., Squires, E.L. and Graham, J.K. (2005a) Effect of seminal plasma on the cryopreservation of equine spermatozoa. *Theriogenology* 63, 2372–2381.

Moore, A.L., Squires, E.L. and Graham, J.K. (2005b) Adding cholesterol to the stallion sperm plasma membrane improves cryosurvival. *Cryobiology* 51, 241–249.

Moran, D.M., Jasko, D.J., Squires, E.L. and Amann, R.P. (1992) Determination of temperature and cooling rate which induce cold-shock in stallion spermatozoa. *Theriogenology* 38, 999–1012.

Morehead, J.P., Colon, J.L. and Blanchard, T.L. (2001) Clinical experience with native GnRH therapy to hasten follicular development and first ovulation of the breeding season. *Journal of Equine Veterinary Science* 21, 54–84.

Moreno, D., Bencharif, D., Amirat-Briand, L., Neira, A., Destrumelle, S., and Tainturier, D. (2013) Preliminary results: the advantages of low-density lipoproteins for the cryopreservation of equine semen. *Journal of Equine Veterinary Science* 33(12), 1068–1075.

Morgenthal, J.L. and Van Niekerk, C.H. (1991) Plasma progestagen levels in normal mares with luteal deficiency during early pregnancy and in twinning habitual aborters. *Journal of Reproduction and Fertility, Supplement* 44, 728–729.

Morley, S.A. and Murray, J. (2014) Effects and body condition on the reproductive physioogy of the broodmare. A Review. *Journal of Equine Veterinary Science* 34(7), 842–853.

Moros-Nicolás, C., Douet, C., Reigner, F. and Goudet, G. (2019) Effect of cumulus cell removal and sperm pre-incubation with progesterone on in vitro fertilization of equine gametes in the presence of oviductal fluid or cells. *Reproduction in Domestic Animals* 54(8), 1095–1103.

Morrell, J.A. (2011) Artificial Insemination: Current and Future Trends. In: Manafi, M. (ed.) *Artificial Insemination in Farm Animals.* InTech, Available from: http://www.intechopen.com/books/artificial-insemination-in-farm-animals/artificial-insemination-current-andfuture-trends (accessed 1 May 2020).

Morrell, J.M. (2012) Applications of colloid centrifugation in Assisted Reproduction. In: Paresh, C.R. (ed.) *Colloids: Classification, Properties and Applications.* Nova Science Publishers Inc., Hauppauge, New York, pp. 75–99.

Morrell, J.M. and Geraghty, R.J. (2006) Effective removal of equine arteritis virus from stallion semen. *Equine Veterinary Journal* 38, 224–229.

Morrell, J.A. and Wallgren, M. (2014) Alternatives to antibiotics in semen extenders: A review. *Pathogens* 3(4), 934–946.

Morresey, P.R. (2005) Prenatal and perinatal indicators of neonatal viability. *Clinical and Technical Equine Practice* 4, 238–249.

Morresey, P.R. (2011a) Oxytocin, inhibin, activin, relaxin and prolactin. In: McKinnon, A.O., Squires, E.L, Vaala, W.E. and Varner, D.D. (eds) *Equine Reproduction* 2nd edn. Wiley-Blackwell, Philadelphia, London, pp. 1679–1686.

Morresey, P.R. (2011b) The placenta. In: McKinnon, A.O., Squires, E.L, Vaala, W.E. and Varner, D.D. (eds) *Equine Reproduction* 2nd edn. Wiley-Blackwell, Philadelphia, London, pp. 84–97.

Morris, L.H. (2004) Low dose insemination in the mare: an update. *Animal Reproduction Science* 82–83, 625–632.

Morris, L.H.A. (2005) Challenges facing sex preselection of stallion spermatozoa. *Animal Reproduction Science* 89(1–4), 147–157.

Morris, L.H.A. (2011) Sex-sorted spermatozoa. In: McKinnon, A.O., Squires, E.L., Vaala, E. and Varner, D.D. (eds) *Equine Reproduction*, 2nd edn. Wiley-Blackwell, Philadelphia, London, pp. 3042–3050.

Morris, L.H.A. and Allen, W.R. (2002a) An overview of low dose insemination in the mare. *Reproduction in Domestic Animals* 37, 206–210.

Morris, L.H.A. and Allen, W.R. (2002b) Reproductive efficiency of intensively managed Thoroughbred mares in Newmarket. *Equine Veterinary Journal* 34, 51–60.

Morris, L.H.A. and Lyle, S.K. (2011) Low dose insemination. In: McKinnon, A.O., Squires, E.L., Vaala, W.E. and Varner, D.D. (eds) *Equine Reproduction*, 2nd edn. Wiley-Blackwell, Philadelphia, London, 3036–3041.

Morris, L.H.A., Hunter, R.H.F. and Allen, W.R. (2000) Hysteroscopic insemination of small numbers of spermatozoa at the uterotubal junction of preovulatory mares. *Journal of Reproduction and Fertility* 118, 95–100.

Morris, L.H.A., Tiplady, C. and Allen, W.R. (2002) The in vitro fertility of caudal epididymal spermatozoa in the horse. *Theriogenology* 58, 643–646.

Morris, L.H.A., Tiplady, C. and Allen, W.R. (2003) Pregnancy rates in mares after a single fixed time hysteroscopic insemination of low numbers of frozen-thawed spermatozoa onto the uterotubal junction. *Equine Veterinary Journal* 35, 197–201.

Morris, R.P., Rich, G.A., Ralston, S.L., Squires, E.L. and Pickett, B.W. (1987) Follicular activity in transitional mares as affected by body condition and dietary energy. In: *Proceedings of the 10th Equine Nutrition and Physiology Symposium, Colorado State University, Colorado.* Equine Nutrition and Physiology Society, pp. 93–99.

Mortensen, C.J., Choi, Y.H., Hinrichs, K., Ing, N.H., Kraemer, D.C., Vogelsang, S.G. and Vogelsang, M.M. (2009) Embryo recovery from exercised mares *Animal Reproduction Science* 110(3–4), 237–244.

Mortimer, D. (2000) Sperm preparation methods. *Journal of Andrology* 21, 357–366.

Moussa, M., Duchamp, G., Mahla, R., Bruyas, J.-F. and Daels, P.F. (2002) Comparison of pregnancy rates for equine embryos cooled for 24 h in Ham's F-10 and emcare holding solutions. *Theriogenology* 58(2/4), 755–757.

Moussa, M., Duchamp, G., Mahla, R., Bruyas, J.-F. and Daels, P.F. (2003) In vitro and in vivo comparison of Ham's F-10, Emcare holding solution and ViGro Holding Plus for the cooled storage of equine embryos. *Theriogenology* 59, 1615–1625.

Moussa, M., Tremoleda, J.L., Duchamp, G., Bruyas, J.-F., Colenbrander, B., Bevers, M.M. and Daels, P.F. (2004) Evaluation of viability and apoptosis in horse embryos stored under different conditions at 5°C. *Theriogenology* 61, 921–932.

Moussa, M., Duchamp, G., Daels, P.F. and Bruyas, J.F. (2006) Effects of embryo age on the viability of equine embryos after cooled storage using two transport systems. *Journal of Equine Veterinary Science* 26, 529–534.

Mugnier, S., Dell'Aquila, M.E., Pelaez, J., Douet, C., Ambruosi, B., De Santis, T., Lacalandra, G.M., Lebos, C., Sizaret, P.Y., Delaleu, B., Monget, P., Mermillod, P., Magistrini, M., Meyers, S.A. and Goudet, G. (2009) New insights into the mechanisms of fertilization. Comparison of the fertyilization steps, composition, and structure of the zona pellucida between horses and pigs. *Biology of Reproduction* 81, 856–870.

Muller, Z. and Cunat, L. (1993) Special surgical transfers of horse embryos. *Equine Veterinary Journal, Supplement* 15, 113–115.

Mumford, E.L., Squires, E.L., Peterson, K.D., Nett, T.M. and Jasko, D.J. (1994) Effect of various doses of gonadotrophin releasing hormone analogue on induction of ovulation in anostrus mares. *Journal of Animal Science* 72, 178–183.

Mumford, E.L., Squires, E.L., Jochle, E., Harrison, L.A., Nett, T.M. and Trigg, T.E. (1995) Use of deslorelin short term implants to induce ovulation in cycling mares during 3 consecutive estrous cycles. *Animal Reproduction Science* 39, 129–140.

Mumford, J.A., Hannant, D. and Jessett, D.M. (1996) Abortigenic and neurological disease caused by experimental infection with equine herpes virus. In: *Equine Infectious Diseases VII, Proceedings of the 7th International Conference.* R.W. Publications, Newmarket, UK, pp. 261–275.

Murase, H., Saito, S., Amaya, T., Sato, F., Ball, B.A. and Nambo, Y. (2015) Anti-Müllerian hormone as an indicator of hemi-castrated unilateral cryptorchid horses. *Journal of Equine Science* 26(1), 15–20.

Murcia-Robayo, R.Y., Jouanisson, E., Beauchamp, G. and Diaw, M. (2018) Effects of staining method and clinician experience on the evaluation of stallion sperm morphology. *Animal Reproduction Science* 188, 165–169.

Murchie, T. (2005) Stallion infertility. *Proceedings of the North American Veterinary Conference. Large animal.* Orlando, Florida 19, 267–269.

Murphy, B.A. (2019) Circadian and circannual regulation in the horse: internal timing in an elite athlete. *Journal of Equine Veterinary Science* 76, 14–24.

Murphy, B.A., Walsh, C.M., Woodward, E.M., Prendergast, R.L., Ryle, J.P., Fallon, L.H. and Troedsson, M.H.T. (2014) Blue light from individual light masks directed at a single eye advances the breeding season in mares. *Equine Vet Journal* 46 (5), 601–605.

Murphy, J.E., Frazer, G., Munsterman, A., Weisbrode, S., Kohn, C. and Beard, W. (2005) Endometrial stromal hyperplasia and mass formation in a yearling Quarter Horse. *Equine Veterinary Education* 17(3), 59–162.

Muyan, M., Roser, J.F., Dybdal, N. and Baldwin, D.M. (1993) Modulation of gonadotrophin releasing hormone modulated luteinising hormone release on cultured male equine anterior pituitary cells by gonadal steroids. *Biology of Reproduction* 49, 340–345.

Naden, J., Amann, R.R. and Squires, E.L. (1990) Testicular growth, hormone concentrations, seminal characteristics and sexual behaviour in stallions. *Journal of Reproduction and Fertility, Supplement* 88, 167–176.

Nafis, I.A. and Pandey, A.K. (2012) Endometritis by Corynebacterium sp. in mares. *Indian Veterinary Journal* 89(10), 136–137.

Nagamine, N., Nambo, Y., Nagata, S., Nagaoka, K., Tsunoda, N., Taniyama, H., Tanaka, Y., Tohei, A., Watanabe, G., and Taya, K. (1998) Inhibin Secretion in the Mare: Localization of Inhibin, ßA, and ßB Subunits in the Ovary. *Biology of Reproduction* 59, 1392–1398.

Nagata, S.I. (2000) Endocrine profiles of testicular functions in the stallion. *Journal of Reproduction and Development* 46, Suppl j13–j24.

Nagata, S., Tsunoda, N., Nagamine, N., Tanaka, Y., Taniyama, H., Nambo, Y., Watanabe, G. and Taya, K. (1998) Testicular inhibin in the stallion: cellular source and seasonal changes in its secretion. *Biology of Reproduction* 58, 62–68.

Nagata, S., Kurosawa, M., Mima, K., Nambo, Y., Fuiji, Y., Watanabe, G. and Taya, K. (1999) Effects of anabolic steroid (19-nortestosterone) on the secretion of testicular hormones in the stallion. *Journal and Reproduction and Fertility* 115, 373–379.

Nagata, S.I., Nagaoka, K., Shinbo, H., Nagamine, N., Tsunoda, N., Taniyama, H., Nambo, Y., Groome, N.P., Watanabe, G. and Taya, K. (2000) Inhibin pro-αC as the marker of testicular function in the stallion. *Journal of Reproduction and Development* 46(3), 201–206.

Nagel, C., Aurich, J. and Aurich, C. (2010) Determination of heart rate and heart rate variability in the equine fetus by fetomaternal electrocardiography. *Theriogenology* 73(7), 973–983.

Nagel, C., Erber, R., Bergmaier, C., Wulf, M., Aurich, J., Möstl, E. and Aurich, C. (2012) Cortisol and progestin release, heart rate and heart rate variability in the pregnant and post partum mare, fetus and newborn foal. *Theriogenology* 78(4), 759–767.

Nagel, C., Erber, R., Ille, N., von Lewinski, M., Aurich, J., Möstl, E. and Aurich, C. (2014) Parturition in horses is dominated by parasympathetic activity of the autonomous nervous system. *Theriogenology* 82(1), 160–168.

Nagy, P., Huszenicza, G., Juhasz, J., Kulcsar, M., Solti, L., Reiczigel, J. and Abavary, K. (1998) Factors influencing ovarian activity and sexual behavior of postpartum mares underfarm conditions. *Theriogenology* 50(7),1109–1119.

Nagy, P., Guillaume, D. and Daels, P. (2000) Seasonality in mares. *Animal Reproduction Science* 60/61, 245–262.

Nagy, P., Duchamp, G., Chavatte-Palmer, P., Daels, P.F. and Guillaume, D. (2002) Induction of lactation in mares with a dopamine antagonist needs ovarian hormones. *Theriogenology* 58, 2–4.

Nagy, P., Huszenicza, G., Reiczigel, J., Juhasz, J., Kulcsar, M., Abavary, K. and Guillaume, D. (2004) Factors affecting plasma progesterone concentration and retrospective determination of time of ovulation in cyclic mares. *Theriogenology* 61(2–3), 203–214.

Nambo, Y., Nagaoka, K., Tanaka, Y., Nagamine, N., Shinbo, H., Nagata, S., Yoshihara, T., Watanbe, G., Groome, N.P. and Taya, K. (2002) Mechanisms responsible for increase in circulating inhibin levels at the time of ovulation in mares. *Theriogenology* 76(6), 1707–1717.

Nam BoRa, Mekuria, Z., Carossino, M., Li GanWu, Zheng Ying, JianQiang, Z., Cook, R.F., Shuck, K.M., Campos, J.R., Squires, E.L., Troedsson, M.H.T., Timoney, P.J. and Balasuriya, U.B.R. (2019) Intrahost selection pressure drives equine arteritis virus evalution during persistent infection in the stallion reproductive tract. *Journal of Virology* 93(12), e00045–19.

Nash D.M., Paddison, J., Davies Morel, M.C.G. and Barnea, E.R. (2018) Preimplantation factor modulates acute inflammatory responses of equine endometrium. *Veterinary Medicine and Science* 4, 351–356.

Nath, L.C., Anderson, G.A. and McKinnon, A.O. (2010) Reproductive efficiency of Thoroughbred and Standardbred horses in northern Victoria. *Australian Veterinary Journal* 88, 169–175.

Nathanielsz, P.W. (1998) Comparative studies on the initiation of labor. *European Journal of Obstetrics and Reproductive Biology* 78, 127–132.

Nathanielsz, P.W., Grussani, D.A. and Wu, W.X. (1997) Stimulation of the switch in myometrial activity from contractures to contractions in the pregnant sheep and non human primate. *Equine Veterinary Journal, Supplement* 24, 83–88.

National Research Council (1989) *Nutritient Requirements of Horses,* 5th edn. Revised. National Academy Press, Washington DC, pp. 100.

National Research Council (2007) *Nutrient Requirements of Horses*, 6th edn. Revised. The National Academies Press, Washington, DC, pp. 315.

Naumenkov, A. and Romankova, N. (1981) An improved semen diluent. *Konevodstvoi Konnyi Sport* 4, 34 (*Animal Breeding Abstracts* (1981) 49, 6207).

Naumenkov, A. and Romankova, N. (1983) Improving diluent composition and handling for stallion sperm. *Nauchnye Trudy. Vsesoyuznyi Nauchno Issledovatel'skii Institut Konevodstva*, 38–47 (*Animal Breeding Abstracts* (1983) 51, 6370).

Neely, D.P. (1983) Evaluation and therapy of genital disease in the mare. In: Hughes, J.P. (ed.) *Equine Reproduction*. Hoffman-LaRoche, Nutley, New Jersey, pp. 40–56.

Neild, D.M., Chaves, M.D., Flores, M., Mora, N., Beconi, M. and Aguero, A. (1999) Hyposmotic test in equine sperm. *Theriogenology* 51, 721–727.

Neild, D.M., Chaves, M.G., Flores, M., Miragaya, M.H., Gonzalez, E. and Agüero, A. (2000) The HOS test and its relationship to fertility in the stallion. *Andrologia* 32(6), 351–5.

Neild, D.M., Gadella, B.M., Chaves, M.G., Miragaya, M.H., Colenbrander, B. and Aguero, A. (2003) Membrane changes during different stages of a freeze-thaw protocol for equine cryopreservation. *Theriogenology* 59(8), 1693–1705.

Neild, D.M., Brouwers, J.F., Colenbrander, B., Aguero, A. and Gadella, B.M. (2005a) Lipid peroxidase formation in relation to membrane stability of fresh and frozen thawed stallion spermatozoa. *Molecular Reproductive Development* 72(2), 230–238.

Neild, D.M., Gadella, B.M., Aguero, A., Stout, T.A. and Colenbrander, B. (2005b) Capacitation, acrosome function and chromatin structure in stallion sperm. *Animal Reproduction Science* 89(1–4), 47–56.

Neilson, J.M. (2005) Endometritis in mares: A diagnostic study comparing cultures from swab and biopsy. *Theriogenology* 64, 510–518.

Nielsen, J.M., Troedsson, M.H., Pedersen, M.R., Bojesen, A.M., Lehn-Jensen, H., Zent, W.W. (2010) Diagnosis of Endometritis in the Mare Based on Bacteriological and Cytological Examinations of the Endometrium: Comparions of Results Obtained by Swabs and Biopsies. *Journal of Equine Veterinary Science* 30(1), 27–30.

Nielsen, M.K. (2016) Equine tapeworm infections – disease, diagnosis, and control. *Equine Veterinary Education* 28(7), 388–395.

Nielsen, M.K., Kaplan, R.M., Thamsborg, S.M., Monrad, J. and Olsen, S.N. (2007) Climatic influences on development and survival of free-living stages of equine strongyles: Implications for worm control strategies and managing anthelmintic resistance. *Veterinary Journal* 174, 23–32.

Nequin, L.G., King, S.S., Johnson, A.L., Gow, G.M. and Ferreira-Dias, G.M. (1993) Prolactin may play a role in stimulating the equine ovary during the spring reproductive transition. *Equine Veterinary Science* 13, 631–635.

Nervo, T., Nebbia, P., Bertero, A., Robino, P., Stella, M.C., Rota, A. and Appino, S. (2019) Chronic endometritis in subfertile mares with presence of Chlamydial DNA. *Journal of Equine Veterinary Science* 73, 91–94.

Neto, C.R., Monteiro, G.A., Zanzarini, D.J.D., Farras, M.C., Dell'aqua, J.A. Papa, F.O. and Alvarenga, M.A. (2013) The relationships between scrotal surface temperature, age and sperm quality in stallions. *Livestock Science* 157(1), 358–363.

Nett, T.M. (1993a) Estrogens. In: McKinnon, A.O. and Voss, J.L. (eds) *Equine Reproduction*. Lea and Febiger, Philadelphia, Pennsylvania, pp. 65–68.

Nett, T.M. (1993b) Reproductive peptide and protein hormones. In: McKinnon, A.O. and Voss, J.L. (eds) *Equine Reproduction*. Lea and Febiger, Philadelphia, Pennsylvania, pp. 109–114.

Nett, T.M. (1993c) Reproductive endocrine function testing in stallions. In: McKinnon, A.O. and Voss, J.L. (eds) *Equine Reproduction*. Lea and Febiger, Philadelphia, Pennsylvania, pp. 821–824.

Neuhauser, S., Gösele, P. and Handler, J. (2018a) The effect of four different commercial semen extenders on the motility of stallion epididymal sperm. *Journal of Equine Veterinary Science* 62, 8–12.

Neuhauser, S., Handler, J., Schelling, C. and Pieńkowska-Schelling, A. (2018b) Disorder of Sexual development in a mare with an unusual tetnative mosaic karyotype: 63,X/64,Xdel(Y). *Sexual Development* 12(5), 232–238.

Neuhauser, S., Bollwein, H., Siuda, M. and Handler, J. (2019a) Comparison of the effects of five semen extenders on the quality of frozen-thawed equine epididymal sperm. *Journal of Equine Veterinary Science* 79, 1–8.

Neuhauser, S., Handler, J., Schelling, C. and Pieńkowska-Schelling, A. (2019b) Fertility and 63,X mosaicism in a Haflinger sibship. *Journal of Equine Veterinary Science* 78, 127–133.

Neuhauser, S., Gösele, P. and Handler, J. (2019c) Postthaw addition of autologous seminal plasma improves sperm motion characteristics in fair and poor freezer stallions. *Journal of Equine Veterinary Science* 72, 117–123.

Neuschaefer, A., Bracher, V. and Allen, W.R. (1991) Prolactin secretion in lactating mares before and after treatment with bromocryptine. *Journal of Reproduction and Fertility, Supplement* 44, 551–559.

Neves, A.P., Keller, A., Trein, C.R., Moller, G., Jobim, M.I., Castilho, L.F., Cardoso, M.R., Leibold, W., Zerbe, H., Klug, E., Gregory, R.M. and Mattos, R.C. (2007) Use of leucocytes as treatment for endometritis in mares experimentally infected with *Streptococcus equi* subsp. *zooepidemicus*. *Animal Reproduction Science* 97, 314–322.

Newcombe, J.R. (1994a) A comparison of ovarian follicular diameter in Thoroughbred mares between Australia and the UK. *Journal of Equine Veterinary Science* 14, 653–654.

Newcombe, J.R. (1994b) Conception in a mare to a single mating 7 days before ovulation. *Equine Veterinary Education* 6, 27–28.

Newcombe, J.R. (1995) Incidence of multiple ovulation and multiple pregnancy in mares. *Veterinary Record* 137, 121–123.

Newcombe, J.R. (1997) The incidence of ovulation during the luteal phase from Day 4 to Day 20 in pregnant and non-pregnant mares. *Journal of Equine Veterinary Science* 17, 120–122.

Newcombe, J.R. (2000a) Embryonic loss and abnormalities of early pregnancy. *Equine Veterinary Education* 12(2), 88–101.

Newcombe, J.R. (2000b) The probable identification of monozygous twin embryos in mares. *Journal of Equine Veterinary Science* 20(4), 269–274.

Newcombe, J.R. (2002) Field observations on the use of a progesterone-releasing intravaginal device to inuce estrus and ovulation in seasonally anestrous mares. *Journal of Equine Veterinary Science* 22, 378–382.

Newcombe, J.R. (2004) The relationship between the number, diameter, and survival of early embryonic vesicles. *Pferdeheilkunde* 20(3), 214–220.

Newcombe, J.R. (2011a) Human Chorionic Gonadotrophin In: McKinnon, A.O., Squires, E.L., Vaala, W.E. and Varner, D.D. (eds) *Equine Reproduction* 2nd edn. Wiley-Blackwell, Philadelphia, London, pp. 1805–1810.

Newcombe, J.R. (2011b) Why are mares with pneumovagina susceptible to bacterial endometritis? A personal opinion. *Journal of Equine Veterinary Science* 31(4), 174–179.

Newcombe, J. and Cuervo-Arango, J. (2008) The effect of interval from mating to ovulation on pregnancy rates and the incidence of intra-uterine fluid inthe mare. *Reproduction in Domestic Animals* 43, 109.

Newcombe, J. and Cuervo-Arango, J. (2016) Comparison of the efficacy of different single doses of buserelin with hCG for timed ovulation induction in the mare. *Journal Equine Veterinary Science* 41, 57.

Newcombe, J.R. and Nout, Y.S. (1998) Apparent effect of management on the hour of parturition in mares. *Veterinary Record* 142, 221–222.

Newcombe, J. and Peters, A.J. (2014) The Buserelin Enigma. How does treatment with this GnRH analogue decrease embryo mortality? *Journal of Veterinary Science and Technolgy* 5(151), 1–7.

Newcombe, J.R. and Wilson, M.C. (1997) The use of progesterone releasing intravaginal devices to induce estrus and ovulation in anoestrus standardbred mares in Australia. *Equine Practice* 19(6), 13–21.

Newcombe, J.R. and Wilson, M.C. (2005) Age, Body Weight and pregnancy loss. *Journal of Equine Veterinary Science* 25(5), 188–194.

Newcombe, J.R. and Wilson, M.C. (2007) The effect of repeated treatment with human chorionic gonadotrophin to induce ovulation in mares. *Proceedings of the 46th Congress British Equine Veterinary Association, Edinburgh, 12–15 Sept 2007. Equine Veterinary Journal* pp. 291.

Newcombe, J.R., Martinez, T.A. and Peters, A.R. (2001) The effect of the gonadotropin releasing hormone analog, buserelin, on pregnancy rates in horse and pony mares. *Theriogenology* 55(8), 1619–1631.

Newcombe, J.R., Handler, J., Klug, E., Meyers, P.J. and Jochle, W. (2002) Treatment of transition phase mares with progesterone intravaginally and with deslorelin or hCG to asist ovulation. *Journal of Equine Veterinary Science* 22(2), 57–64.

Newcombe, J.R., Lichtwark, S. and Wilson, M.C. (2005) Case report: the effect of sperm number, concentration, and volume of insemination dose chilled, stored and transported semen on pregnancy rate in Standardbred mares. *Journal of Equine Veterinary Science* 25(12), 1–6.

Newcombe, J.R., Jochle, W. and Cuervo-Arango, J. (2008) Effect of dose of chloprostenol on the interval to ovulation in the dioestrus mare. A retrospective study. *Journal of Equine Veterinary Science* 28, 532–539.

Nicol, C.J., Davidson, H.P., Harris, P.A., Waters, A.J. and Wilson, A.D. (2002) Study of crib-biting and gastric inflammation and ulceration in young horses. *Veterinary Record* 151(22), 658–662.

Nicol, C.J., Badnell-Waters, A.J., Bice, R., Kelland, A., Wilson, A.D. and Harris, P.A. (2005) The effects of diet and weaning method on the behaviour of young horses. *Applied Animal Behaviour Science* 95(3–4), 205–221.

Nie, G.J. and Wenzel, J.G.W. (2001) Adaptation of the hypoosmotic swelling test to assess functional integrity of stallion spermatozoa membranes. *Theriogenology* 55, 1005–1018.

Nie, G.J., Goodin, A.N., Braden, T.D. and Wenzel, J.G.W. (2001a) Luteal and clinical response following administration of dinoprost tromethamine or cloprostenol at standard intramuscular sites or at the lumbosacral acupuncture points in mares. *American Journal of Veterinary Research* 62, 1285–1289.

Nie, G.J., Johnson, K.E. and Wenzel, J.G.W. (2001b) Use of glass ball to suppress behavioural estrus in mares. In: *Proceedings of American Association of Equine Practitioners* 47, 246–252.

Nie, G.J., Johnson, K.E., Braden, T.D. and Wenzel, J.G.W. (2003) Use of intra-uterine glass ball protocol to extend luteal function in mares. *Journal of Equine Veterinary Science* 23(6), 266–272.

Nielsen, M.K., Kaplan, R.M., Thamsborg, S.M., Monrad, J. and Olsen, S.N. (2007) Climatic influences on development and survival of free-living stages of equine strongyles: Implications for worm control strategies and managing anthelmintic resistance. *Veterinary Journal* 174, 23–32.

Nikolakopoulos, E. and Watson, E.D. (2000) Effect of infusion volume and sperm numbers on persistence of uterine inflammation in mares. *Equine Veterinary Journal* 32(2), 164–166.

Nikolakopoulos, E., Kindahl, H., Gilbert, C.L., Goode, J. and Watson, E.D. (2000a) Release of oxytocin and prostaglandin F2 alpha around teasing, natural service and associated events in the mare. *Animal Reproduction Science* 63, 89–99.

Nikolakopoulos, E., Kindahl, H. and Watson, E.D. (2000b) Oxytocin and PGF2 alpha release in mares resistant and susceptible to persistent mating-induced endometritis. *Journal of Reproduction and Fertility, Supplement* 56, 363–372.

Nilsson, E., Parrott, J.A. and Skinner, M.K. (2001) Basic fibroblast growth factor induces primordial follicle development and initiates folliculogenesis. *Molecular and Cellular Endocrinology* 175, 123–130.

Nishikawa, Y. (1975) Studies on the preservation of raw and frozen semen. *Journal of Reproduction and Fertility, Supplement* 23, 99–104.

Niswender, K.D., Alvarenga, M.A., McCue, P.M., Hardy, Q.P. and Squires, E.L. (2003) Superovulation in cycling mares using equine follicle stimulating hormone (eFSH). *Journal of Equine Veterinary Science* 23, 497–500.

Nogueira, G.P., Barnabe, R.C. and Verreschi, I.T.N. (1997) Puberty and growth rate in Thoroughbred fillies. *Theriogenology* 48, 581–588.

Nolan, M.B., Walsh, C.M., Duff, N., McCrarren, C., Prendergast, R.L. and Murphy, B.A. (2017) Artificially extended photoperiod administered to pre partum mares via blue light to a single eye: Observations on gestation length, foal birth weight and foal hair coat at birth. *Theriogenology* 100, 126–133.

Nonno, R., Capsoni, S., Lucini, V., Mooler, M., Fraschini, F. and Stankoz, B. (1995) Distribution and characterisation of the melatonin receptors in the hypothalamus and pituitary gland of domestic ungulates. *Journal of Pineal Research* 18(4), 207–216.

Norman, S.T., Larsen, J.E. and Morton, J.M. (2006) Oestrous response and follicular development in mares after treatment with an intravaginal progesterone releasing device in association with single injections of oestradiol benzoate and PGF2alpha. *Australian Veterinary Journal* 84, 47–49.

Norris, H.Y., Taylor, W.B. and Garner, F.M. (1968) Equine ovarian granular tumours. *Veterinary Record* 82, 419–420.

Nouri, H., Towhidi, A., Zhandi, M. and Sadeghi, R. (2013) The effects of centrifuged egg yolk used with INRA plus soybean lecithin extender on semen quality to freeze miniature Caspian horse semen. *Journal of Equine Veterinary Science* 33(12), 1050–1053.

Nouri, H., Shojaeian, K., Samadian, F., Lee SooJung, Kohram, H. and Lee JeongIk (2018) Using resveratrol and epigallocatechin-3-gallate to improve cryopreservation of stallion spermatozoa with low quality. *Journal of Equine Veterinary Science* 70 18–25.

Nout-Lomas, Y.S. and Beacom, C.K. (2015) Granulosa cell tumours: Examining the 'moody' mare. *Equine Veterinary Education* 27(10), 515–524.

Oba, E., Bicudo, S.D., Pimentel, S.L., Lopes, R.S., Simonetti, F. and Hunziker, R.A. (1993) Quantitative and qualitative evaluation of stallion semen. *Revista Brasileira de Reproducao Animal* 17(1–2), 57–74.

Oberstein, N., O'Donovan, M.K., Bruemmer, J.E., Seidel Jr, G.E., Carnevale, E.M. and Squires, E.L. (2001) Cryopreservation of equine embryos by open pull straw, cryoloop, or conventional slow cooling methods. *Theriogenology* 55, 607–613.

O'Donnell, L.J., Sheerin, B.R., Hendry, J.M., Thatcher, M.J., Thatcher, W.W. and LeBlanc, M.M. (2003) 24-hour secretion patterns of plasma oestradiol 17beta in pony mares in late gestation. *Reproduction in Domestic Animals* 38, 233–235.

Oetjen, M. (1988) Use of different acrosome stains for evaluating the quality of fresh and frozen semen. PhD thesis, Tierarztliche Hochschule Hannover, German Federal Republic.

Oftedal, O.T. and Jenness, R. (1988) Interspecies variation in milk composition among horses, zebras and asses (Perisodactyla: Equidae). *Journal of Dairy Research* 55, 57–66.

Oftedal, O.T., Hints, H.F. and Schryver, H.F. (1983) Lactation in the horse: milk composition and intake by foals. *Journal of Nutrition* 113, 2096–2106.

O'Grady, S. (1995) Umbilical care in foals. *Journal of Equine Veterinary Science* 15, 12–14.

Oguri, N. and Tsutsumi, Y. (1972) Non surgical recovery of equine eggs and an attempt at non surgical embryo transfer in the horse. *Journal of Reproduction and Fertility* 31, 187–195.

Oguri, N. and Tsutsumi, Y. (1974) Non-surgical egg transfer in mares. *Journal of Reproduction and Fertility, Supplement* 41, 313–317.

Oguri, N. and Tsutsumi, Y. (1980) No surgical transfer of equine embryos. *Archives of Andrology* 5, 108.

Ohnuma, K., Yokoo, M., Kazuei, I., Nambo, Y., Miyake, Y-I., Komatsu, M. and Takahashi, J. (2000) Study of Early Pregnancy Factor (EPF) in equine. *American Journal of Reproductive Immunology* 43, 174–179.

Okada, C.T.C., Andrade, V.P., Freitas-Dell'Aqua, C.P., Nichi, M., Fernandes, C.B., Papa, F.O. and Alvarenga, M.A. (2019) The effect of flunixin meglumine, firocoxib and meloxicam on the uterine mobility of equine embryos. *Theriogenology* 123, 132–138.

Okamura, H., Yamamura, T. and Wakabayashi, Y. (2013) Kisspeptin as a master player in the neural control of reproduction in mammals: an overview of kisspeptin research in domestic animals. *Animal Science Journal* 84, 369–381.

Oliveira Neto, I.V., Canisso, I.F., Segabinazzi, L.G., Dell'Aqua, C.P.F., Alvarenga, M.A., Papa, F.O. and Dell'Aqua Júnior, J.A. (2018) Synchronization of cyclic and acyclic embryo recipient mares with donor mares. *Animal Reproduction Science* 190 1–9.

Olivera, R., Moro, L.N., Jordan, R., Luzzani, C., Miriuka, S., Radrizzani, M., Donadeu, F.X. and Vichera, G. (2016) In vitro and in vivo development of horse cloned embryos generated with iPSCs, mesenchymal stromal cells and fetal or adult fibroblasts as nuclear donors. *PLoS ONE*, 11, e0164049.

Olivera, R., Moro, L.N., Jordan, R., Pallarols, N., Guglielminetti, A., Luzzani, C., Miriuka, S.G., and Vichera, G. (2018). Bone marrow mesenchymal stem cells as nuclear donors improve viability and health of cloned horses. *Stem Cells and Cloning: Advances and Applications* 11, 13–22.

Onuma, H. and Ohnami, Y. (1975) Retention of tubal eggs in mares. *Journal of Reproduction and Fertility, Supplement* 23, 507–511.

Oriol, J.G. (1994) The equine capsule. *Equine Veterinary Journal* 26(3), 184–186.

Oriol, J.G., Sharom, F.J. and Betteridge, K.J. (1993) Developmentally regulated changes in the glycoproteins of the equine embryonic capsule. *Journal of Reproduction and Fertility* 99, 653–664.

Ortiz-Escribano, N., Bogado Pascottini, O., Woelders, H., Vandenberghe, L., De Schauwer, C., Govaere, J., Van den Abbeel E., Vullers, T., Ververs, C., Roels, K., Van De Velde, M., Van Soom, A. and Smits, K. (2018) An improved vitrification protocol for equine immature oocytes, resulting in a first live foal. *Equine Veterinary Journal* 50, 391–397.

Osborne, V.E. (1975) Factors influencing foaling percentages in Australian mares. *Journal of Reproduction and Fertility, Supplement* 23, 477–483.

Osterman, L.E.O., Kuzmina, T., Uggla, A., Waller, P.J. and Hoglund, J. (2007) A field study on the effect of some anthelmintics on cyathostomins of horses in Sweden. *Veterinary Research Communications* 124, 34–37.

Ott, E.A. (2001) Energy, protein and amino acids requirements for growth of young horses. In: Pagan, J.D. and Guer, R.J. (eds) *Advances in Equine Nutrition II*. Nottingham University Press, Nottingham, UK, pp. 153–159.

Ousey, J.C. (1997) Thermoregulation and energy requirement of the newborn foal, with reference to prematurity. *Equine Veterinary Journal, Supplement* 24, 104–108.

Ousey, J. (2002) Induction of parturition in the healthy mare. *Equine Veterinary Education Manual* 5, 83–87.

Ousey, J. (2006) Hormone profiles and treatments in the late pregnant mare. *Veterinary Clinics Equine* 22, 727–747.

Ousey, J.C. (2011a) Endocrinology of pregnancy. In: McKinnon, A.O., Squires, E.L, Vaala, W.E. and Varner, D.D. (eds) *Equine Reproduction* 2nd edn. Wiley-Blackwell, Philadelphia, London, pp. 2222–2233.

Ousey, J.C. (2011b) Endocrinological adaptation. In: McKinnon, A.O., Squires, E.L, Vaala, W.E. and Varner, D.D. (eds) *Equine Reproduction* 2nd edn. Wiley-Blackwell, Philadelphia, London, pp. 69–83.

Ousey, J.C. and Fowden, A.L. (2012) Prostaglandin and the regulation of parturition in mares. *Equine Veterinary Jounrnal* 44(s42), 140–148.

Ousey, J.C., Dudan, F. and Rossdale, P.D. (1984) Preliminary studies of mammary secretions in the mare to assess foetal readiness for birth. *Equine Veterinary Journal* 16, 259–263.

Ousey, J.C., McArthur, A.J. and Rossdale, P.D. (1991) Metabolic changes in Thoroughbred and pony foals during the first 24 hours post partum. *Journal of Reproduction and Fertility, Supplement* 44, 561–570.

Ousey, J.C., McArthur, A.J. and Rossdale, P.D. (1996) How much energy do sick foals require compared to healthy ones? *Pferdeheikunde* 12, 231–237.

Ousey, J.C., Rossdale, P.D., Dudan, F.E. and Fowden, A.L. (1998) The effects of intrafetal ACTH administration on the outcome of pregnancy in the mare. *Reproduction, Fertility and Development* 10, 359–367.

Ousey, J.C., Freestone, N., Fowden, A.L., Mason, W.T. and Rossdale, P.D. (2000) The effects of oxytocin and progestagens on myometrial contractility in vitro during equine pregnancy. *Journal of Reproduction and Fertility, Supplement.* 56, 681–689.

Ousey, J.C., Rossdale, P.D., Fowden, A.L., Palmer, L., Turnbull, C. and Allen, W.R. (2004) Effects of manipulating intrauterine growth on post natal adrenocortical development and other parameters of maturity in neonatal foals. *Equine Veterinary Journal* 36(7), 616–621.

Ousey, J.C., Houghton, E., Grainger, L., Rossdale, P.D. and Fowden, A.L. (2005) Progestagen profiles during the last trimester of gestation in Thoroughbred mares with normal or compromised pregnancies. *Theriogenology* 63, 1844–1856.

Ousey, J.C., Kolling, M. and Allen, W.R. (2006) The effects of maternal dexamethasone treatment on gestation length and foal maturation in Thoroughbred mares. *Animal Reproduction Science* 94, 436–438.

Ousey, J.C., Fowden, A.L., Wilsher, S. and Allen, W.R. (2008) The effects of maternal health and body condition on the endocrine responses of neonatal foals. *Equine Veterinary Journal* 40, 673–679.

Ousey, J.C., Palmer, L., Cash, R.S.G., Grimes, K.J., Fletcher, A.P., Barrelet, A., Foote, A.K., Manning, F.M. and Ricketts, S.W. (2009) An investigation into the suitability of a commercial realtime PCR assay to screen for *Taylorella equigenitalis* in routine prebreeding equine genital swabs. *Equine Veterinary Journal* 41, 878–882.

Ousey, J.C., Kölling, M., Kindahl, H. and Allen, W.R. (2011) Maternal dexamethasone treatment in late gestation induces precocious fetal maturation and delivery in healthy Thoroughbred mares. *Equine Veterinary Journal* 43, 424–429.

Ousey, J.C., Kölling, M., Newton, R., Wright, M. and Allen, W.R. (2012) Uterine haemodynamics in young and aged pregnant mares measured using Doppler ultrasonography. *Equine Veterinary Journal* 44(s41), 15–21.

Overbeck, W., Witte, T.S. and Heuwieser, W. (2011) Comparison of three diagnostic methods to identify subclinical endometritis in mares. *Theriogenology* 75, 1311–1318.

Overstreet, J.W., Yanagimachi, R., Katz, D.F., Hayashi, K. and Hanson, F.W. (1980) Penetration of human spermatozoa into the human zona pellucida and the zona-free hamster egg: a study of fertile donors and infertile patients. *Fertility and Sterility* 33, 534–542.

Oxender, W.D., Noden, P.A. and Hafs, H.D. (1977) Estrus, ovulation and serum progesterone, estradiol and LH concentrations in mares after increased photoperiod during winter. *American Journal of Veterinary Research* 38, 203–207.

Ozgur, N., Bagcigil, A., Ikiz, S., Kilicarslan, M., Carioglu, B. (2003) Isolation of *Klebsiella pneumoniae* from mares with metritis and stallions, detection of biotypes and capsule types. *Turkish Journal of Veterinary and Animal Science* 27, 241–247.

Paccamonti, D.L. (2001) Milk electrolytes and induction of parturition. *Pferdeheilkunde* 17, 616–618.

Paccamonti, D.L. and De Vries, P.J. (2011) Reproductive Parameters from Miniature stallions. In: McKinnon, A.O., Squires, E.L., Vaala, E. and Varner, D.D. (eds) *Equine Reproduction*, 2nd edn. Wiley-Blackwell, Philadelphia, London, pp. 1377–1381.

Padilla, A.W. and Foote, R.H. (1991) Extender and centrifugation effects on the motility patterns of slow cooled spermatozoa. *Journal of Animal Science* 60, 3308–3313.

Padilla, A.W., Tobback, C. and Foote, R.H. (1991) Penetration of frozen-thawed, zona-free hamster oocytes by fresh and slow-cooled stallion spermatozoa. *Journal of Reproduction and Fertility, Supplement* 44, 207–212.

Padmanabhan, V., Battaglia, D., Brown, M.B., Karsch, F.J., Lee, J.S., Pan, W., Phillips, D.J. and Van Cleeff, J. (2002) Neuroendocrine control of follicle-stimulating hormone (FSH) secretion: II. Is follistatin-induced suppression of FSH secretion mediated via changes in activin availability and does it involve changes in gonadotropin-releasing hormone secretion? *Biology of Reproduction* 66(5), 1395–1402.

Pagan, J.D. and Hintz, H.F. (1986) Composition of milk from pony mares fed various levels of digestible energy. *Cornell Veterinarian* 76(2), 139–148.

Pagan, J.D. (2005) The role of nutrition in the management of Developmental Orthopaedic Disease. In: *Advances in Equine Nutrition III*. Nottingham University Press, Nottingham, UK, pp. 417–431.

Paget, S., Ducos, A., Mignotte, F., Raymond, I., Pinton, A., Seguela, A., Berland, H.M., Brun-Baronnat, C., Darre, A. and Darre, R. (2001)

XO/65, XY mosaicism in a case of equine male pseudohermaphroditism. *Veterinary Record* 148, 24–25.

Pagl, R., Aurich, J.E., Muller-Schlosser, F., Kankofer, M. and Aurich, C. (2006a) Comparison of an extender containing defined milk protein fractions with a skim milk-based extender for storage of equine semen at 5°C. *Theriogenology* 66, 1115–1122.

Pagl, R., Aurich, C. and Kanofer, M. (2006b) Anti-oxidative status and semen quality during cooled storage in stallions. *Journal of Medical Anatomy, Physiology, Pathology and Clinical Medicine* 53(9), 486–489.

Paidas, M.J., Krikun, G., Huang, S.J., Jones, R., Romano, M., Annunziato, J. and Barnea, E.R. (2010) A genomic and proteomic investigation of the impact of preimplantation factor on human decidual cells. *American Journal Obstetrics and Gynecology* 202(5), 459.

Palmer, E., Draincourt, M.A. and Ortavant, R. (1982) Photoperiodic stimulation of the mare during winter anoestrus. *Journal of Reproduction and Fertility* 32, 275–282.

Palmer, E., Domerg, D., Fauquenot, A. and de Sainte-Marie, T. (1984) Artificial insemination of mares: results of five years of research and practical experience. In: *Le Cheval. Reproduction, Selection, Alimentation, Exploitation.* Institut National de la Recherche Agronomique, Paris, pp. 133–147.

Palmer, E., Bezard, J., Magistrini, M. and Duchamp, G. (1991) In vitro fertilisation in the horse. *A retrospective study Journal of Reproduction and Fertility Supplement* 44, 375–384.

Panchal, M.T., Gujarati, M.L. and Kavani, F.S. (1995) Study of some of the reproductive traits of kathi mares in Gujarat state. *Indian Journal of Animal Reproduction* 16, 47–49.

Pantaleon, M., Scott, J. and Kaye, P.L. (2008) Nutrient sensing by the early mouse embryo: hexosamine biosynthesis and glucose signaling during preimplantation development. *Biology of Reproduction* 78, 595–600.

Pantke, P., Hyland, J., Galloway, D.B., Maclean, A.A. and Hoppen, H.O. (1991) Changes in luteinising hormone bioactivity associated with gonadotrophin pulses in the cycling mare. *Journal of Reproduction and Fertility, Supplement* 44, 13–20.

Pantke, P., Hyland, J.H., Galloway, D.B., Liu, D.Y. and Baker, H.W.G. (1992) Development of a zona pellucida sperm binding assay for the assessment of stallion fertility. *Australian Equine Veterinarian* 10(2), 91.

Pantke, P., Hyland, J.H., Galloway, D.B., Liu, D.Y. and Baker, H.W.G. (1995) Development of a zona pellucida sperm binding assay for the assessment of stallion fertility. *Biology of Reproduction Monograph Equine Reproduction VI* 1, 681–687.

Panzani, D., Zicchino, I., Taras, A., Marmorini, P., Crisci, A., Rota, A. and Camillo, F. (2011) Clinical use of dopamine antagonist sulpiride to advance first ovulation in transtional mares. *Theriogenology* 75, 138–143.

Papa, F.O., Alvarenga, M.A., Lopes, M.D. and Campos Filho, E.P. (1990) Infertility of autoimmune origins in a stallion. *Equine Veterinary Journal* 22, 145–146.

Papa, F.O., Melo, C.M., Monteiro, G.A., Papa, P.M., Guasti, P.N., Maziero, R.R.D., Derussi, A.A.P., Magalhães, L.C.O., Martin, J.C. and Martin, I. (2014) Equine Perineal and Vulvar Conformation Correction Using a Modification of Pouret's Technique. *Journal of Equine Vet Science* 34, 459–464.

Papaioannou, K.Z., Murphy, R.P., Monks, R.S., Hynes, N., Ryan, M.P., Boland, M.P. and Roche, J.F. (1997) Assessment of viability and mitochondrial function of equine spermatozoa using double staining and flow cytometry. *Theriogenology* 48, 299–312.

Parker, E., Tibary, A., and Vanderwall, D.K. (2005) Evaluation of a new early pregnancy test in mares. *Journal of Equine Veterinary Science* 25, 66–69.

Parker, W.G., Sullivan, J.J. and First, N.L. (1975) Sperm transport and distribution in the mare. *Journal of Reproduction and Fertility, Supplement* 23, 63–66.

Parkes, R.D. and Colles, C.M. (1977) Fetal electrocardiography in the mare as a practical aid to diagnosing singleton and twin pregnancies. *Veterinary Record* 100, 25–26.

Parks, J.E. and Lynch, D.V. (1992) Lipid composition and thermotropic phase behaviour of boar, bull, stallion and rooster sperm membrane. *Cryobiology* 29(2), 255–266.

Parlevliet, J.M. (2000) Pre-seasonal breeding evaluation of the stallion. *Pferdeheilkunde* 15(6), 523–528.

Parlevliet, J.M. and Colenbrander, B. (1999) Prediction of first season fertility in three year old Dutch Warmbloods with prebreeding assessment of morphologically live sperm. *Equine Veterinary Journal* 31(3), 248–251.

Parlevliet, J.M. and Samper, J.C. (2000) Disease transmission through semen. In: Samper, J.C. (ed.) *Equine Breeding Management and Artificial Insemination.* W.B. Saunders, Philadelphia, Pennsylvania, pp. 133–140.

Parlevliet, J.M., Kemp, B. and Colenbrander, B. (1994) Reproductive characteristics and semen quality in maiden Dutch Warmblood stallions. *Journal of Reproduction and Fertility* 101, 183–187.

Parlevliet, J.M., Bleumink-Pluym, N.M.C., Houwers, D.J., Remmen, J.L.A.M., Sluijter, F.J.H. and Colenbrander, B. (1997) Epidemiologic aspects of *Taylorella equigenitalis. Theriogenology* 47, 1169–1177.

Pascoe, J.R., Ellenburg, T.V., Culbertson, M.R. and Meagher, D.M. (1981) Torsion of the spermatic cord in a horse. *Journal of American Veterinary Medical Association* 178, 242–245.

Pascoe, R.R. (1979) Observations of the length of declination of the vulva and its relation to fertility in the mare. *Journal of Reproduction and Fertility, Supplement* 27, 299–305.

Pascoe, R.R. (1995) Effects of adding autologous plasma to an intrauterine antibiotic therapy after breeding on pregnancy rates in mares. *Biology of Reproduction Monograph* 1, 539–543.

Pashan, R.L. (1984) Maternal and foetal endocrinology during late pregnancy and parturition in the mare. *Equine Veterinary Journal* 16, 233–238.

Pashan, R.L. and Allen, R. (1979) The role of the fetal gonads and placenta in steroid production, maintenance of pregnancy and parturition. *Journal of Reproduction and Fertility, Supplement* 27, 499–509.

Pasolini, M.P., Del Prete, C., Fabbri, S. and Auletta, L. (2016) Endometritis and Infertility in the Mare – The Challenge in Equine Breeding Industry–A Review. In: Darwish, A.F. (ed) *Genital Infections and Infertility.* IntechOpen, DOI: 10.5772/62461. https://www.intechopen.com/books/genital-infections-and-infertility/endometritis-and-infertility-in-the-mare-the-challenge-in-equine-breeding-industry-a-review.

Pattle, R.E., Rossdale, P.D., Schock, C. and Creasey, J.M. (1975) The developments of the lung and its surfactant in the foal and other species. *Journal of Reproduction and Fertility, Supplement* 23, 651–657.

Peaker, M., Rossdale, P.D., Forsyth, I.A. and Falk, M. (1979) Changes in mammary development and composition of secretion during late pregnancy in the mare. *Journal of Reproduction and Fertility, Supplement* 27, 555–561.

Pearce, S.G., Firth, E.C., Grace, N.D. and Fennessy, P.F. (1998) Effect of copper supplementation on the evidence of developmental orthopaedic disease in pasture-fed New Zealand Thoroughbreds. *Equine Veterinary Journal* 30, 211–218.

Pearson, H. and Weaver, B.M. (1978) Priapism after sedation, neuroleptanalgesia and anaesthesia in the horse. *Equine Veterinary Journal* 10, 85–90.

Pearson, R.C., Hallowell, A.C., Bayley, W.M., Torbeck, R.L. and Perryman, L.E. (1984) Times of appearance and disappearance of colostral IgG in the mare. *American Journal of Veterinary Research* 45, 186–190.

Pelehach, L.M., Greaves, H.E., Porter, M.B. and Desvousges, A. (2002) The role of oestrogen and progesterone in the indiction of uterine oedema in mares. *Theriogenology* 58(2), 441–444.

Peregrine, A.S., Molento, M.B., Kaplan, R.M. and Nielsen, M.K. (2014) Anthelmintic resistance in important parasites of horses: does it really matter? *Veterinary Parasitology* 201, 1–8.

Perez, C.C., Rodriguez, I., Mota, J., Dorado, J., Hidalgo, M., Felipe, M. and Sanz, J. (2003) Gestation length in Cathusian Spanish mares. *Livestock Production Science* 82, 181–187.

Pérez-Marín, C.C., Vizuete, G., Vazquez-Martinez, R. and Galisteo, J.J. (2018) Comparison of different cryopreservation methods for horse and donkey embryos. *Equine Veterinary Journal* 50(3), 398–404.

Perkins, N.R. and Grimmett, J.B. (2001) Pregnancy and twinning rates in Thoroughbred mares following administration of human chorionic gonadotrophin (hCG). *New Zealand Veterinary Journal* 49, 94–100.

Perkins, N.R. and Threlfall, W.R. (1993) Mastitis in the mare. *Equine Veterinary Education* 5, 192–194.

Perry, E.J. (1968) *The Artificial Insemination of Farm Animals,* 4th edn. Rutgers University Press, New Brunswick, New Jersey.

Perry, J.D. and Freydiere, A.M. (2007) The application of chromogenic media in clinical microbiology.

Journal of Applied Microbiology 103(6), 2046–2055.

Pesch, S., Bostedt, H., Failing, K. and Bergmann, M. (2006) Advanced fertility diagnosis in stallion semen using transmission electron microscopy. *Animal Reproduction Science* 91, 285–298.

Pessoa, M., Cannizza, A., Reghini, M. and Alvarenga, M. (2011) Embryo efficiency of Quater horse athletic mares. *Journal Equine Vet Science* 31(12), 703–705.

Petersen, M.M., Wessel, M.T., Scott, M.A., Liu, I.K.M. and Ball, B.A. (2002) Embryo recovery rates in mares after deep intrauterine insemination with low numbers of cryopreserved spermatozoa. In: Evans, M.J. (ed.) *Equine Reproduction VIII. Theriogenology.* Vol. 58. Lea and Febiger, Philadelphia, Pennsylvania, pp. 663–666.

Petry, S., Breuil, M., Duquesne, F. and Laugier, C. (2018) Towards European harmonization of contagious equine metritis diagnosis through interlaboratory trials. *Veterinary Record* 183(3), 96–103.

Phetudomsinsuk, K. (2017) Investigation into the effect of prostaglandin F2a, GnRh analogie and hCG on induction of ovulation in mares. *Thaie Journal of Veterinary Medicine* 47(4), 493–499.

Philpott, M. (1993) The danger of disease transmission by artificial insemination and embryo transfer. *British Veterinary Journal* 149, 339–369.

Phillips, D.J. (2005) Activins, inhibins and follustatins in the large domestic species. *Domestic Animal Endocrinology* 28, 1–16.

Piao, S. and Wang, Y. (1988) A study on the technique of freezing concentrated semen of horses (donkeys) and the effect of insemination. In: *Proceedings of the International Congress for Animal Reproduction and Artificial Insemination* 3, 286a–286c.

Pickerel, T.M., Crowell-Davis, S.L., Cundle, A.B. and Estep, D.Q. (1993) Sexual preferences of mares (*Equus caballus*) for individual stallions. *Applied Animal Behaviour Science* 38, 1–13.

Pickett, B.W. (1993a) Factors affecting sperm production and output. In: McKinnon, A.O. and Voss, J.L. (eds) *Equine Reproduction.* Lea and Febiger, Philadelphia, Pennsylvania, London, pp. 689–704.

Pickett, B.W. (1993b) Collection and evaluation of stallion semen for artificial insemination. In: McKinnon, A.O. and Voss, J.L. (eds) *Equine Reproduction.* Lea and Febiger, Philadelphia, Pennsylvania, London, pp. 705–714.

Pickett, B.W. (1993c) Seminal extenders and cooled semen. In: McKinnon, A.O. and Voss, J.L. (eds) *Equine Reproduction.* Lea and Febiger, Philadelphia, Pennsylvania, London, pp. 746–754.

Pickett, B.W. (1993d) Reproductive evaluation of the stallion. In: McKinnon, A.O. and Voss, J.L. (eds) *Equine Reproduction.* Lea and Febiger, Philadelphia, Pennsylvania, London, pp. 755–768.

Pickett, B.W. and Amann, R.P. (1993) Cryopreservation of semen. In: McKinnon, A.O. and Voss, J.L. (eds) *Equine Reproduction.* Lea and Febiger, Philadelphia, Pennsylvania, London, pp. 769–789.

Pickett, B.W. and Shiner, K.A. (1994) Recent developments in AI in horse. *Livestock Production Science* 40, 31–36.

Pickett, B.W. and Voss, J.L. (1972) Reproductive management of stallions. In: Milne, F.J. (ed.) *Proceedings of the 18th Annual Convention of the American Association of Equine Practitioners, San Francisco, California.* American Association of Equine Practitioners, 18, 501–531.

Pickett, B.W. and Voss, J.C. (1998a) Management of shuttle stallions for maximum reproductive efficiency – Part 1. *Journal of Equine Veterinary Science* 18, 212–227.

Pickett, B.W. and Voss, J.L. (1998b) Management of shuttle stallions for maximum reproductive efficiency – Part 2. *Journal of Equine Veterinary Science* 18, 280–287.

Pickett, B.W., Faulkner, L.C. and Voss, J.L. (1975) Effect of season on some characteristics of stallion semen. *Journal of Reproduction and Fertility, Supplement* 23, 25.

Pickett, B.W., Voss, J.L., Squires, E.L. and Amann, R.P. (1981) Management of the stallion for maximum reproductive efficiency. *Animal Reproduction Laboratory General Series Bulletin No. 1005*, Colorado State University, Fort Collins, Colorado.

Pickett, B.W., Amann, R.P., McKinnon, A.O., Squires, E.L. and Voss, J.L. (1989) Management of the stallion for maximum reproductive efficiency II. *Bulletin of the Colorado State University Agriculture Experimental Station Animal Reproduction Laboratory General Series Bulletin No. 05.* Colorado State University, Fort Collins, Colorado, pp. 121–125.

Pickett, B.W., Voss, J.L. and Jones, R.L. (1999) Control of bacteria in stallions and their semen. *Journal of Equine Veterinary Science* 19(7), 424–469.

Pickett, B.W., Voss, J.L., Squires, E.L., Vanderwall, D.K., McCue, P.M. and Bruemmer, J.E. (2000) Collection, preparation and insemination of stallion semen. *Bulletin No 10 Animal Reproduction and Biotechnology Laboratory*. Colorado State University, Fort Collins, Colorado, pp. 1–15.

Pieppo, J., Huntinen, M. and Kotilainen, T. (1995) Sex diagnosis of equine preimplantation embryos using the polymerase chain reaction. *Theriogenology* 44(5), 619–627.

Pierce, S.W. (2003) Foal care from birth to 30 days : a practioners perspective. In: *Proceedings of the 49th Annual Convention of the American Association of Equine Practioners*, New Orleans, Louisiana, Lexington, Kentucky, pp. 13–21.

Pierson, R.A. (1993) Folliculogenesis and ovulation. In: McKinnon, A.O. and Voss, J.L. (eds) *Equine Reproduction*. Lea and Febiger, Philadelphia, Pennsylvania, pp. 161–171.

Pietrani, M., Losinno, L. and Arango, J.C. (2019) Effect of the Interval from Prostaglandin F2alpha treatment to ovulation on reproductive efficiency rates in a commercial equine embryo transfer program. *Journal of Equine Veterinary Science* 78, 123–126.

Pillet, E., Duchamp, G., Batellier, F., Beaumal, V., Anton, M., Desherces, S., Schmitt, E. and Magistrini, M. (2011) Egg yolk plasma can replace egg yolk in stallion freezing extenders. *Theriogenology* 75(1), 105–114.

Pillet, E., Labbe, C., Batellier, F., Duchamp, G., Beaumal, V., Anton, M., Desherces, S., Schmitt, E. and Magistrini, M. (2012) Liposomes as an alternative to egg yolk in stallion freezing extender. *Theriogenology* 77(2), 268–279.

Pinto, C.R.F. (2011) Proestagens and Progsterone. In: McKinnon, A.O., Squires, E.L, Vaala, W.E. and Varner, D.D. (eds) *Equine Reproduction* 2nd edn. Wiley-Blackwell, Philadelphia, London, pp. 1811–1819.

Pinto, M.R., Miragaya, M.H., Burns, P., Douglas, R. and Neild, D.M. (2017) Strategies for increasing reproductive efficiency in commercial embryo transfer program with high performance mares under training. *Journal of Equine Veterinary Science* 54, 93–97.

Piquette, G.N., Kenney, R.M., Sertich, P.L., Yamoto, M. and Hsueh, A.J.W. (1990) Equine granulosa theca cell tumours express inhibin α and βA subunit messenger ribonucleic acids and proteins. *Biology of Reproduction* 43, 1050–1057.

Pitra, C., Schafer, W. and Jewgenow, K. (1985) Quantitative measurement of the fertilising capacity of deep-frozen stallion semen by means of the hamster egg penetration test. *Monatschefte fur Veterinarmedizin* 40(7), 235–237.

Plata-Madrid, H., Youngquist, R.S., Murphy, C.N., Bennett-Wimbrush, K., Braun, W.F. and Loch, W.E. (1994) Ultrasonographic characteristics of the follicular and uterine dynamics in Belgium mares. *Journal of Equine Veterinary Science* 14, 421–423.

Plewinska-Wierzobska, D. and Bielanski, W. (1970) The methods of evaluation the speed and sort of movement of spermatozoa. *Medycyna Weterynaryjna* 26, 237–250.

Polge, C., Smith, A.U. and Parkes, A.S. (1949) Revival of spermatozoa after vitrification and dehydration at low temperature. *Nature* 164, 666.

Pollark, P. (2017) Approach to the cryptorchid horse. *In Practice* 39(6), 284–290.

Pollock, P.J. and Russell, T.M. (2011) Inguinal hernias. In: McKinnon, A.O., Squires, E.L., Vaala, E. and Varner, D.D. (eds) *Equine Reproduction*, 2nd edn. Wiley-Blackwell, Philadelphia, London, pp. 1540–1545.

Pommer, A.C., Linfor, J.J. and Meyers, S.A. (2002) Capacitation and acrosomal exocytosis are enhanced by incubation of stallion spermatozoa in a commercial semen extender. *Theriogenology* 57(5), 1493–1501.

Ponthier, L., van de Weerdt, M. and Deleuze, S. (2008) Pregnancy diagnosis in the mare by semiquantitative relaxin quick assay kit. *Reproduction in Domestic Animals* 43, 11.

Pook, J.F., Power, M.L., Sangster, N.C., Hodgson, J.L. and Hodgson, D.R. (2002) Evaluation of tests for anthelmintic resistance in cyaathostomes. *Veterinary Parasitology* 106, 331–343.

Pool, K.C., Charneco, R. and Arns, M.J. (1993) The influence of seminal plasma from fractionated ejaculation on the cold storage of equine spermatozoa. In: *Proceedings of the 13th Conference of the Equine Nutrition and Physiology Symposium,*

Gainesville, Florida. Equine and Physiology Society, pp. 395–396.

Popescu, S. and Diugan, E.A. (2017) The relationship between the welfare quality and stress index in working and breeding horses. *Research in Veterinary Science* 115, 442–450.

Popescu, S., Lazar, E.A., Borda, C., Niculae, M., Sandru, C.D. and Spinu, M. (2019) Welfare quality of breeding horses under different housing conditions. *Animals* 9(3), 81.

Pouret, E.J.M. (1982) Surgical techniques for the correction of pneumo and uro vagina. *Equine Veterinary Journal* 14, 249–250.

Power, S.G.A. and Challis, R.G. (1987) Steroid production by dispersed cells from fetal membranes and intrauterine tissue of sheep. *Journal of Reproduction and Fertility* 81(1), 65–76.

Pozor, M. (2017) Understanding how your ultrasound machine works. *Proceedings of the 63rd Annual Convention of the American Association of Equine Practitioners*, San Antonio, Texas, pp. 335–339.

Pozor, M. and McDonnell, S. (2002) Ultrasonographic measurement of accessory sex glands, ampullae and urethra of normal stallions of various size and type. *Theriogenology* 58, 1425–1430.

Pozor, M. and McDonnell, S. (2004) Colour Doppler ultrasound evaluation of testicular blood flow in stallions. *Theriogenology* 61, 799–810.

Pozor, M.A., McDonnell, S.M., Kenney, R.M. and Tischner, M. (1991) GnRH facilitates the copulatory behaviour in geldings treated with testosterone. *Journal of Reproduction and Fertility, Supplement* 44, 666–667.

Pozor, M., Morrissey, H., Albanese, V., Khouzam, N., Deriberprey, A., Macpherson, M.L. and Kelleman, A.A. (2017) Relationship between echotextural and histomorphometric characteristics of stallion testes. *Theriogenology* 99, 134–145.

Pozor, M., Conley, A.J., Roser, J.F., Nolin, M., Zambrano, G.L., Runyon, S.P., Kelleman, A.A. and Macpherson, M.L. (2018) Anti-Müllerian hormone as a biomarker for acutetesticular degeneration caused by toxic insults to stallion testes. *Theriogenology* 116, 95–102.

Price, S., Aurich, J., Davies Morel, M. and Aurich, C. (2007) Effects of oxygen exposure and gentamicin on stallion semen stored at 5°C and 15°C. *Reproduction in Domestic Animals* 43(3), 261–266.

Price, S.B.P. (2008) Effects of storage conditions on cooled-stored stallion semen. MSc thesis, University of Wales, Aberystwyth, UK.

Pricking, S., Spilker, K., Martinsson, G., Rau, J., Tönissen, A., Bollwein, H. and Sieme, H. (2019) Equine fetal gender determination in mid- and advanced-gestation by trans abdominal approach – comparative study using 2D B-Mode ultrasound, Doppler sonogrophy, 3D B-Mode and following tomographic ultrasound imaging. *Pferdeheilkunde* 35(1), 11–19.

Proudman, C.J. and Matthews, J.B. (2000) Control of Intestinal Parasites in Horses. *In Practice* 22, 90–97.

Proudman, C.J. and Trees, A. (1996) Correlation of antigen specific IgG and IgG(T) responses with *Anoplocephala perfoilata* infection intensity in the horse. *Parasite Immunology* 18, 499–506.

Province, C.A., Amann, R.P., Pickett, B.W. and Squires, E.L. (1984) Extenders for preservation of canine and equine spermatozoa at 5°C. *Theriogenology* 22, 409–415.

Province, C.A., Squires, E.L., Pickett, B.W. and Amann, R.P. (1985) Cooling rates, storage temperature and fertility of extended equine spermatozoa. *Theriogenology* 23, 925–934.

Pruitt, J.A., Arns, M.J. and Pool, K.C. (1993) Seminal plasma influences recovery of equine spermatozoa following *in vitro* culture (37°C) and cold storage (5°C). *Theriogenology* 39, 291.

Pugh, D.G. (1985) Equine ovarian tumours. *Compendium of Continuing Education, Practice Veterinarian* 7, 710–715.

Pugh, D.G. and Schumacher, J. (1990) Management of the broodmare. In: Royer, M.G. (ed.) *Proceedings of the 36th Annual Convention of the American Association of Equine Practitioners, Lexington, Kentucky* pp. 61–78.

Pugliesi, G., Fürst, R. and Carvalho, G.R., 2014. Impact of using a fast-freezing technique and different thawing protocols on viability and fertility of frozen equine spermatozoa. *Andrologia* 46(9), 1055–1062.

Purohit, G.N. (2011) Intra-partum conditions and their management in the mare *Journal of Livestock Science* 2, 20–37

Pycock, J.F. (2000) Breeding management of the problem mare. In: Samper, J.C. (ed.) *Equine*

Breeding Management and Artificial Insemination. W.B. Saunders, Philadelphia, Pennsylvania, pp. 195–228.

Pycock, J.F. (2011) Ultrasonography. In: McKinnon, A.O., Squires, E.L., Vaala, E. and Varner, D.D. (eds) *Equine Reproduction*, 2nd edn. Wiley-Blackwell, Philadelphia, London, pp. 1914–1921.

Pycock, J.F. and Newcombe, J.R. (1996) Assessment of the effects of three treatments to remove intrauterine fluid on pregnancy rates in the mare. *Veterinary Record* 138(14), 320–323.

Pycock, J.F., Dieleman, S., Drifhout, P., van der Brug, Y., Oei, C. and Van Der Weijden, G.C. (1995) Correlations of plasma concentrations of progesterone and oestradiol with ultrasound characteristics of the uterus and duration of oestrus behaviour in the mare. *Reproduction in Domestic Animals* 30, 224–227.

Pyn, O. (2014) Managing mare dystocia in the field. *In Practice* 36(7), 347–354.

Quinn, G.C. and Woodford, N.S. (2005) Infertility due to a uterine leiomyoma in a Thoroughbred mare: clinical findings, treatment and outcome. *Equine Veterinary Education* 17(3), 150–152.

Quinn, B.A., Hayes, M.A., Waelchli, R.O., Kennedy, M.W. and Betteridge, K.J. (2007) Changes in major proteins in the embryonic capsule during immobilisation (fixation) of the conceptus in the third week of pregnancy in the mare. *Reproduction* 134, 161–170.

Raeside, J.I., Liptrap, R.M., McDonnell, W.N. and Milne, E.J. (1979) A precursor role for dihydroepiandrosterone DHA in feto-placental unit for oestrogen formation in the mare. *Journal of Reproduction and Fertility, Supplement* 27, 493–497.

Raeside, J.L., Gofton, N., Liptrap, R.M. and Milne, F.J. (1982) Isoloation and identification of steroids from gonadal vein blood of the fetal horse *Journal of Reproduction and Fertility, Supplement* 32, 383–387.

Raeside, J.I., Ryan, P.L. and Lucas, Z. (1991) A method for the measurement of oestrone sulphate in faeces in feral mares. *Journal of Reproduction and Fertility, Supplement* 44, 638.

Rahaley, R.S., Gordon, B.J., Leipold, H.W. and Peter, J.E. (1983) Sertoli cell tumour in a horse. *Equine Veterinary Journal* 15(1), 68–70.

Ralston, S.L. (1997) Feeding the rapidly growing foal. *Journal of Equine Veterinary Science* 17(12), 634–636.

Ralston, S.L., Rich, G.A., Jackson, S. and Squires, E.L. (1986) The effect of vitamin A supplementation on sexual characteristics and vitamin A absorption in stallions. *Journal of Equine Veterinary Science* 6(4), 203–207.

Rambags, B.P. and Stout, T.A. (2005) Transcervical endoscope-guided emptying of a transmural cyst in a mare. *Veterinary Record* 156, 679–682.

Rambags, B.P., Stout, T.A. and Rijkenhuizen, A.B. (2003) Ovarian granulosa cell tumours adherent to other abdominal organs; surgical removal from 2 warmblood mares. *Equine Veterinary Journal* 35(6), 627–632.

Rambags, B.P., Krijtenburg, P.J., Drie, H.F., Lazzari, G., Galli, C., Pearson, P.L., Colebrander, B. and Stout, T.A. (2005) Numerical chromosomal abnormalities in equine embryos produced in vivo and in vitro. *Molecular Reproduction and Development* 72, 77–87.

Rambags, B.P.B., van Boxtel, D.C.J., Tharasnit, T., Lenstra, J.A., Colenbrander, B. and Stout, T.A.E. (2006) Maturation in vitro leads to mitochondrial degeneration in oocytes recovered from aged but not young mares. *Animal Reproduction Science* 94, 359–361.

Rantanen, N.W. and Kinkaid, B. (1989) Ultrasound guided fetal cardiac puncture: a method of twin reduction. In: *Proceedings of the American Association of Equine Practitioners* 34, 173–179.

Rasmussen, C.D., Haugaard, M.M., Petersen, M.R., Nielsen, J.M., Pedersen, H.G. and Bejesen, A.M. (2013) *Streptococcus equi* subsp. *zooepidemicus* isolates from equine infectious endometritis belong to a distinct genetic group. *Veterinary Research* 44(2013), 26.

Rathi, R., Colenbrander, B., Bevers, M.M. and Gadella, B.M. (2001) Evaluation of in vitro capacitation of stallion spermatozoa. *Biology of Reproduction* 65(2), 426–430.

Raub, R.H., Jackson, S.G. and Baker, J.P. (1989) The effect of exercise on bone growth and development in weanling horses. *Journal of Animal Science* 67, 2508–2514.

Rauterberg, H. (1994) Use of glasswool sephadex filtration for the collection of fresh semen from horses. Laboratory studies and field trials. PhD thesis, Tierarztliche Hochschule, Hannover, Germany.

Raz, T., Carley, S. and Card, C. (2009) Comparison of the effects of eFSH and deslorelin treatment regimes on ovarian stimulation and embryo production of donor mares in early vernal transition. *Theriogenology* 71, 1358–1366.

Raz, T., Carley, S.D., Green, J.M. and Card, C.E. (2011) Evaluation of two oestrus synchranization regimens in eFSH-treated donor mares. *Veterinary Journal* 188(1), 105–109.

Rebordao, M.R., Galvao, A., Pinto-Bravo, P., Pinheiro, J., Gamboa, S., Silva, E., Mateus, L. and Ferreira-Dias, G. (2017) Endometrial prostaglandin synthases, ovarian steroids, and oxytocin receptors in mares with oxytocin-induced luteal maintenance. *Theriogenology* 87, 193–204.

Reef, V.B. (1993) Diagnostic ultrasonography of the foal's abdomen. In: McKinnon, A.O. and Voss, J.L. (eds) *Equine Reproduction.* Lea and Febiger, Philadelphia, Pennsylvania, pp. 1088–1094.

Reef, V.B. (1998) Fetal ultrasonography. In: Reef, V.B. (ed.) *Equine Diagnostic Ultrasound.* W.B. Saunders, Philadelphia, Pennsylvania, pp. 425–445.

Reef, V., Vaala, W. and Worth, L. (1995) Ultrasonographic evaluation of the fetus and intrauterine environment in healthy mares during gestation. *Veterinarian Radio Ultrasound* 1995, 256–258.

Reghini, M.F.S., Ramires Neto, C., Segabinazzi, L.G., Chaves, M.M.B.C., Dell'Aqua, C. de P.F., Bussiere, M.C.C., Dell'Aqua, J.A. Jr., Papa, F.O. and Alvarenga, M.A. (2016) Inflammatory response in chronic degenerative endometritis mares treated with platelet rich plasma. *Theriogenology* 86(2), 516–522.

Reichart, M., Lederman, H., Hareven, D., Keden, P. and Bartoov, B. (1993) Human sperm acrosin activity with relation to semen parameters and acrosomal ultrastructure. *Andrologia* 25(2), 59–66.

Reichmann, P., Moure, A. and Gamba, C.G. (2004) Bone mineral content of the third metacarpal bone in quarter horse foals from birth to one year of age. *Journal of Equine Veterinary Science* 24(9), 391–396.

Reifenrath, H. (1994) Use of L4 leucocyte absorption membrane filtration in AI in horses, using fresh or frozen semen. PhD thesis, Tierarztliche Hochschule Hannover, German Federal Republic.

Reilas, T. and Katila, T. (2002) Proteins and enzymes in uterine lavage fluid of post partum and non parturient mares. *Reproduction in Domestic Animals* 37, 261–268.

Reinfenrath, H., Jensen, A., Sieme, H. and Klug, E. (1997) Ureteroscopic catheterisation of the vesicular glands in the stallion. *Reproduction in Domestic Animals* 32, 47–49.

Reis, A.P. (2015) Acceptability of Biotechnologes in the Horse Industry in Europe. *Proceedings of the IETS Equine Reproduction Symposium.* Paris. pp. 34–35.

Reppert, S.M. and Weaver, D.R. (2002) Coordination of circadian timing in mammals. *Nature* 418, 935–941.

Resende, H.L., Carmo, M.T., Ramires Neto, C. and Alvarenga, M.A. (2014) Determination of equine fetal sex by Doppler ultrasonography of the gonads. *Equine Veterinary Journal* 46(6), 756–758.

Revell, S.G. (1997) A sport horse for the future. In: *Proceedings of the British Society for Animal Science Equine Conference, Cambridge.* British Society for Animal Science, Nottingham University Press, Nottingham, UK.

Revell, S.G. and Mrode, R.A. (1994) An osmotic resistance test for bovine semen. *Animal Reproduction Science* 36, 77–86.

Rezac, P., Pospisilova, D., Slama, P. and Havlicek, Z. (2013) Different effects of month of conception and birth on gestation lengths in mares. *Journal of Animal and Veterinary Advances* 12, 731–735.

Rezende, M.L., Ferris, R.A., Leise, B.S., Mama, K.R., Scofield, D.A. and McCue, P.M. (2014) Treatment of intraoperative persistent penile erection in a stallion. *Journal of Equine Veterinary Science* 34(3), 431–435.

Ribeiro, B.I., Love, L.B., Choi, L.H. and Hinrichs, K. (2008) Transport of equine ovaies for assisted reproduction. *Animal Reproduction Science* 108, 171–179.

Ricker, J.V., Linfor, J.J., Delfino, W.J., Kysar, P., Scholtz, E.L., Tablin, F., Crowe, J.H., Ball, B.A. and Meyers, S.A. (2006) Equine sperm membrane phase behaviour: the effects of lipid-based cryoprotectants. *Biology of Reproduction* 74(2), 359–365.

Ricketts, S.W. (1978) Histological and histopathological studies of the endometrium of the mare. Fellowship thesis, Royal College of Veterinary Surgeons, London.

Ricketts, S.W. (1993) Evaluation of stallion semen. *Equine Veterinary Education* 5(5), 232–237.

Ricketts, S.W. (2011) Uterine and clitoral cultures. In: McKinnon, A.O., Squires, E.L., Vaala, E. and

Varner, D.D. (eds) *Equine Reproduction*, 2nd edn. Wiley-Blackwell, Philadelphia, London, pp. 1963–1978.

Ricketts, S.W. and Alonso, S. (1991) The effect of age and parity on the development of equine chorionic endometrial disease. *Equine Veterinary Journal* 23, 189–192.

Ricketts, S.W. and Barrelet, A. (1997) A retrospective review of the histopathological features seen in a series of 4241 endometrial biopsy samples collected from UK Thoroughbred mares over a 25 year period. *Pferdeheilkunde* 13(5), 525–530.

Ricketts, S.W. and Mackintosh, M.E. (1987) Role of anaerobic bacteria in equine endometritis. *Journal of Reproduction and Fertility, Supplement* 35, 343–351.

Ricketts, S.W., Young, A. and Medici, E.B. (1993) Uterine and clitoral cultures. In: McKinnon, A.O. and Voss, J.L. (eds) *Equine Reproduction*. Lea and Febiger, Philadelphia, Pennsylvania, London, pp. 234–245.

Ricketts, S.W., Barrelet, A. and Whitwell, K.E. (2003) Equine abortion. *Equine Veterinary Education* 6, 18–21.

Riddle, W.T. (2003) Preparation of the mare for normal parturition. *49th Annual Convention of the American Association of Equine Practitioners*, New Orleans. Louisiana, pp. 601–1103.

Riddle, W., LeBlanc, M. and Stromberg, A. (2007) Relationships between uterine culture, cytology and pregnancy rates in Thoroughbred practice. *Theriogenology* 68, 395–402.

Ridman, R. and Keiper, R.R. (1991) Body Condition of feral ponies on Assateague Island. *Equine Veterinary Journal* 23(6), 435–456.

Riera, F.L., Roldan, J.E., Gomez, J. and Hinrichs, K. (2016) Factors affecting the efficiency of foal production in a commercial oocyte tranfer program. *Theriogenology* 85, 1053–1062.

Rigby, S., Love, C., Carpenter, K., Varner, D. and Blanchard, T. (1998) Use of prostaglandin E2 to ripen the cervix of the mare prior to parturition. *Theriogenology* 50, 897–904.

Rigby, S., Derczo, S., Brinsko, S., Blanchard, T.L., Taylor, T., Forrest, D. and Varner, D. (2000) Oviductal sperm numbers following proximal uterine horn or uterine body insemination. *Proceedings, 46th Annual American Association of Equine Practitioners Convention, San Antonio, Texas, 26–29 November*. American Association of American Practitioners, pp. 332–334.

Rigby, S.L., Barhoumi, R., Burghardt, R.C., Colleran, P., Thompson, J.A., Varner, D.D., Blanchard, T.L., Brinsko, S.P., Taylor, T., Wilkerson, M.K. and Delp, M.D. (2001a) Mares with delayed uterine clearance have an intrinsic defect in myometrial function. *Biology of Reproduction* 65(3), 740–747.

Rigby, S.L., Brinsko, S.P., Cochran, M., Blanchard, T.L., Love, C.C. and Varner, D.D. (2001b) Advances in cooled semen technologies: seminal plasma and semen extender. *Animal Reproduction Science* 68(3–4), 171–180.

Riggs, L.M. (2006) How to perform non surgical correction of acute uterine torsion. *Proceedings of the American Association of Equine Practionners* 52, 256–258.

Rispoli, L.A. and Nett, T.M. (2005) Pituitary gonadotrophin releasing hormone (GnRH) receptor: structure, distribution and regulation of expression. *Animal Reproduction Science* 88, 57–74.

Risvanli, A. (2011) Reproductive Immunology in Mares. *Asian Journal of Animal and Veterinary Advances* 6, 547–554.

Rivera, R.M., and Ross, J.W. (2013) Epigenetics in fertilization and preimplantation embryo development. *Progress in Biophysics and Molecular Biology* 113, 423–432.

Rivera Del Alamo, M.M., Reilas, T., Kindahl, H. and Katila T. (2008) Mechanisms behind intrauteine device-induced luteal persistence in mares. *Animal Reproduction Science* 7(12), 94–106.

Rizzo, M., Ducheyne, K.D., Deelen, C., Beitsma, M., Cristarella, S., Quartuccio, M., Stout, T.A.E. and Ruijter-Villani, M. de (2019) Advanced mare age impairs the ability of invitro-matured oocytes to correctly align chromosomes on the metaphase plate. *Equine Veerinary Journal* 51(2), 252–257.

Roberts, K., Hemmings, A.J., McBride, S.D. and Parker, M.O. (2017) Causal factors of oral verses locomoter stereotypy in horses. *Journal of Veterinary Behaviour* 20, 37–43.

Roberts, S.J. (1986) Infertility in male animals (andrology). In: Roberts, S.J. (ed.) *Veterinary Obstetrics and Genital Diseases (Theriogenology)*, 3rd edn. Edwards Brothers, North Pomfret, Vermont, pp. 752–893.

Roberts, S.M. (1993) Ocular disorders. In: McKinnon, A.O. and Voss, J.L. (eds) *Equine Reproduction*. Lea and Febiger, Philadelphia, Pennsylvania, pp. 1076–1087.

Robinson, G., Porter, M.B., Peltier, M.R., Cleaver, B.C., Farmerie, T.A., Wolfe, M.W., Nilson, J.H. and Sharp, D.C. (1995) Regulation of luteinising hormone β and α messenger ribonucleic acid by estradiol or gonadotrophin-releasing hormone following pituitary stalk section in ovarectomised pony mares. *Biology of Reproduction Monographs* 1, 373–383.

Robinson, J.A., Allen, G.K., Green, E.M., Fales, W.H., Loch, W.E. and Wilkerson, G. (1993) A prospective study of septicaemia in colostrums deprived foals. *Equine Veterinary Journal* 25(3), 214–219.

Robinson, S.J., Neal, H. and Allen, W.R. (2000) Modulation of oviductal transport in mares by local application of prostaglandin E2. *Journal of Reproduction and Fertility, Supplement* 56, 587–92.

Robles, M., Peugnet, P.M., Valentino, S.A., Dubois, C., Dahirel, M., Aubrière, C., Reigner, F., Serteyn, D., Wimel, L., Tarrade, A. and Chavatte-Palmer, P. (2018) Placental structure and function in different breeds in horses. *Theriogenology* 108, 136–145.

Rochat, M.C. (2001) Priapism: a review. *Theriogenology* 56, 713–722.

Rode, K., Sieme, H., Richterich, P., and Brehm, R. (2015) Characterization of the equine blood-testis barrier during tubular development in normal and cryptorchid stallions. *Theriogenology* 84, 763–72.

Rode, K., Sieme, H., Otzen, H., Schwennen, C., Lüpkee, M., Richterich, P., Schrimpf, R., Distl, O. and Brehm, R. (2016). Effects of repeated testicular biopsies in adult warmblood stallions and their diagnostic potential. *Journal of Equine Veterinary Science* 38, 33–47.

Rodgerson, D.H. (2011) Prepubic and abdominal wall. In: McKinnon, A.O., Squires, E.L., Vaala, E. and Varner, D.D. (eds) *Equine Reproduction*, 2nd edn. Wiley-Blackwell, Philadelphia, London, pp. 2428–2431.

Rogers, C.W., Gee, E.K. and Faram, T.L. (2004) The effect of two different weaning procedures on the growth of pasture reared Thoroughbred foals in New Zealand. *New Zealand Veterinary Journal* 52(6), 401–403.

Rogers, C.W., Firth, E.C., McIlwraith, C.W., Barneveld, A., Goodship, A.E., Smith, R.K.W. and Van Weeren, P.R. (2008) Evaluation of a new straegy to modulate skeletal development in Thoroughbred performance horses by imposing track-based exercise during growth. *Equine Vet Journal* 40, 111–118.

Rohrbach, B., Sheerin, P., Steiner, J., Mathews, P., Cantell, C. and Dodds, L. (2006) Use of *Propionibacterium acnes* as adjunct therapy in treatment of persistent endometritis in the broodmare. *Animal Reproduction Science* 94, 259–60.

Roizen, J., Luedke, C.E., Herzog, E.D. and Muglia, L.J. (2007) Oxytocin in the circadian timing of birth. *PLos One* 2, e922. Doi: 10,1371/journal.pone.0000922.

Rollins, W.C. and Howell, C.E. (1951) Genetic sources of variation in gestation length of the horse. *Journal of Animal Science* 10, 797–805.

Rook, J.S., Braselton, W.E., Nachreiner, R.F., Lloyd, J.W., Shea, M.E., Shelle, J.E. and Hitzler, P.R. (1997) Multi-element assay of mammary gland secretions and sera from periparturient mares by inductively coupled argon plasms emission spectroscopy. *American Journal of Veterinary Research* 58, 376–378.

Rophia, R.T., Mathews, R.G., Butterfield, R.M., Moss, G.E. and McFalden, W.J. (1969) The duration of pregnancy in Thoroughbred mares. *Veterinary Record* 84, 552–555.

Rose, B.V., Firth, M., Morris, B., Roach, J.M., Verheyn, K.L.P. and de Mestre, A.M. (2018) Descriptive study of current therapeutic practices, clinical reproductive findings and incidence of pregnancy loss in intensively managed thoroughbred mares. *Animal Reproduction Science*, 188, 74–84.

Rose, R.J. (1988) Cardiorespiratory adaptations in neonatal foals. *Equine Veterinary Journal*, Supplement 5, 11–13.

Roser, A.J. (1995) Endocrine profiles in fertile, subfertile and infertile stallions. Testicular response to human chorionic gonadotrophin in infertile stallions. *Biology of Reproduction, Monograph, Equine Reproduction. VI* 1, 661–669.

Roser, J.F. (1997) Endocrine basis for testicular function in the stallion. *Theriogenology* 48(5), 883–892.

Roser, J.F. (2001a) Endocrine and paracrine control of sperm production in stallion. *Animal Reproduction Science* 68, 139–151.

Roser, J.F. (2001b) Endocrine diagnostics for stallion infertility. In: Ball, B.A. (ed.) *Recent Advances in Equine Reproduction* International Veterinary Information Service (IVIS), Ithaca, New York.

Roser, J.F. (2008) Regulation of testicular function in the stallion: an intricate network of endocrine, paracrine and autocrine systems. *Animal Reproduction Science* 107, 179–196.

Roser, J.F. (2011) Endocrin-Paracrine–Autocrine regulation of reproductive function in the stallion. In: McKinnon, A.O., Squires, E.L., Vaala, E. and Varner, D.D. (eds) *Equine Reproduction*, 2nd edn. Wiley-Blackwell, Philadelphia, London, pp. 996–1014.

Roser, J.F. and Hughes, J.P. (1991) Prolonged pulsatile administration of gonadotrophin releasing hormone (GnRH) to fertile stallions. *Journal of Reproduction and Fertility, Supplement* 44, 155–168.

Roser, J.F. and Hughes, J.P. (1992a) Seasonal effects on seminal quality, plasma hormone concentrations, and GnRH-induced LH response in fertile and subfertile stallions *Journal of Andrology* 13, 214–223.

Roser, J.F. and Hughes, J.P. (1992b) Dose-response effects of gonadotropin-releasing hormone on plasma concentrations of gonadotropins and testosterone in fertile and subfertile stallions. *Journal of Andrology* 13, 543–550.

Roser, J.F. and Lofstedt, R.M. (1989) Urinary eCG patterns in the mare during pregnancy. *Theriogenology* 32(4), 607–622.

Roser, J.F. and Meyers-Brown, G. (2012) Superovulation in mares: a work in progress. *Journal of Equine Veterinary Science* 32, 376–386.

Roser, J.F., McCue, P. and Hoye, E. (1994) Inhibin activity in the mare. *Domestic Animal Endocrinology* 11, 87–100.

Ross, J., Palmer, J.E. and Wilkins, P.A. (2008). Body wall tears during delayed pregnancy in mare: 13 cases (1995–2006). *Journal of the American Veterinary Medicine Association* 232, 257–261.

Rossdale, P.D. (1967) Clinical studies on the newborn thoroughbred foal. 1. Perinatal behaviour. *British Veterinary Journal* 123, 470–481.

Rossdale, P.D. (2004) The maladjusted foal: influence of intrauterine growth retardation and birth trauma. *Proceedings of the 50th Annual Convention of the American Association of Equine Practitioners, Denver, Colorado. 4–8 December 2004*. American Association of Equine Practitioners, pp. 75–126.

Rossdale, P.D. and Ousey, J.C. (2002) Fetal programming for athletic performance in the horse: potential effects of IUGR. *Equine Veterinary Education* 14, 98–112.

Rossdale, P.D. and Ricketts, S.W. (1980) *Equine Stud Farm Medicine*, 2nd edn. Balliere Tindall, London.

Rossdale, P.D. and Short, R.V. (1967) The time of foaling of Thoroughbred mares. *Journal of Reproduction and Fertility, Supplement* 13, 341–343.

Rossdale, P.D., Silver, M., Comline, R.S., Hall, L.W. and Nathanielsz, P.W. (1973) Plasma cortisol in the foal during the late foetal and early neonatal period. *Research in Veterinary Science* 15(3), 395–397.

Rossdale, P.D., Pashan, R.L. and Jeffcote, L.B. (1979) The use of prostaglandin analogue (fluprostenol) to induce foaling. *Journal of Reproduction and Fertility, Supplement* 27, 521–529.

Rossdale, P.D., Ousey, J.C., Silver, M. and Fowden, A.L. (1984) Studies on equine prematurity, guidelines for assessment of foal maturity. *Equine Veterinary Journal* 16, 300–302.

Rossdale, P.D., Ousey, J.C., Cottrill, C.M., Chavatte, P., Allen, W.R. and McGladdery, A.J. (1991) Effects of placental pathology on maternal plasma progestagen and mammary secretion calcium concentrations and on neonatal adrenocortical function in the horse. *Journal of Reproduction and Fertility, Supplement* 44, 579–590.

Rossdale, P.D., McGladdery, A.J., Ousey, J., Holdstock, N., Grainger, C. and Houghton, E. (1992) Increase in plasma progestagen concentrations in the mare after foetal injection with CRH, ACTH or beta methasone in late gestation. *Equine Veterinary Journal* 24(5), 347–350.

Rossdale, P.D., Ousey, J.C. and Chavatte, P. (1997) Readiness for birth: an endocrinological duet between fetal foal and mare. *Equine Veterinary Journal, Supplement* 24, 96–99.

Rota, A., Furzi, C., Panzani, D. and Camillo, F. (2004) Studies on motility of cooled stallion spermatozoa.

Reproduction in Domestic Animals 39(2), 103–109.

Rousset, H., Chanteloube, P., Magistrini, M. and Palmer, E. (1987) Assessment of fertility and semen evaluations of stallions. *Journal of Reproduction and Fertility Supplement* 35, 25–31.

Rowley, M.S., Squires, E.L. and Pickett, B.W. (1990) Effect of insemination volume on embryo recovery in mares. *Equine Veterinary Science* 10, 298–300.

Roy, S.K. and Greenwald, G.S. (1987) In vitro steroidogenesis by primary to antral follicles in the hamster during the periovulatory period. Effects of follicle stimulating hormone, luteinising hormone and prolactin. *Biology of Reproduction* 37(1), 39–46.

Rudak, E., Jacobs, P. and Yanagimachi, R. (1978) Direct analysis of chromosome constitution of human spermatozoa. *Nature (London)* 174, 911–913.

Saastamoinen, M.T., Lahdekorpi, M. and Hyppa, S. (1990) Copper and zinc levels in the diet of pregnant and lactating mares. In: *Proceedings of the 41st Annual Meeting of the European Association for Animal Production*. Wageningen Academic Publishers, Wageningen, The Netherlands, pp. 1–9.

Sabbagh, M., Danvy, S. and Richard, A. (2014) Genetic and environmental analysis of dystocia and still births in draft horses. *Animal* 8(1), 184–191.

Sack, W.O. (1991) Isolated male organs. *Rooney's Guide to the Dissection of the Horse*, 6th edn. Veterinary Textbooks, Ithaca, New York, pp. 75–78.

Saini, S.N., Mohindroo, J., Mahajan, S.K., Raghunath, M., Sangwan, V., Kumar, A., Anand, A., Singh, T. and Singh, N. (2013a) Surgical management of third degree perneal laceration in young mares. *Indian Journal of Animal Sciences* 83(5), 525–526.

Saini, N.S., Mohindroo, J., Mahajan, S.K., Ragunath, M., Kumar, A., Sangwan, V., Singh, T., Singh, N., Sing, S.S., Anand, A. and Singh, K. (2013b) Surgical correction of uterine torsion and mare-foal survival in advance pregnant equine patients. *Journal of Equine Veterinary Science* 33, 31–34.

Salamone, D.F., Canel, N.G. and Rodríguez, M.B. (2017) Intracytoplasmic sperm injection in domestic and wild mammals. *Reproduction* 154, F111–F124.

Salisbury, G.W., Van Denmark, N.L. and Lodge, J.R. (1978) Part 2. The storage and the planting. *Physiology of Reproduction and AI of Cattle*, 2nd edn. W.H. Freeman, San Francisco, California, pp. 187–578.

Samper, J.C. (1991) Relationship between the fertility of fresh and frozen stallion semen and semen quality. *Journal of Reproduction and Fertility, Supplement* 44, 107–114.

Samper, J.C. (1995a) Diseases of the male system. In: Kobluk, C.N., Ames, T.R. and Goer, R.J. (eds) *The Horse, Diseases and Clinical Management*. Vol. 2. W.B. Saunders, Philadelphia, Pennsylvania, pp. 937–972.

Samper, J.C. (1995b) Stallion semen cryopreservation: male factors affecting pregnancy rates. In: *Proceedings of the Society for Theriogenology*, San Antonio, Texas, pp. 160–165.

Samper, J.C. (1997) Reproductive anatomy and physiology of breeding stallion. In: Youngquist, R.S. (ed.) *Current Therapy in Large Animal Theriogenology*. W.B. Saunders, Philadelphia, Pennsylvania, pp. 3–12.

Samper, J.C. (2000) *Equine Breeding Management and Artificial Insemination*. W.B. Saunders, Philadelphia, Pennsylvania, pp. 306.

Samper, J.C. (2008) Induction of estrus and ovulation: Why some mares respond and others do not. *Theriogenology* 70, 445–447.

Samper, J.C. (2009a) Artificial Insemination. In: Samper, J.C. (ed.) *Equine Breeding Managment and Artificial Insemination* 2nd ed. Saunders, St Louis, Missouri, pp. 165–174.

Samper, J.C. (2009b) Embryo transfer. In: Samper, J.C. (ed.) *Equine Breeding Managment and Artificial Insemination* 2nd ed. Saunders, St Louis, Missouri, pp. 185–199.

Samper, J.C. (2011) Breeding with cooled transported semen. In: McKinnon, A.O., Squires, E.L., Vaala, E. and Varner, D.D. (eds) *Equine Reproduction*, 2nd edn. Wiley-Blackwell, Philadelphia, London, pp. 1316–1322.

Samper, J.C. and Crabo, B.G. (1988) Filtration of capacitated spermatozoa through filters containing glass wool and/or Sephadex. In: *Proceedings of the 11th International Congress on Animal Production and Artificial Insemination, University College Dublin*. Vol. 3, paper 294. University College Dublin, Dublin, Republic of Ireland.

Samper, J.C. and Plough, T.A. (2012) How to deal with dystocia and retained placenta in the field. *Proceedings of the American Association of Equine Practionners* 58, 359–361.

Samper, J.C. and Pycock, J.F. (2007) The normal uterus in estrous. In: Samper, J.C., Pycock, J.F., McKinnon, A.O. (eds) *Curent therapy in Equine Reproduction*. Saunders Elsevier, St Louis, Missouri, pp. 32–35.

Samper, J.C. and Tibary, A. (2006) Disease transmission in horses. *Theriogenology* 66, 551–559.

Samper, J.C., Loseth, K.J. and Crabo, B.G. (1988) Evaluation of horse's spermatozoa with Sephadex filtration using three extenders and three dilutions. In: *Proceedings of the 11th International Congress on Animal Production and Artificial Insemination, University College Dublin*. Vol. 3, brief communications 294. University College Dublin, Dublin, Republic of Ireland.

Samper, J.C., Behnke, E.J., Byers, A.P., Hunter, A.G. and Crabo, B.G. (1989) *In vitro* capacitation of stallion spermatozoa in calcium-free Tyrode's medium and penetration of zona-free hamster eggs. *Theriogenology* 31(4), 875–884.

Samper, J.C., Hellander, J.C. and Crabo, B.G. (1991) The relationship between the fertility of fresh and frozen stallion semen and semen quality. *Journal of Reproduction and Fertility, Supplement* 44, 107–114.

Samper, J.C., Jensen, S., Sergeant, J. and Estrada, A. (2002) Timing of induction of ovulation in mares treated with Ovuplant or Chorulon. *Journal of Equine Veterinary Science* 22, 320–323.

Sanchez, R.A., von Frey, G.W. and de los Reyers, S.M. (1995) Effect of semen diluents and seminal plasma on the preservation of refrigerated stallion semen. *Veterinaria Argentina* 12(113), 172–178.

Sánchez, R., Blanco, M., Weiss, J., Rosati, I., Herrera, C., Bollwein, H., Burger, D. and Sieme, H. (2017) Influence of embryonic size and manipulation on pregnancy rates of mares after transfer of cryopreserved equine embryos. *Journal of Equine Veterinary Science* 49, 54–59.

Sang Kyu, L. DongHoon, L. and HyunGu, K. (2009) Surgical treatment and postoperative management of third-degree perineal laceration occurring at the time of foaling in a Thoroughbred horse. *Journal of Veterinary Clinics* 26(3), 286–289.

Sang, L., Yang, W.C., Han, L., Liang, A.X., Hua, G.H., Xiong, J.J., Huo, L.J. and Yang, L.G. (2011) An immunological method to screen sex-specific proteins of bovine sperm. *Journal of Dairy Science* 94, 2060–2070.

Sanocka, D. and Kurpisz, M. (2004) Reactive oxygen species and sperm cells. *Reproductive Biology and Endocrinology* 2, 12.

Santos, A, and Silvestre, A. (2008) A sudy of Lusitano mare lactation curve with Wood's model. *Journal of Dairy Science* 91(2), 760–766.

Santos, V.G., Beg, M.A., Bettencourt, E.M. and Ginther, O.J. (2013) Role of PGF2α in lutolysis based on inhibition of PGF2α synthesis in the mare. *Theriogenology* 80(7), 812–20.

Saragusty, J. and Arav, A (2011) Current progress in oocyte and embryo cryopreservation by slow freezing and vitrification. *Reproduction* 141(1), 1–19.

Saragusty, J., Gacitua, H., Pettit, M.T. and Arav, A. (2007) Directional freezing of equine semen in large volumes. *Reproduction in Domestic Animals* 42, 610–615.

Sarnecky, B.A., Vanderwall, D.K., Mason, H.M., Kirschner, S.M., Ambrose, B. and Parker, T.L. (2019) Evaluation of a proprietary slow-release oxytocin formulation on corpus luteum function in mares. *Journal of Equine Veterinary Science* 77, 28–30.

Satoh, M., Higuchi, T., Inoue, S., Gotoh, T., Murase, H. and Nambo, Y. (2017) Factors affecting the prognosis for uterine torsion: the effect of treatment based on measurements of setrum progesterone and estradiol concentrations after surgery. *Journal of Equine Science* 28(4), 163–167.

Satué, K. and Gardón, J.C. (2013) A Review of the Estrous Cycle and the Neuroendocrine Mechanisms in the Mare. *Journal of Steroids and Hormonal Science*, 4, 115.

Satué, K. and Gardón, J.C. (2016) Infection and Infertility in Mares, Genital Infections and Infertility. Atef M. Darwish, IntechOpen, DOI: 10.5772/63741. Available from: https://www.intechopen.com/books/genital-infections-and-infertility/infection-and-infertility-in-mares

Satue, K., Felipe, M., Mota, J. and Munoz, A. (2011) Factors influencing gestation length in mares: A Review. *Livestock Science* 136, 287–294.

Sauberli, D.S. (2013) Effectiveness and efficiency of ovulation induction agents in mares. MSc thesis University of Illinois, Illinois.

Saunders, C.M., Larman, M.G., Parrington, J., Cox, L.J., Royse, J., Blayney, L.M., Swann, K. and Lai, F.A. (2002) PLC zeta: A sperm-specific trigger of Ca(2+) oscillations in eggs and embryo development. *Development* 129, 3533–3544.

Savage, C. and Lewis, L.D. (2002) The role of nutrition in musculoskeletal development and disease. In: Stashak, T.S. (ed.) *Adams' Lameness in Horses* (5th edn). Lipincott Williams and Wilkins, Philadelphia, Pennsylvania.

Savage, C., McCarthy, R.N. and Jeffcote, L.B. (1993) Effects of dietary phosphorous and calcium on induction of dyschondroplasia in foals. *Equine Veterinary Journal (Supplement)* 16, 80–83.

Savage, C.J. (2011) abnormalities of the cardiovascular system. In: McKinnon, A.O., Squires, E.L., Vaala, E. and Varner, D.D. (eds) *Equine Reproduction*, 2nd edn. Wiley-Blackwell, Philadelphia, London, pp. 511–523.

Scarlet, D., Wulf, M., Kuhl, J., Köhne, M., Ille, N., Conley, A.J. and Aurich, C. (2018) Anti Müllerian hormone profiling in prepubertal horses and its relationship with gonadal function. *Theriogenology* 117, 72–77.

Scaramuzzi, R.J. and Martin, G.B (2008) The importance of interactions among nutrition, seasonality and socio-sexual. Factors in the development of hormone-free methods for controlling fertility. *Reproduction in Domestic Animals* 43 (Supplement 2), 129–136.

Scheffrahn, N.S., Wiseman, B.S., Vincent, D.L., Harrison, P.C. and Kesler, D.J. (1980) Ovulation control in pony mares during early spring using progestins, PGF2x, hCG and GnRH. *Journal of Animal Science, Supplement* 1(51), 325.

Scherbarth, R., Pozvari, M., Heilkenbrinker, T. and Mumme, J. (1994) Genital microbial flora of the stallion – microbiological examination of presecretion samples between 1972 and 1991. *Deutsche Tierarztliche Wochenschrift* 101(1), 18–22.

Scherzer, J., Davis, C. and Hurley, D.J. (2011) Laser assisted vitrification of large equine embryos. *Reproduction in Domestic Animals* 46, 1104–1106.

Schlafer, D.H. (2004). Postmortem examination of the equine placenta, fetus, and neonate: methods and interpretation of findings. *Proceedings of the 50th Annual Convention of the American Association of Equine Practitioners*, Denver, Colorado and Lexington, Kentucky, pp. 144–161.

Schlafer, D.H. (2007) Equine endometrial biopsy: enhancement of clinical value by more extensive histopathology and application of new diagnostic techniques? *Theriogenology* 68(3), 413–422.

Schlafer, D.H. (2011a) Examination of the placenta. In: McKinnon, A.O., Squires, E.L, Vaala, W.E. and Varner, D.D. (eds) *Equine Reproduction* 2nd edn. Wiley-Blackwell, Philadelphia, London, pp. 99–110.

Schlafer, D.H. (2011b) Non-neoplastic abnormalities. In: McKinnon, A.O., Squires, E.L, Vaala, W.E. and Varner, D.D. (eds) *Equine Reproduction* 2nd edn. Wiley-Blackwell, Philadelphia, London, pp. 2697–276.

Schober, D., Aurich, C., Nohl, H. and Gille, L. (2007) Influence of cryopreservation on mitochondrial functions in equine spermatozoa. *Theriogenology* 68(5), 745–754.

Schoon, H.A. and Schoon, D. (2003) The category 1 mare (Kenney and Doig 1986): Expected foaling rate 80–90% – fact or ficton? *Pferdeheilkunde* 19, 698–701.

Schryver, H.F., Ofledal, O.T., Williams, J., Soderholm, L.V. and Hintz, H.F. (1986) Lactation in the horse: the mineral composition of mare's milk. *Journal of Nutrition* 116, 2142–2147.

Schuler, G. (1998) Indirect pregnancy diagnosis in the mare: determination of oestrone sulphate in blood and urine. *Praktische Tierarzt* 79(1), 43–49.

Schumacher, J. and Varner, D.D. (1993) Neoplasia of the stallion's reproductive tract. In: McKinnon, A.O. and Voss, J.L. (eds) *Equine Reproduction*. Lea and Febiger, Philadelphia, Pennsylvania, pp. 871–878.

Schumacher, J. and Varner, D.D. (2011a) Abnormalities of the penis and prepuce. In: McKinnon, A.O., Squires, E.L, Vaala, W.E. and Varner, D.D. (eds) *Equine Reproduction* 2nd edn. Wiley-Blackwell, Philadelphia, London, pp. 1130–1144.

Schumacher, J. and Varner, D.D. (2011b) Abnormalities of the spermatic cord. In: McKinnon, A.O.,

Squires, E.L, Vaala, W.E. and Varner, D.D. (eds) *Equine Reproduction* 2nd edn. Wiley-Blackwell, Philadelphia, London, pp. 1145–1155.

Schumacher, J., Varner, D.D., Schmitz, D.G. and Blanchard, T.L. (1995) Urethral defects in geldings with hematuria and stallions with haemospermia. *Veterinary Surgery* 24(3), 250–254.

Schutten, K.J. (2016) Successful foaling by a Standardbred mare with a ruptured prepubic tendon. *Canadian Veterinary Journal* 57, 1287–1289.

Schutzer, W.E. and Holton, D.W. (1995) Novel progestin metabolism by the equine utero-fetal-placental unit. *Biology of Reproduction* 52 (Supplement 1), 188.

Schwab, C.A. (1990) Prolactin and progesterone concentrations during early pregnancy and relationship to pregnancy loss prior to day 45. *Journal of Equine Veterinary Science* 10(4), 280–283.

Scott, M.A. (2000) A glimpse at sperm function in vivo: sperm transport and epitheial interaction in the female reproductive tract. *Animal Reproduction Science* 60–61, 337–348.

Scott, M.A., Liu, I.K.M., Overstreet, J.W. and Enders, A.C. (2000) The structural morphology and epithelial association of spermatozoa at the utero-tubal junction: a descriptive study of equine spermatozoa in situ using scanning electron microscopy. *Journal of Reproduction and Fertility, Supplement* 56, 415–421.

Scott, T.J., Carnevale, E.M., Maclellan, L.J., Scoggin, C.F. and Squires, E.L. (2001) Embryo development rates after transfer of oocytes matured *in vivo, in vitro,* or within oviducts of mares. *Theriogenology* 55, 705–715.

Scraba, S.T. and Ginther, O.J. (1985) Effect of lighting programs on the ovulatory season in mares. *Theriogenology* 24, 607–679.

Seamens, M.C., Roser, J.F., Linford, R.L., Liu, I.K.M. and Hughes, J.P. (1991) Gonadotrophin and steroid concentrations in jugular and testicular venous plasma in stallions before and after GnRH injection. *Journal of Reproduction and Fertility, Supplement* 44, 57–67.

Searle, D., Dart, A.J., Dart, C.M. and Hodgson, D.R. (1999) Equine castration: review of anatomy, approaches, techniques and complications in normal, cryptorchid and monorchid horses. *Australian Veterinary Journal* 77(7), 428–471.

Seidel, J. (2003) Sexing mammalian sperm – intertwining of commerce, technology and biology. *Animal Reproduction Science* 79, 145–156.

Seidel Jr, G.E., Herickhoff, L.A., Schenk, J.L., Doyle, S.P. and Green, R.D. (1998) Artificial insemination of heifers with cooled, unfrozen sexed semen. *Theriogenology* 49(1), 365.

Seki, Y., Seimiya, Y.M., Yaegashi, G., Kumagai, S., Sentsui, H., Nishimori, T. and Ishihara, R. (2004) Occurance of equine coital exanthema in pastured draft horses and isolation of equine herpesvirus 3 from progenital lesions. *Journal of Veterinary Medical Science* 66, 1503–1508.

Sellon, D.C. (2006) Neonatal immunity. In: Paradise, M.R. (ed.) *Equine Neonatal Medicine.* Elsevier Saunders, Philadelphia, Pennsylvania, pp. 31–38.

Seltzer, K.L., Divers, T.J., Vaala, W.E., Byars, T.D. and Rubin, J.L. (1993) The urinary system. In: McKinnon, A.O. and Voss, J.L. (eds) *Equine Reproduction.* Lea and Febiger, Philadelphia, Pennsylvania, pp. 1030–1040.

Senger, P.L. (2011) *Pathways to Pregnancy and Parturition,* 2nd edn. Current Conceptions Inc.

Serafini, R., Longobardi, V., Spadetta, M., Neri, D., Ariota, B., Gasparrini, B. and Di Palo, R. (2013) Trypan blue/giemsa staining to assess sperm membrane integrity in Salernitano stallions and its relationship to pregnancy rates. *Reproduction in Domestic Animals* 49(1), 41–47.

Sertich, P.L. (1993) Cervical problems in the mare. In: McKinnon, A.O. and Voss, J.L. (eds) *Equine Reproduction.* Lea and Febiger, Philadelphia, Pennsylvania, London, pp. 404–407.

Sertich, P.L. (1998) Ultrasonography of the genital tract of the mare. In: Reef, V.B. (ed.) *Equine Diagnostic Ultrasound.* W.B. Saunders, Philadelphia, Pennsylvania, pp. 405–424.

Sertich, P.L. (2011) Examination of External Genitalia. In: McKinnon, A.O., Squires, E.L, Vaala, W.E. and Varner, D.D. (eds) *Equine Reproduction* 2nd edn. Wiley-Blackwell, Philadelphia, London, pp. 1458–1461.

Sertich, P.L., Love, L.B., Hodgson, M.R. and Kenny, R.M. (1988) 24 hour cooled storage of equine embryos. *Theriogenology* 30(5), 947–952.

Sessions-Bresnahan, D.R., Graham, J.K. and Carnevale, E.M. (2014) Validation of a heterologous fertilization assay and comparison of fertilization rates of equine oocytes using in vitro fertilization, perivitelline, and intracytoplasmic sperm injections. *Theriogenology* 82(2), 274–282.

Setchell, B.P. (1991) Male reproductive organs and semen. In: Cupps, P.T. (ed.) *Reproduction in Domestic Animals*, 4th edn. Academic Press, London, pp. 221–249.

Sevinga, M., Hesselink, J.W. and Barkema, H.W. (2002) Reproductive performance of Friesian mares after retained placenta and manual removal of the placenta. *Theriogenology* 57(2), 923–930.

Shand, N., Alexander, S.L. and Irvine, C.H.G. (1995) Oxytocin secretion patterns in normal stallions as measured in pituitary venous blood: Correlation with gonadotrophn secretion and effect of sexual arousal. *Biology of Reproduction, Monographs*, pp. 565–575.

Shannon, P. (1972) The effect of egg yolk level and dose rate on conception rate of semen diluted in caprogen. In: *Proceedings of the 7th International Congress of Animal Reproduction and AI, Munich*. International Congress Animal Reproduction, pp. 279–280.

Sharma, R., Hogg, J. and Bromham, D. (1993) Is spermatozoan acrosin a predictor of fertilisation and embryo quality in the human? *Fertility and Sterility* 60(5), 881–887.

Sharma, S., Davies Morel, M.C.G., Dhaliwal, G.S. and Dadarwal, D. (2010) The pattern of embryonic fixation and its relationship to pregnancy loss in Thoroughbred mares. *Reproduction in Domestic Animals* 45, 361–367.

Sharp, D.C. (1993) Maternal recognition of pregnancy. In: McKinnon, A.O. and Voss, J.L. (eds) *Equine Reproduction*. Lea and Febiger, Philadelphia, Pennsylvania, pp. 473–485.

Sharp, D.C. (2011a) Melatonin. In: McKinnon, A.O., Squires, E.L, Vaala, W.E. and Varner, D.D. (eds) *Equine Reproduction*, 2nd edn. Wiley-Blackwell, pp. 1689–1678.

Sharp, D.C. (2011b) Vernal transition into the breeding season. In: McKinnon, A.O., Squires, E.L, Vaala, W.E. and Varner, D.D. (eds) *Equine Reproduction*, 2nd edn. Wiley-Blackwell, Philadelphia, London, pp. 1704–1715.

Sharp, D.C. (2011c) Photoperiod. In: McKinnon, A.O., Squires, E.L, Vaala, W.E. and Varner, D.D. (eds) *Equine Reproduction*, 2nd edn. Wiley-Blackwell, Philadelphia, London, pp. 1771–1777.

Sharpe, J.C. and Evans, K.M. (2009) Advances in flow cytometry for sperm sexing. *Theriogenology* 71, 4–10.

Shaw, E.B., Houpt, K.A. and Holmes, D.F. (1988) Body temperature and behaviour of mares during the last two weeks of pregnancy. *Equine Veterinary Journal* 20, 199–200.

Shaw, F.D. and Morton, H. (1980) The immunological approach to pregnancy diagnosis: a review. *Veterinary Record* 106, 268–270.

Sheoran, A.S., Karenski, S.S., Whalen, J.W., Chrisman, M.V., Powell, D.G. and Timoney, J.F. (2000) Prepartum equine rotavirus including strong specific IgG in mammary secretion *Veterinary Record* 146, 672–673.

Shepherd, M. (2015) Protecting your investment: nutrition for the foal. *Clinical Theriogenology* 7(3), 275–278.

Shideler, R.K. (1993a) History. In: McKinnon, A.O. and Voss, J.L. (eds) *Equine Reproduction*. Lea and Febiger, Philadelphia, Pennsylvania, London, pp. 196–198.

Shideler, R.K. (1993b) External examination. In: McKinnon, A.O. and Voss, J.L. (eds) *Equine Reproduction*. Lea and Febiger, Philadelphia, Pennsylvania, London, pp. 199–203.

Shideler, R.K. (1993c) Rectal palpation. In: McKinnon, A.O. and Voss, J.L. (eds) *Equine Reproduction*. Lea and Febiger, Philadelphia, Pennsylvania, pp. 204–210.

Shideler, R.K. (1993d) The prefoaling period. In: McKinnon, A.O. and Voss, J.L. (eds) *Equine Reproduction*. Lea and Febiger, Philadelphia, Pennsylvania, pp. 955–963.

Shiner, K.A., Pickett, B.W., Juergens, T.D. and Nett, T.M. (1993) Clinical approach to diagnosis and treatment of subfertile stallions: opinions. *Proceedings of the American Association of Equine Practionners* 149–157.

Shoemaker, C.F., Squires, E.L. and Shideler, R.K. (1989) Safety of altrenogest in pregnant mares and on health and development of offspring. *Journal of Equine Veterinary Science* 9, 67–72.

Shoemaker, R., Bailey, J., Janzen, E. and Wilson, D.G. (2004) Routine castration in 568 draught colts: incidence of evisceration and omental herniation. *Equine Veterinary Journal* 36, 336–340.

Siciliano, P.D. (2011) Feeding the growing horse to avoid developmental orthopedic disease. In: McKinnon,

A.O., Squires, E.L., Vaala, E. and Varner, D.D. (eds) *Equine Reproduction*, 2nd edn. Wiley-Blackwell, Philadelphia, London, pp. 782–793.

Siciliano, P.D., Wood, C.H., Lawrence, L.M. and Duren, S.D. (1993) Utilization of a field study to evaluate digestible energy requirements of breeding stallions. In: *Proceedings of the 13th Equine Nutrition and Physiology Society Symposium, Gainesville, Florida*. Equine and Physiology Society, 293–298.

Sieme, H. (2011a) Semen extenders for frozen semen. In: McKinnon, A.O., Squires, E.L., Vaala, E. and Varner, D.D. (eds) *Equine Reproduction*, 2nd edn. Wiley-Blackwell, Philadelphia, London, pp. 2964–2971.

Sieme, H. (2011b) Freezing semen. In: McKinnon, A.O., Squires, E.L., Vaala, E. and Varner, D.D. (eds) *Equine Reproduction*, 2nd edn. Wiley-Blackwell, Philadelphia, London, pp. 2972–2982.

Sieme, H., Martinsson, G., Rauterberg, H., Walter, K., Aurich, C., Petzoldt, R. and Klug, E. (2003a) Application of techniques for sperm selection in fresh and frozen-thawed stallion semen. *Reproduction in Domestic Animals* 38(2), 134–140.

Sieme, H., Bonk, A., Ratjen, J., Klug, E. and Rath, D. (2003b) Effect of sperm number and site/technique of insemination on pregnancy in mares. *Pferdeheilkunde* 19(6), 677–683.

Sieme, H., Schafer, T., Stout, T.A., Klug, E. and Waberski, D. (2003c) The effects of different insemination regimes on fertility in mares. *Theriogenology* 60, 1153–1164.

Sieme, H., Katila, T. and Klug, E. (2004a) Effect of semen collection practices on sperm characteristics before and after storage and on fertility of stallions. *Theriogenology* 61(4), 769–784.

Sieme, H., Bonk, A., Hamann, H., Klug, E. and Katila, T. (2004b) Effects of different artificial insemination techniques and sperm doses on fertility of normal mares and mares with abnormal reproductive history. *Theriogenology* 62, 915–928.

Sieme, H., Topfer-Petersen, E., Bader, H. and Petzold, R. (2019) AI – Sperm of the stallion: Evaluation criteria and minimal standards – A survey. *Pferdeheilkunde* 17(2), 145–154.

Siemieniuch, M.J., Gajos, K., Kozdrowski, R. and Nowak, M. (2017) Advanced age in mares affects endometrial secretion of arachidonic acid metabolites during equine subclinical endometritis. *Theriogenology* 103, 191–196.

Silberzahn, P., Pouret, E.J.M. and Zwain, I. (1989) Androgen and estrogen response to a single injection of hCG in cryptorchid horses. *Equine Veterinary Journal* 21, 126–129.

Silva, L.A. and Ginther, O.J. (2006) An early endometrial vascular indicator of completed orientation of the embryo and the role of dorsal endometrial encroachment in mares. *Biology of Reproduction* 74, 337–343.

Silva, L.A., Gastal, E.L., Beg, M.A. and Ginther, O.J. (2005) Changes in vascular perfusion of the endometrium in association with changes in location of the embryonic vesicle in mares. *Biology of Reproduction* 72(3), 755–761.

Silva, P.F. and Gadella, B.M. (2006) Detection of damage in mammalian sperm cells. *Theriogenology* 65(5), 958–978.

Silver, M. (1990) Prenatal maturation, the timing of birth and how it may be regulated in domestic animals. *Experimental Physiology* 75(3), 285–307.

Silver, M. and Fowden, A.L. (1994) Prepartum adrenocortical maturation in the fetal foal: responses to ACTH 1–24. *Journal of Endocrinology* 142, 417–425.

Silver, M., Steven, D.H. and Comline, R.S. (1973) Placental exchange and morphology in ruminants and mares. In: Comline, R.S., Cross, K.W., Davies, G.S. and Nathanielsz, P.W. (eds) *Foetal and Neonatal Physiology*. Cambridge University Press, Cambridge, UK, pp. 245–262.

Silver, M., Barnes, R.J., Comline, R.S., Fowden, A.L., Clover, L. and Mitchell, M.D. (1979) Prostaglandins in maternal of foetal plasma and in allantoic fluid during the second half of gestation in the mare. *Journal of Reproduction and Fertility, Supplement* 27, 531–539.

Silver, M., Ousey, J.C., Dudan, F.E., Fowden, A.L., Knox, J., Cash, R.S. and Rossdale, P.D. (1984) Studies on equine prematurity 2: Post natal adrenocortical activity in relation to plasma adrenocorticotrophic hormone and catecholamine levels in term and premature foals. *Equine Veterinary Journal* 16(4), 278–286.

Simmons, H.A., Cox, J.E., Edwards, G.B., Neal, P.A. and Urquhart, K.A. (1985) Paraphimosis in seven debilitated horses. *Veterinary Record* 116, 126–127.

Simpson, B.S. (2002) Neonatal foal handling. *Applied Behaviour Science* 78, 303–317.

Sinnemaa, L., Jarvimaa, T., Lehmonen, N., Makela, O., Reilas, T., Sankari, S. and Katila, T. (2003) Effect of insemination volume on uterine contractions and inflammatory response and on elimination of semen in the mare's uterus – scintigraphic and ultrasonographic studies. *Theriogenology* 60(4), 727–733.

Sirosis, J., Ball, B.A. and Fortune, J.E. (1989) Patterns of growth and regression of ovarian follicles during the oestrous cycle and after hemiovarectomy in mares. *Equine Veterinary Journal, Supplement* 18, 43–48.

Sissener, T.R., Squires, E.L. and Clay, C.M. (1996) Differential suppression of endometrial prostaglandin F2 alpha by the equine conceptus. *Theriogenology* 45, 541–546.

Sist, M.D. (1987) Fecal oestrone sulphate assay for pregnancy. *Veterinary Medicine* 82, 1036–1043.

Sist, M.D., Williams, J.F., Alma, M. and Geary, B.S. (1987) Pregnancy diagnosis in the mare by immunoassay of estrone sulfate in serum and milk, *Journal of Equine Veterinary Science* 7(1), 20–23.

Skidmore, J., Boyle, M., Cran, D. and Allen, W. (1989) Micromanipulation of equine embryos to produce monozygotic twins. *Equine Veterinary Journal* 21(S8), 126–128.

Skidmore, J.A., Boyle, M.S. and Allen, W.R. (1990) A comparison of two different methods of freezing horse embryos. *Journal of Reproduction and Fertility, Supplement* 44, 714–716.

Slusher, S.H. (1997) Infertility and diseases of the reproductive tract in stallions. In: Youngquist, R.S. (ed.) *Current Therapy in Large Animal Theriogenology.* W.B. Saunders, Philadelphia, Pennsylvania, pp. 16–23.

Smith, J.A. (1973) The occurrence of larvae of *Strongylus edentatus* in the testicles of stallions. *Veterinary Record* 93, 604–606.

Smith, M. (2006) Management of umbilical disorders in the foal. *In Practice* 28, 280–287.

Smith, R.L., Vernon, K.L., Kelley, D.E., Gibbons, J.R. and Mortensen, C.J. (2012) Impact of moderate exercise on ovarian blood flow and early embryonic outcomes in mares. *Journal of Animal Science* 90, 3770–3777.

Smith, S., Marr, C., Menzies-Gow, N., (2015) The effect of obesity and endocrine function on foal birthweight in Thoroughbred mares. Clinical Research Abstracts. British Equine Veterinary Association Congress. *Equine Veterinary Journal* 47(48), 2.

Smits, K., Govaere, J., Hoogewijs, M., Piepers, S. and Van Soom, A. (2012) A pilot comparison of laser-assisted vs Piezo drill ICSI for in vitro production of horse embryos. *Reproduction in Domestic Animals* 47(1), 1–3.

Smolders, E.A.A., Van Der Veen, N.G. and Van Polanen, A. (1990) Composition of horse milk during the suckling period. *Livestock Production Science* 25, 163–171.

Sondergaard, E. and Jago, J. (2010) The effect of early handling of foals on their reaction to handling, humans and novelty, and the foal-mare relationship. *Applied Animal Science* 123, 93–100.

Snow, D.H., (1993) Anabolic steroids. *Veterinary Clinics of North America Equine Practionners* 9(3), 563–576.

Søndergaard, E. and Ladewig, J. (2004) Group housing exerts a positive effect on the behaviour of young horses during training. *Applied Animal Behavior Science* 87, 105–118.

Spencer, T.E. and Bazer, F.W. (2004) Uterine and placental factors regulating conceptus growth in domestic animals. *Journal of Animal Science* 82 (E-Suppl.), E4–13.

Spensley, M.S. and Markel, M.D. (1993) Management of rectal tears. In: McKinnon, A.O. and Voss, J.L. (eds) *Equine Reproduction.* Lea and Febiger, Philadelphia, Pennsylvania, pp. 464–472.

Spirito, M.A. and Sprayberry, K.A. (2011) Uterine prolapse. In: McKinnon, A.O., Squires, E.L., Vaala, E. and Varner, D.D. (eds) *Equine Reproduction,* 2nd edn. Wiley-Blackwell, Philadelphia, London, pp. 2431–2434.

Squires, E.L. (1993a) Progesterone. In: McKinnon, A.O. and Voss, J.L. (eds) *Equine Reproduction.* Lea and Febiger, Philadelphia, Pennsylvania, pp. 57–64.

Squires, E.L. (1993b) Progestin. In: McKinnon, A.O. and Voss, J.L. (eds) *Equine Reproduction.* Lea and Febiger, Philadelphia, Pennsylvania, London, pp. 311–318.

Squires, E.L. (1993c) Estrus detection. In: McKinnon, A.O. and Voss, J.L. (eds) *Equine Reproduction.* Lea and Febiger, Philadelphia, Pennsylvania, pp. 186–195.

Squires, E.L. (2008) Hormone manipulation of the mare: A review. *Journal of Equine Veterinary Science* 28(11), 624–627.

Squires, E.L. (2009) Changes in equine reproduction: have they been good or bad for the horse industry? *Journal of Equine Veterinary Science* 29, 268–273.

Squires, E.L. (2011a) Reproductive parameters from light horse stallions. In: McKinnon, A.O., Squires, E.L., Vaala, E. and Varner, D.D. (eds) *Equine Reproduction*, 2nd edn. Wiley-Blackwell, Philadelphia, London, pp. 1367–1376.

Squires, E.L. (2011b) Progesterone. In: McKinnon, A.O., Squires, E.L., Vaala, E. and Varner, D.D. (eds) *Equine Reproduction*, 2nd edn. Wiley-Blackwell, Philadelphia, London, pp. 1778–1781.

Squires, E.L. (2019) Perspectives on the development and incorporation of assisted reproduction in the equine industry. *Reproduction and Fertility* 31(12), 1753–1757.

Squires, E.L. and McCue, P.M. (2007) Superovulation in mares. *Animal Reproduction Science* 99(1–2), 1–8.

Squires, E.L. and McCue, P.M. (2011) Superovulation. In: McKinnon, A.O., Squires, E.L., Vaala, E. and Varner, D.D. (eds) *Equine Reproduction*, 2nd edn. Wiley-Blackwell, Philadelphia, London, pp. 1836–1845.

Squires, E.L. and McCue, P.M. (2016) Cryopreservation of equine embryos. *Journal of Equine Veterinary Science* 41, 7–12.

Squires, E.L. and Seidel, G.E. (1995) *Collection and Transfer of Equine Embryos*. Colorado State University, Fort Collins, Colorado, pp. 11–16.

Squires, E.L., Todter, G.E., Berndtson, W.E. and Pickett, B.W. (1982) Effect of anabolic steroids on reproductive function of young stallions. *Journal of Animal Science* 54, 576–582.

Squires, E.L., Voss, J.L. and Villahoz, M.D. (1983) Immunological methods for pregnancy detection in mares. In: Milne, F.J. (ed.) *Proceedings of the 28th Annual Convention of the American Association of Equine Practitioners, Atlanta, Georgia*. American Association of Equine Practitioners, pp. 45–51.

Squires, E.L., Garcia, R.H. and Ginther, O.J. (1985a) Factors affecting the success of equine embryo transfer. *Equine Veterinary Journal, Supplement* 3, 92–95.

Squires, E.L., Voss, J.L., Maher, J.M. and Shideler, R.K. (1985b) Fertility of young mares after long-term anabolic steroid treatment. *Journal of the American Veterinary Medical Association* 186, 583–587.

Squires, E.L., McClain, M.G., Ginther, O.J. and McKinnon, A.O. (1987) Spontaneous multiple ovulation in the mare and its effect on the incidence of twin embryo collections. *Theriogenology* 28, 609–614.

Squires, E.L., Seidel Jr, G.E. and McKinnon, A.O. (1989) Transfer of cryopreserved equine embryos to progestin treated ovarectomised mares. *Equine Veterinary Journal, Supplement* 8, 89–95.

Squires, E.L. Wilson, J.M., Kato, H. and Blaszczyk, A. (1996) A pregnancy after intracytoplasmic sperm injection into equine oocytes matured in vitro. *Theriogenology* 45, 306.

Squires, E.L., Badzinski, S.L., Amann, R.P., McCue, P.M. and Nett, T.M. (1997) Effects of altrenogest on scrotal width, seminal characteristics, concentration of LH and testosterone and sexual behaviour of stallions. *Theriogenology* 48(2), 313–328.

Squires, E.L., McCue, P.M. and Vanderwall, D. (1999) The current status of equine embryo transfer. *Theriogenology* 51, 91–100.

Squires, E.L., Carnevale, E.M., McCue, J.E. and Bruemmer, J.E. (2003) Embryo technologies in the horse. *Theriogenology* 59, 151–170.

Squires, E.L., Keith, S.L. and Graham, J.K. (2004) Evaluation of alternative cryoprotectants for preserving stallion spermatozoa. *Theriogenology* 62, 1056–1065.

Squires, E.L., Hughes, S.E., Ball, B.A., Troedsson, M.H.T. and Stowe, J. (2013) Effect of season and reproductive status on the incidence of equine dystocia. *Journal of Equine Veterinary Science* 33(5), 375.

Stabenfeldt, G.H., Hughes, J.P., Evans, J.W. and Neely, D.P. (1974) Spontaneous prolongation of luteal activity in the mare. *Equine Veterinary Journal* 6, 158–163.

Stabenfeldt, G.H., Hughes, J.P., Kennedy, P.C., Meagher, D.M. and Neely, D.P. (1979) Clinical findings, pathological changes and endocrinological secretory patterns in mares with ovarian tumours. *Journal of Reproduction and Fertility, Supplement* 27, 277–285.

Stabenfeldt, G.H., Daels, P.F., Munro, C.J., Kindahl, H., Hughes, J.P. and Lasley, B. (1991) An oestrogen conjugate enzyme immunoassay for monitoring pregnancy in the mare: limitations of the assay between days 40 and 70 of gestation. *Journal of Reproduction and Fertility, Supplement* 44, 37–44.

Staempfli, S.A. (2011) Prostaglandins. In: McKinnon, A.O., Squires, E.L, Vaala, W.E. and Varner, D.D. (eds) *Equine Reproduction*, 2nd edn. Wiley-Blackwell, Philadelphia, London, pp. 1797–1803.

Staniar, W.B., Akers, R.M., Williams, C.A., Kronfeld, D.S. and Harris, P.A. (2001) Plasma insulin-like growth factor-I (IGF-I) in growing Thoroughbred foals fed a fat and fiber versus a sugar and a starch supplement. In: *Proceedings of the 17th Equine Nutrition and Physiology Symposium, North Lexington, Kentucky*. Equine and Physiology Society, pp. 176–177.

Staniar, W.B., Kronfeld, D.S., Akers, R.M. and Harris, P.A. (2007) Insulin-like growth factor I in growing Thoroughbreds. *Journal of Animal Physiology and Animal Nutrition* 91, 390–399.

Stamatkin, C.W., Roussev, R.G., Stout, T., Absalon-Medina, V., Ramu, S., Goodman, C., Colam C.B.O., Gilbert, R., Godke, R.A. and Barnea, E.R. (2011) PreImplantation Factor (PIF) correlates with early mammalian embryo development-bovine and murine models. *Reproductive Biology and Endocrinology* 9, 63.

Stanton, M.E. (2011a) Uterine involution. In: McKinnon, A.O., Squires, E.L., Vaala, E. and Varner, D.D. (eds) *Equine Reproduction*, 2nd edn. Wiley-Blackwell, Philadelphia, London, pp. 2291–2293.

Stanton, M.E. (2011b) Uterine cysts. In: McKinnon, A.O., Squires, E.L., Vaala, E. and Varner, D.D. (eds) *Equine Reproduction*, 2nd edn. Wiley-Blackwell, Philadelphia, London, pp. 2665–2668.

Stanton, M.B., Steiner, J.V. and Pugh, D.G. (2004) Endometrial cysts in the mare. *Journal of Equine Veterinary Science* 24, 14–19.

Starbuck, G.R., Stout, T.A.E., Lamming, G.E., Allem, W.R. and Flint, A.P.R. (1998) Endometrial oxytocin receptor and uterine prostaglandin secretion in mares during the oestrous cycle and early pregnancy. *Journal of Reproduction and Fertility* 113, 173–179.

Stashak, T.S. (1993) Inguinal hernia. In: McKinnon, A.O. and Voss, J.L. (eds) *Equine Reproduction*. Lea and Febiger, Philadelphia, Pennsylvania, London, pp. 925–932.

Stashak, T.S. and Vandeplassche, M. (1993) Cesarean section. In: McKinnon, A.O. and Voss, J.L. (eds) *Equine Reproduction*. Lea and Febiger, Philadelphia, Pennsylvania, pp. 437–443.

Stecco, R., Paccamonti, D., Gutjahr, S., Pinto, C.R.F. and Eilts, B. (2003) Day of cycle affects changes in equine intrauterine pressure in response to teasing. *Theriogenology* 60(4), 727–733.

Steiner, J.N. (2000) Breeding management of the Thoroughbred stallion. In: Samper, J.C. (ed.) *Equine Breeding Management and Artificial Insemination*. W.B. Saunders, Philadelphia, Pennsylvania, pp. 67–72.

Steiner, J.N., Antczak, D.F., Wolfsdorf, K., Saville, K., Brooks, S., Millere, D., Bailey, E. and Zent, W. (2006) Persistent endometrial cups. *Animal Reproduction Science* 94, 274–275.

Stevenson, K.R., Parkinson, T.J. and Wathes, D.C. (1991) Measurements of oxytocin concentration in plasma and ovarian extracts during the oestrus cycle of mares. *Journal of Reproduction and Fertility, Supplement* 93, 437–441.

Stewart, D.R., Stabenfeldt, G.H. and Hughes, J.P. (1982) Relaxin activity in foaling mares. *Journal of Reproduction and Fertility, Supplement* 32, 603–609.

Stewart, D.R., Addiego, L.A., Pascoe, D.R., Haluska, G.J. and Pashen, R. (1992) Breed differences in circulating equine relaxin. *Biology of Reproduction* 46, 648–652.

Stewart, F., Charleston, B., Crossett, B., Baker, P.J. and Allen, W.R. (1995) A novel uterine protein that associates with the embryonic capsule in equids. *Journal of Reproduction and Fertility* 105, 65–70.

Stewart, J.H., Rose, R.J. and Barko, A.M. (1984) Respiratory studies in foals from birth to seven days old. *Equine Veterinary Journal* 16, 323–328.

Stone, R. (1994) Timing of mating in relation to ovulation to achieve maximum reproductive efficiency in the horse. *Equine Veterinary Education* 6, 29–31.

Stoneham, S.J. (1991) Failure of passive transfer of colostral immunity in the foal. *Equine Veterinary Education* 3, 43–44.

Stoneham, S.J., (2006) Assessing the newborn foal. In: Paradise, M.R. (ed.) *Equine neonatal medicine*. Elsevier Saunders, Philadelphia, Pennsylvania, pp. 1–10.

Stoneham, S.D.L. (2011) The normal post partum foal. In: McKinnon, A.O., Squires, E.L., Vaala, E. and Varner, D.D. (eds) *Equine Reproduction*, 2nd edn. Wiley-Blackwell, Philadelphia, London, pp. 63–68.

Storer, W.A., Thompson Jr, D.L., Gilley, R.M. and Burns, P.J. (2009) Evaluation of injectable sustained release progestin formulations for the suppression of estrus and ovulation in mares. *Journal of Equine Veterinary Science* 39, 33–36.

Stout, T.A.E. (2003) Selection and management of the embryo transfer donor mare. *Pferdheilkunde* 19, 685–688.

Stout, T.A. (2005) Modulating reproductive activity in stallions: a review. *Animal Reproduction Science* 89(1–4), 93–103.

Stout, T.A. (2006) Equine embryo transfer: review of developing potential. *Equine Veterinary Journal* 38(5), 467–478.

Stout, T.A. (2011) Prostaglandins. In: McKinnon, A.O., Squires, E.L., Vaala, E. and Varner, D.D. (eds) *Equine Reproduction*, 2nd edn. Wiley-Blackwell, Philadelphia, London, pp. 1642–1647.

Stout, T.A.E (2012a) How to Manage Early Embryonic Death. *Proceedings of the American society for Equine Practionners* 58, 331–333.

Stout, T.A.E. (2012b) Cryopreservation of Equine Embryos: Current State-of-the-Art. *Reproduction in Domestic Animals* 47 (Suppl 3), 84–89.

Stout, T. (2016) Embryo–maternal communication during the first 4 weeks of equine pregnancy. *Theriogenology*, 86(1), 349–354.

Stout, T.A. and Allen, W.R. (2001) Role of prostaglandins in intrauterine migration of the equine conceptus. *Reproduction* 121(5), 771–775.

Stout, T.A.E. and Allen, W.R. (2002) Prostaglandin E2 and F2α production of equine conceptuses and concentrations in conceptus fluids and uterine flushings recovered from early pregnant and dioestrus mares. *Reproduction* 123, 261–268.

Stout, T.A. and Colenbrander, B. (2004) Suppressing reproductive activity in horses using GnRH vaccines, antagonists or agonists. *Animal Reproduction Science* 82–83, 633–643.

Stout, T.A and Colenbrander, B. (2011) Reproductive parameters of draft horse, fresian and warmblood stallions. In: McKinnon, A.O., Squires, E.L., Vaala, E. and Varner, D.D. (eds) *Equine Reproduction*, 2nd edn. Wiley-Blackwell, Philadelphia, London, pp. 1362–1366.

Stout, T.A.E., Lamming, G.E. and Allen, W.R. (1999) Oxytocin administration prolongs luteal function in cyclic mares. *Journal of Reproduction and Fertility*, 116, 315–320.

Stout, T.A.E., Lamming, G.E. and Allen, W.R. (2000) The uterus as a source of oxytocin in cyclic mares. *Journal of Reproduction and Fertility, Supplement* 56, 281–287.

Stout, T.A.E., Meadows, S. and Allen, W.R. (2005) Stage-specific formation of the equine blastocyst capsule is instrumental to hatching and to embryonic survival in vivo. *Animal Reproduction Science* 87, 269–281.

Stradaioli, G., Chiacchiarini, P., Monaci, M., Verini Supplizi, A., Martion, G. and Piermati, C. (1995) Reproductive characteristics and seminal plasma carnitine concentration in maiden maremmano stallions. In: *Proceedings of the 46th Annual Meeting of the European Association for Animal Production, Prague.* European Association for Animal Production.

Strzemienski, P.J., Sertich, P.L., Varner, D.D. and Kenney, R.M. (1987) Evaluation of cellulose acetate/ nitrate filters for the study of stallion sperm motility. *Journal of Reproduction and Fertility, Supplement* 35, 33–38.

Suarez, S.S. and Ho, H.C. (2003) Hyperactivation of mammaliam sperm. *Cellular Molecular Biology* 49, 351–356.

Sudderth, A.K., Kiser, A.M., Brinsko, S.P., Love, C.C., Varner, D.D., Burns, P.J. and Blanchard, T.L. (2013) Efficacy of long-acting formulations of estradiol or progesterone plus estradiol on estrous synchronisation in broodemares. *Journal of Equine Veterinary Science* 33(8), 670–672.

Suire, S., Stewart, F., Beauchamp, J. and Kennedy, M.W. (2001) Uterocalin, a lipocalin provisioning the preattachment equine conceptus: fatty acid and retinol binding properties, and structural characterization. *Biochemistry Journal.* 356(Pt 2), 369–376.

Sundberg, J.P., Burnstein, T., Page, E.H., Kirkham, W.W. and Robinson, F.R. (1977) Neoplasms of equidae. *Journal of the American Veterinary Medical Association* 170, 150–152.

Sutton, E.I., Bowland, J.P. and Rattcliff, W.D. (1977) Influence of level of energy and nutrient intake by mares on reproductive performance and on blood serum composition of the mares and foals. *Canadian Journal of Animal Science* 57, 551–558.

Swinker, A.M., Squires, E.L., Mumford, E.L., Knowles, J.E. and Kniffen, D.M. (1993) Effect of body weight and body condition score on follicular development and ovulation in mares treated with GnRH analogue. *Journal of Equine Veterinary Science* 13, 519–520.

Takagi, M., Nishimura, K., Oguri, N., Ohnuma, K., Ito, K., Takahashi, J., Yasuda, Y., Miyazawa, K. and Sato, K. (1998) Measurement of early pregnancy factor activity for monitoring the viability of the equine embryo. *Theriogenology* 50, 255–262.

Takahaski, J.S. (2004) Finding new clock components past and future. *Journal of Biological Rhythms* 19, 339–347.

Talluri, T.R., Arangasamy, A., Singh, J., Ravi, S.K., Pal, Y., Legha, R.A., Raj, M.A., Chopra, A., Singh, R.K. and Trpathi, B.N. (2016) Factors affecting length of gestation in artificially inseminated Marwari mares in India. *Asian Journal of Reproduction* 5(6), 481–489.

Tamilselvan, S., Sivagnanam, S., Iniya, K., Jayachitra, S., Balasundaram, K. and Lavanya, C. (2015) Gross Morphology of Placenta in Mare. *International Journal of Currents and Microbiology and Applied Science* 4(4), 197–200.

Tanaka, Y., Nagamine, N., Nambo, Y., Nagata, S., Nagaoka, K., Tsunoda, N., Taniyama, H., Yoshihara, T., Oikawa, M., Watanbe, G. and Taya, K. (2000) Ovarian secretion of inhibin in mares. *Journal of Reproduction and Fertility, Supplement* 56, 239–245.

Tarapour, N. (2014) The effect of mare age at conception and mating to ovulation interval on foal gender, live foal rate and pregnancy rate in Thoroughbred horses. MSc thesis, Aberystwyth University, UK.

Tayade, C., Cnossen, S., Wessels, J., Linton, N., Quinn, B., Waelchi, R., Croy, A.B., Hayes, M. and Betteridge, K. (2008) IFN-δ, a Type I interferon is expressed by both the conceptus and endometrium during early equid pregnancy. In: Proceedings of the 41st Annual Meeting of the Society for the Study of Reproduction, Kona, Hawaii. SSR, Madison, Wisconsin, Abstr 83.

Taylor, M.J., Evans, J.W., Housholder, D.D., Potter, G.D. and Varner, D.D. (1997) Reproductive parameters of breeding stallions in response to a moderate physical conditioning program. In: *Proceedings of the 15th Equine Nutrition and Physiology Symposium Fort Worth, Texas*. Equine and Physiology Society, pp. 104–108.

Tetzke, T.A., Ismail, S., Mikuckis, G. and Evans, J.W. (1987) Patterns of oxytocin secretion during the oestrous cycle of the mare. *Journal of Reproduction and Fertility, Supplement* 35, 245–252.

Teubner, A., Müller, K., Bartmann, C.P., Sieme, H., Klug, E., Zingrebe, B., and Schoon, H.A (2015) Effects of an anabolic steroid (Durateston) on testicular angiogenesis in peripubertal stallions. *Theriogenology* 84(3), 323–332.

Teuscher, C., Kenney, R.M., Cummings, M.R. and Catten, M. (1994) Identification of two stallion sperm specific proteins and their autoantibody response. *Equine Veterinary Journal* 26(2), 148–151.

Thackare, H., Nicoholson, H.D. and Whittington, K. (2006) Oxytocin: its role in male reproduction and new potential therapeutic uses. *Human Reproduction Update* 12, 437–448.

Tharasanit, T., Colenbrander, B. and Stout, T.A. (2005) Effect of cryopreservation on the cellular integrity of equine embryos. *Reproduction* 129, 789–798.

Tharasanit, T., Colenbrander, B. and Stout, T.A. (2006) Effect of maturation stage at cryopreservation on post-thaw cytoskeleton quality and fertilizability of equine oocytes. *Molecular Reproductive Development* 73(5), 627–637.

Thein, P. (2012) Infectious abortions in mare; etiology, prevention and defense. *Pferdeheilkunde* 28(2), 171–186.

Thomas, P.G.A. and Ball, B.A. (1996) Cytofluorescent assay to quantify adhesion of equine spermatozoa to oviduct epithelial cells in vitro. *Molecular Reproduction and Development* 43(1), 55–61.

Thomas, P.G.A., Ball, B.A., Miller, P.G., Brinsko, S.P. and Sothwood, L. (1994) A subpopulatipon of morphologically normal, motile spermatozoa attach to equine oviduct epithelial cells in vitro. *Biology of Reproduction* 51, 303–309.

Thomas, P.G.A., Ignotz, G.G., Ball, B.A., Brinsko, S.P. and Currie, W.B. (1995) Effect of coculture with stallion spermatozoa on de novo protein synthesis and secretion by equine oviduct epithelial cells. *American Journal of Veterinary Research* 56(12), 1657–1662.

Thomassen, R. (1991) Use of frozen semen for artificial insemination in mares, results in 1990. *Norsk Veterinaertidsskrift* 103(3), 213–216.

Thompson Jr, D.L. (1992) Reproductive physiology of stallions and jacks. In: Warren Evans, J. (ed.) *Horse Breeding and Management*. Elsevier, Amsterdam, pp. 237–261.

Thompson, D.L. (1994) Breeding management of stallions: breeding soundness evaluations. *Journal of Equine Veterinary Science* 14(1), 19–20.

Thompson, D.L. (2011) Anestrus. In: McKinnon, A.O., Squires, E.L., Vaala, W.E. and Varner, D.D. (eds) *Equine Reproduction*, 2nd edn. Wiley-Blackwell, pp. 1696–1703.

Thompson, Jr. D.L., Johnson, L. and Wiest, J.J. (1987) Effect of month and age on prolactin concentrations in stallion semen. *Journal of Reproduction and Fertility (Suppl)* 35, 67–70.

Thompson Jr, D.L., DePhew, C.L., Oritz, A., Sticker, L.S. and Rahmanian, M.S. (1994) Growth hormone and prolactin concentrations in plasma of horses: sex differences and effects of acute exercise and administration of growth hormone releasing hormone. *Journal of Animal Science* 72, 2911–2918.

Thompson, J.A., Love, C.C., Stich, K.L., Brinsko, S.P., Blanchard, T.L. and Varner, D.D. (2004) A Bayesian approach to prediction of stallion daily sperm output *Theriogenology* 62, 1607–1617.

Thompson, K.N. (1995) Skeletal growth of weanling and yearling Thoroughbred horses. *Journal of Animal Science* 73, 2513–2517.

Thompson, K.N., Baker, J.P. and Jackson, S.G. (1988a) The influence of supplemental feed on growth and bone development of nursing foals. *Journal of Animal Science* 66, 1692–1696.

Thomson, C.H., Thompson Jr, D.L., Kincaid, L.A. and Nadal, M.R. (1996) Prolactin involvement with increase in seminal volume after sexual stimulation in stallions. *Journal of Animal Science* 74(10), 2468–2472.

Threlfall, W.R. (1993) Retained placenta. In: McKinnon, A.O. and Voss, J.L. (eds) *Equine Reproduction*. Lea and Febiger, Philadelphia, Pennsylvania, pp. 614–621.

Threlfall, W.R. (2011) Retained fetal membranes. In: McKinnon, A.O., Squires, E.L., Vaala, E. and Varner, D.D. (eds) *Equine Reproduction*, 2nd edn. Wiley-Blackwell, Philadelphia, London, pp. 2520–2529.

Threlfall, W.R. and Carleton, C.L. (1996) Mare's genital tract. In: Traub-Dargatz, J.L. and Brown, C.M. (eds) *Equine Endoscopy*, 2nd edn. Mosby, St. Louis, Missouri, pp. 204–217.

Threlfall, W.R., Carelton, C.L., Robertson, J., Rosol, T. and Gabel, A. (1990) Recurrent torsion of the spermatic chord and scrotal testis in a stallion. *Journal of American Veterinary Association* 196, 1641–1643.

Tibary, A. (2004) Testicular disease in the stallion. Large animal. *Proceedings of the North American Veterinary Conference*, Orlando, Florida, 18 pp. 234–237.

Tibary, A. (2011a) Dopamine antagonists. In: McKinnon, A.O., Squires, E.L., Vaala, E. and Varner, D.D. (eds) *Equine Reproduction*, 2nd edn. Wiley-Blackwell, Philadelphia, London, pp. 1789–1793.

Tibary, A. (2011b) Failure to dilate. In: McKinnon, A.O., Squires, E.L., Vaala, E. and Varner, D.D. (eds) *Equine Reproduction*, 2nd edn. Wiley-Blackwell, Philadelphia, London, pp. 2724–2732.

Tibary, A., Pearson, L.K. and Fite, C.L. (2014) Reproductive tract infections. In: Sellon, D.C., Long, M.T., (eds) *Equine infectious diseases*, 2nd ed. Saunders Elsevier; St. Louis, Missouri: pp. 84–105.

Tilbrook, A.J. and Clarke, I.J. (2001) Negative feedback regulation of the secretion and actions of gonadotrophin-releasing hormone. *Biology of Reproduction* 44, 735–742.

Timoney, P.J. (2011a) Equine herpesvirus. In: McKinnon, A.O., Squires, E.L., Vaala, E. and Varner, D.D. (eds) *Equine Reproduction*, 2nd edn. Wiley-Blackwell, Philadelphia, London, pp. 2391–2398.

Timoney, P.J. (2011b) Equine viral arteritis. In: McKinnon, A.O., Squires, E.L., Vaala, E. and Varner, D.D. (eds) *Equine Reproduction*, 2nd edn. Wiley-Blackwell, Philadelphia, London, pp. 2391–2398.

Timoney, P.J. (2011c) Contagious equine metritis. In: McKinnon, A.O., Squires, E.L., Vaala, E. and Varner, D.D. (eds) *Equine Reproduction*, 2nd edn. Wiley-Blackwell, Philadelphia, London, pp. 2399–2409.

Timoney, P.J. (2011d) Diseases potentially transmitted with frozen or cooled semen. In: McKinnon, A.O., Squires, E.L., Vaala, E. and Varner, D.D. (eds) *Equine Reproduction*, 2nd edn. Wiley-Blackwell, Philadelphia, London, pp. 3015–3028.

Timoney, P.J. (2011e) Contagious equine metritis: an insidious threat to the horse breeding industry in the United States. *Journal of Animal Science* 89, 1552–1560.

Timoney, P.J. and McCollum, W.H. (1993) Equine viral arteritis. *Veterinary Clinics of North America – Equine* 9, 295–309.

Timoney, P.J. and McCollum, W.H. (1997) Equine viral arteritis: essential facts about the disease. In: Norwood, G. *Proceedings of the 43rd Annual American Association of Equine Practitioners Convention, Phoenix, Arizona.* American Association of Equine Practitioners 43, 189–195.

Tischner, M., Kosiniak, K. and Bielanski, W. (1974) Analysis of ejaculation in stallions. *Journal of Reproduction and Fertility* 41, 329–335.

Toal, R. (1996) *Ultrasound for Practitioners.* PSI, Effingham, UK, pp. 211.

Torres-Bogino, F., Sato, K., Oka, A., Kamo, Y., Hochi, S.I., Oguri, N. and Braun, J. (1995) Relationship among seminal characteristics, fertility and suitability for semen preservation in draft stallions. *Journal of Veterinary Medical Science* 57(2), 225–229.

Trantz-Williams, L., Physick-Sheard, P., McFarlane, H., Pearl, D.L., Martin, S.W. and Peregrine, A.S. (2008) Occurrence of *Anoplocephala perfoilata* infection in horses in Ontario, Canada and associations with colic and management practices. *Veterinary Parasitiology* 153, 73–84.

Traub-Dargatz, J.L., Salman, M.D. and Viss, J.L. (1991) Medical problems of adult horses, as ranked by equine practioners. *Journal of the American Veterinary Medical Association* 198(10), 1745–1747.

Traub-Dargatz, J.L. (1993a) Post natal care of the foal. In: McKinnon, A.O. and Voss, J.L. (eds) *Equine Reproduction.* Lea and Febiger, Philadelphia, Pennsylvania, pp. 981–984.

Traub-Dargatz, J.L. (1993b) Disorders of the digestive tract. In: McKinnon, A.O. and Voss, J.L. (eds) *Equine Reproduction.* Lea and Febiger, Philadelphia, Pennsylvania, pp. 1023–1029.

Traversa, D., Klei, T.R., Iorio, R., Pooletti, B., Lia, R.P., Otranto, D., Sparagano, O.A.E. and Giangaspero, A. (2007) Occurrence of anthelmintic resistant equine cyathostome populations in central arid southern Italy. *Preventative Veterinary Medicine* 82, 314–320.

Troedsson, M.H.T. (1999) Uterine clearance and resistance to persistent endometritis in the mare. *Theriogenology* 52, 461–471.

Troedsson, M.H.T. (2006) Breeding-Induced Endometritis in Mares. *Veterinary Clinics of North American Equine Practice* 22, 705–712.

Troedsson, M.H.T. (2011) Endometritis. In: McKinnon, A.O., Squires, E.L., Vaala, E. and Varner, D.D. (eds) *Equine Reproduction*, 2nd edn. Wiley-Blackwell, Philadelphia, London, pp. 2608–2619.

Troedsson, M.H.T., Lee, C.S., Franklin, R.K. and Crabo, B.G. (2000) Post-breeding uterine inflammation: The role of seminal plasma. *Journal of Reproduction and Fertility* 56, 341–349.

Troedsson, M.H.T., Alghamdi, A.S. and Mattisen, J. (2002) Equine seminal plasma protects fertility of spermatozoa in an inflamed uterine environment. *Theriogenology* 58, 453–456.

Troedsson, M.H., Desvousges, A., Alghamdi, A.S., Dahma, B., Dow, C.A., Hayna, J., Valesco, R., Collhan, P.T., Macpherson, M.L., Pozor, M. and Buhi, W.C. (2005) Components in seminal plasma regulateng sperm transport and elimination. *Animal Reproduction Science* 89(1–4), 171–186.

Troedsson, M.H.T., Paprocki, A.M., Koppang, R.W., Syverson, C.M., Griffin, P., Klein, C., and Dobrinski, J.R. (2010) Transfer success of biopsied and vitrified equine embryos. *Animal Reproduction Science* 121S, 295–296.

Tucker, K.E., Henderson, K.A. and Duby, R.T. (1991) In vitro steroidogenesis by granulosa cells from equine preovulatory follicles. *Journal of Reproduction and Fertility, Supplement* 44, 45–55.

Turkstra, J.A., Van der Meer, F.J.U.M., Knaap, J., Rottier, P.J.M., Teerds, K.J., Colenbraner, B. and Melon, R.H. (2005) Effects of GnRH immunization in sexually mature pony stallions. *Animal Reproduction Science* 86, 247–259.

Turner, J.W., Jr. and Kirkpatrick, J.F. (1982) Steroids. Behaviour and fertility control in feral stallions in the field. *Journal of Reproduction and Fertility, Supplement* 32, 79–87.

Turner, A.S. and McIlwraith, C.W. (1982) Umbilical herniorrhaphy in the foal. In: Turner, A.S. and McIlwraith, C.W. (eds) *Techniques in Large Animal Surgery.* Lea and Febiger, Philadelphia, Pennsylvania, pp. 254–259.

Turner, J.E. and Irvine, C.H.G. (1991) The effect of various gonadotrophin releasing hormone regimens on gonadotrophins, follicular growth and ovulation in deeply anoestrus mares. *Journal of Reproduction and Fertility Supplement* 44, 213–225.

Turner, R.M. (1998) Ultrasonography of genital tract of stallion. In: Reef, V.B. (ed.) *Equine Diagnostic*

Ultrasound. W.B. Saunders, Philadelphia, Pennsylvania, pp. 446–479.

Turner, R.M.O. (2007) Pathogenesis, Diagnosis, and Management of Testicular Degeneration in Stallions. *Clinical Techniques in Equine Practice* 6(4), 278–284.

Turner, R.M. (2011a) Abnormalities of the Ejaculate. In: McKinnon, A.O., Squires, E.L., Vaala, E. and Varner, D.D. (eds) *Equine Reproduction*, 2nd edn. Wiley-Blackwell, Philadelphia, London, pp. 1119–1129.

Turner, R.M. (2011b) Ultrasonography of the genital tract. In: McKinnon, A.O., Squires, E.L., Vaala, E. and Varner, D.D. (eds) *Equine Reproduction*, 2nd edn. Wiley-Blackwell, Philadelphia, London, pp. 1469–1490.

Turner, R.M. (2018) Understanding and managing age-related subfertility in the stallion. *Clinical Theriogenology* 10(3), 295–302.

Turner, R.M. (2019) Declining testicular function in the aging stallion: management options and future therapies. *Animal Reproduction Science* 207, 171–179.

Turner, R.M. and McDonnell, S.M. (2007) Mounting expectations for Thoroughbred stallions. *Journal of the American Veterinary Medicine Association* 230, 1458–1460.

Turner, R.M., McDonnell, S.M., Feit, E.M., Grogan, E.H. and Foglia, R. (2006) Real-time ultrasound measure of the fetal eye (vitreous body) for prediction of parturition date in small ponies. *Theriogenology* 66(2), 331–337.

Tyznik, W.J. (1972) Nutrition and disease. In: Catcott, E.J. and Smithcors, J.R. (eds) *Equine Medicine and Surgery*, 2nd edn. American Veterinary Publications, Santa Barbara, California, pp. 239–250.

Ullrey, D.E., Struthers, R.D., Hendricks, D.G. and Brent, B.E. (1966) Composition of mare's milk. *Journal of Animal Science* 25, 217–222.

Umphenour, N.W., Sprinkle, T.A. and Murphy, H.Q. (1993) Natural service. In: Mckinnon, A.O. and Voss, J.L. (eds) *Equine Reproduction*. Lea and Febiger, Philadelphia, Pennsylvania, pp. 798–820.

Umphenour, N.W., McCarthy, P. and Blanchard, T.L. (2011) Management of stallions in natural-service programs. In: McKinnon, A.O., Squires, E.L., Vaala, E. and Varner, D.D. (eds) *Equine Reproduction*, 2nd edn. Wiley-Blackwell, Philadelphia, London, pp. 1208–1227.

Utt, M.D., Acosta, T.J., Wiltbank, M.C. and Ginther, O.J. (2007) Acute effectos of Prostaglandin F2 (alpha) on systemic oxytocin and progesterone concentrations during the mid- or late- luteal phase in mares. *Journal of Reproduction and Fertility, Supplement* 56, 289–296.

Vaala, W.E. (1993) The cardiac and respiratory systems. In: McKinnon, A.O. and Voss, J.L. (eds) *Equine Reproduction*. Lea and Febiger, Philadelphia, Pennsylvania, pp. 1041–1059.

Vaala, W. (2000). How to stabilize a critical foal prior to and during referral. *Proceedings of the 46th Annual Convention of the American Association of Equine Practitioners*, San Antonio, Texas and Lexington, Kentucky, pp. 182–187.

Vaala, W.E. (2011) Enteral and parenteral nutrition for the neonatal foal. In: McKinnon, A.O., Squires, E.L., Vaala, E. and Varner, D.D. (eds) *Equine Reproduction*, 2nd edn. Wiley-Blackwell, Philadelphia, London, pp. 263–279.

Vaillencourt, D., Gucy, P. and Higgins, R. (1993) The effectiveness of gentamicin or polymixin B for the control of bacterial growth in equine semen stored at 20°C or 5°C for up to forty eight hours. *Canadian Journal of Veterinary Research* 57(4), 277–280.

Valenzuela, O.A., Couturier-Tarrade, A., Choi, Y.H., Aubriere, M.C., Ritthaler, J., Chavatte-Palmer, P. and Hinrichs, K. (2017). Impact of equine assisted reproductive technologies (standard embryo transfer or intracytoplasmic sperm injection (ICSI) with in vitro culture and embryo transfer) on placenta and foal morphometry and placental gene expression. *Reproduction, Fertility and Development* 30, 371–379.

Van Buiten, A., Zhang, J. and Boyle, M.S. (1989) Integrity of plasma membrane of stallion spermatozoa before and after freezing. *Journal of Reproduction and Fertility* 4, 18–22.

Van Buiten, A., Van der Broek, J., Schukken, Y.H. and Colenbrander, B. (1999) Validation of non-return rates as a parameter for stallion fertility. *Livestock Production Science* 60, 13–19.

Van Camp, S.D. (1993) Uterine abnormalities. In: McKinnon, A.O. and Voss, J.L. (eds) *Equine Reproduction*. Lea and Febiger, Philadelphia, Pennsylvania, London, pp. 392–396.

Vandeplassche, M. (1975) Uterine prolapse in the mare. *Veterinary Record* 97, 19.

Vandeplassche, M. (1993) Dystocia. In: McKinnon, A.O. and Voss, J.L. (eds) *Equine Reproduction*. Lea and Febiger, Philadelphia, Pennsylvania, pp. 578–587.

Vandeplassche, M., Spincmaille, J. and Bouters, R. (1976) Dropsy of the fetal sac in mares: induced and spontaneous abortion. *Veterinary Record* 99, 67–69.

Van der Holst, W. (1984) Stallion semen production in AI programs in the Netherlands. In: Courot, M. (ed.) *The Male in Farm Animal Production*. Martinus Nijhoff, Boston, Massachusetts, pp. 195–201.

Van der Kolk, J.H. (1997) Equine Cushing's disease. *Equine Veterinary Education* 9, 209–214.

Van der Veldon, M. (1988) Surgical treatment of acquired inguinal hernia in the horse: a review of 39 cases. *Equine Veterinary Journal* 20, 173–177.

Vanderwall, D.K. (2011) Progesterone. In: McKinnon, A.O., Squires, E.L., Vaala, E. and Varner, D.D. (eds) *Equine Reproduction*, 2nd edn. Wiley-Blackwell, Philadelphia, London, pp. 1637–1641.

Vanderwall, D.K. and Woods, G.L. (2003) Effect on fertility of uterine lavage performed immediately prior to insemination in mares. *Journal of the American Veterinary Association* 222(8), 1108–1110.

Vanderwall, D.K., Woods, G.L., Freeman, D.A., Weber, A., Roch, R.W. and Tester, D.F. (1993) Ovarian follicles, ovulations and progesterone concentrations in aged versus young mares. *Theriogenology* 40, 21–32.

Vanderwall, D.K., Silvia, W.J. and Fitzgerald, B.P. (1998) Concentrations of oxytocin in the intercavernous sinus of mares during luteolysis: temporal relationship wit concentrations of 13,14-dihydro-15-keto-prostaglandin *F2α*. *Journal of Reproduction and Fertility* 112, 337–346.

Vanderwall, D.K., Juergens, T.D. and Woods, G.L. (2001) Reproductive performance of commercial broodmares after induction of ovulation either hCG or ovuplant (Deslorelin). *Journal of Equine Veterinary Science* 21, 539–542.

Vanderwall, D.K., Woods, G.L., Aston, K.I., Bunch, T.D., Meerdo, L.N. and White, K.L. (2004) Cloned horse pregnancies produced using adult cumulus cells. *Reproduction Fertilization and Development* 16(7), 675–679.

Van Dierendonck, M. and Goodwin, G. (2005) Human animal relationship. *Animals in Philosophy and Science* 4(2), 25–35.

Van Gall, C., Stehl, J.H. and Weaver, D.R. (2002) Mammalian melatonin receptors: molecular biology and signal transduction. *Cell Tissue Research* 309, 151–162.

Van Huffel, X.M., Varner, D.D., Hinrichs, K., Garcia, M.C., Stremienski, P.J. and Kenney, R.M. (1985) Photomicrographic evaluation of stallion spermatozoal motility characteristics. *American Journal of Veterinary Research* 46(6), 1272–1275.

Van Maanen, C., Bruin, G., de Boer-Luijtze, E., Smolders, G. and de Boer, G.F. (1992) Interference of maternal antibodies with the immune response of foals after vaccination against equine influenza. *Veterinary Quaterly* 14(1), 13–17.

Van Niekerk, C.H. and Morgenthal, J.C. (1982) Foetal loss and the effect of stress on plasma progesterone levels in pregnant Thoroughbred mares. *Journal of Reproduction and Fertility, Supplement* 32, 453–457.

Van Niekerk, C.H. and Van Heerden, J.S. (1972) Nutritional and ovarian activity of mares early in the breeding season. *Journal of the South African Veterinary Medicine Association* 43(4), 351–360.

Van Niekerk, C.H. and Van Heerden, J.S. (1997) The effect of dietary protein on reproduction in the mare. III. Ovarian and uterine changes during the anovulatory season, transitional and ovulatory periods in the non-pregnant mare. *Journal of the South African Veterinary Association* 68, 86–92.

Van Niekerk, F.E. and Van Niekerk, C.H. (1997) The effect of dietary protein on reproduction in the mare. III Growth of foals, body weight of mares and serum protein concentration of mares during the anovulatory, transitional and pregnant periods. *Journal of the South African Veterinary Association* 68, 81–85.

Van Weeren, P.R., Knapp, J. and Firth, E.C. (2003) Influence of copper status of mare and new born foal on the development of osteochondrotic lesions. *Equine Veterinary Journal* 35, 67–71.

Varner, D.D. (1983) Equine perinatal care, part 1. Prenatal care of the dam. *Compendium of Continuing Education Practical Vet* 5, S356–S362.

Varner, D.D. (1986) Collection and preservation of stallion spermatozoa. In: *Proceedings of the Annual Meeting (1986) of the Society of Theriogenology*. Society of Theriogenology, pp. 13–33.

Varner, D.D. (1991) Composition of seminal extenders and its effect on motility of equine spermatozoa.

In: *Proceedings of the Annual Meeting of the Society for Theriogenology*. Society of Theriogenology, 146–150.

Varner, D.D. (2005) Handling the breeding stallion. In: *Proceedings of the 51st Annual Convention of the American Association of Equine Practioners* 498–505.

Varner, D.D. (2008) Development in stallion semen evaluation. *Theriogenology* 70, 448–462.

Varner, D.D. (2011) Handling the breeding stallion. In: McKinnon, A.O., Squires, E.L, Vaala, W.E. and Varner, D.D. (eds) *Equine Reproduction* 2nd edn. Wiley-Blackwell, Philadelphia, London, pp. 1391–1395.

Varner, D.D. (2016) Approaches to breeding soundness examination and interpretation of results. *Journal of Equine Veterinary Science* 43, 37–44.

Varner, D.D. and Johnson, L. (2007) From a sperm's eye view: revisiting our perception of this intriguing cell. *American Association of Equine Practitioners* 53, 104–177.

Varner, D.D. and Schumacher, J. (1991) Diseases of the reproductive system: the stallion. In: Colahan, P.T., Mayhew, I.G., Merritt, A.M. and Moore, J.N. (eds) *Equine Medicine and Surgery*. Vol. 2, 4th edn. American Veterinary Publication Incorporated, Goleta, California, pp. 847–948.

Varner, D.D. and Schumacher, J. (1999) Diseases of the scrotum. In: Colahan, P.T., Merritt, A.M. and Moore, J.N. (eds) *Equine Medicine and Surgery*, 5th edn. Mosby, Philadelphia, Pennsylvania, pp. 1034–1035.

Varner, D.D. and Schumacher, J. (2011) Abnormalities of the accessory sex glands. In: McKinnon, A.O., Squires, E.L., Vaala, E. and Varner, D.D. (eds) *Equine Reproduction*, 2nd edn. Wiley-Blackwell, Philadelphia, London, pp. 1113–1129.

Varner, D.D., Blanchard, T.L., Meyers, P.S. and Meyers, S.A. (1989) Fertilizing capacity of equine spermatozoa stored for 24 hours at 5°C or 20°C. *Theriogenology* 32, 515–525.

Varner, D.D., Schumacher, J., Blanchard, T.L. and Johnson, L. (1991) *Diseases and Management of Breeding Stallions*. American Veterinary Publications, Goleta, California.

Varner, D.D., McIntosh, A.L., Forrest, D.W., Blanchard, T.L. and Johnson, L. (1992) Potassium penicillin G, amikacin sulphate or a combination in seminal extenders for stallions: effects on spermatozoal motility. In: *Proceedings of the International Congress of Animal Reproduction and AI 12*. International Congress of Animal Reproduction, luprositol University of Dublin, Dublin, 1496–1498.

Varner, D.D., Taylor, T.S. and Blanchard, T.L. (1993) Seminal vesiculitis. In: McKinnon, A.O. and Voss, J.L. (eds) *Equine Reproduction*. Lea and Febiger, Philadelphia, Pennsylvania, pp. 861–863.

Varner, D.D., Blanchard, T.L., Brinsko, S.P., Love, C.C., Taylor, T.S. and Johnson, L. (2000) Techniques for evaluating selected reproductive disorders of stallions. *Animal Reproduction Science* 60–61, 493–509.

Varner, D.D., Love, C.C., Blanchard, T.L., Bliss, S.B., Carroll, B.S. and Macpherson, M.L. (2010) Breeding management strategies and semen handling techniques for stallions – Case scenarios *Proceedings of the American Association of Equine Practioners* 56, 215–226.

Varner, D.D., Gibb, Z. and Aitkin, A.J. (2015) Stallion fertility; A focus on the spermatozoon. *Equine Veterinary Journal* 47, 16–24.

Vasey, J.R. (1993) Uterine torsion. In: McKinnon, A.O. and Voss, J.L. (eds) *Equine Reproduction*. Lea and Febiger, Philadelphia, Pennsylvania, pp. 456–460.

Vasey, J.R. and Russell, T. (2011) Uterine torsion. In: McKinnon, A.O., Squires, E.L., Vaala, E. and Varner, D.D. (eds) *Equine Reproduction*, 2nd edn. Wiley-Blackwell, Philadelphia, London, pp. 2435–2440.

Vaughan, J.T. (1993) Penis and prepuce. In: McKinnon, A.O. and Voss, J.L. (eds) *Equine Reproduction*. Lea and Febiger, Philadelphia, Pennsylvania, pp. 885–894.

Vasquez, J.J., Garcia, A., Kass, P.H., Liu, I.K.M. and Ball, B.A. (2010) Influence of environmental temperature, exercise, semen type and ovulation characteristics on reproductive performance in a commercial embryo transfer program. *Animal Reproduction Science* 121, 284–285.

Vecchi. I., Sabbioni, A., Bigliardi, E., Morini, G., Ferrari, L., De Ianni, F., Superchi, P. and Parmigiani, E. (2010) Relationship between body fat and body condition score and their effects on estrous cycles of the Standardbred maiden mare. *Veterinary Research Communications* 34 (Supplement 1) S41–45.

Veeramachaneni, D.N.R. (2011) Spermatozoal morphology. In: McKinnon, A.O., Squires, E.L., Vaala, E. and Varner, D.D. (eds) *Equine Reproduction*, 2nd edn. Wiley-Blackwell, Philadelphia, London, pp. 1297–1307.

Veeramachaneni, D.N.R, Moeller, C.L. and Sawyer, H.R. (2006) Sperm morphology in stallions: ultrastructure as a functional and diagnostic tool. *Veterinary Clinics of North America, Equine Practioners* 22, 683–692.

Velde, M. van de, Roels, K., Ververs, C., Gerits, I. and Govaere, J. (2018) Equine foetal geder determination in mid- to late gestational mares: a practical inquiry. *Reproduction in Domestic Animals* 53(5), 1027–1032.

Vera, L., Decloedt, A., Steenkiste, G. van, Clercq, D. de, Govaere, J. and Loon, G. van (2018) Electrocardiographic confirmation of a twin pregnancy in a mare at 8 months of gestation. *Journal of Veterinary Cardiology* 20(4), 294–299.

Verberckmoes, S., Van Soom, A., Dewulf, J. and de Kruir, A. (2005) A comparison of three diluents for the storage of fresh bovine semen. *Theriogenology* 63, 912–922.

Veronesi, M.C., Battocchio, M., Faustini, M., Gandini, M. and Cairoli, F. (2003) Relationship between pharmacological induction of estrous and/or ovulation and twin pregnancy in the Thoroughbred mare. *Domestic Animal Endocrinology* 25, 133–140.

Vick, M.M., Sessions, D.R., Murphy, B.A., Kennedy, E.L., Reedy, S.E. and Fitzgerald, B.P. (2006) Obesity is associated with altered metabolic and reproductive activity in the mare. *Reproduction, Fertility and Development* 18, 609–617.

Vidament, M., Dupere, A.M., Julienne, P., Evain, A., Noue, P. and Palmer, E. (1997) Equine frozen semen: freezability and fertility field results. *Theriogenology* 48(6), 907–917.

Vilar, J.M., Batista, M., Carrillo, J.M., Rubio, M., Sopena, J. and Álamo, D. (2018) Histological, cytogenetic and endocrine evaluation in twenty-five unilateral cryptorchid horses. *Journal of Applied Animal Research* 46(1), 441–444.

Villani, C., Sighieri, C., Tedeschi, D., Gazzano, G., Sampieri, G.U., Ducci, M. and Martelli, F. (2000) Serial progesterone measurements in early pregnancy diagnosis in the mare. *Selezione Vetinaria, Supplement* s287–s291.

Villani, M. and Romano, G. (2008) Induction of parturition with daily low-dose oxytocin injections in pregnant mares at term: clinical applications and limitations. *Reproduction in Domestic Animals* 43(4), 481–483.

Visser, E.K., Ellis, A.D. and Van Reenen, C.G. (2008) The effect of two different housing conditions on the welfare of young horses stabled for the first time. *Applied Animal Behaviour Science* 114, 521–533.

Vita, M.E. and Necchi, D. (2019) Selection and management of embryo recipient mares. *Revista Acadêmica: Ciência Animal* 17(Supl. 2), 78–81.

Vivrette, S.L., Reimers, T.J. and Knook, L. (1990) Skeletal diseases in a hypothyroid foal. *Journal of the American Veterinary Association* 197, 1635–1638.

Vivrette, S.L., Kindahl, H., Munro, C.J., Roser, J.F. and Stabenfeldt, G.H. (2000) Oxytocin release and its relationship to dihydro-15-keto PGF2alpha and arginine vasopressin release during parturition and to suckling in postpartum mares. *Journal of Reproduction and Fertility* 119, 347–357.

Voge, J.L., Sudderth, A.K., Brinsko, S.P., Burns, P.J. and Blanchard, T.L. (2012) Comparison of efficacy of two dose rates of histrelin to human chorionic gonadotropin for inducing ovulation in broodmares. *Journal of Equine Veterinary Science* 32, 208–210.

Vogelsang, S.G., Sorensen Jr, A.M., Potter, G.D., Burns, S.J. and Dreamer, D.C. (1979) Fertility of donor mares following non-surgical collection of embryos. *Journal of Reproduction and Fertility, Supplement* 27, 383–386.

Volkmann, D.H., Botschinger, H.J. and Schulman, M.L. (1995) The effect of prostaglandin E2 on the cervices of dioestrus and pre-partum mares. *Reproduction in Domestic Animals* 30, 240–244.

Voss, J.L. (1993) Human chorionic gonadotrophin. In: McKinnon, A.O. and Voss, J.L. (eds) *Equine Reproduction*. Lea and Febiger, Philadelphia, Pennsylvania, pp. 325–328.

Voss, J.L. and McKinnon, A.O. (1993) Hemospermia and urospermia. In: McKinnon, A.O. and Voss, J.L. (eds) *Equine Reproduction*. Lea and Febiger, Philadelphia, Pennsylvania, pp. 864–870.

Voss, J.L. and Pickett, B.W. (1975) The effect of rectal palpation on the fertility of cyclic mares. *Journal of Reproduction and Fertility, Supplement* 23, 285–290.

Voss, J.L. and Pickett, B.W. (1976) *Reproductive Management of Broodmare*. Animal Reproduction Laboratory General Series Bulletin No. 961. Colorado State University, Fort Collins, Colorado.

Vullers, T. (2004) Recovery and freezing of embryos for use in commercial equine embryo transfer programme. In: Muller, J., Muller, Z. and Wafe, J.F. (eds.) *Proceedings of the 3rd meeting of the European Equine Gamete Group,* Pardubice, Havemeyer Foundation Monograph Series No 13, R and W Publications pp. 54–56.

Waelchi, R.O. (2011) Hydrops. In: McKinnon, A.O., Squires, E.L., Vaala, E. and Varner, D.D. (eds) *Equine Reproduction*, 2nd edn. Wiley-Blackwell, Philadelphia, London, pp. 2367–2372.

Waelchi, R.O., Gerber, D., Volkmann, D.H. and Betteridge, K.J. (1996) Changes in the osmolarity of the equine blastocyst fluid between days 11 and 25 of pregnancy. *Theriogenology* 45, 290.

Wagner, B., Flaminio, J.B., Hillegas, J., Leibold, W., Erb, H.N. and Antczak, D.F. (2006) Occurrence of IgE in foals: evidence for transfer of maternal IgE by the colostrums and late onset of endogenous IgE production in the horse. *Veterinary Immunology and Immunopathology* 110(3–4), 269–278.

Waite, J.A., Love, C.C., Brinsko, S.P., Teague, S.R., Salazar Jr, J.L., Mancill, S.S. and Varner, D.D. (2008) Factors impacting equine sperm recovery rate and quality following cushioned centrifugation. *Theriogenology* 70, 704–714.

Walbornn, S.R., Love, C.C., Blanchard, T.L., Brinsko, S.P. and Varner, D.D. (2017) The effect of dual-hemisphere breeding on stallion fertility. *Theriogenology* 94, 8–14.

Walsh, C.M., Prendergast, R.L., Sheridan, J.T. and Murphy, B.A. (2013) Blue light from light emitting diodes directed at a single eye elicits a dose dependent suppression of melatonin in horses. *The Veterinary Journal* 196, 231–235.

Walt, M.L., Stabenfeldt, G.H., Hughes, J.P., Neely, D.P. and Bradbury, R. (1979) Development of the equine ovary and ovulation fossa. *Journal of Reproduction and Fertility, Supplement* 27, 471–477.

Walter, I., Handler, J., Reifinger, M. and Aurich, C. (2001) Association of endometrosis in horses with differentiation of periglandular myofibroblasts and changes of extracellular matrix proteins. *Reproduction* 121, 581–586.

Walter, J., Neuberg, K.P., Failing, K. and Wehrend, A. (2012) Cytological diagnosis of endometritis in the mare: Investigations of sampling techniques and relation to bacteriological results. *Animal Reproduction Science* 132, 178–186.

Waran, N.K., Clarke, N. and Farnsworth, M. (2008) The effects of weaning on the domestic horses (*Equus caballus*). *Applied Animal Behaviour Science* 110, 42–57.

Warren, L.K., Lawrence, L.M., Griffin, A.S., Parker, A.L., Barnes, T. and Wright, D. (1997) The effect of weaning age on foal growth and bone density. In: *Proceedings of the 15th Equine Nutrition and Physiology Society* 15, 65–70.

Warren, L.K., Lawrence, L.M., Griffin, A.S., Parker, A.L., Barnes, T. and Wright, D. (1998a) Effect of weaning on foal growth and radiographic density. *Journal of Equine Veterinary Science* 18(5), 335–342.

Warren, L.K., Lawrence, L.M., Parker, A.L., Barnes, T. and Griffin, A.S. (1998b) The effect of weaning age on foal growth and radiographic bone density. In: *Proceedings of 16th Equine Nutrition and Physiology Society* 18(5), 335–340.

Warszawsky, L.F., Parker, W.G., First, N.L. and Ginther, O.J. (1972) Gross changes of internal genitalia during the estrous cycle in the mare. *American Journal of Veterinary Research* 33(1), 19–26.

Waters, A.J., Nicol, C.J. and French, N.P. (2002) Factors influencing the development of stereotypic and redirected behaviours in young horses: findings of a four year prospective epidemiological study. *Equine Veterinary Journal* 34(6), 572–579.

Watson, E.D. (1997) Fertility problems in stallions. *In Practice* 19(5), 260–269.

Watson, E.D. (2000) Post-breeding endometritis. *Animal Reproduction Science* 60–61, 221–232.

Watson, E.D. and Nikolakopoulos, E. (1996) Sperm longevity in the mare's uterus. *Journal of Equine Veterinary Science* 16(9), 390–392.

Watson, E.D., Clarke, C.J., Else, R.W. and Dixon, P.M. (1994a) Testicular degeneration in three stallions. *Equine Veterinary Journal* 26(6), 507–510.

Watson, E.D., McDonnell, A.M. and Cuddeford, D. (1994b) Characteristics of cyclicity in maiden thoroughbred mares in the United Kingdom. *Veterinary Record* 135, 104–106.

Watson, E.D., Nikolakopoulos, E., Gilbert, C. and Goode, J. (1999) Oxytocin in the semen and gonads of stallions. *Theriogenology* 51, 855–865.

Watson, E.D., Buckingham, J., Bjorksten, T.S. and Nikolakopoulos, E. (2000) Immunolocalisation of oxytocin in the uterus of the mare. *Journal of Reproduction and Fertility, Supplement* 56, 289–296.

Watson, E.D., Pedersen, H.G., Thomson, S.R. and Fraser, H.M. (2000b) Control of follicular developmemt and luteal function in the mare: effects of a GnRH antagonist. *Theriogenology* 54(4), 599–609.

Watson E.D., Thomassen, R., Steele, M., Heald, M., Leask, R., Groome, N.P. and Riley, S.C (2002a) Concentrations of inhibin, progesterone and oestradiol in fluid from dominant and subordinate follicles from mares during spring transition and the breeding season. *Animal Reproduction Science* 74, 55–67.

Watson, E.D., Heald, M., Tsigos, A., Leask, R., Steele, M., Groome, N.P. and Riley, S.C. (2002b) Plasma FSH, inhibin A and inhibin isoforms containing pro- and -αC during winter anoestrus, spring transition and the breeding season in mares. *Reproduction* 123, 535–542.

Watson, E.D., Thomassen, R. and Nikolakopoulos, E. (2003) Association of uterine edema with follicle waves around the onset of the breeding season in pony mares. *Theriogenolgy* 59(5–6), 1181–1187.

Watson, P.F., (1981) The roles of lipid and protein in the protection of ram spermatozoa at 5 degrees-C by egg yolk lipoprotein. *Journal of Reproduction and Fertility* 62, 483–492.

Watson, P.F., (1990) AI and the preservation of semen. In: Lamming, G.E. (ed.) *Marshall's Physiology of Reproduction, Volume 2, Male Reproduction.* Churchill Livingston, London, pp. 747–869.

Webb, G.W., Arns, M.J. and Pool, K.C. (1993) Spermatozoa concentration influences the recovery of progressively motile spermatozoa and the number of inseminates shipped in conventional containers. *Journal of Equine Veterinary Science* 13, 486–489.

Webb, R.L., Evans, J.W., Arns, M.J., Webb, G.W., Taylor, T.S. and Potter, G.D. (1990) Effects of vesiculectomy on stallion spermatozoa. *Journal of Equine Veterinary Science* 10(3), 218–223.

Weber, J. and Woods, G. (1992) Transrectal ultrasonography for the evaluation of stallion accessory sex glands. *Veterinary Clinic of North America Equine Practice* 8, 183–190.

Weber, J.A. and Woods, G.L. (1993) Ultrasonic measurements of stallion accessory glands and excurrent ducts during seminal emission and ejaculation. *Biology of Reproduction* 49(2), 267–273.

Weber, J.A., Geary, R.T. and Woods, G.L. (1990) Changes in accessory sex glands of stallions after sexual preparation and ejaculation. *Journal of the American Veterinary Medical Association* 186(7), 1084–1089.

Weber, J.A., Freeman, D.A., Vanderwall, D.K. and Woods, G.L. (1991) Prostaglandin E2 hastens oviductal transport of equine embryos. *Biology of Reproduction* 45, 544–546.

Weber, J.A., Woods, G.L. and Lichtenwalner, A.B. (1995) Relaxatory effect of prostaglandin E2 on circular smooth muscle isolated from equine oviductal isthmus. *Biology of Reproduction, Monograph* 1, 125–130.

Weedman, P.J., King, S.S., Newmann, K.R. and Nequin, L.G. (1993) Comparison of circulating oestradiol 17β and folliculogenesis during the breeding season, autumn transition and anestrus in the mare. *Journal of Equine Veterinary Science* 13, 502–505.

Weems, C.W., Weems, Y.S. and Randel, R.D. (2006) Prsotaglandins and reproduction in female farm animals. *Veterinary Journal* 171, 206–228.

Welch, G.R. and Johnson, L.A. (1999) Sex preselection: laboratory validation of the sperm sex ratio of flow sorted X-and Y-sperm by sort reanalysis for DNA. *Theriogenology* 52, 1343–1352.

Weiermayer, P. and Richter, B. (2009) Simultaneous presence of a seminoma and a leiomoma in the testes of a horse. *Equine Veterinary Education* 21(4), 172–176.

Welsch, B.B. (1993) The neurologic system. In: McKinnon, A.O. and Voss, J.L. (eds) *Equine Reproduction.* Lea and Febiger, Philadelphia, Pennsylvania, pp. 1017–1022.

Wen, D., Banaszynski, L.A., Rosenwaks, Z., Allis, C.D. and Rafii, S. (2014) H3.3 replacement facilitates epigenetic reprogramming of donor nuclei in somatic cell nuclear transfer embryos. *Nucleus* 5, 369–375.

Wespi, B., Sieme, H., Wedekind, C. and Burger, D. (2014) Exposure to stallion accelerates the onset of mares's cyclicity. *Theriogenology* 82, 189–194.

Wessel, M. (2005) Staging and predicting parturition in the mare. *Clinical techniques in Equine Practice* 4(3), 219–227.

Wesson, J.A. and Ginther, O.J. (1981) Influence of season and age on reproductive activity in pony mares on the basis of a slaughterhouse survey. *Journal of Animal Science* 52(1), 119–129.

Whitmore, H.L., Wentworth, B.C. and Ginther, O.J. (1973) Circulating concentrations of luteinising hormone during estrous cycles of mares as determined by radioimmunoassay. *American Journal of Veterinary Research* 34, 631–636.

Whitwell, K.E. (1975) Morphology and pathology of the equine umbilical cord. *Journal of Reproduction and Fertility, Supplement* 23, 599–603.

Whitwell, K.E. and Jeffcote, L.B. (1975) Morphological studies on the fetal membranes of the normal singleton foal at term. *Research in Veterinary Science* 19, 44–55.

Wilhelm, K.M., Graham, J.K. and Squires, E.L. (1996) Comparison of the fertility of cryopreserved stallion spermatozoa with sperm motion analyses, flow cytometry evaluation and zona-free hamster oocyte penetration. *Theriogenology* 46(4), 559–578.

Wilkins, P.A. (2003) Lower respiratory problems of the neonate. *Veterinary Clinics of North America: Equine Practice* 19(1), 19–33.

Williams, G.L., Thorson, J.F., Prezotto, L.D., Velez, T.C., Cardoso, R.C. and Amstalden, M. (2012) Reproductive seasonality in the mare: neuroendocrine basis and pharmacological control. *Domestic Animal Endocrinology* 43, 103–115.

Willmann, C., Schulerc, G., Hoffmann, B., Parvizid, N. and Aurich, C. (2011) Effects of age and altrenogest treatment on conceptus development and secretion of LH, progesterone and eCG in early–pregnant mares. *Theriogenology* 75, 421–428.

Wilsher, S. and Allen, W.R. (2003) The effects of maternal age and parity on placental and fetal development in the mare. *Equine Veterinary Journal* 35(5), 476–483.

Wilsher, S. and Allen, W.R. (2004) Special article, an improved method for nonsurgical embryo transfer in the mare. *Equine Veterinary Education* 16(1), 39–44.

Wilsher, S. and Allen, W.R. (2011a) Factors influencing equine chorionic gonadotrophin production in the mare. *Equine Veterinary Journal* 43, 430–438.

Wilsher, S. and Allen, W.R. (2011b) Development and Morphology of the Placenta. In: McKinnon, A.O., Squires, E.L., Vaala, E. and Varner, D.D. (eds) *Equine Reproduction*, 2nd edn. Wiley-Blackwell, Philadelphia, London, pp. 2234–2244.

Wilsher, S. and Allen, W.R. (2012) Factors influencing placental structure and function in the mare. *Equine Veterinary Journal* 44(s41), 113–119.

Wilsher, S., Ball, M. and Allen, W.R. (1999) The influence of maternal size on placental area and foal birth weights in the mare. *Pferdeheilkunde* 15, 599–602.

Wilsher, S., Clutton-Brock, A. and Allen, W. (2010) Successful transfer of day 10 horse embryos: influence of donor–recipient asynchrony on embryo development. *Reproduction* 139(3), 575–585.

Wilsher, S., Lefranc, A.C. and Allen, W.R. (2012) The effects of an advanced uterine environment on ebryonic survival in the mare. *Equine Veterinary Journal* 44(4), 432–439.

Wilson, C.G., Downie, C.R., Hughes, J.P. and Roser, J.F. (1990) Effects of repeated hCG injection on reproductive efficiency in mares. *Journal of Equine Veterinary Science* 10, 301–308.

Wilson, J.H. (1987) Eastern equine encephalomyelitis. In: Robinson, N.E. (ed.) *Current Therapy on Equine Medicine*, 2nd edn. W.B. Saunders, Philadelphia, pp. 345–347.

Wilson, K.E., Dascanio, J. J., Duncan, R., Delling, U. and Ladd, S.M. (2007) Orchitis, epididymitis and pampiniform phlebitis in a stallion. *Equine Veterinary Education* 19(5), 239–243.

Wilson, W.D. (2005) Strategies for vaccinating mares, foals and weanlings. *Proceedings of the 51st Annual Convention of the American Association of Equine Practitioners*, Seattle, Washington, 3–7 December, pp. 421–438.

Wilson, W.D. (2011) Vaccination of mares, foals and weanlings. In: McKinnon, A.O., Squires, E.L., Vaala, E. and Varner, D.D. (eds) *Equine Reproduction*, 2nd edn. Wiley-Blackwell, Philadelphia, London, pp. 302–330.

Wilson, W.D., Mihalyi, J.E., Hussey, S. and Lunn, D.P. (2001) Passive transfer of maternal immunoglobulin isotype antibodies against tetanus and influenza and their effect on the response of foals to vaccination. *Equine Veterinary Journal* 33, 644–650.

Windsor, D.P., Evans, G. and White, I.G. (1993) Sex predetermination by separation of X and Y chromosome-bearing sperm: a review. *Reproduction, Fertility and Development* 5, 155–171.

Winskill, L.C., Warren, N.K. and Young, R.J. (1996) The effect of a foraging device (a modified Edinburgh football) on the behaviour of the stabled horse. *Applied Animal Behaviour Science* 48, 25–35.

Witherspoon, D.H. and Talbot, R.B. (1970) Noctural ovulation in the equine animal. *Veterinary Record* 87, 302–304.

Witkowski, M. and Pawłowski, K. (2014) Clinical observations on the course of oxytocin- or prostaglandin E2 oxytocin-induced parturition in mares. *Polish Journal of Veterinary Sciences* 17(2), 347–351.

Witkowski, M., Katkiewicz, M., Kochan, J. and Panzani, D. (2017) Uterine glands agenesia in the mare. *Journal of Equine Veterinary Science* 58, 47–50.

Witte, T.S., Melkus, E., Walter, I., Senge, B., Schwab, S., Aurich, C. and Heuwieser, W. (2012) Effects of oral treatment with N-acetylcysteine on the viscosity of intrauterine mucus and endometrial function in estrous mares. *Theriogenology* 78(6), 1199–1208.

Wockener, A. and Collenbrander, B. (1993) Liquid storage and freezing of semen from New Forest and Welsh pony stallions. *Deutsche Tierarztliche Wochenschrift* 100(3), 125–126.

Wockener, A. and Schuberth, H.J. (1993) Freezing of maiden stallion semen – motility and morphology findings in sperm cells assessed by various staining methods including a monoclonal antibody with reactivity against an antigen in the acrosomal ground substance. *Reproduction in Domestic Animals* 28(6), 265–272.

Wolf, C.A., Maslchitzky, E., Gregory, R.M., Jobim, M.I. and Mattos, R.C. (2012) Effect of corticotherapy on proteomics of endometrial fluid from mares susceptible to persistent post breeding endometritis. *Theriogenology* 77, 1351–1359.

Wood, J.L., Chirnside, E.D., Mumford, J.A. and Higgins, A.J. (1995) First recorded outbreak of equine viral arteritis in the United Kingdom. *Veterinary Record* 136, 381–385.

Wooding, F.B., Morgan, G., Fowden, A.L., Allen, W.R. (2001) A structural and immunological study of chorionic gonadotrophin production by equine trophoblast girdle and cup cells. *Placenta* 22, 749–767.

Woods, G.L., White, K.L., Vanderwall, D.K., Aston, K.I., Bunch, T.D. and Campbell, K.D. (2002) Cloned mule pregnancies produced using nuclear transfer. *Theriogenology* 58, 779–782.

Woods, G.L., White, K.L., Vanderwall, D.K., Li, G.P., Aston, K.I., Bunch, T.D., Meerdo, L.N. and Pate, P.L. (2003) A mule cloned from fetal cells by nuclear transfer. *Science* 301, 1063–1065.

Woods, J., Bergfeldt, D.R. and Ginther, O.J. (1990) Effects of time of insemination relative to ovulation on pregnancy rate embryonic loss rate in mares. *Equine Veterinary Journal* 22, 410–415.

Woodward, E.M. and Troedsson, M.H. (2013) Equine breeding induced endometritis: A Review. *Journal Equine Vet Science* 33, 673–682.

Woodward, E.M., Christoffersen, M., Campos, J., Squires, E.L and Troedsson, M.H. (2012) Susceptibility to persistent breeding-induced endometritis in the mare: relationship to endometrial biopsy score and age, and variations between seasons. *Theriogenology* 78(3), 495–501.

Worthy, K., Escreet, R., Renton, J.P., Eckersall, P.D., Douglas, T.A. and Flint, D.J. (1986) Plasma prolactin concentrations and cyclic activity in pony mares during parturition and early lactation. *Journal of Reproduction and Fertility* 77(2), 569–574.

Wrench, N., Pinto, C.R.F., Klinefelter, G.R., Dix, D.J., Flowers, W.L. and Farin, C.E., 2010. Effect of season on fresh and cryopreserved stallion semen. *Animal Reproduction Science* 119(3–4), 219–227.

Wright, P.J. (1980) Serum sperm agglutinins and semen quality in the bull. *Australian Veterinary Journal* 56(1), 10–13.

Wu, W. and Nathanielsz, P.W. (1994) Changes in oxytocin receptor messenger RNA in the endometrium, myometrium, mesometrium and cervix of sheep in late gestation and during spontaneous and cortisol induced labour. *Journal of the Society of Gynaecological Investigation* 1(3), 191–196.

Wu, W., Zheng, X., Luo, Y., Huo, F., Dong, H., Zhang, G., Yu, W., Tian, F., He, L. and Chen, J. (2015) Cryopreservation of stallion spermatozoa using different cryoprotectants and combinations of cryoprotectants *Animal Reproduction Science* 163, 75–81.

Wulf, M., Erber, R., Ille, N., Beythien, E., Aurich, J. and Aurich, C. (2017) Effects of foal sex on some perinatal characteristics in the immediate neonatal period in the horse. *Journal of Veterinary Behavior: Clinical Applications and Research* 18, 37–42.

Wulf, M., Beythien, E., Ille, N., Aurich, J. and Aurich, C. (2018) The stress response of 6 month-old horses to abrupt weaning is influenced by their sex. *Journal of Veterinary Behavior* 23, 19–24.

Xiao, H., Zhang, L., Tuohut, A., Shi, G. and Li, H. (2015) Effect of Weaning Age on Stress-Related Behavior in Foals (*Equus caballus*) by Abrupt – Group Weaning Method. *Journal of Phylogenetics and Evolutionary Biology* 3, 151.

Yadav, S.K., Gangwar, D.K., Singh, J., Tikadar, C.K., Khanna, V.V., Saini, S., Dhopria, S., Palta, P., Manik, R.S., Singh, M.K. and Singla, S.K. (2017) An immunological approach of sperm sexing and different methods for identification of X- and Y-chromosome bearing sperm *Veterinary World.* 10(5), 498–504.

Yamamoto, K., Yasuda, J. and Too, K. (1992) Arrhythmias in newborn Thoroughbred foals. *Equine Veterinary Journal* 23, 169–173.

Yamamoto, Y., Oguri, N., Tsutsumi, Y. and Hachinohe, Y. (1982) Experiments in freezing and storage of equine embryos. *Journal of Reproduction and Fertility, Supplement* 2, 399–403.

Yanagimachi, R. (1989) Sperm capacitation and gamete interactions. *Journal of Reproduction and Fertility* 38, 27–33.

Yanagimachi, R., Yanagimachi, H. and Roger, B.J. (1976) The use of a zona-free animal ova as a test system for the assessment of the fertilising capacity of human spermatozoa. *Biology of Reproduction* 15, 471–472.

Yasine, A., Daba, M., Ashenafi, H., Geldhof, P., Brantegem, L., van. Vercauteren, G., Dmissie, T., Bekana, M., Tola, A., Soom, A., van Duchateau, L., Goddeeris, B. and Govaere, J. (2019) Tissue (re) distribution of Trypanosoma equiperdum in venereal infected and blood transfused horses. *Veterinary Parasitology* 268, 87–97.

Yoon, M. (2012) The oestrous cycle and induction of ovulation in mares. *Journal of Animal Science and Technology* 54, 165–174.

Yoon, M.J., Boime, I., Colgin, M., Niswender, K.D., King, S.S., Alvarenga, M., Jablonka-Shariff, A., Pearl, C.A. and Roser, J.F. (2007) The efficacy of a single chain recombinant equine luteinizing hormone (reLH) in mares: induction of ovulation,

hormone profiles and nter-ovulatory intervals. *Domestic Animal Endocrinology* 33, 470–479.

Yorke, E.H., Caldwell, F.J. and Johnson, A.K. (2012) Uterine torsion in mares. *Compendium of Continuing Education Veterinary* 34(12), E2.

Yoshinaga, K. and Toshimori, K. (2003) Organisation and modifications of sperm acrosomal molecules during spermatogenesis and epididymal maturation. *Microscopic Research and Technology* 61, 39–45.

Young, C.A., Squires, E.L., Seidel, G.E., Kato, H. and McCue, P.M. (1997) Cryopreservation procedures for day 7–8 equine embryos. *Equine Veterinary Journal, Supplement* 25, 98–102.

Youngquist, R.S. and Threlfall, W.R. (2007) Clinical Reproductive Anatomy and Physiology of the Mare. In: Youngquist, R.S. and Threlfall, W.R. (eds) *Large Animal Theriogenology.* Saunders Elsevier, St Louis, Missouri, pp. 47–67.

Ytrehus, B., Carlson, C.S. and Ekman, S. (2007) Etiology and pathogenesis of osteochondrosis. *Veterinary Pathology* 44, 429–448.

Yurdaydin, N., Tekin, N., Gulyuz, F., Aksu, A. and Klug, E. (1993) Field trials of oestrus synchronisation and artificial insemination results in Arab broodmare herd in the National Stud Hasire/Eskisehir (Turkey). *Deutsche Tierarztiche Wochenschrift* 100(11), 432–434.

Zafracas, A.M. (1975) Candida infection of the genital tract in thoroughbred mares. *Journal of Reproduction and Fertility, Supplement* 23, 349.

Zafracas, A.M. (1994) The equines in Greece nowadays. *Bulletin of Veterinary Medical Society* 45(4), 333–338.

Zaniboni, A., Merlo, B., Zannoni, A., Bernardini, C., Lavitrano, M., Forni, M., Mari, G. and Bacci, M. L. (2013) Expression of fluorescent reporter protein in equine embryos produced through intracytoplasmic sperm injection mediated gene transfer (ICSI-MGT). *Animal Reproduction Science* 137, 53–61.

Zavos, P.M. and Gregory, G.W. (1987) Employment of the hyposmotic swelling (HOS) test to assess the integrity of the equine sperm membrane. *Journal of Andrology* 8, 25.

Zavy, M.T., Vernon, M.W., Sharp, D.C. and Bazer, F.W. (1984) Endocrine aspects of early pregnancy in pony mares. A comparison of uterine luminal and peripheral plasma levels of steroids during the oestrous cycle and early pregnancy. *Endocrinology* 115, 214–219.

Zent, W.W. (2011) History. In: McKinnon, A.O., Squires, E.L., Vaala, E. and Varner, D.D. (eds) *Equine Reproduction*, 2nd edn. Wiley-Blackwell, Philadelphia, London, pp. 1897–1899.

Zent, W.W. and Steiner, J.V. (2011) Vaginal Examination. In: McKinnon, A.O., Squires, E.L., Vaala, E. and Varner, D.D. (eds) *Equine Reproduction*, 2nd edn. Wiley-Blackwell, Philadelphia, London, pp. 1900–1903.

Zerbe, H., Engelke, F., Klug, E., Schoon, H.-A. and Leibold, W. (2004) Degenerative endometrial changes do not change the functional capacity of immigrating uterine neutrophils in mares. *Reproduction in Domestic Animals* 39, 94–98.

Zhang, J., Boyle, M.S., Smith, C.A. and Moore, H.D.M. (1990a) Acrosome reaction of stallion spermatozoa evaluated with monoclonal antibody and zona-free hamster eggs. *Molecular Reproduction and Development* 27(2), 152–158.

Zhang, J., Rickett, S.J. and Tanner, S.J. (1990b) Antisperm antibodies in the semen of a stallion following testicular trauma. *Equine Veterinary Journal* 22, 138–141.

Zhao, D., Yu, Y., Shen, Y., Liu, Q., Zhao, Z., Sharma, R. and Reiter, R.J. (2019) Melatonin synthesis and function: evolutionary history in animals and plants *Frontiers in Endocrinology* 10, 1–16.

Zicker, S.C. and Lonnerdal, B. (1994) Protein and nitrogen composition of equine (*Equus caballus*) milk during early lactation. *Comparative Biochemistry and Physiology: Comparative Physiology* 108 (41), 1–421.

Zidane, N., Vaillancourt, D., Guay, P., Poitras, P. and Bigras-Poulin, M. (1991) Fertility of fresh equine semen preserved for up to 48 hours. *Journal of Reproduction and Fertility, Supplement* 44, 644.

Zinaman, M.J., Uhler, M.L., Vertuno, E., Fisher, S.G. and Clegg, E.D. (1996) Evaluation of computer-assissted semen analysis (CASA) with IDENT stain to determine sperm concentration. *Journal of Animal Science* 17(3), 288–292.

Zirkler, H., Gerbes, K., Klug, E. and Sieme, H. (2005) Cryopreservation of stallion semen collected from good and poor freezers using a directional freezing device (Harmony CryoCare –nMultithermal Gradient 516). *Animal Reproduction Science* 89, 291–294.

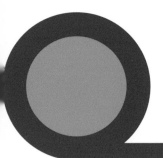

Index

Note: Page numbers in **bold** type refer to **figures**
Page numbers in *italic* type refer to *tables*

CABI – who we are and what we do

Ministry of Agriculture
People's Republic of China

Australian Government
Australian Centre for
International Agricultural Research

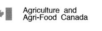 Agriculture and
Agri-Food Canada

Ministry of Foreign Affairs of the
Netherlands

Schweizerische Eidgenossenschaft
Confédération suisse
Confederazione Svizzera
Confederaziun svizra

Swiss Agency for Development
and Cooperation SDC

Discover more

To read more about CABI's work, please visit: **www.cabi.org**

Browse our books at: **www.cabi.org/bookshop**,
or explore our online products at: **www.cabi.org/publishing-products**

Interested in writing for CABI? Find our author guidelines here:
www.cabi.org/publishing-products/information-for-authors/